SIXTH EDITION

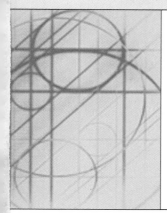

Neurology for the Non-Neurologist

WILLIAM J. WEINER, MD
Professor and Chairman
Department of Neurology
University of Maryland School of Medicine
Director, Maryland Parkinson's Disease and Movement Disorders Center
Baltimore, Maryland

CHRISTOPHER G. GOETZ, MD
Professor of Neurological Sciences and Pharmacology
Rush Medical College
Senior Physician
Rush University Medical Center
Chicago, Illinois

ROBERT K. SHIN, MD
Associate Professor of Neurology
Associate Professor of Ophthalmology and Visual Sciences
University of Maryland School of Medicine
Baltimore, Maryland

STEVEN L. LEWIS, MD
Professor and Associate Chairman
Department of Neurological Sciences
Rush University Medical Center
Chicago, Illinois

Wolters Kluwer | Lippincott Williams & Wilkins
Health
Philadelphia · Baltimore · New York · London
Buenos Aires · Hong Kong · Sydney · Tokyo

Acquisitions Editor: Frances Destefano
Product Manager: Tom Gibbons
Vendor Manager: Bridgett Dougherty
Senior Manufacturing Manager: Benjamin Rivera
Marketing Manager: Brian Freiland
Design Coordinator: Holly McLaughlin
Production Service: MPS Limited, A Macmillan Company

© 2010 by LIPPINCOTT WILLIAMS & WILKINS, a WOLTERS KLUWER business
Two Commerce Square
2001 Market Street
Philadelphia, PA 19103

Sixth Edition

Printed in China

Library of Congress Cataloging-in-Publication Data

Neurology for the non-neurologist/editors, William J. Weiner ... [et al.].—6th ed.
   p. cm.
   Includes index.
   ISBN 978-1-60547-239-3
   1. Neurology. 2. Nervous system—Diseases. I. Weiner, William J.
   RC346.N453 2010
   616.8—dc22

2010010048

Care has been taken to confirm the accuracy of the information presented and to describe generally accepted practices. However, the authors, editors, and publisher are not responsible for errors or omissions or for any consequences from application of the information in this book and make no warranty, expressed or implied, with respect to the currency, completeness, or accuracy of the contents of the publication. Application of the information in a particular situation remains the professional responsibility of the practitioner.

The authors, editors, and publisher have exerted every effort to ensure that drug selection and dosage set forth in this text are in accordance with current recommendations and practice at the time of publication. However, in view of ongoing research, changes in government regulations, and the constant flow of information relating to drug therapy and drug reactions, the reader is urged to check the package insert for each drug for any change in indications and dosage and for added warnings and precautions. This is particularly important when the recommended agent is a new or infrequently employed drug.

Some drugs and medical devices presented in the publication have Food and Drug Administration (FDA) clearance for limited use in restricted research settings. It is the responsibility of the health care provider to ascertain the FDA status of each drug or device planned for use in their clinical practice.

To purchase additional copies of this book, call our customer service department at (800) 638-3030 or fax orders to (301) 223-2320. International customers should call (301) 223-2300.

Visit Lippincott Williams & Wilkins on the Internet: at LWW.com. Lippincott Williams & Wilkins customer service representatives are available from 8:30 am to 6 pm, EST.

10 9 8 7 6 5 4 3 2

CCS1011

For my parents who would have enjoyed the outcome
William J. Weiner

To my family, Monica, Celine, Peter, and Elena
Christopher G. Goetz

To my parents who gave me every opportunity, and to
Tricia who stayed up with me
Robert K. Shin

To Julie, for all of her support, and to David, Michael, Adam, and Elliot
Steven L. Lewis

Contents

Contributors   vi

Preface   ix

Acknowledgments   xi

1. The Neurologic Examination   1
Robert K. Shin and Neil C. Porter

2. An Approach to Neurologic Symptoms   20
Steven L. Lewis

3. Clinical Use of Neurologic Diagnostic Tests   33
Madhu Soni

4. Fundamentals of Neuroradiology   43
Robert E. Morales and Dishant G. Shah

5. Neurologic Emergencies   63
Tricia Y. Ting and Lisa M. Shulman

6. Examination of the Comatose Patient   89
Jordan L. Topel and Steven L. Lewis

7. Cerebrovascular Disease   105
Roger E. Kelley and Alireza Minagar

8. Headache Disorders   127
Amy Wilcox Voigt and Joel R. Saper

9. Epilepsy   143
Donna C. Bergen

10. Sleep Disorders   156
Ružica Kovačević-Ristanović and Tomasz J. Kuźniar

11. Multiple Sclerosis   192
Peter A. Calabresi and Scott D. Newsome

12. Parkinson Disease   222
Bradley J. Robottom, Lisa M. Shulman, and William J. Weiner

13. Hyperkinetic Movement Disorders   241
Gonzalo J. Revuelta, William J. Weiner, and Stewart A. Factor

14. Alzheimer Disease and Other Dementias   287
Neelum T. Aggarwal and Raj C. Shah

15. Behavioral Neurology   307
Robert S. Wilson and Christopher G. Goetz

16. Traumatic Brain Injury   324
Michael J. Makley

17. Neuromuscular Diseases   344
Dianna Quan and Steven P. Ringel

18. Peripheral Neuropathy   375
Joshua Gordon and Morris A. Fisher

19. Neurologic Evaluation of Low Back Pain   398
Megan M. Shanks

20. Dizziness and Vertigo   412
Robert K. Shin and Judd M. Jensen

21. An Approach to the Falling Patient   427
Kathryn A. Chung and Fay B. Horak

22. Neurotoxic Effects of Drugs Prescribed by Non-Neurologists   446
Katie Kompoliti

23. Neurologic Complications of Alcoholism   470
Allison L. Weathers

24. Central Nervous System Infections   486
Larry E. Davis

25. Neurologic Aspects of Cancer   499
Deborah Olin Heros

26. Eye Signs in Neurologic Diagnosis   516
Robert K. Shin and James A. Goodwin

27. Principles of Neurorehabilitation   551
David S. Kushner

28. Medicolegal Issues in the Care of Patients with Neurologic Illness   572
Maria R. Schimer and Lois Margaret Nora

Index   588

Contributors

Neelum T. Aggarwal, M.D.
Associate Professor of Neurological Sciences
Rush University
Clinical Core Leader, Rush Alzheimer's Disease
  Research Center
Rush University Medical Center
Chicago, Illinois

Donna C. Bergen, M.D.
Professor
Department of Neurological Sciences
Rush University Medical Center
Chicago, Illinois

Peter A. Calabresi, M.D.
Professor of Neurology
The Johns Hopkins University School of Medicine
Director, The Johns Hopkins Multiple Sclerosis Center
Baltimore, Maryland

Kathryn A. Chung, M.D.
Assistant Professor
Department of Neurology
Oregon Health and Science University
Portland, Oregon

Larry E. Davis, M.D.
Professor of Neurology
University of New Mexico School of Medicine
Chief, Neurology Service, New Mexico VA Health
  Care System
Albuquerque, New Mexico

Stewart A. Factor, D.O.
Professor of Neurology and Riley Family Chair in
  Parkinson's Disease
Emory University School of Medicine
Director, Movement Disorders Program of Emory
  University
Atlanta, Georgia

Morris A. Fisher, M.D.
Professor of Neurology
Loyola University Medical Center
Maywood, Illinois
Acting Chief of Neurology
Edward Hines, Jr. VA Medical Center
Hines, Illinois

Christopher G. Goetz, M.D.
Professor of Neurological Sciences and Pharmacology
Rush University Medical Center
Chicago, Illinois

James A. Goodwin, M.D.
Associate Professor of Ophthalmology
University of Illinois at Chicago
Director, Neuro-ophthalmology Service
University of Illinois Eye and Ear Infirmary
Chicago, Illinois

Joshua Gordon, M.D.
Assistant Professor of Neurology
Loyola University Medical Center
Chicago, Illinois
Assistant Professor of Neurology
Edward Hines, Jr. VA Medical Center
Hines, Illinois

Deborah Olin Heros, M.D.
Associate Professor of Clinical Neurology and
  Neuro-Oncology
University of Miami Leonard M. Miller
School of Medicine Chief of Neurology
University of Miami Hospital
Miami, Florida

Fay B. Horak, Ph.D., P.T.
Research Professor
Department of Neurology
Oregon Health and Science University
Portland, Oregon

Judd M. Jensen, M.D.
Penobscot Bay Medical Center
Rockport, Maine

Roger E. Kelley, M.D.
Professor and Chair of Neurology
Tulane University School of Medicine
New Orleans, Louisiana

Katie Kompoliti, M.D.
Associate Professor of Neurological Sciences
Rush University Medical Center
Chicago, Illinois

Ružica Kovačević-Ristanović, M.D.
Clinical Associate Professor of Neurology
University of Chicago Medical Center
Chicago, Illinois
Attending Medical Director, Sleep Disorders Center
Evanston Hospital
Evanston, Illinois

David S. Kushner, M.D.
Associate Professor of Rehabilitation Medicine
University of Miami Leonard M. Miller School
*   of Medicine*
Miami, Florida

Tomasz J. Kuźniar, M.D., Ph.D.
Assistant Professor of Medicine
Northwestern University
Chicago, Illinois
Attending Physician
North Shore University Health System
Evanston, Illinois

Steven L. Lewis, M.D.
Professor and Associate Chairman
Department of Neurological Sciences
Rush University Medical Center
Chicago, Illinois

Michael J. Makley, M.D.
Assistant Professor of Neurology
University of Maryland School of Medicine
Director, Traumatic Brain Injury Unit, Kernan
*   Hospital*
Baltimore, Maryland

Alireza Minagar, M.D.
Associate Professor of Neurology
Louisiana State University Health Sciences Center
Shreveport, Louisiana

Robert E. Morales, M.D.
Assistant Professor of Radiology
University of Maryland School of Medicine
Director, Neuroimaging
University of Maryland Medical Center Baltimore,
*   Maryland*

Scott D. Newsome, D.O.
Assistant Professor of Neurology
The Johns Hopkins University School of Medicine
Baltimore, Maryland

Lois Margaret Nora, M.D., J.D.
President and Dean, College of Medicine
Northeastern Ohio Universities Colleges of Medicine
*   and Pharmacy*
Rootstown, Ohio

Neil C. Porter, M.D.
Assistant Professor of Neurology
University of Maryland School of Medicine
Baltimore, Maryland

Dianna Quan, M.D.
Associate Professor of Neurology
University of Colorado Health Sciences Center
Director, Electromyography Laboratory, University
*   of Colorado Hospital*
Denver, Colorado

Gonzalo J. Revuelta, D.O.
Movement Disorders Fellow, Department of
*   Neurology*
Emory University School of Medicine
Atlanta, Georgia

Steven P. Ringel, M.D.
Professor of Neurology
University of Colorado Health Sciences Center
Director, Neuromuscular Unit, University of
*   Colorado Hospital*
Denver, Colorado

Bradley J. Robottom, M.D.
Assistant Professor of Neurology
University of Maryland School of Medicine
*   Baltimore, Maryland*

Joel R. Saper, M.D.
Clinical Professor of Medicine-Neurology
Michigan State University
Director, Michigan Headache & Neurological
*   Institute*
Ann Arbor, Michigan

Maria R. Schimer, M.P.H., J.D.
Associate Professor of Community Health
*   Sciences*
Northeastern Ohio Universities Colleges of
*   Medicine and Pharmacy*
Rootstown, Ohio

Dishant G. Shah, M.D.
Fellow, Diagnostic Neuroradiology
University of Maryland Medical Center
Baltimore, Maryland

Raj C. Shah, M.D.
Assistant Professor
Family Medicine and Rush Alzheimer's Disease
*   Center*
Rush University Medical Center
Chicago, Illinois

Megan M. Shanks, M.D.
Assistant Professor
Department of Neurological Sciences
Rush University Medical Center
Chicago, Illinois

Robert K. Shin, M.D.
Associate Professor of Neurology
Associate Professor of Ophthalmology and Visual
*   Sciences*
University of Maryland School of Medicine
Director, Neuro-Ophthalmology, University
*   Eye Care*
Baltimore, Maryland

Lisa M. Shulman, M.D.
Eugenia Brin Professor of Parkinson's Disease and
*   Movement Disorders and*
the Roslyn Newman Distinguished Scholar in
*   Parkinson's Disease*
University of Maryland School of Medicine
Co-Director, Maryland Parkinson's Disease Center
Baltimore, Maryland

Madhu Soni, M.D.
Assistant Professor
Department of Neurological Sciences
Rush University Medical Center
Chicago, Illinois

Tricia Y. Ting, M.D.
Assistant Professor of Neurology
University of Maryland School of Medicine
Director, Ambulatory Services
University of Maryland Epilepsy Center
Baltimore, Maryland

Jordan L. Topel, M.D.
Associate Professor
Department of Neurological Sciences
Rush University Medical Center
Chicago, Illinois

Amy Wilcox Voigt, M.D.
Fellow
Jefferson Headache Center
Thomas Jefferson University
Philadelphia, Pennsylvania

Allison L. Weathers, M.D.
Assistant Professor
Department of Neurological Sciences
Rush University Medical Center
Chicago, Illinois

William J. Weiner, M.D.
Professor and Chairman
Department of Neurology
University of Maryland School of Medicine
Director,
Maryland Parkinson's Disease and Movement
*   Disorders Center*
Baltimore, Maryland

Robert S. Wilson, M.D., Ph.D.
Professor of Neurological and Behavioral Sciences
Rush Alzheimer's Disease Center
Rush University Medical Center
Chicago, Illinois

Preface

This sixth edition of *Neurology for the Non-Neurologist* carries on a tradition of medical education that began over 20 years ago with the first edition of this book. All editions have been anchored in an ongoing commitment to demystify neurology, so that its principles and ever-growing knowledge base are accessible to nonspecialists. Clearly, brain, spinal cord, nerve, and muscle disorders are encountered by primary care physicians, including internists, family practitioners, hospitalists, and pediatricians. Likewise, because of the interplay of brain and mind function as well as the necessary adaptations that patients endure from neurologic disorders, psychiatrists also see many neurologic patients. As the core group of physicians for whom this book is written, these colleagues have embraced the former editions of *Neurology for the Non-Neurologist*, and we hope this new version will likewise meet their educational and practice-based needs.

Structurally, the new edition is similar to the last edition, but with several significant additions. The major neurologic disorders are covered with an attention to the more commonly encountered diseases, but with careful signaling to signs or symptoms that can suggest more unusual disorders. We begin the textbook with three overview chapters on Neurologic Symptoms, Neurologic Examination, and Diagnostic Tests. These chapters orient readers to the significance of typical patterns of patient descriptions, the different clustering of neurologic signs that help clarify diagnostic categories, and the panoply of neurologic investigations available to define a likely single diagnosis. Subsequent chapters focus on major neurologic dilemmas that non-neurologists will encounter, ranging from Epilepsy, Dementia, Infections, and Sleep Disorders to Peripheral Neuropathy, Neuromuscular Disease, Movement Disorders, including Parkinson's Disease, Multiple Sclerosis, and Cerebrovascular Disease, including stroke. We also cover topics based primarily on patient complaints: Vertigo and Dizziness, Headaches, Low Back Pain, and Falls. Most of these chapters stand as independent discussions, but they are integrated with chapters that cross individual disease-based categories and therefore have broad applications to other chapters: Neuroradiology, Behavioral Neurology, Drug-induced Disorders, Medical-legal Issues, Neurologic Emergencies, Eye Signs in Neurologic Diagnosis, and Rehabilitation. With these different levels and approaches, we hope to cover the major areas of neurology from the perspective of the non-neurologist who is likely to be the first-line physician with primary responsibility for managing neurologic problems within a full medical context.

As editors, we have asked authors to follow a template that is consistent from chapter to chapter. Each chapter begins with a few *Key Points* that can be reviewed before launching into the full text. Each chapter presents the general pattern of neurologic signs pertinent to the topic and this text is interspersed with highlighted *Special Clinical Points* to focus the reader on the most important details. Neurology is anchored in a two-part discipline of defining the anatomy of a syndrome and then establishing an etiology or cause. This principle is carried through each chapter text. Authors alert readers to *Special Considerations in the Hospitalized Patient* and *When a Non-neurologist Should Consider Referring to a Neurologist*. Finally, we close each chapter with a section, termed *Always Remember*, to leave the reader with a few important issues that can be immediately applied in practice. We feel this new arrangement helps to integrate the chapters and allows busy practitioners to read the full text or to scan the chapters with these most important highlights clearly marked. Updated references and a series of self-study questions close each chapter.

We are particularly proud of our list of recruited authors. Some have been part of this textbook since the first edition, some have participated in at least one earlier edition, and some are new. Their commitment to education, a clear writing style, and direct experience with neurologic education have made the editorial management of this edition smooth and efficient. We have also expanded our Editor team to four editors, with the long-term plan that the senior editors will need to pass the baton eventually if this book remains successful and if book publishing remains a viable educational tool. Editorship requires an agile and harmonious team that can work together and at the same time assume individual responsibility; we feel we have achieved both goals very comfortably with the textbook edition. In an era when North American practice patterns and health care may rapidly evolve, we feel that *Neurology for the Non-Neurologist* is particularly important as an educational resource.

William J. Weiner, MD
Christopher G. Goetz, MD
Steven L. Lewis, MD
Robert K. Shin, MD

Acknowledgments

We continue to acknowledge the direction and help that Maynard M. Cohen, MD, PhD, provided when the first edition of this book appeared in 1981. We are also indebted to the very fine support work provided by Cheryl Grant-Johnson, Marilynn Payton, and Janet Gillard.

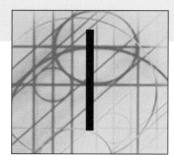

The Neurologic Examination

ROBERT K. SHIN AND NEIL C. PORTER

> **key points**
> - The neurologic examination provides a comprehensive assessment of the function of the human nervous system.
> - When used in conjunction with the history, the neurologic examination can provide information critical to making a correct diagnosis.
> - With practice, the neurologic examination can be performed efficiently and quickly.

he neurologic examination is the foundation of the practice of neurology and an integral part of the physical examination. Unlike some medical disciplines that may emphasize ancillary studies, investigations in neurology are guided primarily by the information gleaned from the neurologic history and examination. Because the neurologic examination is often crucial in establishing the correct diagnosis, all physicians should be able to perform and document a complete evaluation of the nervous system.

At the same time, it is not always practical to perform a detailed neurologic examination on every patient. A focused neurologic examination should be influenced by the information obtained from the interview and guided by the examiner's clinical judgment.

■ **SPECIAL CLINICAL POINT: Not every patient requires a detailed neurologic examination, but physicians should at least be familiar with each component of the comprehensive neurologic examination.**

TABLE 1.1	Organization of the Neurologic Examination

I. Cognition
II. Cranial nerves
III. Motor function
IV. Deep tendon reflexes (DTR)
V. Sensation
VI. Coordination and gait

The neurologic examination is divided into several parts (Table 1.1). These include assessment of cognition, cranial nerves, motor function, reflexes, sensation, and coordination and gait. Each of these parts has multiple components with which all physicians should be familiar.

MENTAL STATUS AND COGNITION

The cognitive examination provides an assessment of the patient's general mental status, evaluating the integrity of the cerebral hemispheres.

A comprehensive mental status examination may begin with a general assessment of the patient's *appearance*, *level of consciousness*, and *mood and affect*. Important primary cognitive domains to be tested include *speech and language*, *memory*, *visuospatial processing*, and *executive functioning* (including judgment and insight). *Disorders of perception* or *disorders of thought form and content* should be noted.

■ **SPECIAL CLINICAL POINT: Important primary cognitive domains include speech and language, memory, visuospatial processing, and executive functioning.**

Often patients with cognitive problems will try to hide their deficiencies or may try to avoid directly answering questions. One can minimize resistance to this testing by reassuring the patient that all of the questions are part of the standard exam (e.g., "These are questions that we ask everybody."). Mistakes on the patient's part should be noted silently or corrected gently by the examiner in order to keep the patient at ease.

Appearance and Behavior

The patient's appearance and general behavior are important indicators of his or her general level of function. The well-dressed, well-organized patient is likely functioning at a higher level than the disheveled, unkempt patient. Additionally, a patient's dress and demeanor are important indicators of underlying psychiatric and psychological disturbances, such as the patient who is inappropriately dressed for the weather or is clearly responding to unseen stimuli.

Level of Consciousness

Level of consciousness is a crucial part of the mental status examination. One should note and document whether the patient is awake, alert, and attentive versus unresponsive or drowsy. A *lethargic* patient appears drowsy but is easily aroused. An *obtunded* patient has a reduced level of consciousness and cannot easily be aroused. An unconscious patient who cannot be fully aroused is *stuporous*. An unconscious patient with no purposeful response to even noxious stimuli is *comatose*.

Mood and Affect

Mood refers to a person's persistent emotional state, while *affect* denotes more immediacy. Mood and affect can be assessed by observing the patient's body language and behavior as well as by verbal report. *Depression* is a state of persistently low mood. A brief screen for depression includes inquiries about reduced "spirits," reduced energy, poor self-attitude, poor appetite, disturbed sleep, anhedonia, thinking difficulty, suicidal ideation, and psychomotor retardation. Conversely, *mania* is a state of persistently elevated mood, increased energy, and heightened self-attitude, sometimes in association with delusions of grandeur, pressured speech, and "flight of ideas." Depression is seen in a number of neurologic disorders including Parkinson disease, Huntington disease, and strokes affecting the dominant hemisphere; mania may be seen occasionally with cerebral lesions of the nondominant hemisphere.

Speech and Language

Speech refers to the articulation of words, while language deals more with the structure and meaning of the spoken and written word. Both provide the examiner valuable insight into the patient's mental state and can be assessed easily during the interview. Important aspects of speech include the amplitude or loudness, volume or amount (paucity vs. overabundance), and prosody or fluidity. Often patients with end-stage dementia will have paucity of speech. Patients with Parkinson disease will often have *hypophonic* or soft speech. Patients with cerebellar disorders may speak in a "choppy" *ataxic* manner. Speech may be slurred or *dysarthric* in a number of different clinical settings.

A patient's language capabilities can be assessed quickly by evaluating spontaneous speech and comparing it to comprehension of spoken and written material. The presence of a language disturbance or *aphasia* should be identified early, as it may preclude an adequate assessment of the rest of the mental status examination. An aphasia may be *expressive* or *receptive*. An expressive or nonfluent aphasia (e.g., Broca aphasia) is characterized by difficulty producing speech with intact comprehension, and typically results from lesions in the inferior frontal region of the dominant (usually left) hemisphere. In contrast, a receptive or fluent aphasia (e.g., Wernicke aphasia) is characterized by poor comprehension without difficulty producing speech. This may result in the production of nonsensical speech ("word salad") and is typically caused by lesions of the posterior temporal area of the dominant hemisphere.

Additonal localizing information can be gleaned by assessing the patient's ability to repeat and write.

Memory

Two components of memory are commonly assessed–*working memory* (also known as primary memory) and *long-term memory* (also known as secondary memory).

Working memory is assessed by measuring *digit span* (most patients can repeat strings of approximately seven digits) or by *backward spelling* ("Please spell WORLD backward."), which are commonly interpreted as tests of attention.

Long-term memory is typically tested using *delayed word recall*. Patients are given a list of three to five words (e.g., "cat, table, apple, purple, and bank") and asked to repeat them back (registration). After being distracted by other tasks (such as tests of working memory or visuospatial processing), the patient is asked to recall the list of words (retrieval). Clues or cues may be given (e.g., "One of the words was an animal," or "One of the words began with the letter C."). Difficulty with this type of delayed

recall can be seen with lesions of the temporal lobe or thalami affecting the hippocampi or other structures within the *Papez loop*. The distinction between "recent long-term memory" (e.g., "What you had for breakfast this morning?") versus "remote long-term memory" (e.g., an event from childhood) is somewhat artificial.

The use of the term *short-term memory* may be confusing as some use it to refer to working memory, while others use it to refer to recent long-term memory (see Chapter 15, Behavioral Neurology).

Visuospatial Processing

Common tests of visuospatial processing include *copying a complex figure* or *clock drawing*. Patients can be asked to copy a design drawn by the examiner (e.g., a drawing of a cube, intersecting pentagons, or the façade of a house), or they may be asked to draw a clock face set to a particular time (e.g., "twenty after eight"). Patients with parietal dysfunction may neglect to draw half of the figure or may have trouble placing the numbers correctly on the clock face.

Executive Function

The integrity of the frontal lobes may be tested in several ways. Poor performance on tests of *executive function*, poor *judgment and insight*, or the presence of *frontal release signs* may all be evidence of frontal lobe impairment.

Some simple tests of executive function include assessment of *verbal fluency* and *oral trail making*. To assess verbal fluency, patients should be asked to generate a list of words from a specific category (e.g., "words that begin with the letter F" or "all of the animals you can think of") in 1 minute. Although normative values vary based on age and level of education, most patients should be able to generate 10 or more items for each list without much difficulty. Oral trail making involves having the patient sequentially alternate between letters and numbers ("A–1–B–2–C–3– etc."). Patients with frontal lobe dysfunction may perform poorly on these tests while doing surprisingly well on other components of the cognitive examination.

A person's *judgment* relies on the value system, making an assessment of judgment the most subjective component of the mental status examination. Clinicians may ask questions such as "What would you do if you found a stamped envelope lying on the ground?" with the expected answer being, "Place the envelope in a mailbox." Such questioning is probably most helpful in the patient who is demented or cognitively impaired. *Insight* refers to the patient's understanding of his or her condition. The patient with Alzheimer disease, for example, may have little awareness of memory loss, often denying any problems in thinking.

When the frontal lobes are damaged due to trauma, tumor, stroke, or dementia, primitive reflexes may resurface. For example, the presence of a *palmar grasp reflex* (reflexive gripping of a finger or object stroking the palm) may signify a lesion of the contralateral frontal lobe. An abnormal *glabellar reflex* (persistent blinking in response to tapping of the forehead) can be noted in the setting of frontal lobe injury, although it may also be present in parkinsonian disorders. Other frontal release signs include the *palmomental reflex* (a twitch of the corner of the mouth when the ipsilateral palm is stroked), *rooting* (turning toward the cheek when stroked), and the *snout reflex* (pursing of the lips when the lips are tapped lightly). The presence or absence of frontal release signs does not, however, correlate well with degree of dementia.

Perceptual Disturbances

Patients who are psychotic or delirious often report bizarre sensory experiences such as hallucinations and illusions. *Hallucinations* are perceptions in the absence of stimuli. These can be elicited by asking the patient if he or she has seen (or heard) things that "weren't really there" or "that others couldn't see (or hear)." *Illusions* are misperceptions, whereby the patient mistakes an object for something else, such as a coat for an intruder. Both hallucinations and illusions can be seen in patients who are delirious or encephalopathic.

Thought Form and Content

Abnormalities of thought form and content are "psychotic features" associated with delirium, dementia, schizophrenia, and severe affective disorders. Abnormalities of thought content consist of bizarre beliefs such as delusions, obsessions, compulsions, and phobias. *Delusions* are fixed, false, idiosyncratic beliefs tenaciously held by patients. *Obsessions* are intrusive, recurring thoughts that disturb patients. Similarly, compulsions are acts that patients feel compelled to perform over and over again. Lastly, *phobias* are irrational fears held by patients. These abnormalities of thought content can be uncovered by simply asking the patient if he or she has "any special powers," or any strong beliefs or practices that others do not share. Paranoid delusions can be specifically detected by asking patients if "anyone is after them" or if "anyone is out to get them."

Abnormalities of thought form consist of disordered thinking such as "thought blocking," "loosening of associations," and "flight of ideas." *Thought blocking* is evident when patients are unable to complete their thoughts while speaking. *Loosening of associations* is seen when patients jump from one subject to another with little connection. Similarly, *flight of ideas* is manifested by patients speaking at a rapid pace, on any number of subjects, without easily identifiable connections. Detecting abnormalities of thought form involves noting the manner in which patients volunteer information or respond to questions. Responses that are clear and concise are easily distinguishable from answers that are difficult to follow.

Mini-Mental Status Examination (MMSE)

The MMSE is a commonly used screen for abnormalities of cognition. The MMSE is a 30-

point instrument that assesses orientation, language, recall, concentration, and some visuospatial skills. Ten points are awarded for varying degrees of orientation in time and space. Three points are given for registration (correctly repeating the names of three objects). Five points are given for concentration, which is tested by having the patient spell "WORLD" backward or sequentially subtracting 7 from 100 five times (e.g., 100, 93, 86, 79, 72, 65). Three points are given for correctly naming two objects and repeating the phrase "No ifs, ands, or buts." Three points are given for following a three-step command. Three points are given for reading and enacting the sentence "close your eyes," writing a sentence, and copying a figure composed of two interlocking pentagons. Finally, three points are given for recalling the three objects mentioned for testing registration.

■ **SPECIAL CLINICAL POINT: The MMSE should not serve as a substitute for the full mental status evaluation, but it may be helpful as a screening tool.**

Other brief neuropsychological batteries have been developed which may be useful in the clinical setting, such as the Montreal Cognitive Assessment (MoCA), which includes measures of frontal lobe/executive functioning in addition to tests of memory, language, and visuospatial processing.

CRANIAL NERVES

There are 12 pairs of cranial nerves, each serving a specific function as illustrated in Table 1.2. A superficial examination of the cranial nerves should be incorporated into any neurologic examination and can be completed

TABLE 1.2	Cranial Nerves and Their Functions	
Cranial Nerve	**Name of the Cranial Nerve**	**Function**
I	Olfactory	Smell
II	Optic	Vision
III	Oculomotor	Elevation, depression, and adduction of the eye; pupillary constriction
IV	Trochlear	Depression of the adducted eye; intorsion of the abducted eye
V	Trigeminal	Sensation of the face and motor control of the muscles of mastication
VI	Abducens	Abduction of the eye
VII	Facial	Muscles of facial expression, taste to the anterior two thirds of the tongue
VIII	Vestibulocochlear	Hearing and balance
IX	Glossopharyngeal	Taste of posterior one third of the tongue, sensation for gag reflex
X	Vagus	Gag reflex motor to soft palate, pharynx, larynx; autonomic fibers to esophagus, stomach, small intestine, heart, trachea; sensation from ear; viscera
XI	Spinal accessory	Motor control of the sternocleidomastoid and trapezius muscles
XII	Hypoglossal	Motor control of the tongue

in just a few minutes. Abnormalities found on the cursory examination may necessitate a more detailed study of that area.

■ **SPECIAL CLINICAL POINT: A systematic examination of the cranial nerves provides "top to bottom" information about the integrity of the brainstem. Remember the "4-4-4" rule: The first four cranial nerves involve the "higher" subcortical structures or *midbrain*. The second four cranial nerves generally localize to the *pons*. The final four cranial nerves originate from the *medulla* or upper cervical cord.**

CN I. The Olfactory Nerve

The olfactory nerve (cranial nerve I) is responsible for the sense of smell. CN I is not tested routinely during the screening neurologic examination, but should be assessed when patients complain of loss of smell. Olfaction is assessed by having the patient identify a fragrant substance such as coffee or cloves. A small vial of the aromatic substance is held under one nostril, while the other nostril is occluded. The patient is asked to breathe through the unobstructed nostril and identify the scent. The exercise is repeated on the other side with a different aromatic substance. Noxious substances such as ammonia or "smelling salts" should be avoided because of the concomitant stimulation of cranial nerve V, the trigeminal nerve. Although reduced olfaction may be due to advanced age, pathologic states such as head trauma, tumors affecting the base of the skull, and certain inflammatory disorders such as sarcoid should also be considered.

CN II. The Optic Nerve

The optic nerve (cranial nerve II) is responsible for vision. Evaluation of the optic nerve includes examination of visual acuity, visual fields, the pupillary light reflex, and funduscopy. Visual acuity is typically tested using a wall chart or handheld "near-card." Each eye should be tested separately with contact lenses or glasses in place (if needed).

The pupillary light reflex is checked by having the patient look into the distance while swinging a bright light from one eye to the other. Normally, both pupils react equally to light shone in either eye (the "consensual response"). A lesion of one optic nerve may result in a weaker pupillary response from one eye when compared to the other. When severe, such a *relative afferent pupillary defect* results in a paradoxical dilation of the pupils when light is swung from the "good eye" to the "bad eye."

Visual fields can be easily tested in the office or at the bedside by confrontation. The patient should be asked to fixate on the examiner's nose while covering one eye. The examiner should hold up one, two, or five fingers in each of the four quadrants of the visual field and ask the patient to count the fingers. One or multiple trials can be conducted, depending on the accuracy of the patient. The other eye should be tested in the same manner.

A visual field defect present only in one eye suggests a lesion within that eye or of the optic nerve. Visual field defects present in both eyes may suggest a lesion farther back along the visual pathway. A *bitemporal hemianopia* (affecting the temporal fields of both eyes) implies a lesion of the optic chiasm. *Quadrantanopias*, lesions of the same quadrant of both eyes (upper right, upper left, lower right, or lower left), suggest a lesion of the optic radiations. A *homonymous hemianopia*, a field cut involving the same side of both eyes (meaning the temporal field of one eye and the nasal field of the other eye), suggests a lesion of the contralateral optic tract or occipital cortex. With experience, additional visual field defects such as central scotomas, macular sparing, or incongruous hemianopias can be detected as well (see Chapter 26, Eye Signs in Neurologic Diagnosis).

For many examiners, the funduscopic examination is the most challenging aspect of the neurologic examination. Proficiency with ophthalmoscopy requires careful instruction and practice. Items that can be evaluated with a direct handheld ophthalmoscope include the optic disc, the retinal vessels that emanate from the disc, the macula, and the peripapillary retina. The optic disc lies slightly nasal to midline and is best visualized by approaching the patient slightly from the side with the same eye (i.e., use the right eye to look in a patient's right eye, and the left eye to look in a patient's left eye). Normally, the optic disc has a sharp border, but in the setting of papilledema or optic neuritis, the margins appear blurred. Optic atrophy due to optic nerve damage results in a pale disc. Arteries and veins generally run together, with veins appearing thicker than arteries. The forklike branching of retinal arteries and veins "point to" the disc. A number of medical conditions, such as diabetes and hypertension, produce characteristic findings on the funduscopic examination. The macula can be visualized by asking the patient to "look directly at the light."

CN III. Oculomotor Nerve, CN IV. Trochlear Nerve, and CN VI. Abducens Nerve

The oculomotor nerve (cranial nerve III), trochlear nerve (cranial nerve IV), and abducens nerve (cranial nerve VI) control eye movements. The oculomotor nerve (CN III) supplies the superior, inferior, and medial rectus muscles as well as the inferior oblique muscle. These muscles elevate, depress, and adduct the eye. The trochlear nerve supplies the superior oblique muscle. Contraction of this muscle results in depression of the adducted eye and intorsion of the abducted eye. The abducens nerve supplies the lateral rectus muscle. Contraction of this muscle results in abduction of the eye.

These three cranial nerves are assessed together during testing of eye movements. The patient should follow the examiner's finger or pen vertically and horizontally into the cardinal directions of gaze (up, down, left, and right). Normally, the eyes should move together (conjugate gaze). A monocular limitation of abduction may suggest a sixth palsy. A monocular limitation in vertical gaze could be consistent with a third or fourth nerve palsy. Myasthenia gravis and thyroid eye disease can

be associated with eye movement abnormalities. Nystagmus may be noted during the eye movement examination, which can suggest vestibular or cerebellar dysfunction.

The third nerve also controls elevation of the upper eyelid (via the levator palpebrae superioris) muscle and pupillary constriction via parasympathetic fibers to the pupilloconstrictor and ciliary muscles. A complete lesion of the cranial nerve III will result in ptosis and an eye that is abducted and depressed ("down and out"), with a dilated pupil (*mydriasis*). A lesion of cranial nerve VI will result in *esotropia* ("crossed eyes") and an inability to abduct the affected eye. A lesion of cranial nerve IV may result in the patient having a head tilt and head turn away from the affected eye (see Chapter 26, Eye Signs in Neurologic Diagnosis).

CN V. The Trigeminal Nerve

The trigeminal nerve is responsible for sensory information from the skin of the face and anterior scalp, providing motor innervation to the muscles of mastication (masseter, temporalis, and pterygoid), and mediating the *jaw jerk reflex*. The trigeminal nerve is divided into three branches, V_1 (ophthalmic branch), V_2 (maxillary branch), and V_3 (mandibular branch) (Fig. 1.1). V_1 innervates the forehead and anterior scalp down to the lateral corner of the eye; V_2 innervates the cheek down to the corner of the mouth; and V_3 innervates the jaw including the underside of the chin, but excluding the angle of the jaw.

The sensory function of the trigeminal nerve can be tested using a safety pin for pain sensation, a cool tuning fork for temperature sensation, and a fingertip or cotton swab for light touch. The corneal reflex also can be used to evaluate CN V, particularly in an unresponsive patient. To test the corneal reflex, the examiner touches a wisp of cotton to the cornea over the iris, avoiding the pupil or central visual axis.

Jaw strength can be tested by asking the patient to forcibly clench his or her teeth against the resistance of the examiner or by forcibly

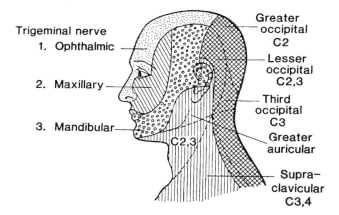

FIGURE 1.1 Distribution of the three divisions of the trigeminal nerve. The sensory portion of the trigeminal nerve has three divisions: I, ophthalmic; II, maxillary; III, mandibular. Their approximate locations are illustrated. (From members of the Department of Neurology, Mayo Clinic, and Mayo Foundation for Medical Education and Research. *Clinical Examinations in Neurology.* 6th ed. St. Louis: Mosby Year Book; 1991:270, with permission.)

opening the jaw against resistance. The jaw jerk reflex is mediated solely by the trigeminal nerve and is elicited by placing one's index finger across the relaxed jaw of the patient and tapping that finger with a reflex hammer. A normal response is a brisk but slight contraction of the muscles of mastication causing partial jaw closure. An exaggerated response may be a sign of cerebral pathology (an upper motor neuron sign originating above the foramen magnum), but an absent response has little clinical significance.

CN VII. The Facial Nerve

The facial nerve provides innervation to the muscles of facial expression and also supplies taste to the anterior two thirds of the tongue via the *chorda tympani*. Integrity of the facial nerve can be assessed by having the patient perform various maneuvers such as forcibly closing his or her eyes, smiling, puffing air into the cheeks, and wrinkling the forehead muscles. Weakness is indicated by an inability to "bury" the eyelashes, an asymmetric smile, inability to hold air fully in the cheeks, and reduced forehead wrinkling. Facial weakness also can be assessed by simple observation. A downturned mouth,

sagging cheek (flattened nasolabial fold), or sagging lower eyelid (widened palpebral fissure) are all indicators of facial weakness. Peripheral lesions of the facial nerve produce eyelid retraction and not ptosis, so that the eye on the affected side appears "larger" than the normal eye. Facial weakness can occur on the basis of disturbances in the central or peripheral nervous systems. Involvement of the frontalis muscles (responsible for wrinkling the forehead) can reliably distinguish between these two possibilities. The forehead is spared with central lesions such as strokes but is affected by peripheral lesions as in *Bell palsy*.

The sense of taste may be affected by a peripheral disturbance if the lesion is proximal to the chorda tympani. To test the sense of taste, the patient is asked to protrude his or her tongue and identify sweet or sour substances, although this is not commonly tested as a part of a routine neurologic examination.

CN VIII. The Vestibulocochlear Nerve

The vestibulocochlear, or acoustic, nerve (cranial nerve VIII) is a compound nerve composed of the cochlear nerve, responsible for hearing, and the vestibular nerve, involved in balance. Although a number of techniques can be used to assess hearing, a simple screen consists of gently rubbing one's fingers together near the patient's ear to check for gross hearing defects.

Additional methods to test function of cranial nerve VIII include the Rinne and Weber tests. In the Rinne test, the base of a vibrating tuning fork (256 Hz) is held against the mastoid bone. When the sound disappears, the head of the tuning fork then is placed beside the patient's ear. Normally, air conduction is greater than bone conduction. If bone conduction is greater than air conduction, a blockage of the external ear or a defect within the middle ear should be suspected. In the Weber test, a vibrating tuning fork is pressed firmly against the middle of the patient's forehead. Normally, sound is perceived equally in both ears and the sound of the vibration is appreciated as being in the midline. With conductive hearing loss, the sound lateralizes to the abnormal ear. In contrast, with sensorineural hearing loss, the sound lateralizes to the opposite ear with the intact nerve.

Dysfunction of the vestibular component of the acoustic nerve is suggested by complaints of vertigo and a unidirectional jerk nystagmus on examination of eye movements. Advanced testing of vestibular function might include the head thrust maneuver and testing of dynamic visual acuity.

CN IX. Glossopharyngeal Nerve and CN X. Vagus Nerve

The glossopharyngeal nerve is responsible for providing sensation to the pharynx and taste to the posterior tongue. The vagus nerve performs a number of functions within the body, including supplying parasympathetic innervation to the heart and gut and contributing to the normal motor function of the oropharynx.

Cranial nerve IX mediates the sensory limb of the *gag reflex*, and cranial nerve X mediates its motor limb. Typically, a gag reflex is elicited by gently stimulating the soft palate with a cotton swab or tongue blade. Normally,

a gag response is elicited by stimulation of either side. A unilateral cranial nerve lesion may suppress the gag reflex on one side. A wide range of variability exists for the normal gag reflex. Some patients will start to gag as soon as they see the tongue blade, while others will have no gag reflex. In the appropriate clinical setting (e.g., the patient with swallowing difficulties), an apparently abnormal gag reflex may assume greater significance. Oftentimes clinicians forgo formal testing of the gag reflex, assessing simply the motor aspect by having the patient say "aah."

Normally, the soft palate and uvula elevate symmetrically with stimulation of the soft palate or when a subject says "aah." With a unilateral lesion of the vagus nerve, the uvula and palate deviate away from the lesion. With bilateral lesions, no movement may be seen.

CN XI. Spinal Accessory Nerve

The accessory nerve innervates the trapezius and sternocleidomastoid muscles. It arises from the upper five cervical segments of the spinal cord, ascends through the foramen magnum, and exits through the jugular foramen. The accessory nerve is tested by having the patient shrug his or her shoulders or turn his or her head against resistance (the examiner's hand pressed against the subject's jaw). A unilateral lesion causes weakness of shoulder shrugging on the same side or impaired head turning toward the opposite side.

CN XII. Hypoglossal Nerve

The hypoglossal nerve (cranial nerve XII) provides motor innervation to the tongue. Testing of CN XII includes examination of the bulk of the tongue, the ability of the patient to protrude the tongue in the midline, and the ability of the patient to rapidly move the tongue from side to side. Normally, the tongue should appear symmetrical and the patient should be able to protrude the tongue straight ahead and move the tongue rapidly from side to side.

With unilateral lesions of CN XII, the tongue may appear atrophied with evident fasciculations (muscle twitches) on one side. Furthermore, on protrusion, the tongue will deviate toward the weak side.

MOTOR EXAMINATION

The motor examination consists of assessment of muscle bulk, tone, strength, and dexterity, with notation of any abnormal movements. Muscle bulk simply refers to the normal size and contour of the muscle and is assessed by simple inspection. Muscle wasting or atrophy is a "lower motor neuron sign" seen in disorders of the peripheral nervous system such as radiculopathies and neuropathies; muscle hypertrophy is rarely seen, but may be noted in specific disorders (e.g., calf hypertrophy in Duchenne muscular dystrophy).

Muscle tone is defined as the resistance to passive movement. In the arm, one assesses muscle tone by supporting the patient's relaxed upper arm, grasping the patient's fingers, and then quickly flexing, extending, pronating, and supinating the arm at the elbow. Normal tone is negligible, but increased tone can be appreciated as marked resistance to movement. The increased tone may have a "ratchety" quality that is intermittent (i.e., "cogwheel" rigidity of Parkinson disease), a give-way quality reminiscent of one opening a pocket or "clasp knife" (i.e., spasticity seen in upper motor neuron lesions), or a more diffuse, persistent quality (i.e., "lead-pipe" rigidity seen with disorders of the basal ganglia). In the leg, one assesses tone with the patient supine and relaxed. The examiner grasps the patient's knee with two hands and quickly lifts the knee into the air noting whether the patients heel drags along the bed (normal) or comes off the bed (indicative of increased tone).

■ **SPECIAL CLINICAL POINT: Upper motor neuron signs (increased tone, brisk reflexes, Babinski sign) signify pathology of the central nervous system (brain or spinal cord). Lower motor neuron signs (decreased tone, muscle atrophy and fasciculations, depressed reflexes) signify pathology of the peripheral nervous system (nerve roots or peripheral nerves). A mix of upper and lower motor neuron signs may be seen in motor neuron disease (e.g., amyotrophic lateral sclerosis) or in spinal cord lesions that involve the anterior horn.**

Muscle power or strength refers to the force that muscles are able to generate. The examiner assesses muscle strength through manual muscle testing. Proper technique dictates that the examiner "isolate" the muscle being tested, using two hands to "stabilize" the limb proximal to the joint of interest and apply force to the limb distal to that joint. One should avoid testing across multiple joints to guard against involving unwanted muscles. Sufficient force must be applied to detect even mild weakness, yet not hurt the patient. Muscles that are commonly tested in the upper extremities include the deltoids, biceps, triceps, wrist extensors and flexors, and finger flexors and extensors. In the lower extremities, the hip flexors, knee flexors and extensors, and ankle dorsiflexors and plantarflexors are commonly tested.

Muscle strength is graded on a scale from 0 to 5: 0 = absence of movement; 1 = a flicker of movement; 2 = movement in the horizontal plane, removing the effect of gravity; 3 = movement against gravity; 4 = movement against some resistance; and 5 = normal strength (Table 1.3). Various patterns of weakness help one determine the origin of the disturbance.

TABLE 1.3	Medical Research Council (MRC) Grading of Muscle Strength
0/5	No movement
1/5	Flicker of movement
2/5	Moves with gravity removed but not against gravity
3/5	Moves against gravity
4/5	Movement against resistance
5/5	Normal strength

Weakness of muscle groups on one side of the body would suggest a cerebral disturbance. Weakness of the proximal muscles suggests a myopathy, while weakness of distal muscles suggests a neuropathic process (see Chapter 17, Neuromuscular Disorders).

Testing for a *pronator drift* is an easy method to detect subtle arm weakness. The patient holds up both arms, extended at the elbows, with the palms facing upward. When the patient closes his or her eyes, both arms should stay in place, next to each other. In the case of subtle arm weakness, however, the weaker arm will begin to pronate and drop toward the ground. A pronator drift is an extremely sensitive test, especially for subtle weakness of central origin.

To test the speed and dexterity of movement, patients are asked to open and close their hands rapidly, to tap their index finger and thumb together, or to pat their feet on the floor. The examiner is looking for the speed, amplitude, and regularity of these movements. Slowed movements suggest a problem within the pyramidal tracts or the extrapyamidal system.

Abnormal movements such as chorea and tremor are observed while the patient is at rest and while his or her hands are outstretched. These abnormal movements will be discussed in chapter 13, Hyperkinetic Movement Disorders.

DEEP TENDON REFLEXES (DTRs)

The DTRs, or muscle stretch reflexes, are monosynaptic reflexes responsible for preventing overstretching of the muscles and hyperextension of the corresponding joints (Table 1.4).

The afferent limb of each reflex is composed of sensory nerves that transmit information from the muscle spindles to the anterior horn cells within the spinal cord. The efferent limb is composed of motor nerves running from the spinal cord back to the original muscle. Although a number of DTRs have been described, only a few are routinely tested in the neurologic examination. These reflexes are the biceps, brachioradialis, and triceps reflexes in the upper extremities and the patellar (knee jerks) and Achilles reflexes (ankle jerks) in the lower extremities.

■ **SPECIAL CLINICAL POINT: The segmental representation of the commonly tested deep tendon reflexes can be remembering the "1-to-8" rule: The Achilles tendon reflex or "ankle jerk" is mediated by fibers from the S1 and S2 nerve roots. The patellar reflex or "knee jerk" is mediated by fibers from the L3 and L4 nerve roots. The biceps reflex is mediated by the C5 and C6 nerve roots. The triceps reflex is mediated by the C7 and C8 nerve roots.**

The Achilles reflex (ankle jerk) is elicited by striking the Achilles tendon just proximal to the heel and monitoring for subsequent plantarflexion. The patellar reflex (knee jerk) is elicited by striking the patellar tendon just below the kneecap. The biceps reflex is elicited by having the examiner strike his or her own finger that is pressed against the patient's biceps tendon within the antecubital fossa. The triceps reflex is elicited by striking the triceps tendon within the olecranon fossa, just above the elbow.

DTRs may be graded numerically (Table 1.5). Absent reflexes are graded as 0, reduced reflexes

TABLE 1.4	Segmental Innervation of the Various Deep Tendon Reflexes
S1, S2	Achilles reflex
(L2) L3, L4	Patellar reflex
C5, C6	Biceps reflex
(C6) C7, C8	Triceps reflex

TABLE 1.5	Deep Tendon Reflex Grading
1+ Reduced	
2+ Normal	
3+ Increased	
4+ Pathologically increased, clonus	

as 1+, normal reflexes as 2+, and brisk reflexes as 3+. When *clonus* is elicited (rhythmic, oscilatory movements of the joint), a grade of 4+ is given. Unfortunately, the determination of "normal" versus "reduced" versus "brisk" is subjective. To increase reliability, some authors promote the convention of using 3+ when "spread" is seen, whereby the testing of one reflex elicits responses in multiple reflex arcs (e.g., striking the biceps tendon elicits a triceps reflex). Similarly, the grade of 1+ could be reserved for instances in which "augmentation" is necessary (e.g., the patient is asked to "bite down" while the reflex is being elicited to reduce the threshold for the response).

Hyperactive reflexes are considered an "upper motor neuron sign" seen in central nervous system disturbances of the brain or spinal cord. Examples of such disorders include strokes, brain tumors, or spinal cord injuries. Somewhat brisk reflexes, however, can be seen in otherwise healthy young people. Reduced reflexes are seen in disorders of the peripheral nervous system and are considered a "lower motor neuron sign." Asymmetric decrease or loss of a particular reflex may be seen with focal lesions such as radiculopathies, plexopathies, or mononeuropathies. For example, a lesion of the sixth cervical root may lead to ipsilateral loss of the biceps and brachioradialis reflexes, while a femoral neuropathy may result in loss of the knee reflex. Symmetrical loss of reflexes implies a more generalized process. For example, bilaterally decreased or absent DTRs in the legs suggest a peripheral neuropathy, and generalize areflexia is often seen with Guillain–Barré syndrome (see Chapter 18, Peripheral Neurologic Disorders).

Assessment of the plantar response is included under reflex testing. The plantar response is obtained most commonly by stroking the lateral sole of the foot, starting at the heel, and then coming across the ball of the foot. This maneuver can be performed with a blunt but rigid object such as a key, a tongue depressor broken lengthwise, or even one's finger. The normal plantar response is flexion of the great toe with downward curling of the toes. In the setting of a central or upper motor neuron disorder, *Babinski sign* may be noted, in which the great toe extends and the toes fan outward.

SENSORY TESTING

The sensory examination is the most subjective portion of the neurologic examination, relying heavily on accurate reporting by the patient. If the patient is confused, demented, aphasic or delirious, the responses may be invalid and this portion of the examination may need to be omitted.

The primary sensory modalities consist of light touch, pain and temperature sensation, vibratory sensation, and proprioception. More complex cortical sensory processing includes stereognosis, graphesthesia, and appreciation of double simultaneous simulation.

The primary sensory modalities are carried on two separate sets of nerve fibers. In the peripheral nervous system, vibratory sensation and proprioception are carried by "large-fiber" nerves, while pain and temperature sensation are carried by "small-fiber" nerves. This dichotomy is preserved within the spinal cord where vibration and proprioception are conveyed by uncrossed fibers in the dorsal columns, while pain and temperature sensation are carried by crossed spinothalamic tracts. The two pathways eventually converge at the thalamus, which then sends projections to the primary sensory cortex within the parietal lobe. In diabetes and other small-fiber neuropathies, pain and temperature sensation may be more diminished than vibration and proprioception. In large-fiber neuropathies or dorsal column disease, as in vitamin B_{12} deficiency, the opposite pattern of sensory loss is seen with vibration sensation and proprioception being disproportionately affected.

Cortical sensory modalities are the products of the integrated primary sensory modalities. Cortical sensory loss can be evaluated only in the presence of intact primary sensory modalities. Disturbances in the cortical sensory modalities imply a dysfunction within the parietal lobes.

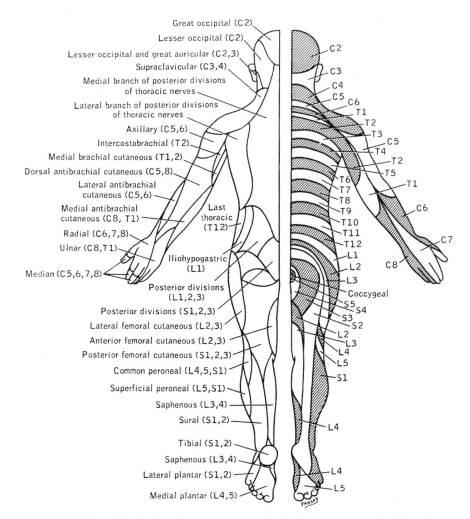

FIGURE I.2 Peripheral distribution of sensory nerves with the dermatomes on the right and cutaneous nerves on the left. (From House EL, Pansky B. *A Functional Approach to Neuroanatomy.* New York: McGraw-Hill; 1960:286, with permission.)

The primary sensory modalities should be evaluated in an organized fashion. Pain sensation is most reliably assessed with a disposable, sharp implement such as a safety pin. A quick assessment of side-to-side and proximal versus distal comparisons usually suffices unless the patient specifically complains of a region of reduced sensation. If a particular area of decreased sensation is identified, careful attention to its boundaries may suggest a disturbance at the level of the peripheral nerve, plexus, or nerve root (dermatomal) sensory loss (Fig. 1.2). Temperature sensation can be quickly tested using a cool tuning fork. As with assessment of pain, side-to-side and proximal versus distal differences should suffice. To test proprioception, the examiner grasps the subject's distal phalanx (tip of the great toe or index finger) on the sides of the digit while stabilizing the proximal digit. The examiner moves the finger or toe upward or downward, asking the patient to correctly identify the direction of movement without looking. The examiner assesses the patient's threshold for detection by initially moving the digit slightly and then progressively using larger movements until the patient can consistently answer correctly. For vibratory testing, the examiner sets the base of a vibrating tuning fork against a bony portion of the patient's digit or more proximal joint.

Testing of cortical sensory functions (graphesthesia, stereoagnosia, and double simultaneous stimulation) can reveal information about parietal lobe function, but only when the primary sensory modalities are intact. *Graphesthesia* is the ability to recognize by touch a number "written" on the skin. With the patient's eyes closed, the examiner traces numbers on the patient's palm using a finger or blunt object. *Stereognosis* is the ability to recognize objects by touch alone. Various items such as safety pins, keys, coins, or pencils are placed in the patient's hand with the patient's eyes closed. He is allowed to move the object around in his hand to fully appreciate the size, shape, and texture. If the hand is paretic, stereognosis still can be evaluated by moving the object around in the patient's palm. Double simultaneous stimulation is useful for detecting *hemispatial neglect*. The examiner alternately touches body parts (e.g., hand, face, or leg) on one side at a time, then on both sides simultaneously, asking the patient to identify which side has been touched. Patients with neglect may be able to appreciate sensation on both sides of the body when each side is tested separately, but will *extinguish* sensation on one side of the body when both sides are touched simultaneously.

COORDINATION AND GAIT

Coordinated movements require the integrated workings of a number of neurologic systems including the sensory pathways, vestibular system, pyramidal tracts, and extrapyramidal system, including the basal bangia and cerebellum. Incoordination in the setting of intact motor and sensory testing argues strongly for a disorder in cerebellar function. The cerebellum integrates proprioceptive information with information from muscles to allow smooth limb and truncal movements. Cerebellar dysfunction often results in *ataxia*. A unilateral lesion within the cerebellum produces dysfunction on the same side of the body.

Tests of coordination include finger-to-nose and heel-to-shin testing, evaluation of rapid alternating movements, station, and gait. The finger-to-nose and heel-to-shin tests assess for limb (appendicular) ataxia as opposed to truncal ataxia. In finger-to-nose testing, the patient is asked to guide his or her finger back and forth from the examiner's finger to his or her own nose with eyes open. The patient should be forced to fully extend his or her arm to touch the examiner's finger so that any tremor at the extreme of arm extension can be seen. Heel-to-shin testing is performed by having the patient run the heel of one foot along the shin, from the knee to the ankle, of the other leg.

Rapid alternating movements can be tested by asking the patient to pat the front and then back of his or her hand into the palm of the other hand or onto the thigh in a rapid, rhythmic fashion. Because rhythmic movements require an intact cerebellum, difficulty with this task suggests ipsilateral cerebellar dysfunction. The inability to perform this specific task is known as *dysdiadochokinesia*.

Midline cerebellar dysfunction often produces ataxia of the trunk, resulting in difficulties with standing or walking. To test stance, the patient first is asked to arise from a chair. A patient with hip weakness may require the use of his or her hands, while an ataxic patient may require the assistance of another individual. Next, the examiner assesses the patient's stance, noting the subject's posture, stability, and foot position. Normally, the patient should stand erect with feet slightly separated. A patient with Parkinson disease may exhibit a stooped posture, while a patient with cerebellar disease may have a widened stance and marked truncal instability. The examiner can further assess postural stability by gently pulling backward or forward on the patient's shoulders, guarding against the possibility of a fall. Normally, the patient should be able to quickly regain their stance, requiring no more than one or two steps. Patients with truncal instability, however, may need multiple steps to avoid falling or have no capacity to catch themselves.

Although often described as a test of balance, *Romberg test* is actually an assessment of proprioception. Patients are asked to stand with their feet together, and then asked to close their eyes. Patients may sway slightly, but they should not fall over or step to the side to catch their balance. Romberg test is positive when the patients lose their balance with their eyes closed, implying dysfunction of the dorsal columns or proprioceptive fibers. If a patient is unable to maintain balance with the eyes open (e.g., in the setting of vestibular dysfunction), then Romberg test cannot be performed.

■ **SPECIAL CLINICAL POINT: If a patient cannot stand with feet together and eyes open, he or she may have cerebellar or vestibular dysfunction. If a patient can stand with feet together and eyes open but falls with eyes closed (a positive Romberg test), then the problem is likely proprioceptive.**

Finally, the patient's ambulation is analyzed for speed, stride length, turning, and associated movements, with particular attention being paid to any asymmetry. Gait testing can be performed in the examination room or the adjacent hallway. Normally, the patient should exhibit a smooth stride with a narrow base and normal sway of the arms. Patients with a cerebellar disease may have an *ataxic gait* with a wide-based wobbly, off-balance ambulation that looks "drunk." Patients with upper motor neuron disease may have *gait spasticity*, exhibiting stiffness while walking reminiscent of "Frankenstein's monster." Patients with weakness of one side may have a *hemiparetic gait*, favoring one side, or perhaps associated with hip hiking or circumduction of the leg to overcome a unilateral foot drop. A patient with early Parkinson disease or mild unilateral arm weakness may have a decreased arm swing on one side with ambulation.

Optional tests include assessment of the patient's heel-walking, toe-walking, and tandem gait. Heel-walking and toe-walking, as their names imply, are performed by having patients walk on their heels and toes, respectively, testing the strength of foot dorsiflexion and plantarflexion. Tandem gait is assessed by having patients walk "heel to toe" as if walking on a tightrope. Impairment of tandem gait may be seen with mild ataxia and leg weakness.

THE NEUROLOGIC EXAMINATION IN PEDIATRIC NEUROLOGY

Performing age-appropriate examinations of infants and children can be a daunting task, given the amazing developmental changes that occur in early childhood. Infants and young children require adaptations of the routine adult neurologic examination including the use of more functional tasks to assess performance. A good working knowledge of normal gross motor, fine motor, and language development is essential. As with other pediatric disciplines, the child's parents can be enlisted to assist with examination. For small children and infants, much of the examination can be performed on the parent's lap to ensure the comfort and safety of the child. Unpleasant tests such as the testing of pain sensation (i.e., with a pin) should be avoided unless there is a specific need.

■ **SPECIAL CLINICAL POINT: The neurologic examination of children must be tailored to a child's age, abilities, and temperament. In order to be most effective, one must establish rapport with the child, be creative in testing, and make the examination fun!**

Mental Status

The mental status examination often centers around the child's behavior with respect to the parents and surroundings. Assessment of receptive and expressive language skills can yield insight into the child's cognitive abilities even in infancy. Knowledge of normal developmental milestones allows the examiner to relate a child's abilities to the normal population.

Cranial Nerves

Most cranial nerves can be tested easily with creative techniques in children. Visual acuity can be assessed roughly by holding colorful or bright objects of varying sizes within an infant's field of vision. For example, one can offer a toddler a small wad of paper within one's hand. The examiner can test visual fields and eye movements by holding attractive objects in the periphery of the child's vision and then having the child follow those objects with his or her eyes. Visual threat also can be used to test visual fields in infants older than 4 months of age, but this technique may be considered too threatening if not performed in a sufficiently playful manner. The funduscopic examination can be challenging but not impossible. The pupillary light reflex can be tested in standard fashion in all age groups. The corneal reflex can be tested in young infants but may be unacceptably irksome to older children. Although not technically proper, a quick puff of air into the eye is better tolerated than a cotton swab. The examiner can assess facial asymmetry by observing the child's repertoire of facial expressions. Observing how children respond to sounds made outside of their field of view can be used to assess hearing. As with the corneal reflex, testing of the gag reflex is well tolerated only by very young infants and older children. On the other hand, most children relish the opportunity to protrude their tongues at an adult.

Motor

Assessment of muscle bulk in children is no different than in adults except that young infants may have more superficial adipose tissue. Tone can be assessed easily in older children if they are at ease or distracted. Assessment of power in infants usually is restricted to opposing their volitional movements. In young children, one must rely on functional assessment of strength, observing the child perform playful tasks. Older children, however, are usually very cooperative in testing "how strong they are."

Deep Tendon Reflexes

Testing of DTRs in children requires no special accommodations other than gentleness, with the major exception being that the ankle jerks are better elicited in infants by grasping the infant's foot and gently tapping on the bottom of that foot. Along similar lines, the Babinski reflex can be elicited with one's finger in younger children and infants. Remember that an extensor plantar response (an upgoing toe) is normal in infants up to 1 year of age.

Sensory

Vibratory sensation can be tested reliably in older but not younger children. Proprioception is tested more reliably in children because the outcomes are directly observable by the examiner. Temperature sensation can be tested with a cool tuning fork. Testing of pin sensation should be avoided because of the inherently uncomfortable nature of the test.

Coordination

Age-appropriate testing of coordination is straightforward. Infants older than a few months can reach for colorful objects. Toddlers can be assessed for their ability to walk and reach for things. Older children can be asked to run, jump, and hop or stand on one leg.

Always Remember

- General principles of organization (e.g., peripheral vs. central, motor vs. sensory, and proximal vs. distal) allow lesion localization that aids in the differential diagnosis of neurologic disorders.
- A focused neurologic examination should be guided by clinical judgment.
- The neurologic examination should be a helpful tool, not a painful burden to be avoided by nonneurologists.

QUESTIONS AND DISCUSSION

1. A 62-year-old man complains of a 3-week history of generalized weakness, difficulty chewing and swallowing, and a change in the quality of speech. Further questioning reveals that he has been suffering from intermittent diplopia and drooping of one eyelid for the past year. The examination reveals ptosis of the left eyelid, impaired abduction of the left eye, weakness of jaw opening, and nasal speech. The gag reflex is present, but the soft palate elevates poorly. Weakness is generalized, affecting both proximal and distal muscles. There are no cognitive findings (including no emotional lability) and no sensory findings. Reflexes are normal and symmetrical, plantar responses are flexor, and tone is normal. The likely site of the lesion is:
   A. Both cerebral hemispheres
   B. The neuromuscular junction
   C. The brainstem affecting cranial nerves III, V, VI, IX, and X
   D. The peripheral nerves in a diffuse fashion as seen in Guillain–Barré syndrome

The correct answer is B. Myasthenia gravis is the most commonly seen disease of the neuromuscular junction. Myasthenia gravis can produce generalized weakness of the limbs as well as weakness of the face, eyes, and neck. Upper motor neuron signs and sensory findings should be absent.

Bilateral hemispheric disturbances should be associated with cognitive changes and even a reduced level of consciousness. Additionally, one should see bilateral upper motor neuron signs such as hyperreflexia, increased tone, and extensor plantar responses, all of which are lacking in this case.

A brainstem event large enough to affect this many cranial nerves should be associated with upper motor neuron signs and sensory abnormalities.

Guillain–Barré syndrome is an acute or subacute process characterized by hyporeflexia or areflexia. Ptosis is not a recognized feature. Sensory complaints are usually present.

2. A 55-year-old woman has noticed gradual loss of dexterity of her left hand and increasing difficulty with ambulation. Examination discloses an atrophied left hand and bilateral lower-extremity spasticity. The left lower extremity is weaker than the right, whereas pinprick is better perceived on that same side. The decrease in sensation to pinprick on the right side extends to the upper trunk. There are no cranial nerve findings, and cognitive function is intact. The likely site of the lesion is:
   A. An asymmetrical neuropathy affecting the left median nerve and both sciatic nerves
   B. A compressive lesion of the cervical cord
   C. Generalized motor neuron disease (amyotrophic lateral sclerosis)
   D. A lesion of the right cerebral hemisphere

The correct answer is B. This patient harbors a clinical picture consistent with Brown–Sequard syndrome, most likely due to cord compression. Originally seen with traumatic hemisection of the spinal cord, Brown–Sequard syndrome is characterized by weakness and dorsal column dysfunction ipsilateral to the lesion and spinothalamic dysfunction contralateral to the lesion. Additionally, upper motor neuron signs are seen ipsilaterally below the level of the lesion, while lower motor neuron signs (e.g., atrophy) are seen at the level of the lesion. In this case, the precise location of the lesion is given by the hand wasting, suggesting involvement of the lower motor neurons at the C8 or T1 root levels.

Polyneuropathy does not cause spasticity, which is an upper motor neuron sign. Motor neuron disease can present with a combination of upper and lower motor neuron signs as is seen in this case, but sensory involvement should be absent.

3. A 35-year-old woman complains of painful, burning feet and difficulty ambulating. On physical examination, she has severe loss of proprioception and vibratory sensation in the lower extremities (distal more than proximal), lower-extremity spasticity, hyperreflexia, and abnormal Babinski responses. The upper extremities show a similar sensory deficits but to a milder degree. Cranial nerves and cognition are intact. The likely site of the lesion is:
A. The dorsal columns and corticospinal tracts at the level of the spinal cord
B. The peripheral nerves, particularly the large myelinated fibers that conduct proprioceptive information
C. The brainstem, affecting the proprioceptive fibers (medial lemnisci) and corticospinal tracts
D. Bilateral spinothalamic tracts within the spinal cord

The correct answer is A. The loss of proprioception can be caused by a peripheral neuropathy affecting large myelinated fibers or to a disturbance of the dorsal columns in the spinal cord. The concurrent presence of upper motor neuron signs (spasticity, hyperreflexia, and Babinski responses) points to the spinal cord as the site of pathology.

A peripheral neuropathy could be associated with selective loss of proprioception and vibratory sensation but not upper motor neuron findings. The patient does not have evidence of cranial nerve involvement to suggest a disturbance in the brainstem.

4. A 25-year-old woman with myopia presents with a 3-day history of blurred vision and mild pain on eye movements in the left eye. Past history reveals that she has been experiencing amenorrhea for the preceding 6 months. There is a very strong family history of glaucoma. The extraocular movements are intact, and there is no ptosis. The eye examination discloses no overt abnormalities of the cornea, iris, or lens. Visual acuity is 20/80 on the left, corrected by glasses, and 20/15 in the right eye. The left pupil dilates when a light is swung from the right eye to the left eye. The visual field of the right eye is full. The patient has a subtle central scotoma in the left eye. Funduscopic examination is normal in both eyes. There are no other findings on neurologic examination. The likely site of the lesion is:
A. The optic chiasm as a result of compression by a pituitary gland tumor
B. The right occipital lobe or right optic radiations
C. The anterior chamber of the eye from an attack of acute glaucoma
D. The left optic nerve

The correct answer is D. The presentation is typical of acute optic neuritis: a decrease of central vision in one eye, associated with an afferent pupillary defect with minimal to no changes of the optic disc.

Although the patient's amenorrhea warrants investigation, a lesion at the level of the optic chiasm is commonly associated with bilateral visual field defects (e.g., a bitemporal hemianopsia).

A lesion of the right occipital lobe or the optic radiations would cause a loss of vision in the nasal field of the right eye and the temporal field of the left eye (i.e., a left homonymous hemianopsia).

Sudden loss of vision as a result of an acute attack of glaucoma would be associated with severe eye pain, redness, and possibly an unreactive pupil. The patient's positive family history for glaucoma proves to be a red herring rather than a clue in this particular case.

SUGGESTED READING

Adams RD, Victor M. *Principles of Neurology*. 5th ed. New York: McGraw-Hill; 1993:5–9.

De Myer WE. *Technique of the Neurological Examination: A Programmed Text*. 4th ed. New York: McGraw-Hill; 1994.

Glaser JS. *Neuro-ophthalmology*. 2nd ed. Philadelphia: J.B. Lippincott; 1990:37–60.

Haerer AF. *DeJong's the Neurologic Examination*. 5th ed. Philadelphia: J.B. Lippincott; 1992.

Kaplan HI, Sadock BJ. *Synopsis of Psychiatry*. 5th ed. Baltimore: Williams & Wilkins; 1988.

Medical Research Council. *Aids to the Examination of the Peripheral Nervous System*. London: HMSO; 1976.

Members of the Department of Neurology, Mayo Clinic, and Mayo Foundation for Medical Education and Research. *Clinical Examinations in Neurology*. 6th ed. St. Louis: Mosby Year Book; 1991:270.

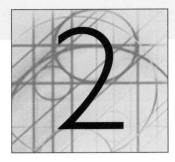

2

An Approach to Neurologic Symptoms

STEVEN L. LEWIS

key points

- A careful neurologic history is the cornerstone of neurologic diagnosis.
- The goal of the neurologic history, followed by the examination and appropriate diagnostic studies, is to determine, first, where in the nervous system the dysfunction lies and, next, how that dysfunction occurred.
- Using neurologic terminology to describe the likely site of neurologic dysfunction can be very helpful in categorizing patients' symptoms and signs.
- Even a very basic and simplified understanding of neuroanatomy can be of great benefit in neurologic diagnosis.
- Recognizing the temporal course of a patient's neurologic illness is critical in determining the likely disease mechanism.

n neurologic diagnosis, individual symptoms and constellations of symptoms can be of telling diagnostic importance both anatomically and etiologically. Thus, a detailed neurologic history that puts together various symptoms and their temporal development can help to define neurologic entities with significant precision; the role of the subsequent neurologic examination is to look for evidence to support, or refute, the diagnostic hypothesis that was generated by analysis of the careful neurologic history.

COMMON NEUROLOGIC TERMS

Before proceeding with a discussion of specific neurologic symptoms, it is worthwhile to define some terms that can be useful in characterizing neurologic symptom complexes. These words are used to indicate certain localizations of pathology (Table 2.1).

Encephalopathy means disease of the brain. Although theoretically the term encephalopathy could refer to any process involving any

TABLE 2.1

Common Terms Used to Describe Localizations of Neurologic Dysfunction

Term	Meaning
Encephalopathy	Disease of brain (usually refers to diffuse brain dysfunction)
Myelopathy	Disease of spinal cord
Radiculopathy	Disease of nerve root
Neuropathy	Disease of nerve
Myopathy	Disease of muscle

part of the brain, it generally is used to mean dysfunction that involves the entirety of both cerebral hemispheres. Thus, the terms encephalopathy and diffuse encephalopathy are synonymous. An example of a common type of encephalopathy is a metabolic encephalopathy, such as that caused by hepatic, uremic, or other metabolic dysfunction.

Myelopathy means disease of the spinal cord. A patient with any symptoms or signs that are caused by spinal cord dysfunction has a myelopathy. An example of a common type of myelopathy is a compressive myelopathy caused by a tumor or other mass lesion compressing the spinal cord, causing weakness, sensory loss, and spasticity below the level of the compression.

Radiculopathy, disease of the nerve roots (radix is Latin for root; a radish is a root vegetable), is the term used for any process involving single or multiple nerve roots in the cervical, thoracic, or lumbar spine. For example, a herniated lumbar disc between the fourth and fifth lumbar spine might cause an L5 radiculopathy; Guillain–Barré syndrome would cause a polyradiculopathy as a result of dysfunction of multiple nerve roots.

Neuropathy means disease of a nerve. The term means dysfunction of one (mononeuropathy), several (mononeuropathy multiplex), or many/diffuse (polyneuropathy) peripheral nerves. Dysfunction of a cranial nerve would be called a cranial neuropathy. Myopathy refers to any disease of muscle.

These generic terms are very helpful to the clinician in categorizing sites of pathology or dysfunction. A specific causative lesion, or causative process, is not conveyed by any of these terms. Unless there is a preceding adjective (e.g., compressive myelopathy or demyelinative polyneuropathy), a cause or mechanism is not implied. Likewise, substitution of the suffix -itis for -pathy (e.g., myositis instead of myopathy) implies, specifically, an inflammatory process, rather than an as-yet-unknown process affecting that region of the nervous system.

AN APPROACH TO SPECIFIC NEUROLOGIC SYMPTOM COMPLEXES

The essential elements of the neurologic diagnostic process are an accurate and detailed history, followed by a neurologic examination. Imaging and laboratory studies follow, as appropriate.

■ **SPECIAL CLINICAL POINT: The goals of neurologic diagnosis are to determine, first, *where* in the nervous system the problem lies, and, next, to determine *how* the dysfunction occurred.**

This section discusses the "where" part of the neurologic formulation using the history and examination to evaluate several specific symptom complexes (mental status changes, weakness, sensory symptoms, and gait disorders). Using the temporal course of the evolution of symptoms to help determine the mechanism of dysfunction (the "what" part) will be discussed later in this chapter.

MENTAL STATUS CHANGES

When confronted with a patient who has had a mental status change, the clinician should try to determine whether there is an alteration in the level of consciousness or an alteration of the content of consciousness. Alterations in the level of consciousness manifest in the continuum between drowsiness and coma. They result either from dysfunction of both cerebral hemispheres, dysfunction of the upper brainstem, or a combination of hemispheric and upper brainstem dysfunction. The clinical approach to the patient who presents with an alteration in level of consciousness is discussed in more detail in Chapter 5.

■ **SPECIAL CLINICAL POINT: A major goal of the neurologic examination of patients with an alteration of the level of consciousness is determining whether there is evidence for focal brainstem dysfunction.**

If brainstem function is intact, the cause of the problem is unlikely to be the result of a focal structural brainstem process; it is more likely the result of a diffuse encephalopathic process. The actual processes that may affect the level of consciousness are vast and are discussed in more detail in Chapter 5.

Neurologic processes can affect the mental status of patients, however, by affecting the content of consciousness without necessarily altering the level of consciousness. Alterations in the content of consciousness are exemplified by psychiatric disorders or by neurologic disorders that affect memory, language, awareness, or global intellectual functioning. Patients with chronic dementing illnesses (Chapter 16) usually have normal alertness despite the deterioration in cognitive functioning. Patients with aphasia—particularly those with fluent aphasias—often appear to be confused. More careful attention to the patient's speech pattern to determine the presence of paraphasic errors and neologisms ("new words" without meaning) often will help the clinician determine that the "confused" patient is actually aphasic; the presence of aphasia is usually a clue to focal dysfunction in the dominant (usually left) hemisphere. Patients with lesions affecting the right hemisphere also may appear to be "confused," neglectful, and unaware, whereas they actually have neglect of the left side of space and may be oblivious of

their deficit (anosagnosia) because of the nondominant hemisphere dysfunction.

WEAKNESS

"Weakness" as a patient complaint may have several possible meanings, besides the usually presumed meaning of a decrease in motor function in one or several extremities. The clinician should keep in mind that some patients might use the term "weakness" to describe generalized fatigue, malaise, or asthenia. Some patients might even describe a symptom such as the generalized bradykinesia of parkinsonism (Chapter 10) as weakness. As in all neurologic diagnosis, an accurate history and examination should help clarify what symptoms the patient is actually describing. Muscular fatigue, although very nonspecific, suggests the possibility of a disorder of the neuromuscular junction, such as myasthenia gravis (see Chapter 19), or a disease of muscle (myopathy), in addition to the many primarily nonneurologic processes that can cause generalized malaise and fatigue.

The following are definitions of some common terms used to describe decreases in motor function. Paresis refers to muscular weakness but not complete paralysis. Plegia is the term used to describe complete paralysis. Monoparesis and monoplegia are terms sometimes used to describe weakness or paralysis in one extremity. Hemiparesis and hemiplegia refer to weakness or paralysis in the arm and leg on one side of the body. Paraparesis and paraplegia describe weakness or paralysis in both legs, and quadriparesis and quadriplegia (sometimes alternatively called tetraplegia) denote weakness or paralysis in all four extremities.

Muscular weakness can occur as a result of dysfunction at any level of the central or peripheral nervous system. To illustrate this, it is worth considering the neuroanatomic pathway for muscle movement. The pathway for muscle movement begins in nerve cells that are located on the precentral gyrus of each frontal lobe (the upper motor neurons). The axons from these nerve cells comprise the corticospinal tract. The corticospinal tracts travel through the white matter of each cerebral hemisphere, through the internal capsule, and further downward into the brainstem, where each corticospinal tract crosses in the low medulla to the opposite side. From the medulla, the corticospinal tracts travel downward through each side of the spinal cord.

Within the spinal cord, the corticospinal tract on each side synapses with nerve cells in the anterior horns located in the spinal cord gray matter (the lower motor neurons). Axons from these second-order neurons become the cervical, thoracic, and lumbosacral nerve roots. The cervical nerve roots then form the brachial plexus, and the nerves that are formed in the brachial plexus travel into the upper extremities and innervate the muscles of the upper extremities. The lumbar nerve roots travel downward within the lumbar spinal canal as the cauda equina, before exiting and forming the lumbosacral plexus and ultimately forming the nerves that innervate the lower-extremity musculature.

■ **SPECIAL CLINICAL POINT: A lesion at any level of the upper and lower motor neuron pathway, from the cerebral cortex to the muscles themselves, can cause weakness.**

The location of this lesion causing weakness, or a history of weakness, is not always immediately obvious, even to an experienced clinician who has performed an accurate history and examination. However, there are typical, or classic, patterns of muscle weakness that lesions at various levels of the pathway for motor function usually will produce. Recognition of these typical patterns can be very helpful in attempting to decide on possible localizations of pathology in patients who present with motor weakness.

Upper Motor Neuron Lesions

Lesions that cause dysfunction of the corticospinal tracts are called upper motor neuron lesions; their distinctive features, in addition to

weakness, include increased or pathologic reflexes, and increased tone and spasticity in chronic lesions. It also should be recognized that these classic findings of upper motor neuron dysfunction might not always be evident. Upper motor neuron syndromes can result from lesions of the corticospinal tract at various levels of the central nervous system. Further clinical details help to specify whether the lesion is cortical, subcortical, or in the spinal cord. When symptoms of transient motor dysfunction occur that have resolved by the time of the examination, however, no abnormalities would be expected on examination, and the site of the lesion must be inferred by the patient's description of the areas of transient weakness and associated symptoms.

Hemispheric motor cortex lesions involving the cortical motor neurons of the lateral surface of one hemisphere usually cause upper motor neuron weakness of the contralateral face and arm, with less weakness of the leg. A lesion in this region, like all corticospinal tract lesions, often will cause predominant weakness in the extensors of the arm and flexors of the leg, with relative preservation of strength in arm flexors and leg extensors. As such, the affected arm is held mildly flexed while walking and the leg is overextended, causing it to drag stiffly, sometimes catching the toe. Hemispheric motor cortex lesions involving the medial aspect of one frontal lobe will predominantly cause contralateral leg weakness. Weakness resulting from cortical lesions often is also accompanied by other signs of cortical dysfunction, giving a clue to the localization of the problem. For example, left hemisphere cortical lesions often are accompanied by abnormalities of language function. Right hemisphere cortical lesions often are accompanied by denial of the left-sided weakness (anosagnosia) or even unawareness of the presence of the left extremities (asomatagnosia). Any complex behavioral change of these types suggests that the upper motor neuron lesion is cortical. Cortical lesions causing weakness are often also accompanied by some contralateral sensory disturbance because of the proximity of the cortical sensory neurons to the motor cortex.

Deep hemispheric or internal capsule lesions also will cause weakness of the contralateral body, but without accompanying signs of cortical dysfunction. Lesions affecting the corticospinal tract fibers in the posterior limb of the internal capsule may produce a characteristic pure motor hemiparesis (or hemiplegia) involving the contralateral face, arm, and leg. This is characterized by significant weakness of one side of the body without sensory disturbance or signs of cortical dysfunction such as aphasia. This distinctive form of isolated weakness occurs because the corticospinal fibers from a large area of the motor cortex all lie close together in the internal capsule, segregated from the sensory fibers, and deep to the cortical structures. In contrast, a hemispheric lesion that would be large enough to cause significant weakness of an entire side of the body most likely also would involve sensory signs or symptoms and signs of cortical dysfunction.

Brainstem lesions that involve the corticospinal tract on one side also will cause weakness of the contralateral side of the body. Some unilateral ventral pontine lesions—affecting only the corticospinal tract but no other brainstem pathways—may even produce an isolated pure motor hemiparesis clinically indistinguishable from an internal capsular lesion. However, many brainstem processes producing weakness also produce brainstem signs or brainstem symptoms such as diplopia, vertigo, nausea, and vomiting, or cranial nerve palsies, which are clues to the brainstem localization of the process.

■ **SPECIAL CLINICAL POINT: One of the pillars of neurologic localization is that a brainstem lesion can cause weakness of the contralateral body (as a result of involvement of the corticospinal tract) and dysfunction of an ipsilateral cranial nerve (as a result of involvement of a cranial nerve nucleus, or the cranial nerve itself, before it exits the brainstem).**

An example would be a right peripheral facial palsy and left body weakness as a result of a right pontine lesion. In addition, because both the right and the left corticospinal tracts are relatively close together in the brainstem, bilateral extremity weakness can be seen in brainstem disease.

Lesions of the corticospinal tracts in the spinal cord cause weakness below the level of the spinal cord lesion. Although it is possible to have unilateral weakness resulting from a spinal cord lesion, many lesions affecting the spinal cord cause bilateral weakness because of involvement of the corticospinal tracts on both sides of the cord. The level of the spinal cord lesion causing the weakness is not always immediately obvious to the examiner, however. The corticospinal fibers destined for arm function end in the lower cervical/first thoracic portion of the spinal cord. The corticospinal tract fibers for leg function need to pass through the cervical and thoracic portions of the spinal cord before ending in the lumbosacral cord. Therefore, weakness of the upper and lower extremities, when the result of a single lesion, must be due to a lesion at least as high as the cervical spinal cord. However, weakness of the legs without weakness of the arms is not necessarily the result of a lesion below the neck; a partial or early process affecting the cervical spinal cord could potentially cause dysfunction primarily affecting that portion of the corticospinal tract destined for lower-extremity function, without obviously affecting those fibers involved in upper-extremity function. This has important implications in the imaging of patients with suspected spinal cord lesions.

Lower Motor Neuron Lesions

Lower motor neuron dysfunction occurs when there is dysfunction at the level of the anterior horn cell, motor nerve root, plexus, peripheral nerve, or neuromuscular junction. Lesions of the lower motor neuron may cause, in addition to weakness, decreased reflexes in the involved limb, if a clinically testable reflex is subserved by the nerve in question. In chronic lesions, lower motor neuron dysfunction may lead to atrophy and fasciculations of muscle because of the trophic influence the lower motor neuron plays in muscle maintenance. In these cases, patients may complain that their muscles are shrinking and have small, visible twitches. Lower motor neuron weakness may be the result of either a focal or diffuse process.

Clinical localization of the source of a patient's weakness to a particular focal lower motor neuron lesion mainly rests in the finding of muscle dysfunction that appears to fit the territory of a specific nerve root (radiculopathy), region of plexus (plexopathy), or peripheral nerve distribution (neuropathy). In addition, when such a lesion also is affecting sensory fibers (as do most lower motor neuron lesions that are distal to the anterior horn cell), the concomitant sensory dysfunction also can be an important clue to the localization of the problem.

Examples of common diffuse lower motor neuron processes include processes that simultaneously affect multiple peripheral nerves (polyneuropathies) or multiple nerve roots (polyradiculopathies). Diffuse polyneuropathies typically predominantly affect the most distal extremities, causing weakness that often is limited to the distal fingers and foot muscles. Distal reflexes (specifically, the ankle jerks) usually are diminished or lost, fairly symmetrically. In most diffuse polyneuropathies, such as diabetic neuropathy, the sensory symptoms are more prominent than the distal motor findings, at least initially. Multifocal, rather than diffuse, polyneuropathies are characterized as a mononeuropathy multiplex. This would be seen clinically by dysfunction in the territories of two or more peripheral nerves. Polyradiculopathic processes clinically resemble (and may be difficult to initially distinguish from) the diffuse polyneuropathies but are suggested by the presence of motor dysfunction that appears to involve multiple motor nerve root territories. Concomitant sensory symptoms such as radicu-

lar pain (see later), when present, are helpful diagnostic clues to the presence of a radicular or polyradicular localization.

Disease of muscle (myopathy) is suggested when a patient presents with weakness that is predominantly proximal in distribution. However, proximal weakness is not pathognomonic for myopathy and also can be seen, for example, in some myelopathic and radiculopathic processes. It also should be noted that some myopathies cause unusual patterns of weakness (e.g., inclusion body myositis) or even predominantly distal weakness (e.g., myotonic dystrophy). Sometimes myopathies cause pain and tenderness in the involved muscles, especially in inflammatory conditions.

PAIN AND SENSORY SYNDROMES

Arguably one can consider all pain to be neurologic in origin because any pain must be transmitted through sensory fibers and perceived in central nervous system structures. However, primary neurologic pain and other neurologic abnormalities of sensation are discussed here and can be defined as pain and other sensory symptoms that are the direct result of dysfunction of nervous system structures. Back pain is discussed in Chapter 21 and headache is discussed in Chapter 7—these topics therefore will not be addressed specifically in this section.

Patients often report "numbness" as a neurologic symptom. However, this term has many potential meanings, including the expected sensory symptoms of decreased sensation (hypoesthesia or anesthesia), a tingling/pins and needles sensation (paresthesias), or very uncomfortable/burning sensations (dysesthesias). Patients, however, sometimes use the word numbness to describe weakness or other nonsensory symptoms. A careful history, specifically asking the patient to explain the symptom of numbness in more detail, usually will suffice for clarification.

The pathways for cutaneous sensation will be summarized here. Sensation starts in the peripheral nerve endings and travels up the sensory nerves to the dorsal nerve roots and into the spinal cord. In the spinal cord, the sensory pathways ascend as the spinothalamic tract (mainly subserving pain and temperature sensation) and the posterior columns (mainly subserving vibration and proprioceptive sensation). These ascending sensory tracts in the spinal cord synapse in the thalamus. From the thalamus, thalamocortical projections send the sensory information to the cerebral cortex.

■ **SPECIAL CLINICAL POINT: Abnormalities at any level of the sensory pathway—peripheral sensory nerve, nerve root, spinal cord, thalamus, or sensory cortex—may produce sensory symptoms.**

Lesions at some of these levels, particularly the sensory nerve, nerve root, or thalamus, also may produce pain.

The sensory symptoms of peripheral nerve lesions generally consist of hypoesthesia, paresthesias, or dysesthesias conforming to the territory of the nerve. When this occurs focally, as a result of a focal peripheral nerve process, the area of numbness is usually well circumscribed, corresponding to a particular peripheral nerve distribution. When the peripheral nerve process is diffuse and symmetric, such as in a distal polyneuropathy, the area of sensory disturbance characteristically occurs in a stocking or stocking-glove pattern.

Like peripheral neuropathic lesions, radiculopathies may cause paresthesias or hypoesthesia in the territory of a nerve root. However, these nerve root lesions often cause characteristic radiculopathic pain, characterized by sharp shooting pain, radiating proximally to distally in the distribution of the root. Radicular pain resulting from cervical or lumbar root processes can occur even in the absence of obvious neck or back pain. The possibility of a cervical or lumbar radiculopathic localization of a patient's symptoms is often apparent given the characteristic symptoms. However, thoracic

radiculopathies are less common and may produce radiating pain, paresthesias, or severe dysesthesias in the territory of one or several thoracic nerve roots. Causes of thoracic radiculopathies include herpes zoster, diabetic thoracic radiculopathies, or structural lesions. Thoracic radiculopathies may mimic serious systemic processes such as intra-abdominal or cardiac pathology. A clue to the primary neurologic, radicular cause of the patient's symptoms would be the presence of clear-cut cutaneous hypoesthesia or dysesthesia on the surface of the skin, conforming to a thoracic dermatomal distribution.

Spinal cord lesions (myelopathies) that affect the ascending sensory tracts cause sensory symptoms (hypoesthesia and paresthesias) below the level of the lesion. Total interruption of these sensory fibers at any level of the cord would cause complete anesthesia below that level. Myelopathies may cause Lhermitte sign, which is an uncomfortable feeling of electricity, vibration, or tingling that radiates down the neck and/or back and sometimes into the extremities, occurring on neck flexion. Lhermitte sign is caused by dysfunction of nerve fibers in the posterior columns. Although it can be seen in multiple sclerosis, it can occur as a result of any process affecting the cord, including compressive lesions. Therefore, when a patient reports a Lhermitte sign, it can be a helpful clue to a spinal cord localization of pathology.

Thalamic lesions may cause decreased sensation and paresthesias over the contralateral body. This may be quite marked, and some patients with thalamic strokes, for example, may have severe sensory dysfunction over an entire half of the body up to the midline. Thalamic lesions, particularly chronic ones, sometimes also cause severe dysesthesias (thalamic pain) in addition to the cutaneous sensory loss. Cortical lesions involving the sensory cortex may cause paresthesias or hypoesthesia in the regions of the contralateral body corresponding to the cortical territory involved. Such sensory cortical lesions also may be associated with motor abnormalities or other signs of cortical dysfunction.

GAIT DISORDERS

Disorders of gait and balance may be caused by nonneurologic or neurologic problems. Nonneurologic causes of gait dysfunction are primarily the result of orthopedic problems such as spine, pelvic, hip, or knee problems. Gait dysfunction resulting from pain in a lower extremity is called an antalgic gait. It is usually, although not always, evident from the history and examination that a disorder of gait is related to an orthopedic, rather than a primary neurologic, process.

The neurologic structures that control gait and balance include the frontal lobes, basal ganglia, cerebellum, and the pathways for motor and sensory function.

■ **SPECIAL CLINICAL POINT: Gait problems can occur as a result of dysfunction in any of the regions that control gait and balance, each of which cause characteristic abnormalities evident on examination.**

Frontal lobe disorders, as can be seen as a result of hydrocephalus or bifrontal mass lesions or as an accompaniment of aging or dementia in some patients, cause a characteristic difficulty with initiation of gait. Patients may complain that their feet are "glued" to the floor. The resulting gait disorder is very similar to a parkinsonian gait, with very short steps, although the way the feet appear to be nearly stuck to the floor, and the absence of other parkinsonian features, help in distinguishing this from parkinsonism. Patients with a frontal lobe gait disorder may or may not have other symptoms of frontal lobe dysfunction such as incontinence or dementia.

When the basal ganglia dysfunction of Parkinson disease (see Chapter 10) affects walking, it causes a characteristic flexed posture and a slow, shuffling, bradykinetic gait, with multiple steps needed for turns, which may be accompanied by impairment of postural reflexes. Patients may complain that they have a difficult time stopping their forward progress while walking (festination of gait).

Disorders of the cerebellum or cerebellar pathways (e.g., in the brainstem) produce an ataxic gait. This is a wide-based unsteady gait indistinguishable from the gait disorder of acute alcohol intoxication.

Unilateral corticospinal tract disease will produce a hemiparetic gait, often with characteristic circumduction of the stiff, overextended, hemiparetic leg, pivoting around the axis of the strong leg. Bilateral corticospinal tract disease such as myelopathy can occur as a result of spinal cord lesions, causes both legs to be stiff, and the resulting spastic gait may include a scissoring motion of each leg around the other while moving forward.

Disorders of the lower motor neuron, or the muscles, of the lower extremities also can affect the gait. The resulting gait abnormality depends on the muscles that are weakened. When there is weakness of extension at the knee joint, the patient may lose the ability to lock the knee, and this may cause buckling and falling. This may be most bothersome in maneuvers that require the knee to lock for stabilization, and patients therefore may note buckling of a leg particularly when walking down stairs. Weakness of foot dorsiflexion may cause the patients to complain of tripping over their toes (foot drop). Severe foot dorsiflexion weakness therefore will produce a steppage gait, with the leg lifted higher than normal to avoid tripping over the toes of the weak foot.

Patients with severely impaired sensation in the lower extremities also may complain of difficulty with gait, even in the absence of motor impairment. Examples include severe peripheral neuropathies or other disorders affecting proprioceptive sensory function in the legs, as can be seen, for example, from vitamin B_{12} deficiency. These patients may not realize that there is an underlying disorder of extremity sensation, and may present to the physician specifically with the complaint of a gait problem, especially when paresthesias or dysesthesias are not prominent. When patients have such a severe loss of proprioceptive sensation in the feet, the resulting wide-based gait disorder is called a sensory ataxia. These patients need to look at their feet while walking, and they often describe a particular tendency to fall when visual cues are lost, such as when standing in the dark or when closing their eyes in the shower (Romberg sign).

ROLE OF THE TEMPORAL COURSE OF NEUROLOGIC ILLNESS IN NEUROLOGIC DIAGNOSIS

An accurate and detailed neurologic history is the cornerstone of neurologic diagnosis. In addition to learning the patient's specific symptoms, another important aspect of the history is the elucidation of the temporal pattern of the neurologic symptoms.

■ **SPECIAL CLINICAL POINT: The time course of neurologic symptoms can give the clinician important clues as to the probable mechanism of nervous system dysfunction.**

In neurologic diagnosis, it is usually most helpful to try to decide which general mechanism of disease is most likely to be present before proceeding further diagnostically. Most neurologic disease processes can be categorized as producing their dysfunction through one of these general mechanisms: compressive, degenerative, epileptic, hemorrhagic, infectious, inflammatory (including demyelinative), ischemic, migrainous, metabolic (including toxic), or traumatic. (Some congenital neurologic processes also may produce disease that results from the congenital absence of certain normal structures or tissues—whether on a subcellular or macroscopic level—thereby leading to abnormal neurologic function.)

These mechanisms of acquired neurologic disease are generic and inclusive; for example,

the compressive mechanism would include such diverse disease processes as a subdural hematoma causing mass effect on the brain, a benign or malignant tumor (with or without associated edema) compressing or infiltrating brain tissue, or a cervical disc compressing the spinal cord. In addition, single pathologic processes can produce clinical symptoms via different potential mechanisms; for example, an intracerebral aneurysm may produce disease because of hemorrhage or because of compression of important structures (e.g., a posterior communicating artery aneurysm causing a compressive oculomotor nerve palsy).

Consideration of the temporal pattern of symptom development, although not specific for a single mechanism, can be most helpful in including or excluding some of these mechanisms; other clues from the history and examination then can be incorporated to narrow the choices of mechanism and specific disease process. The following discussion presents some common temporal patterns of symptomatology and the disease mechanisms they particularly suggest.

■ **SPECIAL CLINICAL POINT: Transient focal neurologic symptoms, which may or may not be recurrent, usually are seen as a result of ischemia, migraine, or seizure.**

Although these three mechanisms may seem to be quite different from each other, they are not always easy to distinguish. Ischemic symptoms, when transient, can produce focal neurologic dysfunction lasting from seconds to hours. Migrainous brain dysfunction can produce a variety of focal neurologic manifestations (even without headache). In addition to the visual scintillations of classic migraine, other neurologic symptoms can be seen as migrainous phenomena, including weakness, paresthesias, and aphasia. These migrainous symptoms typically progress and spread over a period of minutes (e.g., 15 to 30 minutes) before resolving. In contrast, the focal neurologic symptoms of seizures tend to spread somewhat more quickly. The patient's age, associated medical conditions, and other clues from the history and examination may also assist in the delineation of the likely mechanism of transient focal neurologic dysfunction. It should be noted that demyelinating disease (specifically multiple sclerosis) causes focal neurologic dysfunction that can resolve and then recur in a different region of the central nervous system. However, the symptoms of an acute attack of multiple sclerosis usually last at least days to weeks before improving, unlike the more transient symptoms of ischemia, migraine, or epilepsy. Some patients with multiple sclerosis do experience very brief (as short as seconds), repetitive, stereotypical, paroxysmal neurologic symptoms. This is presumably because of "short circuits" (ephaptic transmission) between adjacent demyelinated axons in an acute multiple sclerosis plaque, and the resulting very brief paroxysmal event simply can be considered a kind of white matter electrical event.

Sudden-onset neurologic symptoms suggest ischemia or hemorrhage. A progressive focal neurologic symptom primarily suggests a compressive lesion, but ischemic, inflammatory, or focal infectious processes can progress gradually as well. Degenerative diseases also may produce progressive focal neurologic dysfunction, but the dysfunction is usually more diffuse, even if not symmetric. Ischemic or compressive lesions also can cause waxing and waning focal neurologic symptoms. More diffuse waxing and waning symptoms also would be expected in some toxic or metabolic processes.

Progressive diffuse neurologic symptoms are most suggestive of degenerative processes, infectious or inflammatory processes, or metabolic abnormalities. The specific time course in question can be quite helpful. For example, diffuse neurologic dysfunction that has been progressing over days would more likely be ascribed to a metabolic or infectious process, whereas the same kind of symptoms progressing over years would be more likely caused by a degenerative disease.

Always Remember

- A detailed and thoughtful neurologic history is always the first step in neurologic diagnosis.
- As you take your patient's history and perform your patient's examination, keep basic neuroanatomic concepts in mind.
- Use the clues from the history and examination to determine first the most likely location of the neurologic problem and second the likely cause of the problem.
- Recognition of specific patterns of neurologic symptoms and signs and their temporal development can be very helpful in neurologic diagnosis.

QUESTIONS AND DISCUSSION

1. A 35-year-old man presents to the emergency room with a 3-day history of numbness and tingling from his mid chest down to his legs, and mild weakness in both legs. He describes an unusual sensation like an electric shock whenever he flexes his neck forward. He also has some urinary urgency. Examination shows normal mental status and cranial nerves. There is mild weakness in both legs (4/5). Sensory examination shows that pinprick is diminished below the level of the nipples, including the lower chest, abdomen, and legs. Reflexes are normal in the arms but are brisk in the legs. Babinski signs are present bilaterally. Which of the following terms best describes the localization of this patient's clinical syndrome?
   A. Encephalopathy
   B. Myelopathy
   C. Radiculopathy
   D. Neuropathy
   E. Myopathy

The correct answer is B (myelopathy). This patient has symptoms of spinal cord (myelopathic) dysfunction. Clues to a spinal cord localization of his symptoms include the bi-lateral motor dysfunction in the legs as well as the bilateral sensory dysfunction with a sensory level over the trunk. There are also brisk reflexes in both legs and bilateral Babinski signs, suggestive of bilateral upper motor neuron (corticospinal tract) dysfunc-tion. Although brainstem lesions similarly can cause bilateral motor and sensory symp-toms, the absence of cranial nerve abnormali-ties is evidence that the lesion is below the level of the brainstem. Urinary symptoms, in-cluding urgency, are also commonly associ-ated with spinal cord processes. This patient also describes Lhermitte sign, an electric-like sensation on neck flexion, a finding sugges-tive of a spinal cord process affecting the pos-terior columns. This patient's clinical symptoms and signs are not suggestive of pathology in the brain (encephalopathy), nerve root (radiculopathy), nerve (neuropa-thy), cervical or lumbosacral plexus (plexopa-thy), or muscle (myopathy). Although the cause of this patient's spinal cord dysfunction is not yet clear, the clinical recognition that his symptoms are likely myelopathic is impor-tant and will guide the clinician to the appro-priate choice of imaging and other studies.

2. A 72-year-old woman with a 2-year history of diabetes mellitus comes to the office because of 4 weeks of severe pain. She describes the pain as a severe, sharp, burning sensation that begins in her medial scapula and radiates around her trunk to beneath her right breast. The pain is not worse with breathing, but she notes that the skin in this area is very uncomfortable to touch. Her only medication is an oral hypoglycemic agent. She has seen multiple physicians and has undergone extensive gastrointestinal and cardiac evaluations for the pain, which were unrevealing. Her general physical examination is normal, and there is no skin rash. Neurologic examination shows normal mental status, cranial nerves, and muscle strength.

Sensory testing shows that she has severe discomfort when the skin under the right breast and below the right scapula is touched with either a cotton swab or the point of a pin. This area of sensory abnormality is a strip about 2 cm in height extending from the right mid/upper thoracic spine posteriorly to the lower sternum anteriorly. Reflexes are 1+ and symmetric, and Babinski signs are absent. Which of the following terms best describes the localization of this patient's pain syndrome?

A. Encephalopathy
B. Myelopathy
C. Radiculopathy
D. Neuropathy
E. Plexopathy

The correct answer is C (radiculopathy). This patient has characteristic symptoms and signs of a thoracic radiculopathy. The major clue to a probable nerve root localization of her dis-ease process is the distribution of her sensory symptoms and sensory findings to the cuta-neous territory of a particular nerve root. In this case, her findings map out the territory of either the right T5 or T6 root. Another clue to a radicular localization of her symptoms is the occasional proximal-to-distal shooting pains in the territory of a right thoracic nerve root. The generic diagnosis of a thoracic radiculopathy does not in itself give a specific clinical diagno-sis for this patient. However, the recognition that this is the likely localization of her prob-lem allows the physician to narrow the causative possibilities, and to reasonably ex-clude other possibilities, prior to further inves-tigation. Recognition that this patient's cutaneous sensory symptoms and signs are most compatible with a thoracic radicular process, and not a visceral process, might have saved her from some unnecessary investiga-tion. One caveat, though, is that visceral dis-ease can cause referred pain syndromes suggestive of neurologic or spinal processes, such as mid- or low-back pain from deep chest, abdominal, or retroperitoneal processes. In this patient, the most likely cause of her thoracic radicular syndrome is a diabetic thoracic radiculopathy. Herpes zoster (shingles) in this distribution would cause similar symptoms, but it is less likely given the absence of herpetic skin lesions.

3. Your office nurse tells you that your next patient is complaining of intermittent episodes of dizziness that have been occurring for the last 2 months. The patient is a 54-year-old woman who you have been following for general medical care. She has a history of hypertension but no other previous significant illnesses. Prior to coming to your office today, the patient had a few tests done by another physician, including a magnetic resonance imaging scan of the brain and a 24-hour ambulatory heart monitor test. Which of the following choices would be the most appropriate first step in your evaluation of this patient?
   A. Review the results of the previous workup.
   B. Take a history from the patient.
   C. Perform a general physical examination.
   D. Perform a general neurologic examination.
   E. Check for orthostatic hypotension, and perform a bedside maneuver for positional vertigo.

The correct answer is B (take a history from the patient). Although all of the choices are important and may be helpful, the first step in any neurologic evaluation should be a thorough history. Once the neurologic history is obtained, the clinician usually should have enough clues to determine the likely locations of the lesion (the *where* part of the neurologic diagnostic process) and the possible disease mechanisms involved (the *what* part of the diagnostic process). The neurologic examination can be a very helpful adjunct to the neurologic history, and in many cases it will help exclude or include certain processes that are under considera-tion; however, it should always be performed only after the history has been obtained. The results of ancillary laboratory tests, although often very important in excluding or confirming specific diagnostic considerations, should be ordered and interpreted in light of the clinical history (first) and the neurologic examination (second). Clinical interpretation of a patient's diagnostic studies without regard to the findings of history and examination is fraught with potential hazard. Just as incidental abnormalities may be overinterpreted for clinical importance (red herrings), the clinician also might get false reassurance from the results of normal studies that do not answer the appropriate clinical question at hand.

4. A 25-year-old woman comes to the office because of a 5-year history of intermittent episodes of face and arm numbness and difficulty with vision and speech. The attacks are all very similar, and she has had about two attacks per year. Her symptoms begin with a visual disturbance, which she describes as difficulty seeing the right side of people's faces or the right side of a page, "as if they are covered by heat waves." This then is followed within a few minutes by numbness and tingling in her right hand. This numb sensation then gradually ascends over the next 15 minutes to involve the right arm and cheek. During the attacks, she has difficulty with speech, which she describes as a feeling, "I know what I want to say, but I can't get the words out." The symptoms last a total of about 30 minutes then resolve and usually are followed by a moderately severe throbbing headache over her left temple. Although the majority of her episodes have involved her right vision and body, she recalls having had a few episodes that involved only the left side of her vision, face, and arm, but without the speech disturbance. She has no significant past medical history except for additional

occasional headaches that occur about once a month, located over either or both temples and relieved by over-the-counter analgesics. Her neurologic examination is normal. Which of the following general mechanisms of neurologic dysfunction is the most likely cause of this patient's symptoms?

A. Demyelinative
B. Epileptic
C. Ischemic
D. Metabolic
E. Migrainous

The answer is E (migrainous). This patient has recurrent episodes of transient focal neurologic dysfunction, most likely of migrainous etiology. Recurrent transient focal neurologic symptoms are usually the result of ischemia, epilepsy, or migraine. In this case, migraine is the most likely cause of her visual symptoms, which sound typical of migraine auras. Her other neurologic symptoms, which occur subsequent to the onset of her visual symptom, suggest the focal neurologic symptomatology that migraine sometimes can produce, and they progress with a typical migrainous tempo. The subsequent headache after the neurologic disturbance is also suggestive of migraine, although migrainous neurologic symptoms sometimes can occur without headache, and headache can occur with other neurologic processes, including ischemia and epilepsy. Although ischemia is possible, it is a less likely cause of this patient's symptoms because of the migrainous quality of her symptoms, the number of episodes she has had over many years without obvious sequelae, and her age. A focal seizure is also possible, but it is less likely because of the slow tempo of progression and the fact that her symptoms have occurred on either side. Demyelinating disease is an unlikely cause of this patient's symptoms, as attacks of demyelinating disease typically cause neurologic dysfunction lasting at least days to weeks.

SUGGESTED READING

Brazis PW, Masdeu JC, Biller J. *Localization in Clinical Neurology.* 5th ed. Philadelphia, PA: Lippincott Williams & Wilkins; 2006.

Campbell WW. *DeJong's the Neurologic Examination.* 6th ed. Philadelphia, PA: Lippincott Williams & Wilkins; 2005.

Gelb DJ. *Introduction to Clinical Neurology.* 3rd ed. Boston, MA: Butterworth-Heinemann; 2005.

Gilman S, Newman SW. *Manter & Gatz's Essentials of Clinical Neuroanatomy and Neurophysiology.* 10th ed. Philadelphia, PA: FA Davis; 2002.

Goetz CG. *Textbook of Clinical Neurology.* 3rd ed. Philadelphia, PA: Saunders; 2007.

Lewis SL. *Field Guide to the Neurologic Examination.* Philadelphia, PA: Lippincott Williams & Wilkins; 2004.

Patten JP. *Neurological Differential Diagnosis.* 2nd ed. London: Springer-Verlag; 1998.

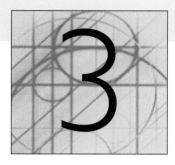

Clinical Use of Neurologic Diagnostic Tests

MADHU SONI

key points

- Computed tomography (CT) is preferred over magnetic resonance imaging (MRI) to visualize hemorrhage and bony structures.
- Posterior fossa structures, such as the brainstem and cerebellum, are not visualized well by CT.
- A routine EEG may be normal in some patients with epilepsy.
- An MRI should not be performed in patients with pacemakers or ferromagnetic devices.
- Nephrogenic systemic fibrosis may occur with MRI dye in patients with renal dysfunction.
- Nerve biopsy is most useful in evaluation of vasculitic neuropathy.
- Ultrasound, computed tomographic angiography, and magnetic resonance angiography have significantly reduced the need for conventional angiography in the routine evaluation of carotid stenosis.

INTRODUCTION

Although the history and physical examination remain the foundation upon which neurologic localization and diagnoses are made, neurologists have an armamentarium of diagnostic tests available to help confirm their clinical impressions. This chapter will highlight the major neurodiagnostic studies, focusing on their indications, benefits, and potential risks (Table 3.1). These tests can be organized into four general categories: neuroimaging tests, vascular imaging studies, neurophysiologic tests, and fluid/tissue studies.

TABLE 3.1 | **Neurodiagnostic Studies**

Neuroimaging tests
    Computed tomography
    Magnetic resonance imaging
    Myelography
Vascular imaging studies
    Ultrasound
    Carotid Doppler
    Transcranial Doppler
    Computed tomographic angiography
    Magnetic resonance angiography
    Magnetic resonance venography
    Catheter angiography
Neurophysiologic tests
    Electroencephalography
    Electromyography
    Evoked potentials
        Visual
        Brainstem
        Somatosensory
Fluid and tissue studies
    Lumbar puncture
    Tissue biopsy
        Brain
        Nerve
        Muscle

NEUROIMAGING TESTS

Computed Tomography (CT)

Perhaps one of the oldest imaging modalities of those that will be described in this chapter, CT remains an important diagnostic tool in the setting of neurologic emergencies. It is widely available, generally accessible in most medical centers at any hour (based on technician availability), and can be performed relatively quickly. Compared to magnetic resonance imaging (MRI), CT is easier to perform in those with claustrophobia or with confusional states.

■ **SPECIAL CLINICAL POINT: CT is preferred over MRI to screen for acute hemorrhage and to visualize bony structures.**

Calcifications in the brain parenchyma, blood vessels, choroid plexus, pineal gland, and within cystic, neoplastic, or infectious lesions are well differentiated on CT. The advent of spiral CT technology also allows three-dimensional reformatted images of the spine. CT additionally provides useful information about ventricular size, the presence of communicating or obstructive hydrocephalus, large mass lesions, and integrity of hemispheric midline structures. Adjacent sinus structures are also visualized on head CT and may provide a clue to the source of a patient's headache or facial pain. Additionally, sinus abnormalities may suggest a site of contiguous spread in the setting of central nervous system infections. Dedicated imaging of the sinuses, however, may be necessary.

■ **SPECIAL CLINICAL POINT: With CT, there are limitations in visualizing posterior fossa structures such as the brainstem and cerebellum and other neuroimaging techniques like MRI are preferred for identifying problems related to these areas.**

If MRI evaluation is not immediately available or when patients are unable to tolerate MRI, requesting thin CT slices through the posterior fossa may be helpful. Due to the associated radiation exposure, CT is not recommended in pregnancy. However, in emergent situations, it may be performed while shielding the abdomen from radiation exposure. The use of contrast dye is helpful in evaluating suspected breaches in the blood–brain barrier as can occur with primary or metastatic brain tumors, meningitis, encephalitis, abscesses and other infections, and active areas of demyelination or inflammation. CT contrast may also help in the evaluation of vascular conditions. In ischemic stroke, a filling defect may be seen due to a thrombosed artery, or in patients with increased intracranial pressure, the classic "empty delta sign" indicates a clot at the confluence of venous sinuses. Aneurysms and arteriovenous malformations (AVMs) are better delineated with the use of contrast and may be missed with a noncontrast study. It is not advisable to administer iodinated contrast to pregnant women, those with renal insufficiency, or if there is an allergy to the contrast agent. If use of contrast is necessary in patients with renal impairment, acetylcysteine and hydration should be used as prophylaxis in attempts to protect the kidneys. Some patients with myasthenia gravis may have an exacerbation of their weakness after the use of CT or MRI contrast and therefore should be monitored closely if use of contrast is necessary.

Magnetic Resonance Imaging

The advent of MRI has provided increased resolution in imaging structures such as soft tissue, cerebral gray and white matter, the brainstem, cerebellum, spinal cord, cranial nerves, spinal nerve roots, peripheral nerves, and muscle without traditional radiation exposure. Generally speaking, T1-weighted images are useful in evaluating the normal anatomy, and cerebrospinal fluid (CSF) appears black. On T2-weighted images, the CSF is white and this sequence highlights abnormalities in the brain or spinal cord parenchyma. In particular, areas of increased water content or edema look bright, or white. Fluid attenuated inversion recovery (FLAIR) sequences also highlight pathology, but the CSF is black, allowing better contrast for lesions around the ventricles, such as in multiple sclerosis, and near the cortical surface. Diffusion-weighted imaging (DWI) has become an important tool in identifying acute stroke and is based on the diffusion properties of water molecules through normal and injured tissue. Although not specific to acute stroke, patterns of restricted water molecule diffusion will appear bright on the DWI sequence. The apparent diffusion coefficient (ADC) is a measure of the mobility of water and if mobility is reduced, as in injured tissue, the corresponding area will appear dark. Therefore, an area that is bright on DWI and dark on ADC corresponds to an area of acute to subacute injury. These changes may persist for 2 weeks.

Orbital MRI is utilized to visualize the optic nerve and extraocular muscles. To optimally visualize these structures, it is important to specify that the study is done with fat suppression. This eliminates the bright artifact from fat within the orbit.

■ **SPECIAL CLINICAL POINT: Patients with pacemakers, mechanical heart valves, brain or spinal cord stimulators, retained bullet or shrapnel fragments, and other ferromagnetic material should not be placed in a magnetic field due to risk of device malfunction and movement of the metal that may result in serious injury or death.**

Aneurysm clips in the current era are designed so that they are compatible with MRI imaging. It is best, however, to verify compatibility prior to ordering an MRI in these patients.

As mentioned earlier, the use of contrast is helpful if a breach of the blood–brain barrier is suspected.

■ **SPECIAL CLINICAL POINT: Although traditionally thought to be safer than iodine-based contrast dye, gadolinium has been associated with nephrogenic systemic fibrosis (NSF; also known as nephrogenic fibrosing dermopathy) when administered to patients with renal dysfunction.**

This condition causes fibrosis of the skin and other organs. It is, therefore, essential to weigh the risk of NSF and renal failure against the diagnostic necessity of using dye in these patients.

Myelography

Evidence for spinal cord or nerve root compression may be evaluated by myelography in patients who are unable to undergo an MRI. Vascular malformations of the cord may also be seen. A lumbar or cervical puncture is performed under fluoroscopic guidance and an iodinated water-soluble contrast agent is injected into the subarachnoid space. X-rays are obtained to visualize the opaque column of dye and to see if there is a block or indentation in the column that may signify an area of compression. Generally, CT is performed after myelography to identify what is causing the compression (i.e., herniated disc, osteophyte, mass) and to increase the diagnostic yield of the procedure. As with lumbar puncture (LP), a post-dural-puncture headache may occur after myelography. Arachnoiditis and idiosyncratic adverse reactions to the dye may occur.

VASCULAR IMAGING STUDIES

Ultrasound

Ultrasonography remains a very useful tool in the evaluation of patients with transient ischemic attacks and stroke, particularly in the evaluation of the extracranial carotid circulation. It provides valuable information about the presence of arterial stenosis by evaluating flow velocities. This imaging modality is portable, widely available, and can be performed relatively quickly. Although not as well known, transcranial Doppler (TCD) offers an evaluation of the intracranial circulation. Performance of the study relies on sonography through bony windows and may be technically limited by cranial hyperostosis. Carotid and TCD studies can help confirm findings on magnetic resonance angiography (MRA) and vice versa, as areas of high-grade stenosis may be overestimated with either modality alone. TCD is also utilized in monitoring for vasospasm after subarachnoid hemorrhage and can help determine the need for transfusion in sickle cell anemia children when the middle cerebral artery flow velocity escalates.

Computed Tomographic Angiography (CTA)

Computed tomographic angiography utilizes spiral CT and allows noninvasive imaging of extracranial and intracranial vessels in a two- and three-dimensional format, utilizing less dye, less time, and less risk compared to conventional angiography. In carotid artery assessment, CTA is comparable to MRA (see below). In detecting occlusive disease, CTA and carotid Doppler studies have the same sensitivity but the specificity is greater for CTA. The intracranial circulation is better visualized and in a shorter period of time with CTA compared to MRA.

Magnetic Resonance Angiography and Magnetic Resonance Venography (MRV)

Arterial and venous vessels may be evaluated without the invasive risks associated with catheter angiography. MRA refers to MRI of arterial vessels, and MRV evaluates venous structures. Small aneurysms (3 mm or less), however, may not be seen with MRA, and arterial stenosis may be overestimated.

Catheter Angiography

Angiography is the gold standard for evaluating arterial and venous structures. This diagnostic study is utilized in the evaluation of cerebral or spinal ischemia due to thrombotic disease or dissection, and in subarachnoid or intracerebral hemorrhage when an aneurysm or AVM is suspected. The procedure is also used for endovascular coiling of aneurysms, embolization of AVM feeder vessels, intra-arterial administration of thrombolytic agents, angioplasty, and stent placement. However, the interventional nature of this procedure is not without risk. These risks include hematoma formation at the site of arterial puncture, vascular injury with a tear in the vessel wall, stroke due to plaque embolism, and an adverse reaction to the contrast agent, including renal dysfunction.

■ **SPECIAL CLINICAL POINT: Noninvasive tests such as ultrasound, computed tomographic angiography (CTA), and magnetic resonance angiography (MRA) have decreased the need for conventional angiography in the evaluation of cerebral ischemia, particularly when at least two of the noninvasive studies show concordant results.**

Individual patient comorbidities, such as cardiopulmonary status and chronic illness, should be considered when deciding whether to accept the risk of conventional arteriography.

NEUROPHYSIOLOGIC TESTS

Electroencephalography (EEG)

Electroencephalography is ordered in patients with spells and altered mental status when there is a concern for seizures. Electrodes are attached with removable adhesive to the scalp and the brain's electrical activity is recorded. Activating procedures such as hyperventilation and photic stimulation are utilized in attempts to trigger a typical spell and increase diagnostic yield. In patients with pulmonary or cardiac conditions in which hyperventilation is contraindicated, specification should be made not to perform the activating procedure. Epileptiform activity may in some cases only be seen during sleep and thus, it is important to record the EEG during both wakefulness and sleep. To ensure sleep is attained, it is recommended that patients limit their sleep prior to the test to half of their usual amount the day before the test.

■ **SPECIAL CLINICAL POINT: A routine EEG may be normal in some patients with epilepsy given the short duration of the study and the paroxysmal nature of epileptic spells that typically do not occur during the EEG. Further, if an epileptic focus is located too deep for detection by the recording scalp electrodes, the EEG will be normal.**

Therefore, the decision to treat patients with anticonvulsants must be based on the clinical syndrome. In patients with nonepileptic spells or pseudoseizures, the EEG is normal during a typical spell. It is important to verify that the event is a characteristic one and may require discussion with family members who have witnessed the spells. Prolonged ambulatory EEG may be necessary to capture these events. Certain EEG patterns may provide etiologic clues

in metabolic and infectious encephalopathies. For example, bilateral triphasic waves classically are seen with hepatic or renal dysfunction. This wave pattern, however, is not specific and may be seen in any condition that causes severe slowing of cerebral activity. Periodic sharp wave complexes in the temporal and frontal lobe regions may be seen with herpes encephalitis or other acute insult. Creutzfeldt–Jakob disease due to prion infection is associated with generalized sharp waves occurring approximately every second, but this may not be seen until later stages of the disease. EEG may also be used as a confirmatory test in evaluating brain death. As with other diagnostic testing methods, clinical correlation is essential in interpreting the significance of electroencephalographic findings.

Electromyography (EMG)

This electrodiagnostic study is used as an extension of the clinical exam to evaluate the peripheral nervous system including the spinal roots, nerves, neuromuscular junction, and muscle. Although the entire test is generically referred to as "EMG," the study consists of two parts: a nerve conduction study (NCS) and needle EMG.

The NCS is performed by applying an electrical impulse over nerve landmarks, recording the generated waveform on a computer screen and analyzing it to determine conduction velocity and amplitude, measures of peripheral myelin, and axon integrity, respectively. Both sensory and motor nerves are tested. Patients should not wear lotions, oils, or ointments to the test as these interfere with the contact between the electrodes and skin and may result in suboptimal or absent waveforms. The presence of edema also technically limits the ability to obtain nerve responses. Nerve conduction slows down with cooler temperatures, so if the patient's limb is cold, appropriate measures must be taken in the lab to warm the limb before interpreting the results. Repetitive nerve stimulation studies are useful in detecting defects in neuromuscular junction transmission as occurs in myasthenia gravis, botulism, and Lambert–Eaton myasthenic syndrome. EMG involves insertion of a thin needle electrode into individual muscles to look for signs of denervation as can occur in motor neuron disease, radiculopathy, plexopathy, or neuropathy. Primary muscle disorders have characteristic patterns that help differentiate them from neurogenic conditions. Diagnostic changes on the needle study may not be seen immediately.

■ **SPECIAL CLINICAL POINT: Because some diagnostic EMG abnormalities take time to develop, it is best to order the test after the patient has had the symptoms for at least 3 weeks.**

Nerve conduction and electromyographic studies will be normal in conditions isolated to the central nervous system.

Evoked Potentials

The three most common evoked potential studies are the visual evoked potential (VEP), brainstem auditory evoked response or brainstem auditory evoked potential (BAER, BAEP), and somatosensory evoked potential (SSEP). These diagnostic studies evaluate the electrical signals generated by the sensory pathways for vision, hearing, and somatic sensation, respectively. Sensory stimuli are provided relevant to the test being performed, for example, a checkerboard pattern for the VEP, auditory clicks for the BAER, and electrical stimulation of a peripheral nerve for the SSEP. Electrodes are strategically placed over the peripheral nerve, spine, scalp, etc. Waveforms are analyzed from the cranial (optic nerve for VEP, vestibulocochlear nerve for BAER) or peripheral nerve (SSEP) to the cerebral cortex. Abnormalities in the waveforms help localize a problem to the peripheral or central nervous system. Using the SSEP as an example, separate waveforms are present for the peripheral nerve, plexus, spinal cord, brainstem, and parietal cortex. A lesion in the brainstem would result in absence/abnormality of the SSEP waveform at that level and at the subsequent cortical level with preservation of the others. In general, evoked potentials are no longer commonly ordered except for the SSEP in intraoperative monitoring, particularly for spine surgery. Prior to the availability of MRI, VEPs and BAERs were commonly done when multiple sclerosis was clinically suspected, to look for evidence of optic nerve dysfunction and multifocal central lesions. There is still a potential role for these tests in patients who are unable to have MRIs due to pacemakers or other metal implants. VEPs are also useful to look for subclinical optic nerve dysfunction in patients suspected of having Devic disease (also called neuromyelitis optica), an aggressive demyelinating condition generally isolated to the spinal cord and optic nerve.

FLUID AND TISSUE STUDIES

Lumbar Puncture

■ **SPECIAL CLINICAL POINT: Although the availability of MRI has significantly decreased the need for diagnostic LPs in patients with multiple sclerosis, analysis of the cerebrospinal fluid (CSF) for the presence of increased intracranial pressure, subarachnoid hemorrhage, infectious or neoplastic meningitis continues to be an important indication for lumbar puncture.**

Cerebrospinal fluid analysis is also used to support or confirm the clinical suspicion of inflammatory demyelinating conditions affecting the central and peripheral nervous system. For example, the presence of oligoclonal bands and intrathecal immunoglobulin synthesis, in the absence of a serologic monoclonal gammopathy, aids the diagnostic probability of multiple sclerosis in patients with a suggestive clinical history and exam findings. An elevated CSF protein with normal cell count (cytoalbuminologic dissociation) is pathognomonic for Guillain–Barré syndrome in patients presenting with acutely progressive limb, facial or oropharyngeal weakness, and areflexia. Chronic inflammatory demyelinating polyradiculoneuropathy (CIDP) is generally associated with an elevated CSF protein, which differentiates it from multifocal motor neuropathy in the appropriate clinical and electrodiagnostic setting. Neuroimaging studies may not detect small areas of subarachnoid hemorrhage and it is therefore imperative to perform an LP, if the head CT is normal, to confirm this suspicion in patients presenting with a sudden, severe, "worst headache of my life." Prior to performing an LP, it is generally recommended that a CT or an MRI of the brain be performed to exclude a contraindication to the procedure, such as the presence of a structural lesion causing elevated intracranial pressure and risk of cerebral or cerebellar herniation. Additionally, patients should be evaluated for the presence of a coagulopathy by checking the PT/INR, PTT, and CBC. Significantly abnormal coagulation studies and thrombocytopenia increase the risk of superficial and deep hematomas, including in the epidural and subdural space, which can lead to nerve root or cord compression. Preparation for LP requires use of sterile technique to minimize the risk of skin, epidural, subdural, or subarachnoid infection. For patients with local back tenderness, fluctuance, fever, history of substance use, or any other "red flags" that raise the concern for a local infection, an imaging study of the spine (preferably, contrasted MRI if no contraindication) should be performed prior to performing or ordering an LP due to the risks of spreading infection by inadvertent needle puncture through an abscess, or adjacent area of discitis or osteomyelitis. A post-dural-puncture or low-CSF-pressure headache may occur in patients after LP, particularly when large diameter spinal needles are used. Occurrence of the headache is not associated with the amount of fluid removed or with the duration the patient is kept supine after the procedure. Clinically, patients are asymptomatic while supine (position of highest CSF pressure) and the headache develops when they sit or stand.

Hydration, caffeine, and rest are recommended for management of these headaches. A blood patch may be required for refractory post-LP headaches. This procedure is generally performed by an anesthesiologist. Approximately 10 cc of the patient's own blood is injected into the epidural space at the same level where the LP was performed. The goal is to create a mechanical seal of the dural tear created by the LP and stop the CSF leak. Patients generally experience prompt relief if the seal is successful. Rarely after LP, epidermoid tumors may form in the spinal canal if epithelial cells from the skin accompany the spinal needle into the subarachnoid space. It is, therefore, important to make sure that while performing an LP, the spinal needle is always inserted and advanced with the stylet in place.

Tissue Biopsy

Brain Biopsy Biopsy of brain tissue is considered when noninvasive studies are insufficient in providing a definitive diagnosis, and patient management would be altered by the results. Neoplastic disease, infection, vasculitis, and rapidly progressive degenerative conditions are situations in which biopsy of a specific brain lesion, the meninges, or functionally affected parenchyma may be considered. Selection of biopsy site is critical to minimize potential loss of function. For example, in cases with multiple lesions, the one most accessible at the surface should be chosen and the language center should be avoided. Computer-assisted stereotactic biopsy allows for tissue retrieval through a burr hole with less risk compared to an open biopsy via craniotomy. As with all invasive tests, risks and benefits must be weighed and discussed with patients and/or family members before proceeding.

Nerve/Muscle Biopsy Nerve or muscle biopsy may be a helpful diagnostic tool in cryptogenic cases of neuropathy and myopathy, respectively. Nerve biopsy is an acceptable diagnostic study if there is a clinical suspicion of an inflammatory, infiltrative, or infectious etiology that would alter management.

■ **SPECIAL CLINICAL POINT: Nerve biopsy is most useful in suspected cases of vasculitis which can present as a mononeuritis multiplex with asymmetric involvement of individual nerves sequentially or at the same time.**

According to a recent practice parameter from the American Academy of Neurology, there is insufficient evidence to recommend when a nerve biopsy would be beneficial in the more common presentation of a symmetric, distal polyneuropathy. A punch biopsy of the skin has been used to evaluate the intraepidermal nerve fiber density, which is reduced in polyneuropathy, including small fiber neuropathy.

■ **SPECIAL CLINICAL POINT: Routine nerve conduction studies only evaluate large nerve fiber function and will be normal in pure small fiber neuropathy cases, in which pain and temperature abnormalities are found with preservation of proprioception and vibration.**

A skin biopsy is therefore helpful in diagnosing small fiber neuropathies but its specific role in the routine evaluation of neuropathy has yet to be established.

Muscle biopsy is utilized in cases of inflammatory myopathy to differentiate inclusion body myositis from polymyositis and dermatomyositis. There are distinguishing pathologic features in each of these conditions and correct classification is important for management and prognostication. For example, dermatomyositis requires periodic surveillance for an underlying malignancy, polymyositis may be associated with interstitial lung disease and connective tissue disease, and there is no specific treatment for inclusion body myositis. Muscle biopsy is also helpful in evaluating potential toxic, metabolic, and infectious causes of otherwise undiagnosed myopathic conditions. Typical muscles used for biopsy are the quadriceps, deltoid, and biceps. The chosen muscle should be clinically or electrodiagnostically affected. Ideally, the muscle should be mildly weak (i.e., grade 4 out of 5 on the Medical Research Council Scale). Biopsy of a severely affected muscle increases the chance of detecting endstage, fibrotic changes that are diagnostically nonspecific. Needle EMG can help identify the site for biopsy. In patients with symmetric weakness, the biopsy site should be contralateral to the studied muscle to avoid needle artifact in the submitted specimen. It is helpful to let the electromyographer know to test only one side if a biopsy is being contemplated.

Always Remember

- CT is preferred over MRI to screen for acute hemorrhage and to visualize bony structures.
- CT is not adequate to visualize the brainstem and cerebellum.
- Check renal function before ordering contrast for CT or MRI.
- Although traditionally thought to be safer than iodine-based contrast dye, gadolinium has been associated with nephrogenic systemic fibrosis when administered to patients with renal dysfunction.
- Patients with pacemakers, mechanical heart valves, brain or spinal cord stimulators, retained bullet or shrapnel fragments, and other ferromagnetic material should not be placed in a magnetic field due to risk of device malfunction and movement of the metal that may result in serious injury or death.
- An area that is bright on DWI MRI sequences and dark on ADC corresponds to an area of acute to subacute injury.
- A normal EEG does not exclude the diagnosis of epilepsy.
- Routine nerve conduction studies only evaluate large nerve fiber function and will be normal in pure small fiber neuropathy.
- To enhance the yield of the EMG study, it is best to perform the test no sooner than 3 weeks after symptom onset.

QUESTIONS AND DISCUSSION

1. A 40-year-old woman presents to the emergency room with the sudden onset of the worst headache of her life. Head CT is normal. What is the most appropriate next step?
   A. Send the patient home with pain medication.
   B. Perform a lumbar puncture.
   C. Order a brain MRI.
   D. Administer subcutaneous sumatriptan.
   E. Consult a neurointerventionalist to perform a cerebral angiogram.

The correct answer is B. In patients with sudden onset of a new, severe headache, it is imperative to evaluate for subarachnoid hemorrhage (SAH). A noncontrast head CT is the appropriate emergent initial diagnostic study. Approximately 10% of hemorrhages, however, either based on size or location, may be missed on CT. MRI is also not 100% sensitive in detecting SAH. In such cases, lumbar puncture is essential to further evaluate the clinical suspicion. Sending the patient home or administering a potent vasoconstrictor such as sumatriptan could potentially be catastrophic. A cerebral angiogram would be appropriate to look for an aneurysm if the CSF shows evidence for SAH.

2. A 23-year-old man presents with recurrent 1 to 2 minute episodes of speech arrest and right facial twitching. He is completely aware of what happens. Which of the following is required to diagnose epilepsy in this patient?
   A. Paroxysmal, stereotypical spells
   B. Loss of consciousness
   C. An abnormal EEG
   D. Convulsions
   E. Tongue biting

The correct answer is A. Since the brain has localized areas of function, seizures may focally emanate from and remain confined to an area outside the motor strip and therefore, not cause convulsions. Loss of consciousness and tongue biting do not occur with all types of seizures. Awareness is retained in simple partial seizures. An abnormal routine EEG is not required to make the diagnosis of epilepsy as scalp electrodes may not pick up a deep or small focus, particularly during the relative short recording time. The diagnosis of epilepsy is a clinical one requiring paroxysmal, stereotypical spells.

3. Which of the following statements is true about magnetic resonance imaging?
   A. It is safe with certain types of pacemakers.
   B. It may be performed if aneurysm clips are ferromagnetic.
   C. It may cause nephrogenic systemic fibrosis if gadolinium is used in the setting of renal dysfunction.
   D. It is readily available and easier to perform than CT in patients with altered mental status.
   E. It is better than CT for detecting acute blood.

The correct answer is C. Gadolinium may induce nephrogenic systemic fibrosis in patients with renal insufficiency. MRI is contraindicated in patients with all types of pacemakers and ferromagnetic material due to the risk of device malfunction and movement that may be fatal. CT is more readily available than MRI and may be performed quicker in confused patients as it does not require the same degree of immobility and cooperation. CT is the imaging study of choice for acute hemorrhage.

4. A 35-year-old woman with hepatitis C presents with painful, burning feet. Examination reveals symmetric, stocking distribution of sensory loss to pain and temperature. Position and vibration are normal. EMG and nerve conduction studies are normal. Which of the following conditions is most likely in this patient?
   A. Lumbar polyradiculopathy
   B. Large fiber polyneuropathy
   C. Mononeuritis multiplex
   D. Small fiber neuropathy
   E. Myositis

The correct answer is D. The patient presents clinically with a small fiber neuropathy. Proprioception and vibration perception are transmitted by large caliber nerve fibers. Of the answers listed, the best choice is small fiber neuropathy as dysfunction of these nerve fibers is not detected on routine nerve conduction/EMG studies.

5. Which of the following features is most consistent with a post-lumbar-puncture headache?
   A. It worsens when patients lie down.
   B. It promptly improves or resolves with standing.
   C. A blood patch may be necessary for treatment.
   D. The CSF opening pressure is high.
   E. It is more likely to occur with use of a small diameter needle.

The correct answer is C. A post-dural-puncture or low-CSF-pressure headache may occur in patients after lumbar puncture, particularly when large diameter spinal needles are used. Occurrence of the headache is not associated with the amount of fluid removed or with the duration the patient is kept supine after the procedure. Clinically, patients are asymptomatic while supine (position of highest CSF pressure) and the headache develops when they sit or stand. Hydration, caffeine, and rest are recommended for management of these headaches. A blood patch may be required for refractory post-LP headaches.

SUGGESTED READING

Bradley WG, Daroff RB, Fenichel GM, et al. *Neurology in Clinical Practice. Volume I: Principles of Diagnosis and Management.* 5th ed. Philadelphia, PA: Butterworth, Heinemann, Elsevier; 2008.

Ellenby MS, Tegtmeyer K, Lai S, et al. Videos in clinical medicine. Lumbar puncture. *N Engl J Med.* 2006;355:e12.

England JD, Gronseth GS, Franklin G, et al. Practice parameter: evaluation of distal symmetric polyneuropathy: role of autonomic testing, nerve biopsy, and skin biopsy (an evidence-based review). *Neurology.* 2009;72:1–8.

Goetz CG. *Textbook of Clinical Neurology.* 3rd ed. Philadelphia, PA: Saunders, Elsevier; 2007.

Osborn AG. *Diagnostic Neuroradiology.* St. Louis, MO: Mosby-Yearbook, Inc.; 1994.

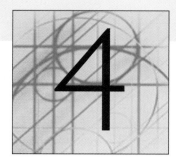

4 Fundamentals of Neuroradiology

ROBERT E. MORALES AND DISHANT G. SHAH

> **key points**
> - Neuroradiologic images must always be evaluated in a systematic fashion with an understanding of fundamental neuroimaging concepts. Otherwise, not only can certain findings be overlooked, but one may quickly proceed down the wrong diagnostic path.
> - Only after these basic concepts are understood, should one focus on specific imaging features of particular disease processes.
> - Once a lesion is identified, it should be initially characterized by its location and by the type of edema that may be present. Only after these features are analyzed, should the CT density characteristics, MR signal characteristics, and possible contrast enhancement patterns be considered.

euroradiology has come a long way from the days when intracranial lesions were indirectly imaged. Air was placed into ventricles and contrast was injected into vessels to look for mass effect on these structures that would then suggest adjacent intracranial pathology. Fortunately, however, times have changed. We now have advanced tools to image lesions directly and less invasively. Magnetic resonance imaging (MRI) and computed tomography (CT) have become powerful instruments that not only depict these lesions but also can further characterize them. Often an abbreviated differential diagnosis can be suggested.

This chapter will review some of the fundamental principles of neuroimaging. Initially, the individual modalities of CT and MRI as well as the utility of contrast administration will be discussed. Basic topics will then be reviewed that form the foundation of image interpretation. These include the imaging findings of herniation and mass effect, hydrocephalus and volume loss, cytotoxic and vasogenic edema, and intra-axial and extra-axial masses. A brief discussion of spinal imaging will follow. Finally, due to their relatively common occurrence and particularly critical clinical implications, intracranial hemorrhage and cerebral ischemia/infarction will be specifically addressed.

COMPUTED TOMOGRAPHY VERSUS MAGNETIC RESONANCE IMAGING

The physics of CT and MRI is complex and beyond the scope of this chapter. In its most basic form, CT uses ionizing radiation to generate cross-sectional images from x-ray absorption of the tissues examined. MR images are generated using principles of in vivo magnetism and capturing signal from water and organic molecules that produce a magnetic field.

When discussing CT, structures are characterized with regard to their *density* or *attenuation* (of the x-ray beam), just as in the interpretation of plain x-ray films. Metal, bone, and calcification are densest (brightest), acute blood is denser than soft tissue, water is denser than fat, and air is the least dense (darkest). The density is measured in Hounsfield units (HU) with water having a HU of zero. Higher HU are measured in bone, blood, and soft tissue, whereas fat and air have HU in the negative range. This is an important fact to remember as HU measurement and density characteristics are often reported in radiology reports while characterizing findings on CT.

In MRI, structures are characterized with regard to their *signal* or *intensity*. There are now more than 20 sequences used in MRI for tissue characterization. In general, the basic sequences are T1 and T2. T1-weighted images are superior in depicting anatomic detail. Postcontrast images are nearly always T1-weighted images. Bright T1 signal is seen in fat, subacute hemorrhage (intracellular and extracellular methemoglobin), proteinaceous fluid, melanin, occasionally calcification and with the use of contrast (gadolinium). Bright T2 signal is seen in substances or tissue with relative higher water content such as cerebrospinal fluid (CSF), edematous/inflamed tissue, gliotic/encephalomalacic tissue, certain stages of hemorrhage (oxyhemoglobin and extracellular methemoglobin), and occasionally fat (if a fast technique of obtaining the T2-weighted images is utilized). FLAIR (fluid attenuated inversion recovery) sequence in basic terms,

nullifies the bright CSF signal (free water) on the T2-weighted images, hence turning the CSF into a dark signal. Thus, pathology seen on T2-weighted images may be more conspicuous on this sequence. This is particularly evident in the periventricular white matter and at the cortex where, on T2-weighted images, the lesions may be somewhat obscured by the bright signal in the ventricles and sulci, respectively (Fig. 4.1).

■ **SPECIAL CLINICAL POINT: A useful approach when interpreting an MRI study is to initially utilize the T1-weighted images to evaluate the anatomy and underlying structure of the brain including the ventricles and CSF spaces. Since many pathologic processes result in surrounding edema, which is very high in signal and more conspicuous on the T2-weighted images, this sequence is then utilized to evaluate for underlying subtle pathology. If a lesion is detected, the signal characteristics on the T1- and T2-weighted images, as well as the possible presence and pattern of contrast enhancement, are then evaluated to more specifically characterize the lesion.**

The T1- and T2-weighted pulse sequences are essentially the foundation of MRI. Other sequences such as FLAIR and diffusion-weighted imaging have been developed to increase the sensitivity of detecting lesions and to add more information when characterizing them.

Diffusion-weighted imaging has revolutionized the ability to image acute infarction. This sequence detects the change in Brownian motion of water molecules in injured tissue. Restricted diffusion signifies cell injury and appears as bright signal on the diffusion-weighted images (with corresponding dark signal on apparent diffusion coefficient [ADC] map images). This sequence generally takes less than a minute to obtain and is highly sensitive in acute infarction. For all practical purposes, diffusion restriction can be seen essentially at the time of onset of an acute infarct. Although diffusion-weighted imaging is usually utilized to evaluate for acute infarction, other lesions/substances, including highly

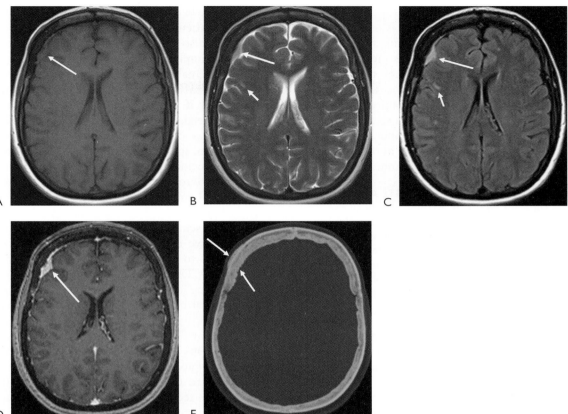

FIGURE 4.1 MR and CT evaluation of a right frontal meningioma. **A:** On T1-weighted MRI, the CSF is low in signal intensity. The white matter is higher in signal intensity than the cortex. The dural-based lesion *(arrow)* is subtle. **B:** On T2-weighted MRI, the CSF is high in signal intensity. The cortex is higher in signal intensity than the white matter. The lesion *(long arrow)* is lower in signal than the adjacent CSF. A small nonspecific subcortical white matter lesion *(short arrow)* is questioned although this may also represent a sulcus. **C:** MR FLAIR imaging is similar to T2-weighted imaging except that free water (CSF) is suppressed and is low in signal intensity. The lesion *(long arrow)* is more conspicuous and the white matter lesion *(short arrow)* is confirmed since the CSF in the sulci is low in signal. **D:** Postcontrast T1-weighted MRI demonstrates enhancement of the lesion (arrow), confirming it is solid. The mass is much more conspicuous. **E:** A CT image with bone windowing demonstrates hyperostosis *(arrows)* of the inner and outer tables of the calvarium adjacent to the mass suggesting a meningioma.

cellular tumors and purulent material can also restrict diffusion. These characteristics can be particularly helpful when evaluating for possible underlying intracranial abscess or purulent collection.

MRI has superior contrast resolution compared to CT, and in all but a few instances, it is superior to CT in evaluating the soft tissues of the central nervous system (CNS). CT is, however, much better in detecting and characterizing osseous abnormalities. CT is superior to MRI in evaluating cortical bone and is used commonly in evaluating trauma patients for underlying fractures. In contrast, MRI is more sensitive in evaluating the marrow spaces for underlying edema or other infiltrating processes. As a result, it is useful in the imaging of infection and neoplasms. For all practical purposes, CT has better spatial resolution than MR and can be used in evaluating structures as small as 0.625 mm with current multislice detector scanners.

■ **SPECIAL CLINICAL POINT: Although MRI is superior to CT at imaging nearly all the nonosseous components of the central nervous system, CT remains the imaging study of choice in the evaluation of acute intracranial hemorrhage, particularly acute subarachnoid hemorrhage. MRI, however, is probably more sensitive if the onset of symptoms was a few days prior.**

Given the increased availability of CT scanners, faster turnaround time in obtaining the study, and cheaper cost, CT remains the mainstay of emergent imaging.

In a few instances, MRI is the initial study of choice. Since MRI is much better in evaluating the thecal sac and spinal cord, emergent MRI of the spine is indicated for the work-up of possible cord compression or intrinsic cord lesion as well as in the evaluation for spinal infection. In some institutions, MRI with limited sequences, including diffusion-weighted imaging, is performed emergently as part of the stroke center "brain attack" protocol.

Although both CT and MRI have tremendous use in the work-up of neurologic disorders, one must be aware of the potential disadvantages and contraindications when ordering a study. CT uses ionizing radiation, and cumulative doses over time may increase the risk of developing cancer. This risk is higher in the pediatric population due to growing cell lines. Every institution has specific imaging protocols, which use lower radiation in the pediatric population; however, this risk must be kept in mind while ordering any study with ionizing radiation. Likewise, there are also guidelines when performing CT and MRI in pregnant patients.

MRI is also usually contraindicated in patients with implanted electronic devices such as cardiac pacemakers, defibrillators, cochlear implants, and nerve stimulators. It is also contraindicated if the patient has ferromagnetic clips or foreign bodies that lay on or in close proximity to delicate structures such as the globes, brain, spinal cord, and nerves. There are resources, including websites, that can be used as a source of reference to determine if a specific device is MR compatible. All patients need to be screened prior to MRI to ensure safety.

Current scanner and postprocessing technologies have enabled us to further advance our abilities to detect CNS pathology. CT angiography (CTA) and MR angiography (MRA) have become essential tools in the imaging evaluation of neurovascular disorders such as in the work-up for infarcts, vascular injury, and vascular lesions, such as arteriovenous malformations (AVM) and aneurysms. Conventional angiography continues to remain the gold standard for neurovascular evaluation if noninvasive techniques do not provide adequate information. CT and MR perfusion imaging are being used more in the setting of acute stroke to evaluate for salvageable tissue. MR perfusion data can also be helpful in distinguishing recurrent neoplasm from radiation necrosis in neuro-oncology. Advanced MR techniques such as MR spectroscopy, functional MRI, and diffusion tensor imaging are now often being used in daily clinical practice to answer specific questions. The ability to detect and characterize CNS pathology rapidly continues to improve with advances in technology and with the development of newer pulse sequences. The trend is always toward obtaining superior images with faster imaging.

CONTRAST VERSUS NONCONTRAST

The question of whether to administer contrast is a common one. Contrast agents used in CT and MRI have risk factors, and screening for possible adverse events must be done before ordering a study with contrast.

■ **SPECIAL CLINICAL POINT: Contrast is not typically necessary when evaluating for acute ischemia or in the setting of trauma. Contrast should be considered when an underlying infectious/inflammatory process or neoplasm is suspected.**

Iodinated contrast agents used with CT have the potential to elicit allergic reactions and can be nephrotoxic in patients with poor renal function. Preventive measures including steroid pretreatment, in patients with a known contrast allergy, and hydration, in patients with compromised renal function, are often performed. The contrast agents used for MRI are molecular forms of gadolinium. Although gadolinium-based contrast agents have a lower propensity to cause allergic reactions, recent literature has associated nephrogenic systemic fibrosis (NSF) with exposure to gadolinium in patients with renal impairment. As a result, an accurate medical history and renal function tests (blood urea nitrogen and creatinine) are often indicated prior to contrast administration of either iodinated CT contrast or gadolinium-based contrast agents.

■ **SPECIAL CLINICAL POINT: Enhancement in abnormal tissue is related to breakdown of the blood–brain barrier with leakage of contrast. Almost any lesion can demonstrate an element of enhancement, particularly mild, linear enhancement along its periphery. However, nodular, solid enhancement is more suggestive of an underlying neoplasm.**

There are, of course, exceptions as certain nonneoplastic lesions can have nodular enhancement such as tumefactive multiple sclerosis. In addition, not all neoplasms enhance. Specifically, low-grade astrocytomas typically do not enhance.

As discussed in the section on CT versus MRI, CTA and MRA are also used to evaluate the vasculature. Of note, MRA can be done without contrast using time of flight (TOF) technique. Contrast-enhanced MRA can be performed in cases where the TOF technique is limited due to artifact or more accurate characterization of a stenosis or lesion is warranted. Another use of contrast is in CT myelography where contrast is injected into the thecal sac followed by CT of the spine. This is particularly useful when MRI is contraindicated or in the postsurgical patient where MRI can be limited due to metallic artifact of underlying hardware.

HERNIATION AND MASS EFFECT

The first step in evaluating the brain is to determine if there is impending herniation that would indicate emergent intervention. On axial imaging, it is useful to evaluate the ventricles and basal cisterns to determine whether they are effaced (compressed), suggesting mass effect or herniation. Sagittal and coronal reconstructions can often also be performed to directly visualize the degree of herniation.

Effacement of the fourth ventricle is a marker for tonsillar herniation, particularly if the process is supratentorial (a lesion in the cerebellum can efface the fourth ventricle without necessarily resulting in overt tonsillar herniation). Evaluation of the posterior fossa with newer CT technology is much better than on older scanners where the foramen magnum was obscured by streak artifact. In addition, if there is any question, sagittal reconstructions can be performed to directly visualize the tonsils. *Effacement of the quadrigeminal plate cistern (behind the superior and inferior colliculi) is a marker for transtentorial herniation.* If the lesion is supratentorial, it signifies downward herniation across the tentorium. If the lesion is infratentorial, it signifies upward herniation across the tentorium. *Effacement of the suprasellar cistern is a marker for uncal herniation (another form of transtentorial herniation), where the medial temporal lobe protrudes into the suprasellar cistern, over the tentorium. Shift of the midline structures and septum pellucidum is usually more obvious with displacement of the lateral ventricles/third ventricle across the midline. This represents subfalcine herniation.* When this is more advanced, the foramen of Monro becomes effaced, and dilatation of the contralateral

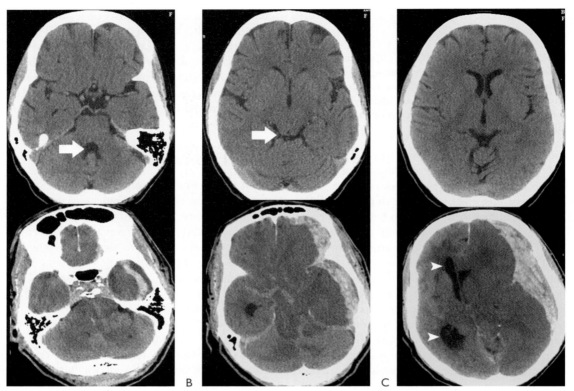

FIGURE 4.2 Comparison of normal anatomy with herniation in a patient with a large subdural hemorrhage. Normal images are on top of each figure. **A:** Tonsillar herniation is evidenced by effacement and obliteration of the fourth ventricle *(arrow)*. **B:** Transtentorial herniation is noted by effacement of the quadrigeminal plate cistern *(arrow)*. **C:** Subfalcine herniation is noted by shift of the lateral and/or third ventricle across the midline. Enlargement of the contralateral lateral ventricle *(arrowheads)* indicates entrapment due to obstruction at the foramen of Monro.

lateral ventricle develops (ventricular trapping) (Fig. 4.2).

Herniation is problematic for a variety of reasons. Parenchyma and other neural structures can be compressed, and vessels can be compromised. Tonsillar herniation compresses the medulla and can depress the centers for respiration and cardiac rhythm control. Transtentorial herniation can compress the posterior cerebral arteries and cause infarction. It can also result in midbrain compression and hemorrhages, likely from tearing of small parenchymal vessels (Duret hemorrhage) (Fig. 4.3).

The mass effect may not be severe enough to result in herniation but can efface local sulci and adjacent cisterns or portions of the ventricles. Although this may be a subtle finding, it is important as it may be the only clue to suggest adjacent pathology that is not otherwise directly visualized. Mass effect in general indicates that the underlying process is active. For example, edema and gliosis/encephalomalacia will both demonstrate decreased density on CT, decreased signal on T1-weighted MRI, and increased signal on T2-weighted MRI. Edema, however, will result in mass effect with displacement/compression of adjacent structures. Gliosis/encephalomalacia will result in the opposite effect with widening of the adjacent CSF spaces due to the loss of parenchymal volume.

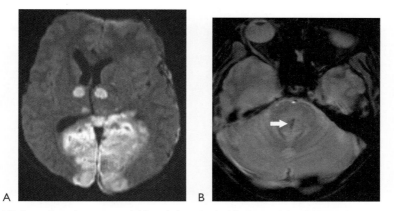

FIGURE 4.3 Sequelae of transtentorial herniation. **A:** A diffusion-weighted image demonstrates acute posterior circulation infarcts in a patient with transtentorial herniation, and compression of the vessels, due to a subdural hemorrhage. There are bilateral posterior cerebral artery territorial infarcts, within the occipital cortex, and bilateral thalamic infarcts. **B:** Gradient echo MRI at the level of the pons demonstrates linear area of susceptibility artifact. This is consistent with a Duret hemorrhage with the low signal due to blood products.

HYDROCEPHALUS VERSUS VOLUME LOSS

After determining whether the ventricles and sulci are effaced or displaced, signifying mass effect, one should make a judgment as to whether the ventricles and sulci in general are normal in size. When the ventricles are enlarged, it can be due to volume loss or hydrocephalus. *If the ventricles are enlarged and the sulci are also enlarged, it suggests volume loss* either due to atrophy or lack of development of the parenchyma (in pediatric patients). In the closed intracranial system, when there is loss of volume of the parenchyma, the CSF spaces diffusely must widen to compensate for the space previously taken up by the parenchyma. *If the ventricles are enlarged but the sulci are not widened, or especially when they are narrow, it suggests hydrocephalus* with the enlarged ventricles taking up space and causing effacement of the surrounding sulci (Fig. 4.4).

If hydrocephalus is established, the next step is to determine whether the cause is noncommunicating (obstructive) or communicating. Obstructive hydrocephalus refers to hydrocephalus where the obstruction of CSF drainage is along the ventricular outflow. Typically this is at the cerebral aqueduct or foramen of Monro, due to the smaller caliber of these passages. Communicating hydrocephalus refers to obstruction at the level of the arachnoid villi as the CSF drains into the dural venous sinuses. This can be due to such etiologies as infectious/inflammatory meningitis, subarachnoid hemorrhage (SAH), and neoplasm (carcinomatous meningitis). In communicating hydrocephalus, all of the ventricles are enlarged.

Once hydrocephalus is diagnosed, a quick method of evaluating for obstructive versus communicating hydrocephalus is to evaluate the fourth ventricle. If the fourth ventricle is normal in size, there is likely obstructive hydrocephalus (Fig. 4.5). If the fourth ventricle is also dilated, communicating hydrocephalus is more likely. Obstructive hydrocephalus from obstruction at the foramen of Luschka and Magendie will result in an enlarged fourth ventricle, but this is uncommon. Normal pressure hydrocephalus appears similar to communicating hydrocephalus. Often it is difficult to determine whether there is an element of mild

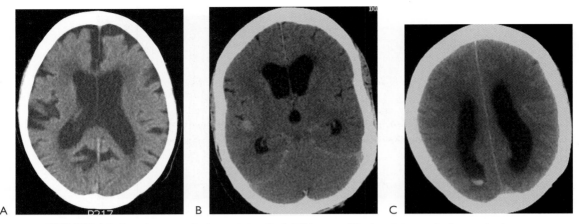

FIGURE 4.4 Atrophy versus hydrocephalus. **A:** A CT image of the head demonstrates cerebral atrophy as noted by prominence of the ventricles and sulci. The CSF spaces diffusely enlarge to occupy the space formed by the parenchymal loss. **B, C:** CT images in a different patient demonstrate widening of the ventricles with effacement of the sulci. The ventricles are enlarged due to communicating hydrocephalus caused by poor functioning arachnoid villi/granulations in this patient with subarachnoid hemorrhage.

communicating hydrocephalus or central volume loss. Widening of the temporal horns, a convex margin of the lateral walls of the third ventricle, and a stretched appearance of the corpus callosum are more suggestive of underlying hydrocephalus.

CYTOTOXIC VERSUS VASOGENIC EDEMA

The identification of edema indicates an acute or active process. It is critical to determine whether cytotoxic edema, vasogenic edema or

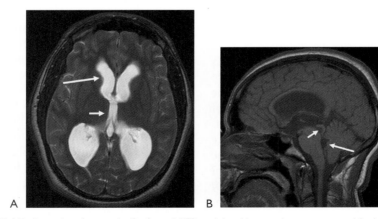

FIGURE 4.5 Aqueductal stenosis. **A:** An axial T2-weighted image demonstrates widening of the lateral *(long arrow)* and third *(short arrow)* ventricles and effacement of the sulci, suggesting hydrocephalus. **B:** A sagittal T1-weighted image demonstrates the fourth ventricle *(long arrow)* to be normal in size, suggesting obstructive hydrocephalus at the level of the cerebral aqueduct of Sylvius. The aqueduct *(short arrow)* is noted to be widened at its superior aspect but narrowed inferiorly without evidence of an underlying mass. This is consistent with aqueductal stenosis.

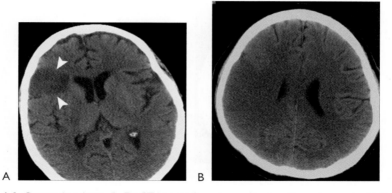

FIGURE 4.6 Cytotoxic edema. **A, B:** CT images from two patients with acute cerebral infarctions (*arrowheads* in **A**) demonstrate cytotoxic edema as noted by "loss of the gray–white matter differentiation," sulcal effacement and also a component of vasogenic edema, with low density within the underlying white matter.

both are present. In its simplest form, cytotoxic edema implies cell injury to the cell body of the neuron in the cortex with failure of the sodium–potassium pump and cell swelling. Vasogenic edema implies breakdown of the blood–brain barrier with fluid extending to the interstitial space and is much less specific with regard to the etiology of the insult.

Cytotoxic edema is swelling of the neurons in the cortex. Normally, the cortex is slighter hyperdense relative to the underlying white matter. *On CT, cytotoxic edema causes the cortical density to decrease, approaching that of the underlying white matter. This is classically described as "loss of the gray–white matter differentiation"* (Fig. 4.6). When there is cytotoxic edema, there is also often a component of vasogenic edema.

Vasogenic edema is interstitial edema within the white matter usually due to breakdown of the blood–brain barrier. The overlying cortex is spared since the neuron itself is not directly injured. *On CT, vasogenic edema appears as decreased density of the fluid tracking along the white matter. This is classically described as a "finger-in-glove" appearance* (Fig. 4.7).

Since many pathologic processes result in breakdown of the blood–brain barrier, resulting in interstitial edema, vasogenic edema is nonspecific and can be associated with essentially any underlying insult. However, if the cortex is involved (cytotoxic edema), the differential diagnosis is much more limited. Diagnostic considerations in this category most commonly include infarction and encephalitis. Although encephalitis is much less common, it is an important process to always consider. In the right clinical context, posttraumatic cortical contusion, edema from seizure activity, and an underlying glioma also can have this appearance. If the etiology of the cytotoxic edema is unclear, and nearly in all cases when vasogenic edema alone is identified, contrast should be administered in order to evaluate for an underlying lesion and to better characterize the findings.

INTRA-AXIAL VERSUS EXTRA-AXIAL

If an intracranial mass is identified, the first step is to determine whether it *is intra-axial* or *extra-axial* in location. *Intra-axial* refers to the lesion being located within the brain parenchyma. *Extra-axial* refers to the lesion being outside the brain but within the confines of the calvarium. *In general, intra-axial lesions are surrounded by brain parenchyma, whereas extra-axial lesions displace brain parenchyma* (Fig. 4.8). Intra-axial lesions rarely produce changes in the adjacent

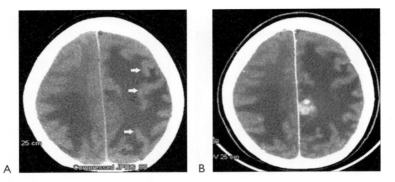

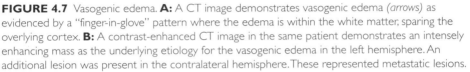

FIGURE 4.7 Vasogenic edema. **A:** A CT image demonstrates vasogenic edema *(arrows)* as evidenced by a "finger-in-glove" pattern where the edema is within the white matter, sparing the overlying cortex. **B:** A contrast-enhanced CT image in the same patient demonstrates an intensely enhancing mass as the underlying etiology for the vasogenic edema in the left hemisphere. An additional lesion was present in the contralateral hemisphere. These represented metastatic lesions.

calvarium, whereas extra-axial lesions can occasionally thin or even thicken it. Meningiomas can cause hyperostosis and thickening of the adjacent osseous cortex as well as thickening of the adjacent dura (dural tail).

Accurately locating the lesion is essential as the differential diagnosis is dependent on this feature. If a lesion is extra-axial, the differential diagnosis is much more limited. If it does not en-

hance, it is typically either an arachnoid cyst, epidermoid/dermoid, or lipoma, unless hematoma or other fluid collection, including an infected collection, is suspected. If it enhances, in a solid fashion, it is typically either a meningioma, schwannoma, meningeal-based metastasis/lymphoma, or occasionally an inflammatory mass from perhaps granulomatous disease. Metastases and lymphoma are often considered together in

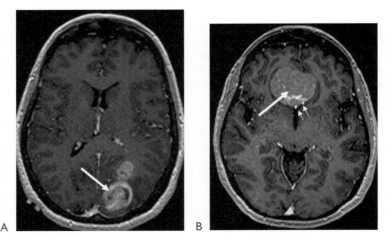

FIGURE 4.8 Intra-axial versus extra-axial masses. **A:** A postcontrast T1-weighted image demonstrates an enhancing intra-axial mass (glioma) *(arrow)* within the left occipital lobe. The mass is surrounded by the parenchyma. **B:** A postcontrast T1-weighted image demonstrates a heterogeneously enhancing extra-axial mass (meningioma) *(long arrow)* within the interhemispheric fissure, displacing the frontal lobes bilaterally. The anterior cerebral arteries *(short arrows)* are displaced posteriorly.

neuroimaging since they are typically included in the differential diagnosis of any enhancing lesion throughout the CNS.

If the lesion is intra-axial, then the differential diagnosis is much more extensive with regard to neoplastic, infectious/inflammatory, congenital, metabolic, posttraumatic and vascular processes. In all of neuroradiology, accurate location of a lesion is perhaps the single most important factor in developing an appropriate differential diagnosis. This is particularly evident in imaging the spine where the differential diagnosis can be significantly narrowed once an accurate location of the lesion is determined.

SPINE IMAGING

Imaging of the spine is discussed briefly. *The spinal cord is essentially an extension of the brain so the differential diagnosis of intramedullary (intra-axial) and extramedullary (extra-axial) lesions is similar. Since the most common lesions of the spine are related to degenerative changes and trauma to the spinal column, which lie outside of the dura, the extramedullary compartment is further divided into two components, the extramedullary intradural and the extradural spaces.* Extradural pathology includes posttraumatic lesions, degenerative changes such as osteophytic spurs and disc herniations, osseous neoplasms, and epidural masses and collections. The extramedullary intradural lesions are the same lesions considered in the intracranial extra-axial space. Lesions within the cord itself are considered intramedullary in location (Fig. 4.9).

The differential diagnosis of intramedullary lesions of the spinal cord is similar to the intra-axial lesions in the brain, although neoplasms are less common within the spinal cord than within the brain. Spinal cord neoplasms usually enhance; in contrast, nonenhancing glial tumors are common in the brain. Demyelinating disease is relatively common in the spinal cord, whereas infarcts are much less common than in the brain. Parenchymal signal abnormality,

from compression by adjacent degenerative changes, is of course specific to the spine.

CT is particularly useful for evaluating the osseous structures, in the setting of trauma, and for evaluating surgical hardware in postoperative patients. MRI is the study of choice when evaluating the spinal cord and nonosseous surrounding structures of the spine such as the intervertebral discs, ligaments, and epidural space. Contrast is useful if infection, neoplasm, or an underlying vascular lesion is suspected. If there has been prior surgery, contrast can help distinguish between epidural scar formation, which enhances, and recurrent disc herniations, which typically do not. This is more of an issue within the lumbar spine since significant scar formation is less common within the cervical spine.

INTRACRANIAL HEMORRHAGE

Evaluating for the presence of intracranial hemorrhage is a common task in neuroimaging. *The four types of hemorrhage, originating from superficial to deep, include epidural, subdural, subarachnoid, and intraparenchymal hemorrhage.* Epidural hematomas are located outside the dura. Subdural hematomas are located between the dura and arachnoid membranes. Subarachnoid hemorrhage (SAH) is located between the arachnoid and pia mater, within the CSF space. Intraparenchymal hemorrhage is located within the parenchymal substance of the brain.

Epidural and subdural hemorrhages are typically due to trauma. The classic epidural hematoma is due to a temporal bone fracture, with injury to the middle meningeal artery. Venous epidural hematoma formation can occur if the dural venous sinuses are torn. This is reportedly more common in pediatric patients. Subdural hemorrhages are typically due to a tear in perforating veins. They are more prone to tearing after less severe trauma if they are already "stretched" due to the presence of volume loss or a preexisting subdural collection. Epidural hematomas exist between the calvarium and the dura with the dura being stripped away from the overlying bone. It usually takes some force to

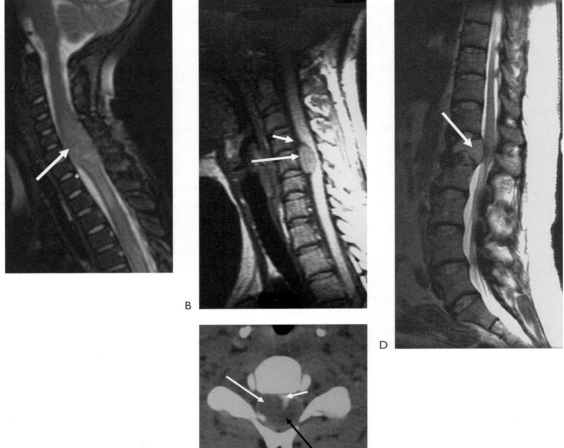

FIGURE 4.9 Intramedullary, extramedullary/intradural, and extradural spine lesions. **A:** A sagittal T2-weighted image demonstrates an intramedullary lesion (astrocytoma) *(arrow)* expanding the cord. **B, C:** A sagittal T1-weighted image **(B)** and an axial image from a CT myelogram **(C)**, demonstrate an extramedullary, intradural mass (meningioma) *(long arrow)* displacing the cord *(black arrow* in **C)** and widening the immediately adjacent subarachnoid space *(short arrows* in **B and C)** as the dura stays on the outside of the lesion. **D:** A sagittal T2-weighted image demonstrates an extradural lesion (osseous metastasis) *(arrow)* displacing the cord and effacing the thecal sac.

accomplish this, with the underlying hematoma being under an element of pressure. As a result, this type of hematoma usually has a convex margin against the brain (Fig. 4.10). Epidural hematomas can cross the midline but typically do not cross the sutures, where the dura is adherent to the calvarium. Subdural hematomas exist within the potential space between the dura and the arachnoid. Since this type of hematoma can more easily extend along this potential space, it usually maintains a concave border along the brain (Fig. 4.11). Since they are deep to the dura, they can cross the sutures, but they are limited by the dural reflections of the falx and tentorium. They do not cross the midline and instead extend along the falx.

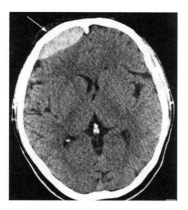

FIGURE 4.10 CT demonstrates an epidural hematoma *(arrow)* in the right frontal region with a convex margin along the brain parenchyma.

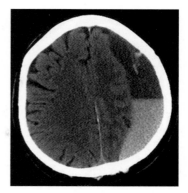

FIGURE 4.11 CT demonstrates a large layering subdural hematoma with a concave margin along the brain parenchyma.

Epidural hematomas tend to cause more focal, local mass effect due to their shape and resistance to diffuse spread. They also can grow rapidly as the patient goes from the "lucid interval" to losing consciousness. However, the overall volume of a subdural hemorrhage along one hemisphere is typically larger and can be underestimated. Even a thin layer of hemorrhage extending along the whole hemisphere cumulatively can result in a large volume of blood.

SAH is most commonly caused by trauma. In cases of spontaneous SAH, aneurysm rupture is the most likely etiology. Since the vast majority of aneurysms are located near the circle of Willis, SAH aneurysm rupture usually presents with some component of the hemorrhage extending into the suprasellar cistern (Fig. 4.12). This is the star-shaped cistern above the sella (pituitary fossa) where the circle of Willis is located.

Intraparenchymal hemorrhage is hemorrhage within the substance of the brain. The etiology for this hemorrhage is more extensive than other types of hemorrhage. If the hemorrhage originates particularly within the basal ganglia or thalamus, or occasionally within the pons or cerebellum, a hypertensive etiology may be initially suspected in the appropriate clinical setting. *An underlying vas-cular or neoplastic lesion, however, should always be considered. If the patient is young or without significant medical history, an underlying AVM needs to be excluded.*

In any intraparenchymal hemorrhage, the differential diagnoses to consider include contusion (if there is a history of trauma and particularly if the hemorrhage is located in the anterior/inferior frontal lobes or anterior temporal lobes), hypertensive hemorrhage (again particularly within the basal ganglia and thalamus) (Fig. 4.13), hemorrhagic conversion of arterial or venous infarcts, underlying vascular

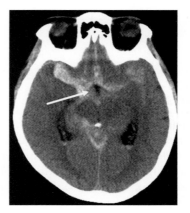

FIGURE 4.12 CT demonstrates subarachnoid hemorrhage *(arrow)* within the suprasellar cistern.

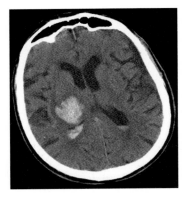

FIGURE 4.13 CT demonstrates a right thalamic intraparenchymal hemorrhage that has extended into the ventricular system.

lesion (including AVM, cavernous angioma, and aneurysm), underlying neoplasm, amyloid angiopathy (if the patient is elderly and has evidence of chronic hemorrhages elsewhere (best seen with special MR sequences [gradient echo])), underlying coagulopathy, and encephalitis.

One must also keep in mind that the jet of blood from a ruptured aneurysm can dissect into the parenchyma and also result in an intraparenchymal hematoma. Typically, in this latter scenario, there is also a component of SAH. Occasionally although this is very minimal such as when a temporal lobe hematoma is caused by a ruptured middle cerebral artery (MCA) aneurysm that is embedded in the sylvian fissure.

INFARCT EVALUATION AND VASCULAR IMAGING

Prior to the advent of MRI, cerebrovascular infarcts were often difficult to visualize within the first 24 hours. From a basic patient management point of view, CT is still the preferred initial study, not only due to the speed and relative ease of acquiring these images, but because the initial primary diagnostic dilemma is to exclude intracranial hemorrhage. Hemor-

rhage may not only be the cause of the neurologic deficit, but may also likely alter therapy. Due to ongoing improvements in developing "stroke centers," the treatment strategies have become more sophisticated, and so have the imaging tools. The goal is to have patients arrive for treatment and be evaluated, as rapidly as possible, for time sensitive treatment. These therapeutic interventions include intravenous tissue plasminogen activator (TPA), intra-arterial thrombolytic therapy, and intra-arterial mechanical thrombectomy.

Although treatment paradigms continue to change and develop, there are basic principles. Initially, if intravenous TPA is to be considered, the main function of imaging (CT) is to exclude intracranial hemorrhage and to see if an infarct is visible in order to determine its size. If the patient is beyond the intravenous therapeutic window and/or intra-arterial therapy is contemplated, one of the roles of imaging is to estimate the risk of hemorrhage after potential clot lysis/mechanical removal and to determine the ischemic *penumbra* (viable, potentially salvageable tissue). With regard to an increased risk of hemorrhage in general, thrombolysis is often not performed in patients with completed infarcts of greater than one third the MCA territory or of significant portions of the basal ganglia.

Currently the treatment protocols are structured around designated time intervals from the onset of symptoms. The goal, however, is to eventually base treatment plans around the physiology of the injured brain parenchyma. For example, hopefully someday treatment decisions will be based on whether there is ischemia to the underlying parenchyma versus completed, irreversible infarction as opposed to the exact time of the onset of the neurologic deficit. Although the current technique of diffusion-weighted MRI can now effectively determine whether an infarct has occurred, almost immediately, it is the task of CT and MR perfusion to estimate the ratio of completed infarction to penumbra. If the volume of parenchyma that has gone on to completed infarction is relatively small and there is a lot of tissue that is ischemic and still viable but at risk for infarction, the interventionalist will likely be more aggressive in pursuing intra-arterial therapy.

Understanding the utility of CT and MRI in evaluating infarcts can be complicated, but there are a few basic principles. Infarcts may be invisible on CT within the first 24 hours. There are some early signs of infarction that can be visualized. The "insular ribbon sign" illustrates early cytotoxic edema of the insular cortex such that there is loss of the normal gray–white matter differentiation between it and the underlying external capsule. Thrombus can also occasionally be seen within the affected vessel as the "hyperdense MCA sign." With improvements in scanner technology thrombus can now occasionally be seen within smaller MCA branches.

With the advent of the diffusion-weighted pulse sequence of MRI, acute infarcts are much more easily detected (Fig. 4.14). This utilizes the parameter of restricted diffusion of water across the cell membrane of acutely infarcted tissue. Without the use of diffusion-weighted imaging, one must rely on the presence or absence of mass effect when determining whether an infarct is recent or chronic, respectively. Edema from recent infarction and gliosis/encephalomalacia from chronic infarction have similar density (CT) and signal intensity (MRI). Edema, however, takes up space and results in mass effect, whereas gliosis/encephalomalacia results in loss of volume, with compensatory widening of the surrounding CSF spaces (Fig. 4.15). With diffusion-weighted imaging, however, new small infarcts can be identified essentially immediately and can be easily separated from chronic infarcts (Fig. 4.16).

CT perfusion imaging can be performed to not only evaluate for infarction but also ischemia. In this technique, a bolus of contrast is tracked as it courses through the brain vasculature. Parameters such as mean transit time, time to peak, cerebral blood flow, and cerebral blood volume can be deduced, and maps can be obtained, depicting areas of infarction and ischemia. MR perfusion serves a similar role.

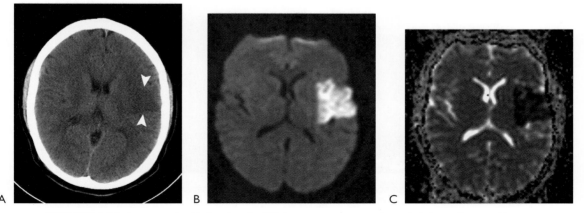

FIGURE 4.14 Acute cerebral infarction. **A:** CT demonstrates somewhat subtle loss of gray–white differentiation and sulcal effacement in the left frontal-temporal region *(arrowheads)*.
B: Diffusion-weighted MRI clearly shows the area of infarction appearing as markedly hyperintense.
C: Corresponding apparent diffusion coefficient (ADC) map shows this area to be darker than surrounding normal brain, thus confirming the finding of true restricted diffusion in this acute infarct.

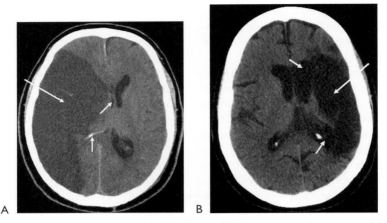

FIGURE 4.15 Recent versus chronic MCA infarction. **A:** CT demonstrates a large recent right MCA infarct *(long arrow)* with marked mass effect, subfalcine herniation, and effacement/compression of the right lateral ventricle *(short arrows)*. **B:** CT demonstrates a chronic left MCA infarct *(long arrow)* with volume loss and compensatory widening of the adjacent sulci and lateral ventricle *(short arrows)*.

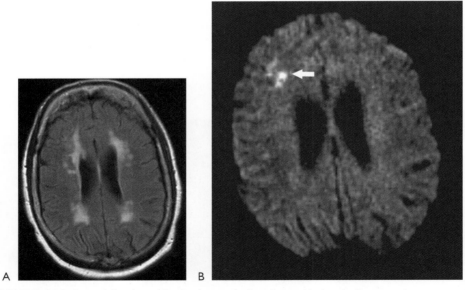

FIGURE 4.16 Acute infarction with a background of small vessel ischemic disease and age indeterminate deep white matter infarcts. **A:** FLAIR MRI demonstrates periventricular white matter disease suggesting chronic small vessel ischemic disease with deep white matter infarcts. This patient had an acute focal neurologic deficit. **B:** On diffusion-weighted MRI, a single hyperintense focus *(arrow)* is identified. This confirms the presence of an acute infarct with the remaining periventricular ischemic changes noted to be chronic.

After establishing the presence of possible cerebral ischemia or infarction, the vasculature will need to be evaluated for underlying thrombus, stenosis, or occlusion. This can be performed with magnetic resonance angiography (MRA), computed tomography angiography (CTA), ultrasound, and/or with conventional angiography. Although conventional angiography remains the gold standard in the evaluation of the vasculature, it carries with it a small but definite risk of infarction and vascular injury.

With MRA and CTA, numerous sequential axial images are obtained maximizing the contrast between the vessels and the surrounding tissues. These "raw data" images can then be manipulated by subtracting out the adjacent tissues and leaving only the vessels. These are then displayed, and can be rotated, in three dimensions (Figs. 4.17 and 4.18). Although CTA requires the administration of intravenous contrast, MRA can be performed without contrast. It can be easily incorporated as part of a comprehensive study of the brain and vasculature in the patient with possible ischemic symptoms or a questioned underlying vascular lesion. If, however, more accurate, detailed evaluation of a stenosis or vascular lesion, such as an aneurysm, is necessary, CTA should be considered. This technique is performed by imaging the region of interest as the contrast bolus traverses the arterial system. The contrast bolus is administered intravenously, similar to any other CT study. The contrast column is directly visualized, like conventional angiography, and is not affected by flow-related artifacts, like MRA.

In general, due to its higher spatial resolution, CTA typically provides a more detailed anatomic evaluation of the vascular system than MRA, other than occasionally at the skull base or where there is marked vascular calcification. It does, however, utilize iodinated contrast and radiation. Since CTA, at this time, is performed by imaging typically during a single vascular phase (e.g., the arterial phase), flow mechanics cannot be evaluated. Flow across luminal narrowing from a dissection or stenosis cannot be characterized. Visualization of an early filling vein, to suggest an underlying fistula or AVM, also cannot be confidently diagnosed. For this type of evaluation, angiography is still often necessary. Newer scanners, however, are now fast enough to image multiple vascular phases. Certain scanners can now image a volume of tissue multiple times, although contrast is in the arterial, capillary, and venous phase, after the administration of a single bolus.

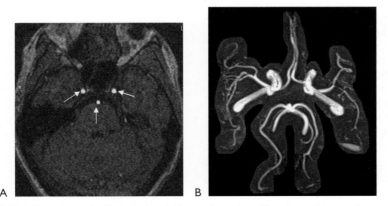

FIGURE 4.17 MR angiography. **A:** A single axial image from the MR angiographic raw data demonstrates increased signal within the patent internal carotid and basilar arteries *(arrows)*. The remainder of the surrounding parenchyma demonstrates relatively low signal. **B:** A three-dimensional reconstructed image of this raw data reveals the circle of Willis.

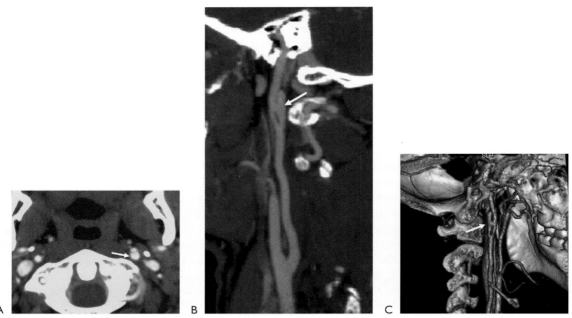

A   B   C

FIGURE 4.18 CT angiography. **A:** A single axial image from the CT angiographic raw data, at the level of the neck, demonstrates dense contrast timed within the arterial structures with a pseudoaneurysm *(arrow)* on the left. **B:** A two-dimensional maximum intensity projection (MIP) image, in the oblique sagittal plane, better demonstrates the extent of the pseudoaneurysm *(arrow)*. **C:** A three-dimensional reconstructed image demonstrates the morphology of the pseudoaneurysm *(arrow)*. Also notice the detailed anatomy of the osseous structures.

■ **SPECIAL CLINICAL POINT: Conventional angiography is still necessary if the smallest vessels need to be evaluated, such as in the work-up of certain aneurysms or when vasculitis is strongly suspected.**

CONCLUSION

Neuroradiology is a rapidly changing field; yet, the fundamental principles of image interpretation remain the same. Detecting a lesion, localizing it to a specific anatomic region within the CNS, characterizing it with regard to its density, signal intensity and the presence or lack of contrast enhancement, and finally developing a differential diagnosis is a common pathway for all image interpretation. As one becomes more experienced, the differential diagnosis becomes more refined, and when the clinical information is applied, a specific diagnosis can often be obtained.

Always Remember

- When evaluating a radiologic study, proceed in a systematic fashion and review the study in the same manner every time. This will decrease the possibility of failing to evaluate a certain anatomic region and overlooking a lesion. One must not jump immediately to the pathologic lesion, ignoring the rest of the study, or hastily come to a diagnosis.
- Although a lesion may be obvious, sometimes only subtle signs of mass effect, such as effacement of sulci, ventricles, or other CSF spaces, are present to suggest an underlying lesion.
- Although the imaging appearance of a lesion can occasionally suggest a specific diagnosis, one should always entertain other differential possibilities.

QUESTIONS AND DISCUSSION

1. Regarding CT and MRI, which of the following is true?
   A. MRI is always better than CT in evaluating for central nervous system pathology
   B. A patient with a metallic hip replacement can have an MRI
   C. FLAIR imaging can demonstrate infarcts earlier than all other MR pulse sequences
   D. Both MRI and CT utilize ionizing radiation

The correct answer is B. Patients with metal that is screwed into bone, such as with hip and knee implants and spinal fusion hardware are able to safely have an MRI study. MRI is better than CT at evaluating most CNS pathology outside of the osseous structures; however, CT is the imaging study of choice in evaluating for acute subarachnoid hemorrhage. CTA also typically gives a more detailed evaluation of the vascular system than MRA. MR diffusion-weighted imaging demonstrates infarcts almost as soon as they happen, earlier than on FLAIR images, T2-weighted images or CT.

2. Regarding hydrocephalus and volume loss, which of the following is false?
   A. Widening of both the ventricles and sulci is suggestive of volume loss
   B. In aqueductal stenosis, the fourth ventricle is typically normal in size
   C. In communicating hydrocephalus, the fourth ventricle is typically normal in size
   D. Meningitis and subarachnoid hemorrhage can cause communicating hydrocephalus

The correct answer is C. In patients with communicating hydrocephalus, the obstruction is at the level of the arachnoid villi. As a result, the fourth ventricle is also enlarged.

3. Regarding patterns of edema, which of the following is false?
   A. Territorial infarcts typically have components of both cytotoxic and vasogenic edema
   B. Metastatic disease typically demonstrates only vasogenic edema
   C. Encephalitis can have cytotoxic edema, vasogenic edema, or both
   D. Loss of the "gray–white junction/interface" implies vasogenic edema

The correct answer is D. Loss of the "gray–white junction/differentiation" suggests cytotoxic edema. On CT, the cortex and deep gray matter structures are more dense than the adjacent white matter. When there is cytotoxic edema, the relative increased density of the cortex is lost, as the cortex becomes lower in density to match the underlying white matter.

4. Regarding intracranial hemorrhage, which of the following is false?
   A. Subdural hematomas do not typically cross the midline as they are limited by the dural reflection of the falx
   B. Aneurysm rupture typically results in subarachnoid hemorrhage
   C. The temporal lobe is a typical location for a hypertensive intraparenchymal hemorrhage
   D. A vascular or neoplastic lesion underlying an intraparenchymal hematoma may be initially obscured by the hemorrhage

The correct answer is C. Although hypertensive hemorrhages can occur anywhere, they are typically located in the basal ganglia or thalamus as well as occasionally in the brainstem and cerebellum. An underlying lesion should always be considered, however, especially when the clinical history is inconsistent. In addition to the multiple etiologies resulting in intracranial hemorrhage, the temporal lobe is a relatively common site for posttraumatic hemorrhagic contusion, hemorrhagic venous infarction from transverse sinus thrombosis and occasionally from a ruptured middle cerebral artery aneurysm, where the jet of blood can be directed predominantly into the parenchyma. Herpes encephalitis can also result in petechial hemorrhage.

5. Regarding extra-axial lesions, which of the following is false?
   A. Epidermoids typically contain fat
   B. Meningiomas can be relatively dark on T2-weighted images, dense on noncontrast CT images and demonstrate hyperostosis and thickening of the adjacent osseous cortex.
   C. Arachnoid cysts should appear similar to CSF on all pulse sequences
   D. Schwannomas are suggested when a mass extends along the expected course of a cranial nerve

The correct answer is A. Epidermoids do not contain fat. If an extra-axial lesion is composed solely of fat, it is likely a lipoma. If it is heterogeneous with fat, areas of typically nonenhancing soft tissue and occasionally calcification, a dermoid should be considered.

SUGGESTED READING

Barkovich AJ, Moore KR, Jones BV, et al. *Diagnostic Imaging Pediatric Neuroradiology.* Canada: Amirsys; 2007.

Castillo M. *Neuroradiology Companion: Methods, Guidelines, and Imaging Fundamentals.* 3rd ed. Philadelphia, PA: Lippincott Williams & Wilkins; 2006.

Grossman RI, Yousem DM. *Neuroradiology: The Requisites.* 2nd ed. Philadelphia, PA: Mosby; 2003.

Harnsberger HR, Osborn AG, Macdonald A, et al. *Diagnostic and Surgical Imaging Anatomy: Brain, Head & Neck, Spine.* Philadelphia, PA: Lippincott Williams & Wilkins; 2006.

Osborn AG, Blaser SI, Salzman KL, et al. *Diagnostic Imaging Brain.* Canada: Amirsys; 2007.

Ross JS, Brant-Zawadzki M, Moore KR, et al. *Diagnostic Imaging Spine.* Canada: Amirsys; 2007.

Willing SJ. *Atlas of Neuroradiology.* Philadelphia, PA: W.B. Saunders Company; 1995.

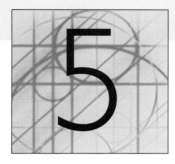

5 Neurologic Emergencies

TRICIA Y. TING AND LISA M. SHULMAN

key points

- Status epilepticus may present with convulsions or nonconvulsive altered mental status. Treatment must be rapidly initiated to achieve early seizure termination for best outcome.

- Delirium, or encephalopathy, may be caused by acute medical conditions that demand emergency medical or surgical treatment for infection (i.e., herpes encephalitis), structural abnormalities (i.e., intracranial hematoma, cerebellar stroke), or toxic-metabolic etiologies (i.e., drug intoxication, thiamine deficiency).

- Other central nervous system emergencies that may require neurosurgical intervention include acute intracranial hypertension and spinal cord compression.

- Increasing weakness in peripheral nervous system disorders, such as myasthenia gravis and Guillain–Barré syndrome, carries the risk of acute respiratory failure. For this reason, inpatient observation and treatment are warranted.

- Neuroleptic malignant syndrome is best treated by discontinuation of dopamine-blocking antipsychotic medications.

Neurologic emergencies are encountered frequently in the practice of medicine, and, if unrecognized, they may progress rapidly to permanent neurologic disability or death. The topics included in this chapter represent the more common and treatable conditions that non-neurologists may likely encounter. Cerebrovascular emergencies are discussed separately in Chapter 7.

CENTRAL NERVOUS SYSTEM

Status Epilepticus

Most epileptic seizures are self-limiting, lasting only seconds to minutes. Seizures that become prolonged or repetitive with impaired recovery of consciousness are at risk of evolving into status epilepticus (SE), a serious medical emergency.

SE is not uncommon, affecting approximately 50 patients per 100,000 population yearly with a mortality rate estimated at up to 20% in adults. Long-term morbidity from SE includes chronic epilepsy, cognitive dysfunction, and focal neurologic deficits.

The point at which a seizure may be defined as SE has been a matter of debate over the past decade. Physiologic evidence for neuronal damage in animal studies formerly led to the definition of SE as any seizure or intermittent seizures without recovery of consciousness lasting for 30 minutes or longer. More recently, however, clinical experience has broadened the definition of SE to continuous or repeated seizure activity without return of consciousness for longer than 5 minutes. The shortened time frame reflects a general push for initiating treatment earlier to minimize the potential morbidity and mortality. Longer seizure duration has been associated with a poorer outcome, and the longer a seizure remains untreated, the more difficult it becomes to abort.

■ **SPECIAL CLINICAL POINT: To optimize patient outcome by earlier treatment, the working definition of SE should be ongoing or repetitive seizures without recovery of consciousness for >5 minutes.**

The most common type of SE carrying the greatest risk of morbidity and mortality is generalized convulsive SE. The seizures are usually easy to recognize clinically as tonic–clonic convulsions of the extremities with complete loss of consciousness. However, generalized convulsive SE may progress over time from overt convulsions to more subtle physical activity such as mild focal twitching or ocular deviation before further evolving to only generalized electrical activity with persistent loss of consciousness but absence of all physical manifestations. There is a risk of delayed recognition of generalized SE when patients present to the emergency room without overt tonic–clonic movements, so clinicians must be aware of the signs of nonconvulsive as well as convulsive SE.

Nonconvulsive SE is a more heterogeneous category that includes absence SE and complex partial SE. Both forms of nonconvulsive SE are characterized by confusion or other altered mental status with minimal motor manifestations. Patients may exhibit blinking, automatisms, or fluctuating bizarre behavior. Evidence from an electroencephalogram (EEG) is important to support the diagnosis of nonconvulsive SE and sometimes, but not always, can help differentiate between absence and complex partial SE. EEG findings may vary from generalized epileptiform discharges to focal discharges or generalized activity with a focal predominance. Absence SE is believed to have little long-term neurologic sequelae. Whether complex partial SE carries a risk of significant neurologic morbidity remains controversial. Although several series documented no lasting neurologic deficits in patients following complex partial SE, there are others that reported long-term morbidity, particularly in those whose seizures were precipitated by acute neurologic disorders. Nevertheless, there is widespread agreement that patients with nonconvulsive SE should be treated quickly and aggressively to avoid potential adverse outcomes.

Morbidity and mortality from SE are a result of multiple factors including central nervous system (CNS) damage from the causative illness or acute insult that precipitated SE, the metabolic consequences of prolonged convulsive SE, and the neuronal excitotoxic effects of prolonged electrical seizure activity. It is recognized that continuous electrical activity for more than 60 minutes, even while correcting for SE-associated metabolic derangements, can result in hippocampal damage and probably in more widespread brain damage as well. Excitotoxic neuronal injury may be compounded by significant systemic manifestations including hypoxemia, metabolic and respiratory acidosis, hyperglycemia, hyperthermia, and blood pressure fluctuation. With more prolonged SE, rhabdomyolysis from prolonged muscle activity and significant sodium and potassium derangements may develop along with renal failure.

Cardiac arrhythmias may occur from CNS dysregulation, electrolyte abnormalities, or even medications used in the treatment of SE. Laboratory investigations commonly demonstrate a peripheral leukocytosis, an acidotic pH, and a mild cerebrospinal fluid (CSF) pleocytosis.

The general principles to minimize the morbidity and mortality associated with SE are early diagnosis, early intervention, and prompt identification and management of concurrent medical and surgical conditions, including potential etiologies. The three most common precipitants of SE in adults are withdrawal from anticonvulsive medications, alcohol withdrawal, and cerebral infarction. Metabolic derangements such as hyponatremia, hyperglycemia or hypoglycemia, hypocalcemia, hepatic failure, and renal failure account for 10% to 15% of the cases reported. Other recognized etiologies of SE include anoxia, hypotension, CNS infections (meningitis, abscess, encephalitis), tumors, trauma, and drug overdose.

Treatment of SE

It has been established that earlier treatment of SE leads to better patient outcome. To this end, the past decade has seen many options investigated for the prehospital treatment of SE and acute repetitive seizures by first-responders—medical personnel and family members of at-risk patients. Concern for respiratory compromise from treatment administered out of the hospital, moreover, has not been substantiated in clinical trials. In fact, a prehospital SE study found the rates of respiratory or circulatory complications after treatment were highest in a placebo group.

Accepted prehospital options for early SE therapy are currently limited to a rectal benzodiazepine gel (diazepam), particularly for nonmedically trained persons, and intravenous (IV) benzodiazepine administration by health care professionals (Table 5.1). Alternative routes of drug administration, including intramuscular (midazolam), buccal, and nasal routes, are under investigation. Prehospital benzodiazepine dosing should be repeated once if necessary to abort continued seizure activity after initial dosing, but activation of emergency services and transfer to an emergency department should then be considered in such cases.

■ **SPECIAL CLINICAL POINT: Rescue therapy that patients can take at home, such a benzodiazepine, can be prescribed for patients with epilepsy who are at high risk for prolonged or acute repetitive seizures and SE.**

Generalized convulsive SE is a medical emergency and should be managed in the emergency department or intensive care unit (ICU) where aggressive measures to provide life support and terminate seizure activity may be best performed. The first steps are to assess vital signs and evaluate oxygenation. An oral or nasopharyngeal airway is inserted, nasotracheal suction is performed, and supplemental oxygen is administered if necessary. Oxygenation is evaluated by clinical examination, pulse oximetry, and arterial blood gas determination. Establishing two intravenous (IV) lines is the next priority, providing a backup IV access as well as allowing parallel delivery of IV glucose, medications, and fluids with IV anticonvulsant therapy. Simultaneously, venous blood is drawn for a complete blood count, electrolytes, glucose, calcium, magnesium, blood urea nitrogen, liver function tests, anticonvulsant drug levels, toxicology screen, and ethanol level. An IV bolus of 50 mL of 50% glucose and thiamine (1 mg/kg) is administered as soon as the IV access is established. Electrocardiographic (ECG) monitoring is instituted immediately, and vital signs are monitored throughout the treatment protocol. Electrographic seizure activity may persist in up to 15% of patients even after anticonvulsant therapy has suppressed all signs of clinical seizure activity. Moreover, seizure activity becomes difficult to assess clinically when patients receive long-acting neuromuscular paralytic agents for endotracheal intubation or when anesthesia is induced for treatment of refractory SE. EEG monitoring, therefore, should begin at the earliest possible opportunity. It should be emphasized, however, that lack of

TABLE 5.1	Management of Status Epilepticus

Objectives	Time Frame	Intervention

Prehospital treatment (nonmedical persons)	>5 minute	1. Recognize SE or acute repetitive seizures
		2. Safety measures, lie patient on side, nothing inserted in mouth
		3. Check blood glucose if appropriate
		4. Treat with rescue benzodiazepine:
		   Adults: Diazepam 10 mg rectally
		   Children: Diazepam 0.5 mg/kg rectally
		Repeat once if needed and activate emergency services for continued seizure activity

Prehospital (medical personnel) or initial in-hospital treatment	5 to 20 minute	1. Recognize SE
		2. Assess vital signs and oxygenation
		3. Insert oral airway and administer oxygen if necessary
		4. Establish two IV lines
		5. Draw blood for CBC, electrolytes, glucose, calcium, magnesium, BUN, LFTs, anticonvulsant levels, toxicology screen, and ethanol level
		6. Begin ECG and EEG[a] monitoring
		7. Administer IV bolus of thiamine 1 mg/kg and 50 mL of 50% glucose
		8. Treat with benzodiazepine:
		   Adults: Lorazepam IV 4 mg bolus or Diazepam IV 10 mg
		   Children: Lorazepam IV 0.1 mg/kg (maximum 4 mg) or
		   Diazepam IV 0.3 mg/kg (maximum 10 mg)

In-hospital treatment/ED setting (second stage SE)	20 to 60 minute	1. Treat with longer-acting AED:
		   Fosphenytoin IV 15–18 mg PE/kg at a rate of 150 PE/min or Phenytoin IV 15–18 mg/kg at maximum rate of 50 mg/min,
		   or in children, Phenobarbital[b] IV 15–20 mg/kg at maximum rate of 100 mg/min
		2. Monitor blood pressure, ECG, and respirations

immediate EEG monitoring should never delay therapy for suspected SE.

Termination of seizure activity is the focus of SE treatment, and benzodiazepines, generally lorazepam or diazepam, are the first-line agents (Table 5.1 details drug dosing). Lorazepam is preferable to diazepam because of a longer duration of action and, consequently, a lower seizure-relapse rate. Benzodiazepine therapy is often followed by treatment with a longer-acting antiepileptic drug (AED), tradi-tionally phenytoin IV. Phenytoin IV should be infused at a rate no faster than 50 mg/min because of the risk of hypotension and cardiac dysrhythmias. ECG and frequent blood pressure monitoring are essential. If hypotension or bradycardia develops, the rate of administration can be decreased or the infusion can be held until the vital signs stabilize. Phenytoin IV should never be delivered by an automatic infusion pump to an unattended patient. Phosphenytoin, a prodrug that is

TABLE 5.1

Management of Status Epilepticus (continued)

Objectives	Time Frame	Intervention
Treatment of refractory SE/ICU setting	>60 minute	1. If seizures persist, consider transfer to an intensive care unit. Perform elective endotracheal intubation 2. Treat with general anesthesia: **Midazolam, 0.2 mg/kg boluses, maximum 2 mg/kg then, infusion rate 0.05–2 mg/kg/hr, or in adults:** **Propofol, 1–2 mg/kg boluses, maximum 10 mg/kg, then infusion rate 2–10 mg/kg/hr, or** **Pentobarbital, 10–15 mg/kg, then infusion rate 0.5–1 mg/kg/hr, or** **Thiopental, 3–5 mg/kg bolus, then infusion rate, 3–5 mg/kg/hr** 3. Titrate anesthetic to burst-suppression pattern on EEG for 24 to 48 hours, then gradually taper infusion rate while monitoring for seizure activity 4. If clinical or electrographic seizure activity is observed, repeat the anesthetic induction
Prevention and treatment of complications of SE	Throughout	1. Monitor vital signs 2. Monitor volume status 3. Maintain airway and prevent aspiration 4. Review laboratory information and treat accordingly
Identification of cause of SE	Throughout	1. Obtain history from relatives and friends 2. Obtain head CT, when indicated 3. Perform lumbar puncture, when indicated 4. Initiate IV antibiotic or antiviral coverage when meningitis or encephalitis is suspected
Prevention of recurrence of SE	Following cessation of seizure activity	1. Monitor anticonvulsant levels 2. Initiate daily therapy with appropriate anticonvulsant(s) 3. Educate patient and family to ensure medication compliance

CBC, complete blood count; BUN, blood urea nitrogen; LFTs, liver function tests; SE, status epilepticus; ICU, intensive care unit; PE, phosphenytoin sodium equivalents.
[a]At earliest availability.
[b]Third-line therapy (after anesthetics) in some protocols.

converted to phenytoin, has gained favor over parenteral phenytoin where available. Dosage is expressed in phosphenytoin sodium equivalents (PE) for ease of transition from more familiar phenytoin dosing. By virtue of its solubility, phosphenytoin does not require the addition of propylene glycol as a vehicle, which is thought to cause most of the clinically significant hypotension, arrhythmias, and local injection reactions of phenytoin administration. Absence of these side effects allows for a faster rate of infusion of phosphenytoin, up to 150 mg PE/min, with peak concentrations within 10 minutes after infusion. Phosphenytoin offers the additional advantage of intramuscular injection in those patients without IV access; therapeutic plasma concentrations are reached within 30 minutes by this route. Phosphenytoin is considerably more expensive than phenytoin, but, in fact, may be more cost-effective as a result of a reduced need for adverse event management.

If seizures persist, phenobarbital IV traditionally has been used as a second-line agent, after benzodiazepines and phenytoin have failed. However, phenobarbital may result in respiratory depression, prolonged sedation, or severe hypotension. This adverse side effect profile has relegated the barbiturate to the status of a third-line agent in some SE treatment algorithms. If phenobarbital IV is used, elective endotracheal intubation is recommended before initiation of the infusion. Valproate IV has become available for use in treating SE, with loading doses of 15 to 20 mg/kg infused at a rate of 3 to 6 mg/kg/min. Its safety profile suggests usefulness as a second-line agent, particularly in patients who are hemodynamically unstable. However, clinical experience with valproate in this capacity remains limited, and it is absent from many standard SE treatment protocols.

Approximately 30% of patients with SE will have ongoing seizures resistant to standard loading doses of anticonvulsant medications, thus requiring therapy for "refractory SE." Anesthetic doses of benzodiazepines, short-acting barbiturates, or propofol are the third-line agents used to treat refractory SE, although some investigators have proposed resorting to these drugs as second-line agents in place of phenobarbital IV. Midazolam is a well-tolerated, short-acting benzodiazepine that causes fewer problems with hypotension. An alternative to more costly midazolam is propofol, a nonbarbiturate, anesthetic agent. A disadvantage of this therapy is the potential for developing "propofol-infusion syndrome," characterized by hypotension, lipidemia, metabolic acidosis, renal failure, and cardiovascular collapse. Finally, pentobarbital and thiopental sodium are short-acting barbiturates that may be used in treating refractory SE. Prolonged elimination and the potential immunosuppressive propensity of these agents are potential disadvantages.

EEG monitoring is important in the management of refractory SE. Although the necessary depth and duration of anesthesia for treatment of refractory SE has not been standardized, anesthetics typically are titrated to produce a burst-suppression pattern on the EEG for 24 to 48 hours. After this time, the infusion rate is decreased gradually. If electrographic or clinical seizures emerge, induction is repeated at progressively longer intervals.

The prevention and management of complications of SE is ongoing throughout the treatment protocol. Hypertension, hyperthermia, and acidosis require attention, but effective treatment of SE should reverse these problems. Hypotension can be a direct consequence of prolonged SE or, alternatively, the effect of anticonvulsant medication, volume depletion, trauma, or cardiovascular disease. The potential risks of rhabdomyolysis, aspiration pneumonia, or traumatic injury as a result of seizure activity also must be recognized and prevented if possible.

The management of SE cannot be separated from the exigency of identifying the underlying cause. Obtaining historical information from the patient's family, friends, or medical records may reveal a pattern of noncompliance with medication or a recurrent history of alcohol withdrawal. Reports of acute neurologic deficits or febrile illness may further help guide appropriate diagnostic evaluation. A head computed tomography (CT) should be considered, with and without contrast (if renal function and allergies permit), to exclude the possibilities of neoplasm, cerebrovascular infarction, intracerebral hemorrhage, and traumatic injury. Following CT, lumbar puncture may be indicated. It should be noted that the CSF can reveal a moderate pleocytosis (up to 150 white blood cells) and an increase in CSF protein (up to 100 mg/dl) following persistent seizure activity. Nonetheless, if there is any suspicion of meningitis, antibiotic therapy should be started promptly and appropriate cultures should be sent for evaluation.

Upon successful treatment of SE, careful attention to initiating a daily dosing schedule of one or more anticonvulsants and monitoring the total and free serum drug levels will help prevent recurrence of seizure activity. In the coming years, the development of novel routes of administration for established drugs as well as new anticonvulsant and neuroprotective agents holds promise for further reducing the morbidity and mortality of SE.

ACUTE ALTERATION OF MENTAL STATUS

An acute alteration of mental status is the most common neurobehavioral disorder seen in hospitalized patients. It is characterized by a sudden change in cognition with impaired attention that may fluctuate; it is potentially reversible; and it is not a result of preexisting dementia.

A well-known form of acute alteration of mental status is **delirium**. The *Diagnostic and Statistical Manual of Mental Disorders*, 4th edition (DSM IV), delineates the following clinical criteria for the diagnosis of delirium: inattention, change in cognition, acute and fluctuating course, and evidence of a medical cause. Subtypes of delirium have been described and categorized by overall psychomotor activity and arousal level. These subtypes include hyperactive, hypoactive, and mixed delirium. Hyperactive delirium is dominated by hyperarousal, hallucinations, and agitation, whereas hypoactive delirium is characterized by lethargy, confusion, and sedation. Although specific etiologies do not consistently coincide with certain subtypes, there do appear to be some trends associating causes with clinical subtypes. For instance, patients with alcohol and benzodiazepine withdrawal typically appear more hyperaroused, whereas those with a metabolic disorder tend toward hypoactivity. Categorizing patients into general subtypes may be helpful prognostically. Investigators found that patients with hypoactive delirium had longer hospitalizations with increased risk of developing pressure ulcers, whereas their hyperactive counterparts incurred an increased risk of falls.

An unexplained acute alteration of mental status due to a medical condition (delirium) must be differentiated from a psychiatric disorder, and even in patients with known psychiatric illness, several evaluations of possible causes of delirium are important to perform. The differential diagnosis of delirium is extensive and can be divided into several broad etiologic categories: infections, structural lesions, toxic-metabolic causes (drug-related, hypoxia, hypoglycemia, hepatic and renal disease, electrolyte abnormalities, thiamine deficiency, etc.), and postictal states. The term "encephalopathy" is frequently substituted for delirium to describe diffusely abnormal brain function from a medical cause (i.e., toxic-metabolic encephalopathy). A psychiatric disorder should only be considered after underlying, potentially life-threatening, medical causes are properly excluded. Several of the more important causes of altered mental status that require special attention are discussed below.

Herpes simplex encephalitis (HSE) is one of the most common, potentially fatal infections of the brain associated with an acute altered mental state. HSE is usually associated with herpes simplex virus (HSV)-1 in adults and children from either primary infection or virus reactivation. The virus causes inflammation of the brain parenchyma, necrosis, and hemorrhage, particularly in the temporal and orbitofrontal lobes. Patients are often ill-appearing with fever, headache, meningitis, focal neurologic deficits such as hemiparesis and aphasia, confusion, and seizures (both partial and secondarily generalized). The clinical course of a patient with HSE may decline precipitously to obtundation, coma, and death if left untreated. For this reason, treatment with IV acyclovir (10 mg/kg every 8 hours for at least 14 days) should be initiated promptly in anyone suspected of having HSE. The risk of acyclovir is low but does include bone marrow suppression, liver and renal toxicities.

■ **SPECIAL CLINICAL POINT: In patients suspected of having herpes simplex encephalitis (HSE), empiric treatment with acyclovir, even prior to completion of diagnostic testing, is warranted due to the high risk of morbidity and mortality from delayed treatment.**

Diagnostic testing for HSE should include a brain magnetic resonance imaging (MRI) (or HCT if not available) and CSF sampling (including HSV PCR analysis). MRI may show edema particularly in the temporal and frontal regions, often with associated hemorrhage. Opening pressure of the lumbar puncture may be elevated, and the CSF may mimic an aseptic meningitis with a mildly decreased glucose, mildly elevated protein, pleocytosis (with lymphocytes and some neutrophils) as well as many red blood cells (RBCs) and xanthrochromia due to hemorrhagic necrosis of the brain parenchyma. A traumatic lumbar puncture may falsely elevate RBCs in the CSF; therefore, cell counts should be sent on the first and last tubes collected to aid interpretation. The sensitivity and specificity of PCR of CSF for HSV is high. It is, therefore, appropriate to consider discontinuation of acyclovir initiated empirically in patients who are later found to have a negative PCR result.

An EEG is frequently indicated in patients with HSE exhibiting overt seizures or an alteration in their mental status without return to their baseline. Seizures are particularly common with temporal lobe lesions, such as seen with HSE. The EEG may show areas of focal slowing or focal epileptiform discharges with temporal predominance, often superimposed upon an abnormal diffusely slowed background. Classically, the focal sharp wave abnormalities in HSE are periodic, lateralized, epileptiform discharges (**PLEDs**), though this is not specific for HSE. Patients who recover from HSE are at somewhat higher risk for later developing epilepsy. AED therapy is appropriate in the management of HSE for the treatment of seizures and in those at high risk for seizures based on the EEG.

Intracranial hematoma should be considered in any patient with a recent history of head trauma and an acute change in mental status, particularly with headache or focal neurologic deficits. A patient with a spontaneous intracerebral or subarachnoid hemorrhage may have a similar acute presentation requiring emergency intervention. These neurologic emergencies, however, are more aptly discussed in the context of cerebrovascular disease (see Chapter 7).

Chronic subdural hematomas, especially in older patients, may result from blunt head trauma and develop slowly over weeks to months, presenting clinically with cognitive decline that can be easily mistaken for dementia. Like the elderly, patients with coagulopathies and alcoholism have a higher risk for subdural hematomas. **Acute epidural** and **subdural hematomas** may develop within just *minutes to hours* after head trauma. Younger patients and those with skull fractures are at greater risk for epidural hematomas, most commonly from tearing arterial vessels. Headache, vomiting, seizures, and focal deficits may progress rapidly to bradycardia, apnea, and coma in a patient with an expanding epidural hematoma coinciding with increasing intracranial pressure and cerebral herniation.

■ **SPECIAL CLINICAL POINT:** A falsely reassuring "lucid interval" may be seen following head injury in a patient with an epidural hematoma who has a transient recovery of mental status after initial impact, only to have rapid neurologic decline minutes to hours later with hematoma expansion.

Patients, thus, presenting after head injury with headache or altered mental status should have an unenhanced head CT as soon as possible and be kept under close surveillance with frequent neurologic evaluations. If necessary, emergency transfer to a trauma center for decompression should be arranged.

Cerebellar stroke, either infarction or hemorrhage, is an acute structural lesion not to be overlooked due to the potentially devastating neurologic outcome. Patients may present with any combination of headache, nausea, vomiting, vertigo, clumsiness, ataxia, and dysarthria, or may present early on in coma. The difficulty in managing acute cerebellar stroke lies in predicting who will deteriorate, deciding which treatment options are needed, and electing when to proceed with surgery. There is as yet no definitive protocol for the management of patients with acute cerebellar stroke. Clinicians generally must rely upon both the overall clinical picture as well as neuroimaging features to guide their decision-making. A deteriorating level of consciousness, gaze palsy, or signs of herniation along with findings on HCT (i.e., effacement of the fourth ventricle, presence of hydrocephalus, size of cerebellar hemorrhage, and evidence of brainstem infarction) may help determine the primary mechanism(s) of clinical decline and, thus, the best therapeutic approach.

■ **SPECIAL CLINICAL POINT: An observation period of 72 to 96 hours in a neurologic intensive care unit is generally recommended for patients with acute cerebellar stroke to enable early detection of a deterioration in neurologic status and, if necessary, emergency surgical intervention.**

Several mechanisms may account for the neurologic deterioration seen in cerebellar stroke. These include obstructive hydrocephalus from fourth ventricle compression, direct brainstem compression from mass effect, upward herniation of the cerebellar vermis through the tentorial notch, and irreversible brainstem infarction. In cases of acute hydrocephalus without brainstem compression (clinically or on imaging), ventriculostomy alone may be adequate. However, if there is no clinical improvement, a posterior fossa decompressive craniectomy may be required as a staged approach following ventriculostomy. In cases of direct brainstem compression or when there is a rapid neurologic decline, a suboccipital craniectomy with hematoma evacuation or resection of infarcted tissue is indicated. Additionally, cerebellar hemorrhages more than 3 cm in diameter usually require surgical evacuation.

Metabolic encephalopathies are common acquired causes of acute alteration in mental status, a diverse group of neurologic disorders defined by an alteration of mental status resulting from failure of organs other than the brain. Cerebral dysfunction may result from three basic mechanisms: deficiency of a necessary metabolic substrate (e.g., hypoglycemia), disruption of the internal environment of the brain (e.g., dehydration), or the presence of a toxin or accumulation of a metabolic waste product (e.g., drug intoxication or uremia). Hepatic and uremic encephalopathies are common metabolic causes of mental status change in hospitalized patients. Disorders of glucose regulation; osmolarity/sodium homeostasis; and derangement of calcium, magnesium, and phosphorous levels are also frequent offenders. Endocrine encephalopathies seen in Cushing syndrome, Addison disease, and thyroid disease are less common and may be overlooked.

A patient with a metabolic encephalopathy may evolve through stages of inattentiveness, disturbed memory, and confusion to lethargy, somnolence, obtundation, and coma. The earlier stages of encephalopathy may go unrecognized because of a patient's concurrent loss of insight and judgment. Of note, an alteration of personality, behavior, cognitive function, or level of alertness may be the only symptom that brings a patient with a metabolic derangement to medical attention.

Drug intoxication and withdrawal are particularly common causes of acute alteration in mental status. At-risk patients typically are taking drugs that have anticholinergic properties, including many antidepressants, neuroleptics, antihistamines, antiparkinsonian agents, and over-the-counter cold preparations. High-dose steroids, narcotic pain medications, and sedatives also may cause acute alterations in mental status, especially in elderly patients. Abused street drugs associated with violent delirium include amphetamines, cocaine, hallucinogens, tranquilizers, sedatives, and alcohol.

Alcoholic patients commonly present to the emergency department with mental status alteration, which should be distinguished clinically from intoxication. A blood ethanol level of 80 to 100 mg/dl correlates with a change in mental status. Sharp declines in blood ethanol levels 12 to 24 hours after intake can result in tremulousness followed by alcohol withdrawal seizures. These seizures are usually brief with return to normal neurologic function. Prolonged or focal seizures, a prolonged postictal state, or a focally abnormal neurologic examination should initiate a search for other causes of seizures. Alcoholic patients are particularly prone to head injury, and brain imaging may reveal epidural or subdural hematomas, intraparenchymal hemorrhage, or traumatic subarachnoid hemorrhage. CNS infection also should be considered, potentially warranting a diagnostic lumbar puncture. Coexistent hepatic failure, hypoglycemia, hyponatremia, or drug ingestion should be screened with appropriate testing. Likewise, nonconvulsive SE should prompt EEG monitoring when suspected.

The clinician should be particularly alert to the possibility of **Wernicke encephalopathy**, a manifestation of thiamine deficiency. It is clinically characterized by an apathetic-confusional state, oculomotor dysfunction (at times evidenced by a subtle nystagmus), and ataxia. Thiamine should be administered routinely, before glucose, at 100 mg/day IV to prevent precipitation and progression of Wernicke encephalopathy to irreversible amnesia. B vitamins also should be supplemented because many patients have concurrent nutritional compromise. Benzodiazepines are the mainstay of management of both alcoholic withdrawal and alcoholic seizures. Although chlordiazepoxide, diazepam, and lorazepam commonly are used, oxazepam may be preferable in patients with liver insufficiency because its clearance is less dependent on hepatic metabolism than other benzodiazepines. Patients should be evaluated for dehydration, hypomagnesemia, and other electrolyte disturbances. Hyponatremia should be corrected slowly, at a rate no faster than 0.5 to 1.0 meq/L/hr, with not more than 12 meq/L correction in 24 hours because rapid correction may lead to the development of central pontine myelinolysis.

■ **SPECIAL CLINICAL POINT: A triad of acute confusion, ophthalmoplegia (eye paralysis) or nystagmus, and gait ataxia,** **especially in the setting of chronic alcohol use, requires immediate treatment with thiamine (IV or IM) for Wernicke encephalopathy to prevent permanent brain injury and coma.**

The general approach to the patient with an acute alteration in mental status involves identification and treatment of the underlying cause, environmental modification, and symptomatic treatment. Historical information should be sought about systemic illness, drug or alcohol use, recent trauma, toxin exposure, baseline mental status, and the temporal course of symptoms. A history of dementia, mental retardation, or pre-existing brain injury may predispose a patient to acute mental status alteration, particularly in the face of undue physical or psychological stress. Unfamiliar surroundings with loss of daily routine, disruption of sleep–wake cycles, and sensory understimulation or overstimulation are common precipitants for these patients. Both the very old and the very young are at special risk, especially older patients with hip fractures (up to 65% incidence) because these patients tend to be more frail; advanced in age; taking multiple medications; and sensitive to electrolyte or metabolic disturbances, infection, and hypotension.

A thorough physical examination includes inspection for stigmata of hepatic, renal, or endocrine disorders. Scrutiny of the state of hydration and nutrition provides important information. Alterations in vital signs may provide clues to a wide diversity of problems, ranging from hypoxia to sepsis to elevated intracranial pressure. Signs of head trauma should be sought in the obtunded or comatose patient.

Examination of mental status should be performed in a reproducible manner to guide subsequent reevaluations of progression and efficacy of therapy. A patient's level of consciousness is best described with a few well-recognized descriptors, such as alert, lethargic (easily aroused), stuporous (difficult to arouse), and comatose (little response to external stimulation). Documentation of patient performance on standardized tests of arousability, orientation, attention, and memory are more reproducible and allow for quantitative comparison. The Folstein Mini-Mental Status Examination or the alternative Montreal Cognitive Assessment (MoCA), and the Glasgow Coma Scale are convenient quantitative scales for this purpose.

The neurologic examination includes tests of pupillary response and ocular motility as well as motor responses to stimulation. Oculocephalic reflexes, oculovestibular reflexes, and respiratory patterns should be noted in comatose patients. Demonstration of intact brainstem function makes a structural lesion of the brainstem, including elevation of intracranial pressure, less likely. Hyperreflexia may be seen in association with metabolic encephalopathy, but other evidence of upper motor neuron dysfunction is usually not demonstrated until advanced stages of disease. Asterixis, generalized tremor, and spontaneous myoclonus often are observed. Toxic encephalopathies should be considered in patients with dysarthria, nystagmus, ataxia, tremor, or dilated pupils.

Diagnostic testing can screen for metabolic abnormalities and toxin exposure. Laboratory tests should include a blood count, platelet count, prothrombin time, partial thromboplastin time, chemistry profile (electrolytes, glucose, blood urea nitrogen, creatinine, calcium, magnesium, phosphorous), liver function tests, ammonia level, thyroid function tests, arterial blood gas, urinalysis, and drug and toxicology screen. Drug levels of prescription medications that may alter mental status should be checked (e.g., anticonvulsants, lithium, theophylline, barbiturates, digoxin). Information gathered during the history and physical examination will guide the choice of additional studies: serum osmolality, plasma cortisol level, syphilis serology, erythrocyte sedimentation rate, antinuclear antibody, vitamin B_{12}, folate, human immunodeficiency virus, ceruloplasmin, serum copper, urinary copper, and urinary porphobilinogen.

Neuroimaging is recommended following an acute change in mental status to exclude a structural lesion resulting in increased intracranial pressure or focal abnormalities. Patients with fluent aphasias from dominant temporoparietal lesions or with nondominant parietal injury can be misdiagnosed as psychotic in the absence of appropriate brain imaging. CSF abnormalities are rare in metabolic encephalopathies. Nevertheless, there should be a low threshold for performing a lumbar puncture to rule out meningitis or encephalitis when previous evaluations have failed to reveal a cause or when there is clinical suspicion of a CNS infection. Brain imaging is recommended prior to lumbar puncture to evaluate for increased intracranial pressure as a result of the risk of provoking herniation.

An EEG can be helpful in patients with metabolic encephalopathy or altered mental status of uncertain etiology. It can provide an objective evaluation of the degree of CNS dysfunction. Loss of the normal EEG patterns and generalized slowing are the most commonly observed changes. Seizure activity, particularly nonconvulsive SE, as well as focal abnormalities may be identified. Often, serial EEG studies are valuable to quantitatively and objectively gauge the degree of cerebral dysfunction. Prognostically, background reactivity on EEG may suggest, in some instances, a potentially reversible encephalopathic process.

Treatment of Delirium

The management of acute alteration in mental status requires medical or surgical treatment targeted at the identified etiologic process. Even with appropriate therapy, mental status alterations, when reversible, can take weeks to months to improve. Controlling a patient's environment can facilitate reorientation. Environmental modifications include instituting regular wake and sleep schedules, diurnal exposure to natural and artificial light, use of clocks and calendars, and frequent reorientation by staff and visitors.

Patients with disorientation, emotional lability, delusions, hallucinations, paranoid ideation, or intoxication may be agitated, aggressive, violent, and resistant to medical evaluation and treatment. Although it is best to avoid the use of drugs that may result in sedation and CNS depression in these patients, symptomatic therapy for delirium is warranted in instances where behavior poses a significant risk to patient or staff safety.

Pharmacologic intervention should be individualized and directed at the specific problem (anxiety, depression, insomnia, disturbance of sleep–wake cycles, agitation, hallucinations, delusions, and aggression). The most commonly used agents are benzodiazepines and neuroleptics. Neuroleptics should be avoided in long-term management of behavior because of the risk of developing irreversible tardive dyskinesia. Moreover, clinicians should be watchful for the symptoms of neuroleptic malignant syndrome, a rare but potentially fatal idiosyncratic drug reaction (see section on Neuroleptic Malignant Syndrome, p. 83). For the patient with acute agitation with psychotic features, haloperidol may be administered in a dosage of 5 mg intramuscularly (IM) every 4 to 8 hours to a maximum of 15 to 30 mg/day. Neuroleptic-induced extrapyramidal symptoms are a significant risk in all patients, particularly the elderly. The atypical neuroleptics, including quetiapine and olanzapine, are less likely to precipitate parkinsonism, acute dystonic reaction, or tardive syndromes (quetiapine 25 to 300 mg/day, olanzapine 2.5 to 10 mg/day). When the predominant feature is anxiety, benzodiazepines (e.g., diazepam, 5 to 10 mg IM) are often sufficient. Rarely, patients may develop paradoxical agitation with benzodiazepines, requiring withdrawal of medication.

Neuroleptics should be used cautiously in patients with mental status alteration, particularly when the underlying etiology is unclear because these drugs can mask evidence of clinical deterioration. Sedation should be, likewise, avoided especially when a patient's level of consciousness is worsening. Intoxication and drug overdose, structural lesions with elevated intracranial pressure, and infections should be excluded. In some situations, the patient's behavior may be a critical index of disease progression, and the use of physical restraints is preferable to sedation.

Although the diagnosis and treatment of delirium may be challenging and difficult in patients with multiple system failure or irreversible brain injury, a significant proportion of these patients are found to have reversible processes. These encounters, when approached with proficiency, can be especially rewarding.

ACUTE INTRACRANIAL HYPERTENSION

The main components of volume in the skull are the brain (1,400 mL), blood (1,400 mL), and CSF (150 mL). Any increase in the volume of one of these components without a corresponding decrease in the volume of the other two will result in **increased intracranial pressure (ICP)**, or intracranial hypertension. Because volume in the cranium cannot change, any volume increase will result initially in a compensatory reduction in intracranial blood volume and displacement of CSF into the lumbar cistern. Once brain compliance is exhausted, small increases in ICP will result in **herniation** of the brain through the foramen magnum. The prompt recognition and treatment of acutely raised intracranial pressure is, thus, vital to preserve brainstem function and life.

Intracranial hypertension poses a risk of cerebral hypoperfusion as well as herniation. Cerebral blood flow (CBF) normally is maintained over a wide range of cerebral perfusion pressures (CPPs). CPP is defined as the difference between mean arterial blood pressure (MAP) (normally 50 to 150 mm Hg) and ICP (normally 3 to 15 mm Hg). A CPP greater than or equal to 70 mm Hg ensures adequate cerebral perfusion. In disease states, the CPP will approximate the CBF in a linear fashion as a result of loss of vascular autoregulation; therefore, any elevation of ICP or decrease in MAP will result in cerebral hypoperfusion.

Understanding the neuroanatomic shifts that evolve with progressive increases in ICP enables better clinical recognition of pending herniation. The cranial vault is divided incompletely into compartments by thick, fibrous bands of dura mater. The tentorium cerebelli is clinically the most important of these structures. It separates the lower brainstem and cerebellum from the cerebral hemispheres and diencephalon, delineating the infratentorial and supratentorial spaces. The midbrain lies within an opening in the tentorium called the tentorial notch and is bound laterally by fascicles of the oculomotor nerve and the medial portion of the temporal lobes (the uncus). Under conditions of increased intracranial pressure, the downward displacement and herniation of the midbrain and uncus can result in compression of the brainstem, compromising vital functions including respiration, maintenance of consciousness, and cardioregulation. Coma and death may ensue.

The two main types of herniation syndromes are uncal and central. Central herniation occurs when diffusely raised supratentorial pressure compresses central brainstem structures and produces a progressive impairment of consciousness, respiratory irregularities, abnormal motor responses (posturing), and symmetric midposition unreactive pupils. Uncal herniation, however, occurs as a unilateral supratentorial mass lesion displaces the medial temporal lobe toward the tentorial notch. Some of the mass lesions that can lead to herniation are listed in (Table 5.2). Early on, the oculomotor (third cranial) nerve becomes compressed between the encroaching uncus and the edge of the tentorial opening, producing a larger and

less reactive pupil on that side. Hemiparesis may occur ipsilateral to the herniating uncus because of the compression of the contralateral cerebral peduncle against the far edge of the tentorial notch as the midbrain is displaced laterally (**Kernohan notch syndrome**). More commonly, however, the hemiparesis is contralateral to the herniating uncus. In either case, hemiparesis is not a good clinical sign for localizing the side of the herniation. The abducens nerve (sixth cranial nerve), by virtue of its extensive intracranial course, is particularly susceptible to traction injury when the intracranial pressure is elevated. Therefore, sixth nerve palsies with inward eye deviation are frequently seen but have little localizing value. A **dilated pupil (third nerve palsy)** is ipsilateral to the herniation 95% of the time and is a more reliable clinical indicator.

Unlike the situation that occurs with mass lesions, raised ICP can be distributed equally among the intracranial compartments with little risk of herniation and brainstem compression. Some of the more common causes of diffuse intracranial hypertension are listed in (Table 5.3).

Symptoms and signs of intracranial hypertension are variable and depend on both the etiology and the rapidity with which the pressure increase develops. Intracranial pressure may increase gradually over an extended

TABLE 5.2	Mass Lesions Associated with Brain Herniation

Neoplasm
Subdural hematoma
Epidural hematoma
Intraparenchymal hemorrhage
Abscess
Infarction

TABLE 5.3	Causes of Diffuse Intracranial Hypertension with Less Risk of Herniation

Hypoxia
Meningitis
Encephalitis
Head trauma without subdural or epidural hematoma
Subarachnoid hemorrhage
Malignant hyperthermia
Cerebral-vein thrombosis
Pseudotumor cerebri
Lead encephalopathy

period or suddenly in a matter of minutes. Headache is more likely to be a prominent symptom in more acute problems, whereas papilledema may be present in subacute or chronic conditions. Patients with large acute hemispheric infarctions may develop signs of herniation between 2 and 5 days of stroke onset, when brain edema typically peaks.

Treatment of Acute Intracranial Hypertension

The primary goal in the management of raised ICP is to reduce ICP while maintaining an adequate CPP (70 mm Hg). Therefore, judicious manipulations of systemic MAP are warranted, as well as reliable measurements of ICP. Although estimations of ICP can be deduced from clinical signs, this is unreliable. The gold standard for ICP monitoring is by direct ventricular pressure measurement through a ventriculostomy. This method is precise and allows for therapeutic CSF drainage to reduce ICP. There are risks, however; parenchymal damage may result from direct penetration during placement of the ventriculostomy, and there is a high incidence of infectious ventriculitis with prolonged insertion of ventricular catheters (particularly after 5 days). Other methods are safer, with fewer infectious complications, but also less precise. They include subarachnoid bolts, epidural transducers, and intraparenchymal fiberoptic transducers. Noninvasive methods with transcranial Doppler are promising but not yet reliable.

The evaluation of patients with suspected intracranial hypertension should begin with a brief history from available informants and a brief physical examination. Patients who are unresponsive and in danger of herniation should be intubated immediately, and emergency treatment should be initiated before diagnostic investigation. Mechanical hyperventilation is the fastest way of reducing intracranial pressure. It is desirable to keep the $PaCO_2$ between 25 and 30 mm Hg. The decreased $PaCO_2$ causes cerebral vasoconstriction, thereby reducing cerebral blood volume and intracranial pressure. Excessive hypocarbia may cause deleterious vasoconstriction. It is also important not to compress the jugular veins with the tape used to secure the endotracheal tube.

Osmotic agents such as mannitol are given to reduce the water content of the brain. The starting dose is 500 mL of 20% mannitol given IV for 20 to 30 minutes (approximately 1 mg/kg). A urinary catheter is recommended. Serum electrolytes and osmolality are monitored closely, using the latter as a guide to further dosing. A mannitol dose of 100 to 250 mg (0.25 mg/kg) can be given every 4 hours as necessary to maintain serum osmolality at 300 to 320 milliosmoles (mOsm) per liter.

Corticosteroids may be administered if vasogenic edema is present. **Vasogenic edema** occurs in conditions with breakdown of the blood–brain barrier and often is seen with brain neoplasms. Steroids are generally not effective for the type of edema that accompanies cerebral infarction (**cytotoxic edema**) and thus are not indicated in large hemispheric strokes. Steroids do not begin working for several hours, so they usually are given concurrently with hyperventilation and hyperosmolar agents in acute situations. Methylprednisolone (Solu-Medrol) 250 mg or dexamethasone (Decadron) 10 mg IV can be used immediately, followed by dexamethasone 4 mg IV every 6 hours.

In situations with rapidly progressing intracranial hypertension, emergency neurosurgery may be necessary. Sizable cerebellar hemorrhages or rapidly expanding epidural or subdural hematomas often require lifesaving evacuation and surgical decompression. Ventricular drainage of CSF can also rapidly decrease ICP and may be performed at the bedside. Decompressive craniotomy for cerebral edema in acute ischemic infarction has shown promise for markedly reducing mortality and morbidity from an otherwise devastating condition. Randomized controlled clinical trials of this treatment are under way to provide more definitive evidence of efficacy. Moderate hypothermia (33 to 36°C) also has been shown to reduce ICP and improve mortality in patients following massive middle cerebral artery infarction. However, increased ICP may rebound with rewarming. Pentobarbital-induced coma may be helpful in the management of refractory intracranial hypertension; but potential adverse effects, including hypotension, reduced cardiac performance, and severe infection, limit its use.

There are a number of other general therapeutic measures that should be undertaken. IV or enteral fluids should be isotonic or hypertonic. Hypotonic solutions such as 5% dextrose or half-normal (0.45) saline can aggravate cerebral edema. Serum osmolarity of less than 280 mOsm/L should be corrected, and mild hyperosmolarity greater than 300 mOsm/L is desired. The composition of fluids replenished is a greater determinant of cerebral edema than the amount of fluids. Blood pressure should be modified to maintain a CPP of 70 to 120 mm Hg. When CPP is greater than 120 and ICP is greater than 20, short-acting antihypertensive medications such as labetalol should be used. Nitroprusside may worsen cerebral edema by dilating the cerebral vasculature. In patients with increased ICP and low CPP, an adequate MAP should be maintained to avoid hypoxic-ischemic injury. Vasopressors sometimes are used in this situation. Sedation may be needed in ventilated patients who become agitated. In these patients, raised intrathoracic pressure may elevate ICP by increasing venous resistance to CSF outflow. Short-acting sedatives are preferred; propofol is gaining popularity in this setting because of its very short half-life, which allows rapid discontinuation, and thus reliable, serial neurologic examinations.

Only after the patient's clinical status has been stabilized should further evaluation with a head CT scan proceed. Because of the risk of precipitating herniation, a lumbar puncture generally should be avoided in a patient suspected of having increased ICP until a mass lesion is excluded by neuroimaging.

ACUTE SPINAL CORD COMPRESSION

Acute compression of the spinal cord often presents insidiously with pain, mild sensory disturbance, weakness, or sphincter or sexual dysfunction, but it may progress rapidly to irreversible paralysis if not corrected. Spinal cord compression is a common complication of metastatic disease, affecting 5% to 10% of patients with cancer, but it also occurs with other conditions (Table 5.4). The most frequent metastatic tumors causing spinal cord compression include multiple myeloma; lymphoma; and carcinomas of the prostate, lung, breast, kidney, and colon.

Pain is the earliest symptom in the vast majority of patients and may be localized to the involved spinal area (96%) or may radiate in a dermatomal pattern (90%) if the dorsal spinal roots are also involved. Pain may be intensified by actions that increase intrathoracic pressure and consequently CSF pressure, such as coughing, sneezing, or straining at stool. Percussion tenderness over the spine is often a valuable clinical sign aiding localization. Thoracic cord compression is the most frequent site of involvement (70%) because it is the narrowest area of the spinal canal. It is followed in frequency by the lumbosacral (20%) and cervical (10%) areas. Up to one fifth of patients have multiple sites of cord compression.

The development of weakness, sensory loss, or erectile or sphincter dysfunction may progress quickly. The distribution of weakness can aid in localizing the level of the lesion. Typically, lesions in the cervical spine region result in paralysis of the legs and varying degrees of

TABLE 5.4	Common Causes of Acute Spinal Cord Compression

Metastatic cancer
Herniated disc
Abscess
Hematoma

weakness in the upper extremities. Less commonly, patients may exhibit weakness that is disproportionately more impaired in the upper extremities than in the lower extremities with bladder dysfunction and varying degrees of sensory loss characteristic of an acute central cervical spinal cord injury. This lesion often results from traumatic hyperextension of the neck causing anterior and posterior cord compression within the spinal canal and subsequent injury to the central substance of the cervical spinal cord.

A rapid diagnosis of acute spinal cord compression is essential for appropriate management and optimal prognosis. This begins with a detailed clinical examination, cervical spinal x-rays to assess vertebral column injury in cases of trauma, and timely MRI of the spinal cord directed at the suspected lesion level(s) to evaluate for intrinsic injury or compression. Plain x-rays of the spine are abnormal in 84% to 94% of cases and may show evidence of bony erosion from metastatic disease, particularly loss of vertebral pedicles; however, they are of little help in imaging the soft-tissue structures that are invading the epidural or subdural spaces and compressing the spinal cord. MRI is the procedure of choice for visualizing the extent of anatomic involvement and spinal cord compression. It is superior to myelography in most instances because it is noninvasive and yields better resolution of anatomic structures. Spinal CT and bone scans play an important role in the diagnostic evaluations of these patients as well.

Treatment of Acute Spinal Cord Compression

Treatment should be started at the first sign of myelopathy. A very high dose of corticosteroids, such as dexamethasone 100 mg IV, is given immediately to reduce the edema caused by the compressing lesion, and this often provides dramatic pain relief and return of some neurologic function. In metastatic epidural cord compression, dexamethasone is continued at 24 mg IV every 6 hours for 24 hours, and then it is tapered over the next 48 hours to 6 mg every 6 hours, until more definite treatment is completed. Lower doses may be as effective. Gastric prophylaxis should be provided concurrently. An indwelling bladder catheter should be inserted. Bladder and bowel function should be monitored, with stool softeners and laxatives given as needed. Patients may require management in the ICU in cases with pulmonary, cardiac, or blood pressure instability.

Specific treatment directed at the underlying process can begin once the etiology and location are defined. In metastatic disease, radiation therapy is started immediately and is especially valuable for the more radiosensitive tumors such as multiple myeloma and lymphoma. Surgical decompression is the treatment of choice for disc disease, epidural abscess, and hematoma, and it sometimes is indicated for metastatic disease in situations in which a tissue diagnosis is needed, spinal stabilization is necessary, or further radiotherapy is not warranted. For acute central cervical spinal cord injury, surgical reduction is warranted for fracture-dislocation injuries, but the benefit of early decompressive surgery is still under investigation. The use of moderate systemic hypothermia (between 33.5 and 34.5° C) to treat acute spinal cord injuries has shown some promise but has not been proven in controlled clinical trials.

The prognosis for meaningful functional recovery depends in large part on the functional state of the patient at presentation. Whereas 80% of patients who are able to walk when they come to medical attention remain ambulatory after treatment, only 30% to 40% of nonambulatory persons with antigravity leg function regain ambulation, and only 5% of people without antigravity leg strength are able to walk after therapy.

A high index of suspicion is required to make the diagnosis of a **spinal epidural abscess,** and a history of recent bacteremia or IV drug use often is obtained. The patient may or may not appear septic at the time of presentation. If epidural abscess is a possibility, high-dose IV antibiotics should be given immediately (after sending blood and other appropriate cultures for analysis), while awaiting radiologic procedures and surgical decompression.

■ **SPECIAL CLINICAL POINT:** If a spinal epidural abscess is suspected, a routine "blind" lumbar puncture (without myelography or enhanced spinal MRI) should be deferred due to the risk of precipitating meningitis or downward spinal coning.

PERIPHERAL NERVOUS SYSTEM

Myasthenic Crisis

Myasthenia gravis is an autoimmune disorder directed against the postsynaptic acetylcholine receptor of striated muscle. Neuromuscular transmission is impaired resulting in weakness and fatigability of voluntary muscles. Classically, a diurnal variation in strength is noted, with strength waning as the day progresses. Diplopia or ptosis is the initial symptom in about one half of the cases. Dysphagia, chewing difficulty, nasal speech, and regurgitation of fluids are the presenting features in one third of patients, reflecting the involvement of bulbar musculature. Proximal limb weakness, without bulbar or ocular involvement, is the least common presentation and is easily misdiagnosed. The outpatient diagnosis and management of myasthenia gravis is described in detail in Chapter 17. This chapter focuses, rather, on the emergency management of myasthenic crisis.

Myasthenic crisis occurs when muscle weakness interferes with vital functions such as breathing and swallowing. Emergency intervention is required. The mortality rate remains approximately 5% to 6%, with cardiac complications and aspiration pneumonia being the leading causes of death. A crisis may be precipitated most commonly by infection, but emotional stress, hypokalemia, thyroid disease, or (rarely) certain drugs (Table 5.5) may trigger a crisis; however, in one third of patients, no

TABLE 5.5	**Drugs That May Exacerbate the Weakness of Myasthenia Gravis**

Aminoglycoside antibiotics
Quinine
Cardiac antiarrhythmics (e.g., quinidine, procainamide, propranolol, lidocaine)
Polymyxin
Colistin

precipitant is identified. A crisis may also be caused by overmedication with anticholinesterase agents, the so-called "cholinergic crisis." A cholinergic crisis may be heralded by an increase in muscarinic symptoms such as abdominal colic and diarrhea, with more severe muscarinic signs such as vomiting, lacrimation, hypersalivation, and miosis indicating impending danger. The differentiation of myasthenic from cholinergic crisis may be more academic than practical, however, because the emergency management is the same—protect the airway and maintain adequate ventilation. Following respiratory stabilization, medications may be adjusted and precipitating factors may be investigated further.

Hospitalization, preferably in an intensive care setting, should be considered in any patient with myasthenia who complains of shortness of breath or difficulty swallowing. Frequent monitoring of the vital capacity is important, with endotracheal intubation performed when the vital capacity is <800 to 1,000 mL (<1 L) or < 15 mL/kg, or if dysphagia is so severe that there is a serious risk of aspiration. Maximal inspiratory and expiratory pressures are more sensitive for detecting ventilatory weakness than vital capacity. A reduction of maximal inspiratory pressure to less than 30% of that predicted for age and weight should alert the physician to impending respiratory failure and the need for mechanical ventilation. Arterial blood gases are *not good predictors* for when to begin mechanical ventilation in a myasthenic crisis because they may be normal up to the onset of respiratory failure.

■ **SPECIAL CLINICAL POINT: A forced vital capacity (FVC) below 1 L should raise concern for the need for intubation. A good bedside estimate of FVC can be made by having the patient count out loud to 25 on one breath. Counting to 25 approximates an FVC of about 2 L while counting to 10 approximates an FVC of only about 1 L.**

When endotracheal intubation is required, nondepolarizing muscle relaxants should be avoided in patients with myasthenia who often have marked sensitivity to these agents leading to difficulty weaning from the ventilator. For this reason, some anesthesiologists depend on deep inhalational anesthesia (i.e., halothane, isoflurane, or sevoflurane) for tracheal intubation. An alternative to mechanical ventilation, bilevel positive airway pressure (BiPAP), may be a useful noninvasive option for the management of acute respiratory failure in patients with myasthenia. Preliminary data suggest that BiPAP may prevent intubation in patients with myasthenia who are not hypercapnic ($PaCO_2$ >50 mm Hg). In addition to respiratory monitoring, oral anticholinesterase agents should be discontinued in all patients and withheld for 48 hours even if cholinergic crisis is not suspected. An increased response to these drugs may occur after this "drug holiday," and often less medication may be needed once resumed.

Treatment of Myasthenic Crisis

Treatment begins with a shorter-acting drug, neostigmine, 0.5 mg IM or 15 mg per nasogastric tube every 2 to 3 hours using the vital capacity or muscle strength as a guide to dosage titration. Once the optimal dose of neostigmine is found, the switch to the longer-acting agent pyridostigmine can be made. Approximately four times the neostigmine dose is required every 3 to 4 hours. Corticosteroids also may be helpful in ending myasthenic crisis, but they should be used cautiously in the presence of infection. Moreover, steroids initially may worsen weakness and result in respiratory failure, particularly in the first few days of use. For

this reason, corticosteroids initially should be administered in a hospital setting, particularly if a high-dose regimen is elected. Because steroids usually are required for several weeks or more following a crisis exacerbation, alternate-day steroid therapy is recommended to minimize long-term side effects. Prednisone 100 mg, or its equivalent, is given on alternate days, with a gradual taper beginning after the patient's status is clearly stabilized, usually several weeks after the crisis is over. Some authors favor giving high-dose IV corticosteroids on a daily basis early in the course before switching to alternate-day prednisone therapy.

Intravenous immune globulins (IVIG) or plasmapheresis are useful adjunctive therapies in myasthenic crisis. Plasmapheresis is directed at removing the acetylcholine receptor antibody that causes myasthenia gravis. However, for unclear reasons, even patients seronegative for the acetylcholine receptor antibody may improve with plasmapheresis. The effects of plasmapheresis alone are temporary, rarely persisting more than 4 to 11 weeks, and may not occur for several days. Thus, concomitant immunosuppressive therapy usually is recommended for more lasting treatment effect. Although plasmapheresis is generally safe, potential complications include hemodynamic instability, hypocalcemia, and dilutional coagulopathy.

IVIG is administered at 400 mg/kg daily for 3 to 5 consecutive days. It has complex immune-modulating effects, potentially involving downregulation of antibody production. Plasma exchange and IVIG are both effective treatments, but the ease of administration of the latter makes it the more commonly used modality. Although IVIG is expensive, costs are comparable with plasma exchange. Moreover, IVIG may be a safer alternative in patients with hypotension, sepsis, or autonomic instability. Potential complications of IVIG include hyperviscosity with possible cardiac or cerebral ischemia, mild aseptic meningitis, acute renal failure, or an allergic reaction. It is important to draw serologic titers before IVIG administration because many of these will be altered by the administration of pooled IVIG. In particular, quantitative immune globulins should be drawn because IgA-deficient individuals can become sensitized and develop adverse responses to repeat administration of IVIG. Plasma exchange has been associated with a better outcome compared to IVIG. However, plasma exchange carries a slightly higher complication rate, especially in hemodynamically unstable patients, and the trend of IVIG use has, in fact, increased compared to plasma exchange.

Because any infection may precipitate a crisis, an infectious source should be sought and treated aggressively. Many patients with myasthenia are iatrogenically immunosuppressed and are highly susceptible to infection. If an infection is suspected, empiric therapy with broad-spectrum antibiotics is started at once after cultures have been sent. The change to more specific drugs is made when the cultures' sensitivities are available. The aminoglycosides are known to interfere with neuromuscular transmission but may be used when necessary. Chest roentgenogram and blood, urine, and sputum cultures on all patients with myasthenia presenting with exacerbation should be checked routinely. In addition, a diligent search for infections is required in elderly or steroid-treated patients who may not manifest the usual systemic signs of infection.

GUILLAIN–BARRÉ SYNDROME

Acute inflammatory polyradiculoneuropathy, commonly referred to as the Guillain–Barré syndrome (GBS), is a rapidly progressive, demyelinating polyneuropathy. This disorder is further described in Chapter 18 within the context of peripheral neuropathies. In its most fulminant form, GBS may lead to sudden respiratory failure and autonomic instability. It, therefore, should be considered a neurologic emergency. The mortality rate remains at 3% to 5% despite modern intensive care management.

The classic presentation is a symmetric, ascending, flaccid paralysis that usually begins in the lower extremities (10% begin in the upper extremities) and progresses upward, with the maximum deficit attained by 4 weeks and partial or complete recovery occurring over weeks to months. In contrast to other more slowly progressive polyneuropathies in which a distal weakness predominates, the greatest weakness in GBS is in proximal muscles. Areflexia is the rule and may precede weakness. Many patients complain of distal paresthesias or dysesthesias initially, but formal testing rarely demonstrates a significant sensory loss. Facial weakness is seen in about one half of the cases. A prior history of a recent (within 4 weeks) respiratory or gastrointestinal illness is obtained in about one half of the patients; however, a fever at onset is atypical. A previous inoculation, surgery, hematologic malignancy, and hepatitis B or mycoplasma infection also have been associated with the syndrome. CSF analysis within the first week may be normal—the classic albuminocytologic dissociation (elevated CSF protein and <10 mononuclear cells) usually appears after the second week of illness.

■ **SPECIAL CLINICAL POINT: The hallmark presentation of GBS is ascending symmetric weakness with loss of deep tendon reflexes.**

Nerve conduction studies may be entirely normal early in the course if the proximal root segments are not studied. The F and H responses, measuring the motor and sensory proximal segments, respectively, may be the only abnormality noted early on. Profound slowing of nerve conduction velocity may appear on routine studies after several weeks of illness. Those cases that show evidence of secondary axonal degeneration with denervation on an electromyogram generally will have a more protracted recovery.

GBS should be differentiated from other causes of rapidly progressive flaccid paralysis (Table 5.6). A brief description of these disorders and their general management follows.

Acute intermittent porphyria can cause a rapidly ascending flaccid paralysis with respiratory and autonomic involvement, but it usually is associated with severe abdominal pain, seizures,

TABLE 5.6	Disorders That Can Mimic Guillain–Barré Syndrome

Acute intermittent porphyria
Diphtheria neuropathy
Botulism
Tick-bite paralysis
Poliomyelitis
Arsenic intoxication

and psychosis. Urine porphobilinogen and delta-aminolevulinic acid are elevated. Unlike in GBS, the CSF protein is usually normal. Attacks of acute intermittent porphyria may be precipitated by certain drugs such as barbiturates, phenytoin, sulfonamides, and some benzodiazepines. Acute attacks are managed supportively. A high carbohydrate intake may help further by suppressing porphyrin synthesis.

Diphtheric neuropathy occurs 1 to 2 months after a characteristic pharyngitis. The onset of weakness usually follows pronounced cranial nerve involvement by several weeks, and it may be associated with myocarditis. Unfortunately, by the time neurologic symptoms appear, specific therapy with antitoxin is ineffective. Thus, the mainstays of treatment are respiratory support and good nursing care.

Botulism may present early on, with blurred vision and diplopia as well as gastrointestinal symptoms. Unlike in GBS, pupillary reflexes are lost and the CSF is normal. Sensation remains intact. The diagnosis is supported by nerve conduction studies with reduced amplitude of compound muscle action potentials and an incremental response following rapid repetitive nerve stimulation. Specific treatment with trivalent botulinum antitoxin is recommended. Nasogastric suctioning and enemas may help remove toxin from the gastrointestinal tract early in the illness. Wound botulism is managed with surgical debridement and penicillin. In food-borne botulism, the role of antibiotics is controversial because of the concern that rapid bacterial destruction might increase the release of toxin.

Tick-bite paralysis is caused by a natural endotoxin that interferes with the release of acetylcholine at the neuromuscular junction. It presents as a rapidly ascending paralysis with respiratory and bulbar involvement. A dramatic improvement can occur after removal of the offending tick.

Poliomyelitis can produce a flaccid paralysis with respiratory involvement. However, the weakness of poliomyelitis is characteristically asymmetric, and the disease usually presents as a febrile illness with gastrointestinal symptoms, myalgias, meningismus, and a CSF pleocytosis. Arsenical neuropathy can present as rapidly developing weakness and areflexia, with CSF and nerve conduction studies indistinguishable from those of GBS. However, the neuropathy usually is accompanied by gastrointestinal, hepatic, and hematologic manifestations of arsenic poisoning. The patient with arsenical neuropathy often complains of burning dysesthesia, a feature not common in GBS.

Treatment of Guillain–Barré Syndrome

GBS is a neurologic emergency because of the life-threatening complications of respiratory failure and cardiovascular collapse that sometimes occur within 24 hours of symptom onset. The patient, therefore, should be monitored in an ICU or an intermediate care unit until the plateau phase of maximal deficit is reached. The vital capacity should be checked every 4 to 6 hours (see **Special Clinical Point** in the Myasthenia Gravis section above); if it is less than 60% of the predicted value (generally below 1 L), endotracheal intubation should be considered. Artificial ventilation may be required in up to 23% of patients. Autonomic instability may be severe, with marked fluctuations in blood pressure, tachycardia, and malignant arrhythmias. Cardiac arrhythmias are probably the main cause of death in the acute period, thus warranting continuous cardiac monitoring. Hypotension is usually mild and can be controlled with IV fluids; vasopressor agents rarely are needed. Extreme caution should be used when treating hypertension. Because of the marked lability in blood pressure, only short-acting, easily titrated drugs such as IV nitroprusside should be used. Sustained tachycardia can be treated with small doses of beta blockers if necessary. Corticosteroids, previously widely used in the acute phase of GBS, are no longer advocated because of compelling evidence of slower recovery and an increased relapse rate associated with steroid use. However, methylprednisolone in combination with IVIG has shown promise in GBS therapy.

IVIG remains the cornerstone of treatment for GBS. Studies comparing high-dose IVIG with plasma exchange indicated a beneficial effect from prompt institution of IVIG, comparable to that seen with plasmapheresis. IVIG has become the treatment of choice for GBS in many centers because of its ease of administration, safety profile, and comparable cost. Despite concerns of early recurrences with IVIG treatment (compared with plasmapheresis), most centers use IVIG as initial treatment of GBS.

Plasmapheresis, if performed within 2 weeks of the onset of symptoms, can significantly shorten the time it takes to attain a functional recovery; however, it does not decrease the incidence of respiratory failure. It is, moreover, contraindicated in patients with severe autonomic instability. Thus, plasmapheresis often is used in patients who do not respond first to IVIG. Waiting 2 weeks before changing to the alternative modality is recommended because the effects of either may not be immediately apparent.

GBS is a self-limiting disease with many patients attaining full recovery; however, some suffer severe residual disabilities including loss of independent ambulation. Studies have identified several clinical predictors of poor outcome for GBS, including advanced age, preceding *Campylobacter jejuni* gastrointestinal illness or cytomegalovirus infection, ventilation requirement, and low compound muscle action potential amplitudes. Whereas the majority of patients with GBS have a demyelinating polyneuropathy, a minority develop axonal

degeneration, which carries a poorer prognosis. Positive anti-ganglioside autoantibodies (anti-GMl IgG), IgG1 subclass, are typically associated with the axonal variant that appears to correlate with slower recovery and more severe residual disability.

NEUROLEPTIC MALIGNANT SYNDROME

NMS is a potentially lethal complication associated with the use of dopamine-blocking agents that act in the CNS. Although NMS is not exclusively associated with neuroleptic drugs, phenothiazines, buty-rophenones, and thioxanthenes are the most commonly implicated agents (Table 5.7). In general, drugs with greater dopamine-blocking potency harbor a greater potential for inducing NMS. Thus, haloperidol, chlorpromazine, and fluphenazine have been associated more frequently with NMS than other less potent dopamine-blocking agents. Even olanzapine, an atypical antipsychotic, has been reported, infrequently, to induce NMS. In addition, the use of a dopamine-depleting agent such as tetrabenazine as well as the abrupt discontinuation of antiparkinsonian dopaminergic medication rarely has been associated with NMS.

TABLE 5.7	Causes of Neuroleptic Malignant Syndrome

Dopamine-blocking agents
   Haloperidol (Haldol)
   Chlorpromazine (Thorazine)
   Fluphenazine (Prolixin)
   Clozapine (Clozaril)
   Thioridazine (Mellaril)
   Thiothixene (Navene)
   Trifluoperazine (Stelazine)
   Metaclopramide (Reglan)
Dopamine-depleting agents (tetrabenazine)
Abrupt discontinuation of antiparkinsonian
   dopaminergic medications
Lithium

The risk of NMS is related neither to the duration of exposure to neuroleptics nor to toxic overdoses of neuroleptics; however, numerous predisposing factors in affected patients have been identified. NMS is associated with the initiation of neuroleptic medications at high doses, the rapid upward titration of dose, as well as the use of long-acting depot neuroleptic preparations. Metabolic factors such as dehydration, physical exhaustion, and acute agitation with excessive sympathetic discharge also have been implicated. The four cardinal features of NMS are hyperthermia, muscle rigidity, altered mental status, and autonomic instability. Hyperthermia is present in all cases of NMS; however, the height of the temperature elevation is variable: >38°C (100.4°F) in 92% and >40°C (104°F) in 40% of patients with NMS. Muscular rigidity, commonly described as "lead pipe" rigidity, is typically generalized and may be severe enough to compromise chest wall compliance, causing hypoventilation and the need for ventilatory support. Dysphagia may occur as a result of the rigidity of the pharyngeal musculature, placing the patient at risk for aspiration. Other commonly reported motor abnormalities include immobility or slowness of movement, and involuntary movements, such as tremor and dystonia. Mental status changes, often described as fluctuating states of consciousness, occur in 75% of affected patients. Progression through stages of agitation to alert mutism, stupor, and coma may be observed. Autonomic dysfunction is universal. Frequently reported manifestations are tachycardia, diaphoresis, blood pressure instability, urinary incontinence, cardiac dysrhythmias, and pallor or flushing of the skin. Infrequent findings include Babinski sign, hyperreflexia, seizures, opisthotonos (body spasm with arching of the back), oculogyric crisis, chorea, and trismus (jaw muscle spasm). The clinical features of NMS typically develop over a 24- to 72-hour period and continue for approximately 5 to 10 days even when the offending agents

are discontinued. Symptoms may persist two to three times longer with depot preparations of neuroleptics.

Although NMS is largely a clinical diagnosis, laboratory investigations can provide supportive data and reveal metabolic alterations that mandate diligent monitoring and treatment. An elevation of the blood creatinine phosphokinase (CPK) level and a polymorphonuclear leukocytosis are consistently found. White blood cell counts between 10,000 and 30,000 cells/mm^3 are present in the majority of cases. Electrolyte levels may reveal dehydration. Lumbar puncture, when performed, demonstrates either normal CSF parameters or nonspecific changes. CT of the head is typically negative, and EEG studies are either normal or consistent with a nonspecific encephalopathy.

The differential diagnosis of NMS includes CNS infection (meningitis, encephalitis, postinfectious encephalomyelitis), malignant hyperthermia (an inherited response to general anesthesia) or heatstroke, anticholinergic toxicity, and idiopathic malignant catatonia (advanced progression of a psychotic disorder). NMS, essentially a drug-induced malignant catatonia, may be difficult to distinguish from idiopathic malignant catatonia. Nevertheless, discontinuation of antipsychotics is necessary in both. Other disorders with a similar presentation include thyrotoxicosis, heat stroke, tetanus, and drug-induced parkinsonism.

Treatment of Neuroleptic Malignant Syndrome

Management of NMS begins as soon as the diagnosis is suspected with the *immediate withdrawal of neuroleptic medications* or other dopamine antagonists. In the acute setting, IV fluids may be indicated for volume repletion, and metabolic abnormalities may need correction. Ice packs and cooling blankets can aid in reducing hyperthermia. In most cases, discontinuation of antipsychotic medication is sufficient as NMS is usually self-limited.

Pharmacologic therapy has not been fully established by controlled trials due to the rarity and heterogenous nature of NMS. For patients with milder and primarily catatonic NMS, lorazepam (1 to 2 mg every 4 to 6 hours IM or IV) may be used as a first-line treatment. The most commonly used medications for NMS are dopaminergic drugs, bromocriptine and amantadine, and dantrolene sodium. Bromocriptine (initiated at 2.5 mg PO every 8 hours, up to a total daily dose of 45 mg as needed) may worsen psychosis and hypotension. Dantrolene (1 to 2.5 mg/kg IV every 6 hours for 48 hours, then tapered), a muscle relaxant, should not be administered with calcium channel blockers due to cardiovascular risks. These medications used alone or in combination promote a reduction of body temperature and serum CPK by reducing skeletal muscle rigidity. If NMS is caused by orally administered neuroleptics, treatment with dantrolene and/or bromocriptine should be continued for at least 10 days because recurrence may develop with early treatment withdrawal. Treatment may even be required for 2 to 3 weeks if depot neuroleptics were used.

The psychiatry literature also supports the use of ECT as second-line treatment for NMS when drug therapy has failed. Recommended ECT regimen (with caution in succinylcholine use for those with rhabdomyolysis) includes 6 to 10 bilateral treatments.

■ **SPECIAL CLINICAL POINT: The primary treatment for NMS is discontinuation of antipsychotics and supportive care. Benzodiazepines, dopaminergic drugs (amantadine or bromocriptine), and dantrolene are not proven but may be helpful in NMS and should be tapered to avoid rebound symptoms.**

Approximately 40% of patients with NMS suffer from medical complications. Respiratory complications arising from diminished chest wall compliance and prolonged immobility include ventilatory failure, aspiration pneumonia, pulmonary edema, and pulmonary embolism. Cardiovascular complications such as phlebitis, dysrhythmias, myocardial infarction,

and cardiovascular collapse may be seen. There is a significant risk of renal failure as a result of the combined effects of volume depletion and myoglobinuria due to rhabdomyolysis.

Mortality may result from the cumulative effects of medical complications. Morbidity and mortality from NMS have decreased over the years: reports document a mortality rate of 25% before 1984 and 11.6% since 1984. The improvement in prognosis is attributed more to early recognition and treatment of the syndrome than to the use of any specific therapeutic agent.

Because many patients who recover from NMS continue to require the use of dopamine-blocking agents, the safety of reintroducing neuroleptics often is raised. Studies have demonstrated that a recurrence of NMS can best be avoided by waiting for a complete resolution of NMS before reintroducing low doses

---

Always Remember

- Early anticonvulsant treatment is associated with the best prognosis for recovery from status epilepticus. Treatment should start if a seizure or series of seizures continue for >5 minutes.
- The risk of acute respiratory failure calls for special observation in patients presenting with GBS or an exacerbation of myasthenia gravis.
- If a diagnosis of herpes encephalitis is suspected in a patient with an acute change in mental status, empiric acyclovir treatment should be initiated even before the diagnostic testing is completed.
- Empiric thiamine therapy for Wernicke encephalopathy should be considered in any patient presenting with a change in mental status and a history of alcohol use.
- Neurosurgical consultation is generally warranted in a patient presenting with a neurologic emergency that may require urgent surgical intervention, such as in the case of intracranial hematoma, cerebellar hemorrhage, increased ICP, or spinal cord compression.

of low-potency neuroleptics and ensuring that the patient is well hydrated and metabolically stable. Rechallenge with antipsychotics should be delayed for at least 2 weeks after recovery from NMS.

The diagnosis of NMS should come to mind when encountering any individual taking neuroleptics who develops unexplained fever with muscle rigidity. Although there are numerous alternate diagnoses, the life-threatening danger of NMS demands that treatment should not be delayed if there is significant clinical suspicion.

QUESTIONS AND DISCUSSION

1. A 21-year-old woman is seen in the emergency room complaining of a feeling of tingling in her feet and hands for 1 day. She has no other neurologic complaints. She denies shortness of breath, exposure to drugs or toxins, or a recent viral illness. An examination reveals diffuse hyporeflexia with absent ankle jerks. Very careful sensory testing is normal despite the patient's complaints. The best course of action would be:
   A. Discharge the patient with the diagnosis of "functional disorder" because of a paucity of objective findings.
   B. Admit her to the hospital for close observation, watching carefully for signs of developing weakness or respiratory difficulty.
   C. Perform a lumbar puncture in the emergency room, suspecting early GBS, with plans to discharge the patient if the results are normal.
   D. Order a brain MRI to rule out a cerebral mass lesion or stroke.

The correct answer is B. Paresthesias without objective sensory findings occur commonly and early in GBS, often before clinical weakness develops. The key features in this case are the sensory complaints in the presence of diffuse hyporeflexia. The typically high CSF protein concentration without

pleocytosis may not occur until after a few weeks of illness.

2. The next day, she complains of difficulty in walking and on examination shows a pulse of 120, diffuse areflexia, and bilateral proximal lower-extremity weakness. The best management at this time would be:
   A. Admit her to an ICU for cardiac monitoring, frequent vital capacities, and lumbar puncture.
   B. Observe her in a general medical ward with daily vital capacities and steroids.
   C. Admit her to an ICU for cardiac monitoring, with monitoring of the vital capacity only if respiratory problems occur.
   D. Admit her to an ICU for vital capacity and cardiac monitoring, and give high-dose steroids.

The correct answer is A. With weakness now developing, it is clear that the patient has GBS. She should be monitored in an ICU setting, and she should be watched closely for the development of cardiac arrhythmias and respiratory compromise. Vital capacities should be checked every 4 to 6 hours, with intubation done if there is less than 60% predicted value. Steroids have not been shown to be effective in GBS.

3. Which of the following statements about generalized SE is true?
   A. Generalized SE should be diagnosed in a patient who within a 2-hour period has a series of seizures, between which he is fully oriented and able to clearly state his medications and dosages.
   B. A patient presents to the clinic with a normal mental status but continuous involuntary twitching of his left thumb, consistent with a diagnosis of generalized SE.
   C. A patient in generalized SE should be immediately intubated and paralyzed with neuromuscular blockade to prevent rhabdomyosis from intense muscular contractions.

D. Generalized SE should be treated with a fast-acting benzodiazepine followed immediately by a loading dose of a long-acting anticonvulsant.

The correct answer is D. Generalized SE is defined by prolonged seizure activity with loss of consciousness or repeated seizures *without recovery of consciousness* between episodes. Statement (A) better describes acute repetitive seizures that may evolve into generalized SE in some patients if left untreated. Focal motor SE, or epilepsia partialis continua, described in statement (B) does not carry the same morbidity or urgency as generalized SE, may persist for weeks without evolving further, and can be very resistant to seizure therapy. Neuromuscular blockade (C) will abolish the motor activity but will not treat the underlying electrical seizure activity. Following preservation of an airway, drawing labs, and the establishment of intravenous access, first-line therapy is aimed at abolishing electrographic seizure activity with anticonvulsants.

4. A 45-year-old man presents to the emergency department confused with an unsteady gait. No additional history was attainable. Neurologic examination further revealed intermittent upbeat nystagmus, horizontal gaze palsy, and severe ataxia. Laboratory evaluation revealed an elevated gamma-glutamyl transpeptidase, serum amylase, and serum lipase, but drug and alcohol testing was negative. The best course of action would be:
   A. Immediately request an EEG to evaluate for nonconvulsive seizure activity while simultaneously initiating a loading dose of intravenous phenytoin.
   B. Stabilize the patient's cervical spine, order cervical spine plain films, and request a psychiatry consultation for further evaluation.
   C. Immediately administer intravenous thiamine followed by glucose and

intravenous fluids, while considering the need for neuroimaging and lumbar puncture.
   D. Order serial neurologic examinations to be done by nursing staff while attempting to contact family members for further historical information.

The correct answer is C. This patient presents with the classic triad of clinical features for Wernicke encephalopathy—ophthalmoplegia, ataxia, and confusion. Immediate infusion of thiamine is warranted because the symptoms are potentially reversible with early treatment. Glucose should be administered for potential hypoglycemia, but it should be given only after thiamine because of the risk of precipitating encephalopathy in those with borderline nutritional status. Pursuing additional evaluative testing including neuroimaging, lumbar puncture, EEG, and cervical spine plain film series may be warranted based on the clinical picture but should not delay early administration of thiamine.

SUGGESTED READING

Alldredge BK, Gelb AM, Isaacs SM, et al. A comparison of lorazepam, diazepam, and placebo for the treatment of out-of-hospital status epilepticus. *N Engl J Med*. 2001;345:631.

Alshekhlee A, Miles JD, Katirji B, et al. Incidence and mortality rates of myasthenia gravis and myasthenic crisis in US hospitals. *Neurology*. 2009;72:1548.

Byrne TN. Spinal cord compression from epidural metastases. *N Engl J Med*. 1992;327:614.

Cappuccino A. Moderate hypothermia as treatment for spinal cord injury. *Orthopedics*. 2008;31(3):243.

Charness ME, Simon RP, Greenberg DA. Ethanol and the nervous system. *N Engl J Med*. 1989;321:442.

DeLorenzo RJ. Status epilepticus: concepts in diagnosis and treatment. *Semin Neurol*. 1990;10:396.

Devinsky O, Leppik I, Willmore LJ, et al. Safety of intravenous valproate. *Ann Neurol*. 1995;38:670.

The Dutch Guillain–Barré Study Group. Treatment of Guillain–Barré syndrome with high-dose immune globulins combined with methylprednisolone: a pilot study. *Ann Neurol*. 1994;35:749.

Factor SA, Singer C. Neuroleptic malignant syndrome. In: Weiner WJ, ed. *Emergent and Urgent Neurology.* Philadelphia: JB Lippincott; 1992.

Gajdos P, Chevret S, Clair B, et al. Clinical trial of plasma exchange and high-dose intravenous immunoglobulins in myasthenia gravis. Myasthenia Gravis Clinical Study Group. *Ann Neurol.* 1997;41:789.

Grant R, Papadopoulos SM, Sandler HM, et al. Metastatic epidural spinal cord compression: current concepts and treatment. *J Neurooncol.* 1994;19:79.

Hadley M. Management of acute central cervical spinal cord injuries. *Neurosurgery.* 2002;50(3 suppl):S166.

Jensen MB, St. Louis EK. Management of acute cerebellar stroke. *Arch Neurol.* 2005;62:537.

Kalviainen R. Status epilepticus treatment guidelines. *Epilepsia.* 2007;48(suppl. 8):99.

Koga M, Yuki N, Hirata K, et al. Anti-GMI antibody IgG subclass: a clinical recovery predictor in Guillain–Barré syndrome. *Neurology.* 2003;60:1514.

Kokontis L, Gutmann L. Current treatment of neuromuscular diseases. *Arch Neurol.* 2000;57:939.

Kwon BK, Mann C, Sohn HM, et al. Hypothermia for spinal cord injury. *Spine J.* 2008;8(6):859.

Leppik IE. Status epilepticus. In: Wyllie E, ed. *The Treatment of Epilepsy: Principles and Practice.* Philadelphia: Lea & Febiger; 1993.

Manno EM. New management strategies in the treatment of status epilepticus. *Mayo Clin Proc.* 2003;78:508.

Meagher DJ. Delirium: optimizing management. *BMJ.* 2001;322:144.

Qureshi AI, Choudhry A, Akbar MS, et al. Plasma exchange versus intravenous immunoglobulin treatment in myasthenic crisis. *Neurology.* 1999;52:629.

Rabinstein A, Wijdicks EE. BiPAP in acute respiratory failure due to myasthenic crisis may prevent intubation. *Neurology.* 2002;59:1647.

Reid RL, Quigley ME, Yen SS. Pituitary apoplexy. *Arch Neurol.* 1985;42:712.

Ropper AH. The Guillain–Barré syndrome. *N Engl J Med.* 1992;326:1130.

Steiner T, Ringleb P, Hacke W. Treatment options for large hemispheric stroke. *Neurology.* 2001;57 (5 suppl 2):S61.

Strawn JR, Keck Jr PE, Caroff SN. Neuroleptic malignant syndrome. *Am J Psychiatry.* 2007;164:870.

Thomas CE, Mayer SA, Gungor Y, et al. Myasthenic crisis: clinical features, mortality, complications, and risk factors for prolonged intubation. *Neurology.* 1997;48:1253.

Van der Meche FG, Schmitz PI, and the Dutch Guillain–Barré Study Group. A randomized trial comparing intravenous immune globulin and plasma exchange in Guillain–Barré syndrome. *N Engl J Med.* 1992;326:1123.

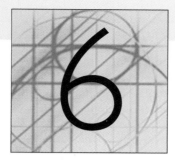

6

Examination of the Comatose Patient

JORDAN L. TOPEL AND STEVEN L. LEWIS

key points

- Coma is not an independent disease entity but a reflection of an underlying disease process.
- Coma results from bilateral, diffuse cerebral hemisphere dysfunction or brainstem (midbrain or pons) involvement of the ascending reticular activating system, or a combination of the two.
- Metabolic or systemic disorders generally cause depressed consciousness without focal neurologic findings.
- Proper management of the unconscious patient includes an aggressive pursuit of the medical history.
- The goal of the neurologic examination of the comatose patient is to determine the presence, location, and nature of the underlying process creating the decreased level of consciousness and also to determine the prognosis of the patient's condition.
- Following the establishment of an airway with stabilization of respiration and maintenance of circulation, certain laboratory tests and therapeutic measures are undertaken that can occur concurrently with the acquisition of a pertinent history and a neurologic examination.

DEFINITIONS AND CLINICAL SYNDROMES

A discussion of the evaluation and treatment of the comatose patient requires one to define certain terms regarding different states and levels of consciousness and unconsciousness. The examination and diagnostic studies must be carried out in an organized and systematic manner with documentation that is clear to all members of the health team. The definitions of different levels of consciousness are, by themselves, often confusing and misleading. When one physician's understanding of terms (e.g., lethargy, stupor, or obtundation) differs from that of his or her colleagues, one may think that a patient's condition has deteriorated, although only the terminology has changed between the observers. It is better to specifically describe a patient's movements, and reactions to painful stimuli, for example, rather than to categorize the patient as being lethargic, semicomatose, or stuporous.

Consciousness is defined as the awareness of one's self and the environment. This is a poor definition, however, because one can argue that a sleeping person is unconscious—that is, unaware of himself or herself and his or her environment. Clinically, however, no one regards a sleeping person as unconscious: he or she can be aroused to appropriate physical and mental activity with appropriate, non-noxious stimuli.

Consciousness comprises a continuum from full alertness to deep coma, or total unresponsiveness. Drowsiness or lethargy is characterized by easy arousal with light stimuli. There may be a verbal response or appropriate limb movements to pain. Stupor reflects arousability by persistent or vigorous stimuli only, and the arousal is incomplete. There is little verbal response, but limb movements still may be appropriate to the stimulus. Mental and physical activities are reduced to a minimum. Coma reflects the state in which the patient cannot be aroused to make purposeful responses. This is subgrouped into light coma, in which there may be reflex, primitive, or disorganized responses to noxious stimuli (e.g., decorticate

and decerebrate responses), and deep coma, in which there is no response to painful stimuli.

Psychogenic unresponsiveness (hysterical coma) is a psychiatric phenomenon in which the patient appears unresponsive but is physiologically awake. The heart and respiratory rates are usually normal. The patient lies with the eyes closed, and the eyelids are frequently difficult to separate (forced eye closure). Muscle tone is normal. Although there may be little resistance to passive movement, suspending the patient's hand over his or her face usually results in its falling to the side instead of directly downward. Pupils are equal and reactive unless certain eyedrops have been used. Ice water caloric testing produces nystagmus, a sign seen only in awake patients. The electroencephalogram (EEG) reveals a waking record.

The "locked-in" syndrome is an important condition to recognize. The patient appears to be in a coma but has essentially all higher mental activities intact. The syndrome most frequently is related to pontine infarction due to basilar artery thrombosis or embolism. There is an interruption of the descending corticobulbar and corticospinal tracts, resulting in quadriplegia and paralysis of lower cranial nerves. The patient is unable to talk, breathe, or move his or her extremities. Because the ascending reticular activating system is spared, however, arousability and wakefulness are present. There also is sparing of fibers controlling eye blinking and vertical eye movements, though horizontal eye movements are almost always impaired. Thus, the patient's only means for communication may be using eye blinks (Morse code). The ramifications of not recognizing this disturbing clinical condition are obvious.

■ **SPECIAL CLINICAL POINT: Every patient, no matter how deep in coma he or she appears to be, should be asked to open and close the eyes and to move them up and down, to assess for the locked-in syndrome.**

The vegetative state is somewhat clinically opposite of the "locked-in" syndrome. The patient appears to be awake with intermittent eye opening but is unable to attain higher mental functions. Simply stated, there is arousal but no awareness. There is no language comprehension or intelligible speech nor responses to visual or auditory stimuli. Sleep–wake cycles may return, but there is no return of higher mental activity.

■ **SPECIAL CLINICAL POINT: The vegetative state occurs in the setting of severe cortical dysfunction with relative brainstem sparing, such as in patients who survive a cardiopulmonary arrest with consequent severe cerebral anoxia. The term "persistent vegetative state" implies that the patient has been in a clinical vegetative state for more than 30 days.**

■ **SPECIAL CLINICAL POINT: The minimally conscious state is seen in patients with marked impairment of consciousness but who have evidence of any awareness of the environment.**

Patients in the minimally conscious state can exhibit some deliberate or cognitively mediated behavior. This may be manifested by the ability to follow very simple commands, show some purposeful behavior, or have minimal verbalization.

It is not uncommon for patients with acute onset of global aphasia to be diagnosed initially as being in coma. The patient is indeed unable to comprehend, communicate, or carry out simple verbal commands. The diagnosis may be established by noting that the patient appears to be awake and alert, often with deviation of the eyes to the left with a right hemiplegia.

COMA

Anatomy

In the evaluation of the comatose patient, it is necessary to consider the physiologic and anatomic abnormalities that result in decreased level of consciousness.

■ **SPECIAL CLINICAL POINT: Coma results from bilateral, diffuse cerebral hemisphere dysfunction or brainstem (midbrain or pons) involvement of the ascending reticular activating system, or a combination of the two.**

Coma is unusual with unilateral cerebral hemisphere disease unless there is a dysfunction of the other hemisphere or secondary pressure or destruction of brainstem structures. Most large cerebral hemisphere infarctions will result in a slightly decreased level of consciousness, but the patient still can be aroused to elicit some purposeful movements or higher mental activity. Rare exceptions may be patients with large, acute lesions affecting the dominant cerebral hemisphere. In contrast, profound coma may result from very small infarctions in the brainstem affecting the ascending reticular activating system.

A unilateral hemispheral mass lesion, such as a tumor, abscess, or expanding hemorrhage, frequently will present with unilateral focal neurologic symptoms and signs. On continued enlargement of the mass, there may be a compression of the contralateral cerebral hemisphere or a downward herniation of the ipsilateral temporal lobe, creating distortion and compression of the brainstem (transtentorial herniation). At this point, coma will ensue. There is also the suggestion that horizontal displacement of the brain at the level of the pineal body may correlate more closely with levels of consciousness than downward displacement with brainstem compression.

Metabolic processes usually affect both brainstem and cerebral hemispheres to produce coma. This likely reflects a direct interference of the metabolic activity of the neurons. Initially, the patient is drowsy, but coma ensues as the metabolic process worsens.

ETIOLOGY

■ **SPECIAL CLINICAL POINT: Coma is not an independent disease entity but a reflection of an underlying disease process.**

The causes of coma can be divided into two main categories: (1) those of primary central nervous system (CNS) disease and (2) those of metabolic or systemic depression (Table 6.1).

TABLE 6.1 Common Causes of Coma

Cause	Comments
	Coma Secondary to Primary Brain Injury or Disease
Infection	
Bacterial meningitis	Nuchal rigidity; CSF shows pleocytosis, increased protein; glucose may be decreased; meningeal enhancement on MRI
Viral encephalitis	May have focal findings; CSF shows increased lymphocytes, increased protein, normal or slightly decreased glucose; positive PCR for HSV; possible focal abnormalities on MRI
Abscess	Focal findings; positive CT or MRI scan; history of ear or sinus infection or HIV or endocarditis; CSF shows mildly increased protein, increased cells, negative cultures
Tumor	
Primary or metastatic	Focal findings; progressive course; may have papilledema
Cerebral infarction	
Basilar occlusion or bilateral internal artery occlusion	Usually no coma unless bilateral or acute, large dominant hemisphere, or involving brainstem reticular activating system
Cerebral hemorrhage	
Subarachnoid	Sudden onset; headache, nuchal rigidity, vomiting; positive CT scan (95%); bloody CSF
Intracerebral	Sudden onset; headache, nuchal rigidity, vomiting; focal findings; abnormal CT scan (100%); history of hypertension or coagulopathy or anticoagulation
Hydrocephalus	
May result from subarachnoid hemorrhage or meningitis	Decreasing level of consciousness; enlarging ventricular size on CT scan
Trauma	
Concussion, contusion	Positive history, evidence of injury on examination; uncomplicated concussion leaves no residual
Subdural hematoma	Depressed level of consciousness can occur before focal findings; may have trivial or no trauma history
Epidural hematoma	Lucid interval; skull fracture over middle meningeal artery
Seizures	
Generalized or focal seizures	Convulsive or nonconvulsive status epilepticus; postictal progressive improvement in level of consciousness unless other factors are involved

The latter group contains the more common causes of a depressed level of consciousness.

Primary central nervous system disorders may or may not produce focal abnormalities on examination.

■ **SPECIAL CLINICAL POINT: Metabolic or systemic disorders generally cause depressed consciousness without focal neurologic findings.**

In these instances, the clinician does not expect to find unequal pupils, signs of weakness on only one side, or asymmetric reflexes. A previous neurologic injury, however, may render certain neurons more susceptible to a metabolic insult and accentuate clinical signs related to the older injury. A metabolic encephalopathy in a patient with an old stroke that had fully resolved thus could produce a reemergence of the former weakness in a focal pattern, even though the cause of the current coma is a metabolic one. With correction of the metabolic abnormality, the focal signs would be expected to disappear

TABLE 6.1

Common Causes of Coma (continued)

Cause	Comments
Coma Secondary to Metabolic and Systemic Diseases	
Exogenous substances	
Sedatives, hypnotics, antidepressants	Positive blood or urine screens; may cause pupillary abnormalities (opiates cause miosis and anticholinergics cause mydriasis)
Alcohol	Breath odor may not be apparent; withdrawal seizures 8 to 48 hours after last drink
Methyl alcohol	Metabolic acidosis; visual symptoms
Heavy metals, cyanide arsenic, lead, salicylates	Lead encephalopathy common in children, not in adults
Endogenous substances	
Hepatic coma	Fetor hepaticus, jaundice, ascites, asterixis; triphasic waves on electroencephalogram
Uremic coma	Uriniferous breath; seizures; asterixis
CO_2 narcosis	Increased P_{CO_2}; abnormal physical chest findings; abnormal electrolytes
Endocrine—pituitary, thyroid, pancreas (diabetes), adrenal glands	Urine and serum osmolalities; thyroid function studies; focal seizures with hyperglycemic nonketotic coma
Hypoxia	
Pulmonary disease, carbon monoxide intoxication, anemia	Abnormal blood gases; elevated carboxyhemoglobin, cherry red lips
Decreased cardiac output	Hypotension, congestive heart failure, myocardial infarction, arrhythmia, cardiopulmonary arrest
Hypertensive encephalopathy	Papilledema; proteinuria; headaches; seizures; posterior reversible encephalopathy syndrome
Hypoglycemia	
Suspect in all comatose patients	Reversed with D50 unless prolonged coma
Thiamine deficiency	
Wernicke encephalopathy	Potentially reversible with IV thiamine
Electrolyte imbalance	
Often multifactorial	Water, sodium, acidosis, alkalosis, calcium
Temperature regulation	
Hypothermia	Exposure; myxedema; circulatory failure
Hyperthermia	Heat stroke; neuroleptic malignant syndrome with muscle rigidity and elevated CK; infection

CSF, cerebrospinal fluid; MRI, magnetic resonance imaging; PCR, polymerase chain reaction; HSV, herpes simplex virus; CT, computed tomography; HIV, human immunodeficiency virus; CK, creatine kinase.

again, unless there was further focal damage superimposed.

HISTORY AND EXAMINATION

A history should be taken, but unfortunately this is often incomplete, nonexistent, or misleading. A search for "less likely" causes for coma is necessary when treatment for the "obvious" cause from the history obtained does not change the patient's clinical status.

■ **SPECIAL CLINICAL POINT: Aggressive management of the unconscious patient includes an aggressive pursuit of the history.**

For example, metabolic abnormalities most often are associated with subacute onset of coma, whereas a history of a more rapid course is suggestive of cardiac or cerebrovascular cause or drug overdose.

There should be a search for evidence of trauma. Battle's sign (purple and blue discoloration of the mastoid skin area), blood in the external auditory canal, or blood noted behind the tympanic membranes may signify a temporal bone or basal skull fracture. Raccoon eyes (purple discoloration of the eyelid and orbital regions) may signify orbital or basal skull fractures. Cerebrospinal fluid rhinorrhea or otorrhea also suggests a skull fracture.

One should check carefully for nuchal rigidity, but several factors must be considered in doing so. If there is any suspicion of a cervical neck fracture, there should be no manipulation of the neck. In deep coma, nuchal rigidity may be lacking despite its presence in a lighter level of consciousness. Finally, some patients with a CNS infection or subarachnoid hemorrhage may not manifest nuchal rigidity initially in the course of their illness.

The odor of the patient's breath may indicate the cause for the coma. Alcohol gives its characteristic smell; hepatic coma is often associated with a musty odor; and a fruity or acetone smell is characteristic of ketoacidosis.

After a screening, general physical examination, an orderly, systematic neurologic examination, is undertaken.

■ **SPECIAL CLINICAL POINT: The goal of the neurologic examination is to determine the presence, location, and nature of the underlying process creating the decreased level of consciousness and also to determine the prognosis of the patient's condition.**

Respiratory patterns yield information regarding the activity of different cerebral areas. When one develops bilateral cerebral hemisphere dysfunction (essentially, functioning at the diencephalic level), Cheyne–Stokes respiration may occur. This respiratory pattern is associated with periods of hyperpnea alternating with periods of apnea. There is a regularity to the respirations: first a gradual buildup of respirations to the level of hyperpnea and then a gradual tapering off of respirations

to apnea. The periods of apnea may last up to 30 seconds or more and may be accompanied by decreased responsiveness and miosis. It is believed that Cheyne–Stokes respiration relates to an abnormal response of carbon dioxide–sensitive respiratory brain centers. There is an increased ventilatory response to carbon dioxide stimulation, creating hyperpnea. After the concentration of carbon dioxide drops below the level at which the centers are stimulated, the apnea phase appears and continues until the carbon dioxide reaccumulates and the cycle repeats itself. Because sleep induces further cerebral-depressing mechanisms, Cheyne–Stokes respiration may be seen in some patients during sleep, whereas they exhibit normal breathing patterns while awake. Cheyne–Stokes respiration is, by itself, not a serious prognostic sign. Although it can be seen in focal primary CNS problems, it also can be seen early in many metabolic and systemic problems.

Central neurogenic hyperventilation appears when lower brain centers are involved; it is noted with dysfunction at the midbrain or the upper pons and often is associated with pulmonary edema. There are continuous, regular, and rapid respirations up to 40 or 50 times per minute. Arterial blood gases reveal a respiratory alkalosis with decreased P_{CO_2} and increased pH. The P_{O_2} must be greater than 70 or 80 mm Hg. If the P_{O_2} is not higher than that level, it raises the possibility of an extracerebral cause (hypoxemia) for the respiratory problem. In reality, most cases of sustained hyperventilation in comatose patients are not central neurogenic hyperventilation. Cardiac, pulmonary, and metabolic (e.g., diabetes, uremia, hepatic, salicylates) problems must be ruled out as possible causes of the hyperventilation.

Apneustic respiration, noted in lower pontine lesions, consists of a prolonged inspiratory phase with a pause at full inspiration. Cluster breathing (short-cycle Cheyne–Stokes respiration), also signifying lower pontine damage, is characterized by a disorderly sequence of closely grouped respirations followed by apnea.

Ataxic respirations signify a lower pontine or medullary respiratory center problem. The breathing pattern is chaotic and haphazard with irregular pauses. It may, and usually does, lead to gasping and eventual cessation of breathing. Ataxic breathing is a forewarner of respiratory arrest, and prompt endotracheal intubation is necessary at the time of its discovery.

An examination of the pupillary responses, eye movements, and fundus must be undertaken. In a patient with a decreased level of consciousness, but who is not yet in coma, visual threat (forceful movements of the hand toward either side of the eyes) may be helpful. Blinking in response to a threat from one side, but not from the other side, suggests a hemianopsia. The abnormality thus would be in the cerebral hemisphere opposite to the side that did not blink. A funduscopic examination may reveal papilledema or retinal hemorrhages suggesting increased intracranial pressure or malignant hypertension.

The pupillary response should be assessed. The light reflex is mediated, in succession, through the optic nerve, the optic chiasm, the optic tract, the posterior diencephalon, and the Edinger–Westphal nuclei of the midbrain and then to the sphincter pupillae by way of the parasympathetic nerve fibers in the oculomotor nerve (cranial nerve III). Thus, it is not surprising that the most significant abnormalities of the pupils are seen with dysfunction at the level of the midbrain or oculomotor nerve.

Diencephalic pupils, the result of bilateral hemispheral dysfunction, are small and reactive. The small size likely reflects sympathetic nerve dysfunction at the level of the takeoff of the sympathetic fibers from the hypothalamus.

Midposition, unreactive (4 to 7 mm) pupils result from direct midbrain (tectal region) damage. The pupillary size likely reflects involvement of both the descending sympathetic fibers and the parasympathetic fibers of the oculomotor complex.

A widely dilated, fixed pupil usually is seen as a result of direct oculomotor nerve involvement, with unopposed dilator sympathetic tone. In addition to the pupillary abnormalities, ptosis and extraocular muscle paralysis (especially paralysis of adduction of the eye) are fre-

quently present. Because the oculomotor nerve is strategically situated at the temporal incisura, temporal lobe herniation may result in a widely dilated, fixed pupil and possibly total cranial nerve III paralysis.

Pinpoint (1 mm) pupils are seen with pontine damage but may be a transient finding for only the first 24 or 48 hours. The pupils are small and can be seen occasionally to react slightly to light if viewed through a magnifying glass. This is thought to relate to damage of the descending sympathetic tracts. Frequently, however, midposition and fixed pupils may be noted with pontine dysfunction.

In general, metabolic causes of coma do not alter pupillary response until late in their course, if at all. For example, a deeply comatose patient with no spontaneous or reflex movements and no respirations, but with reactive pupils, must be considered to be in metabolic coma until proven otherwise. However, certain drugs can alter pupillary size and response. Opiates characteristically produce pinpoint pupils (reversed with naloxone). Atropine may result in widely dilated and fixed pupils. Various eyedrops also may alter pupillary size and reaction.

The position and movements of the eyes are observed, and certain procedures are undertaken to evaluate cerebral hemisphere and brainstem integrity. The neural pathways for the control of horizontal conjugate eye movements are outlined in Figure 6.1. Cortical control originates in the frontal gaze centers (Brodmann's area 8). Descending fibers controlling horizontal conjugate gaze cross the midline in the lower midbrain region and descend to the paramedian pontine reticular formation (PPRF) in the pons. The PPRF is thus the major area of confluence of pathways controlling horizontal eye movements. Neurons from the PPRF project to the nearby abducens nerve (cranial nerve VI) nucleus and thereby stimulate movement in the lateral rectus muscle of the eye ipsilateral to the PPRF and contralateral to the frontal gaze center. In addition, impulses from the abducens nerve nucleus cross the midline and ascend the median longitudinal fasciculus to the medial rectus nucleus of the oculomotor nerve (cranial

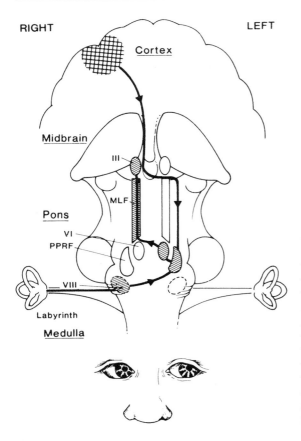

RIGHT

LEFT

Cortex

Midbrain

III

MLF

Pons

VI

PPRF

VIII

Labyrinth

Medulla

FIGURE 6.1 Diagram of the conjugate vision pathways (nuclei and paths are shaded to include those important to left conjugate gaze). Fibers from the right frontal cortex descend and cross the midline, and they synapse in the left paramedian pontine reticular formation (PPRF). Fibers then travel to the nearby left cranial nerve VI nucleus (to move the left eye laterally) and then cross the midline to rise in the right medial longitudinal fasciculus (MLF) to the right cranial nerve III nucleus (to move the right eye medially). In addition to the cortical influence on the left PPRF, there is vestibular influence. With vestibular activation from the right, the left PPRF is stimulated, and the eyes conjugatively move to the left. Instillation of ice water into the right ear canal will test the integrity of this vestibular–PPRF–cranial nerve-VI–cranial nerve-III circuit, and if the eyes move to vestibular stimulation, the brainstem from medulla to midbrain must be functioning.

nerve III) in the midbrain. This stimulates adduction of the eye ipsilateral to the frontal gaze center. Horizontal conjugate gaze thus is completed.

By following these pathways, it can be seen that stimulation of fibers from the frontal gaze center of one cerebral hemisphere results in horizontal, conjugate eye movements to the contralateral side. If one frontal gaze center or its descending fibers are damaged, the eyes will tend to "look" toward the involved cerebral hemisphere because of unopposed action of the remaining frontal gaze center. For example, a destructive lesion in the right cerebral hemisphere, involving descending motor fibers and frontal gaze fibers, will cause a left hemiplegia with head and eyes deviated to the right. In other words, the eyes "look" at a destructive

hemispheral lesion and "look" away from the resulting hemiplegia.

By contrast, a destructive left pontine lesion, for example, will damage the left PPRF. The eyes, therefore, cannot go to the left and will tend to deviate to the right. Because descending pyramidal tract fibers cross the midline in the medulla, damage to the pyramidal tract fibers in the pons on the left results in a right hemiplegia. Thus, the eyes "look" away from a destructive pontine lesion but "look" toward the hemiplegia.

If the abducens nerve or nucleus is destroyed, there will be a loss of abduction of the ipsilateral eye (cranial nerve VI palsy). With destruction of the tract of the medial longitudinal fasciculus, disconjugate gaze results, with loss of adduction of the ipsilateral eye (same side as the tract of the medial longitudinal fasciculus). Abduction of the contralateral eye is preserved, but there is nystagmus. This type of disconjugate gaze abnormality also is termed "internuclear ophthalmoplegia" (see Chapter 22). The pathways for vertical eye movements are less well understood. Lower centers likely exist in the midbrain (pretectal and tectal) regions. Integrity of vertical eye movements can be tested in some patients by gently moving the head back and forth in the vertical plane.

If a patient cannot follow verbal commands, two tests are used to determine brainstem integrity. An oculocephalic (doll's head) maneuver is performed by turning the patient's head rapidly in the horizontal or vertical planes and by noting the movement or position of the eyes relative to the orbits. This maneuver should not be performed if a cervical neck fracture is suspected. If the pontine (horizontal) or midbrain (vertical) gaze centers are intact, the eyes should move in the orbits in the direction opposite to the turning head. An abnormal response (no eye movement with doll's head maneuver) implies pontine or midbrain dysfunction and is characterized by no movement of the eyes relative to the orbits or by an asymmetry of movement.

Horizontal oculocephalic maneuvers are a relatively weak stimulus for horizontal eye movements. If a doll's head maneuver is present, it is not necessary to continue with oculovestibular testing. If, however, a doll's head response is lacking, ice water calorics should be performed because it is a stronger stimulus than oculocephalic maneuvers.

Oculovestibular responses (ice water calorics) are reflex eye movements in response to irrigation of the external ear canals with cold water. The head is raised to 30 degrees relative to the horizontal plane, and the external canals are inspected for the presence of cerumen or a perforated tympanic membrane. Fifty to 100 mL of cold water is instilled into the canal (waiting 5 minutes between ears), and the resulting eye movements are noted. Ice water produces a downward current in the horizontal semicircular canal and decreases tonic vestibular input to the contralateral PPRF. Simplistically, one can

think of this as an indirect means of stimulating the ipsilateral PPRF. Hence, after cold water instillation, there is a slow, tonic, conjugate deviation of the eyes toward the irrigated ear. In a waking patient, there is a correction of the eyes to the opposite side, resulting in a fast nystagmus away from the stimulated ear. In an unconscious patient, there is a loss of the fast-phase nystagmus, and only tonic deviation of the eyes is seen if appropriate pontine–midbrain areas are intact. Thus, if nystagmus is noted in a seemingly unconscious patient, the patient is either in a very light coma or psychogenic unresponsiveness. It is important to be vigilant when performing caloric testing in these states because the stimulation is potentially noxious and can induce vomiting; making certain that the patient is safely positioned so that vomiting would not cause aspiration is paramount.

A lack of oculovestibular responses thus suggests pontine–midbrain dysfunction. Ice water calorics can help to differentiate between the conjugate gaze weakness or paralysis caused by either cortical (cerebral hemisphere) or brainstem (pontine) damage. Oculovestibular responses should not be altered in patients with only hemispheral pathology. Movement of the ipsilateral eye toward the irrigated ear, but no movement of the contralateral eye, suggests an abnormality of the contralateral medial longitudinal fasciculus.

Severe metabolic coma (e.g., after barbiturate overdose) may result in a lack of oculocephalic and oculovestibular responses. Reactive pupils may signify that the coma is of metabolic origin.

Ocular bobbing is characterized by a rapid downward eye movement with a slow return to the horizontal plane. This is seen most often in pontine destruction and is thought to relate to the loss of horizontal eye movements with preservation of midbrain-mediated vertical eye movement pathways. Sustained down gaze can be seen with lesions of the thalamus or pretectum or after cerebral hypoxia.

Roving eye movements signify intact brainstem mechanisms for horizontal gaze. The movements should be distinguished from those seen in patients with seizures. In the latter, the eye movements are of a jerking quality and frequently tend to lateralize to one side. Referring to Figure 6.1, it can be seen that an irritative cortical focus in the area of the frontal gaze center will deviate the eyes away from the side of the lesion (and possibly toward a hemiplegia). Oculovestibular responses usually will be able to overcome the eye deviations because of the strong direct input into the pons, "bypassing" the cortical effects on eye movements.

Asymmetric corneal reflexes may be present in both cortical and brainstem lesions. Metabolic abnormalities and hypoxia can suppress corneal reflexes. It should be noted, however, that corneal responses can be decreased or absent in waking elderly patients.

Motor movements may be spontaneous, induced, reflex, or totally absent. It is important to note not only the type of response but also the symmetry of response. An asymmetric, induced motor movement may be the only indication of an underlying focal problem. Asymmetric muscle tone may also suggest a focal process.

It may be necessary to observe the patient for several minutes to note the presence or lack of spontaneous or reflex motor movements. The position of the extremities (e.g., a persistent externally rotated leg secondary to weakness of that extremity) may indicate focal pathology.

The most favorable prognostic sign related to the motor system is symmetric, spontaneous movements of all four extremities. Appropriate motor response to noxious stimuli (e.g., pain) signifies that sensory pathways are functional and there is at least partial integrity of corticospinal tracts. It is not necessary to use unusually noxious stimuli, but rather mild supraorbital pressure or pinching of the skin of the neck.

Reflex motor movements frequently can be elicited by light, painful stimuli or flexion of the neck or during routine care of the patient, such as tracheal suctioning. Decorticate posturing consists of flexion of the arms, wrists, and fingers and adduction of the upper arms. In the legs, there is extension, internal rotation, and plantar flexion. Decerebrate (extensor) posturing consists of extension, adduction, and hyper-

pronation of the arms. There may be opisthotonic posturing of the neck. The movement of the lower extremities is similar to that seen in decorticate posturing. Although not completely anatomically specific, bilateral decerebrate posturing often is seen in lesions of the midbrain and pons, whereas decorticate posturing often implies a higher corticospinal tract lesion. Decerebrate posturing is generally a poorer prognostic sign than decorticate posturing. However, decerebrate posturing also occasionally can be seen in the setting of severe, although potentially reversible, metabolic encephalopathies.

A common mistake regarding the interpretation of motor responses is that of relating a withdrawal response in the legs as representing an appropriate cortical response. When the bottom of the foot is stroked, or a noxious stimulus is applied to the leg, there may be hip flexion, knee flexion, and dorsiflexion of the foot (triple flexor response). This signifies spinal cord reflex integrity and does not signify an intact cerebral response.

Asymmetric extensor toe signs (i.e., flexion on one side, extensor response on the other) are of moderate value in localizing a focal cerebral lesion. Bilateral extensor toe signs (Babinski signs) can be seen in any form or at any level of coma and are, by themselves, neither prognostic nor localizing. For example, transient extensor toe signs are common in hypertensive encephalopathy.

The Glasgow Coma Scale (Table 6.2) is the most widely used clinical scale for assessment of comatose patients. Although it initially was designed for trauma cases, it is also used now for other causes of coma. It measures the "best responses" of eye opening, motor response, and verbal response. A lower score usually signifies a more serious neurologic problem and possibly a poorer prognosis. However, there can be falsely low scores such as in patients who cannot speak because of mechanical ventilation or aphasia. Recently the FOUR (Full Outline of UnResponsiveness) score has been developed which includes examination of the brainstem reflexes and respiration (Table 6.3).

TABLE 6.2		
	Glasgow Coma Scale	

Eye opening	
Spontaneous	4
To speech	3
To pain	2
None	1
Motor response	
Obeys	6
Localizes	5
Withdraws (flexion)	4
Abnormal reflex (flexion)	3
Extension	2
None	1
Verbal response	
Oriented	5
Confused	4
Inappropriate	3
Incomprehensible	2
None	1

Adapted from Jennett B, Teasdale G, Braakman R, et al. Prognosis of patients with severe head injury. *Neurosurgery.* 1979;4:283.

Although this may be a more accurate coma scale, it is not yet extensively used.

LABORATORY EVALUATION AND TREATMENT

Initial emergency treatment for a comatose patient is the same as for all other medical emergencies. An adequate airway should be established. Endotracheal intubation and artificial ventilation may be necessary. The cardiovascular status must be evaluated promptly, and shock and blood pressure should be controlled. The temperature should be noted because hypothermia or hyperthermia may play a prominent role in the identification of the underlying problem.

▪ **SPECIAL CLINICAL POINT:** Following the establishment of an airway with stabilization of respiration and maintenance of circulation, certain laboratory tests (Table 6.4) and therapeutic measures (Table 6.5) should be undertaken. These measures can occur simultaneously with the acquisition of a medical

TABLE 6.3		
	The FOUR (Full Outline of UnResponsiveness) Score	

Eye response
4 = eyelids open or opened, tracking, or blinking to command
3 = eyelids open but not tracking
2 = eyelids closed but open to loud voice
1 = eyelids closed but open to pain
0 = eyelids remain closed with pain
Motor response
4 = thumbs-up, fist, or peace sign
3 = localizing to pain
2 = flexion response to pain
1 = extension response to pain
0 = no response to pain or generalized myoclonus status
Brainstem reflexes
4 = pupil and corneal reflexes present
3 = one pupil wide and fixed
2 = pupil or corneal reflexes absent
1 = pupil and corneal reflexes absent
0 = pupil, corneal, and cough reflexes absent
Respiration
4 = not intubated, regular breathing pattern
3 = not intubated, Cheyne–Stokes breathing pattern
2 = not intubated, irregular breathing
1 = breathes above ventilator rate
0 = breathes at ventilator rate or apnea

Adapted from Wijdicks EFM, Bamlet WR, Maramattrom BV, et al. Validation of a new coma scale: the FOUR score. *Ann Neurol.* 2005;58:585, with permission of Mayo Foundation for Medical Education and Research. All rights reserved.

history and the performance of the neurologic examination.

Blood is drawn for a complete blood count (CBC), electrolyte, glucose, calcium, blood urea nitrogen (BUN), and creatinine determinations, liver function tests, prothrombin time (PT), partial thromboplastin time (PTT), arterial blood gas determinations, and a drug/toxin screen. Urinalysis and urine drug screening are performed. An electrocardiogram and chest roentgenograms are obtained. If hypoglycemia is suspected, or if the cause of the coma is uncertain, 50 mL (25 g) of 50% dextrose in

TABLE 6.4	Tests in the Evaluation of the Comatose Patient

Blood tests
  Complete blood count
  Glucose, electrolytes, calcium, blood urea nitrogen,
    and creatinine
  Liver function studies and serum ammonia
  Coagulation studies (PT and PTT)
  Arterial blood gases
  Drug/toxin screen
  Thyroid function studies
  Adrenal function studies
  Magnesium
  Serum osmolality
  Carboxyhemoglobin
  Blood cultures
Urine tests
  Urinalysis
  Drug/toxin screen
  Urine osmolality
  Urine culture
Electrocardiogram
Imaging studies
  Chest x-ray
  Computed tomography (CT) brain scan
  Magnetic resonance imaging scan of the brain
Lumbar puncture, if indicated

PT, prothrombin time; PTT, partial thromboplastin time; CT, computed tomography.

water is given intravenously (IV). Hypoglycemia is an extremely important, potentially reversible cause of coma that, if not treated promptly, will lead to irreversible cerebral damage. For suspected opiate overdose, naloxone 0.4 mg IV is given and is repeated every 5 to 15 minutes as needed. Repeated infusions should be instituted if the response to glucose or naloxone is incomplete. Other medications can be given for specific drug overdoses when appropriate, such as intravenous flumazenil for benzodiazepine overdose. If chronic or acute ingestion of alcohol is suspected, or if there is any suggestion of malnutrition, 100 mg of thiamine should be given IV to treat or prevent the Wernicke–Korsakoff syndrome. Thiamine should be given prior to glucose administration. Correction of any other underlying metabolic process (e.g., hyponatremia) must be undertaken. Suspected bacterial meningitis should be treated empirically with appropriate antibiotics (e.g., ceftriaxone and vancomycin), and patients suspected of viral encephalitis should be given acyclovir. If there is significant evidence for increased intracranial pressure, intubation with hyperventilation and the use of mannitol or hypertonic saline must be considered. Corticosteroids may be beneficial to reduce vasogenic edema related to neoplasms, but their effect is not immediate. Neurosurgical intervention should be considered for insertion of an intracranial pressure monitor or possibly surgical decompression. Hypothermia has been shown to improve neurologic outcome and decrease mortality in postventricular fibrillation cardiac arrest patients if started immediately after the patient is stabilized.

Seizure activity may be generalized or focal and necessitates prompt treatment and a search for a cause. Nonconvulsive status epilepticus needs to be considered if the patient does not awaken after appropriate treatment with anticonvulsant drugs. Myoclonus (symmetric or asymmetric rapid, brief movements of the extremities) is frequently seen in metabolic encephalopathies and is common following anoxia (e.g., after cardiac arrest). Unfortunately, myoclonus in the setting of severe anoxic coma is often difficult to treat, and its appearance, especially if multifocal, following anoxia is a poor prognostic sign.

It is urgently necessary to proceed with further neurologic studies if the cause of the coma remains unclear. Computed tomography (CT) will demonstrate intracerebral or extracerebral blood, mass lesions, hydrocephalus, cerebral infarctions (though not always immediately), and abscesses as well as skull fractures. Magnetic resonance imaging (MRI) will show the brain in greater detail and may reveal abnormalities earlier than a CT scan, but it is often difficult to obtain an MRI on a comatose patient. Patients who are unstable will also need to be left unattended for a longer scanning time with MRI than with CT. If a CNS infection or subarachnoid hemorrhage is suspected, a lumbar puncture is indicated, although a CT scan will identify most

TABLE 6.5	
Treatment of the Comatose Patient	

Problem	Comment
Respiration	Immediately obtain an airway and consider intubation; early intubation prevents aspiration, decreases risk of transferring patient to other hospital areas, and allows for more aggressive treatment of seizures
Blood pressure	
Hypotension	Treat with fluids, volume expanders, or pressors; treat sepsis if present
Hypertension	Aggressiveness of treatment depends on etiology and level of elevation of blood pressure; different treatments for ischemic infarction or intracerebral hemorrhage; may need IV labetalol or nicardipine
Arrhythmias	May point to etiology of coma or can be a secondary factor; continuous cardiac monitoring is necessary
Hypoglycemia	50 mL of 50% dextrose in water; risk of worsening hyperglycemia outweighed by benefits of treating hypoglycemia
Thiamine deficiency	To be considered in alcoholic patients or patients who are chronically malnourished or postgastric bypass; glucose load may precipitate Wernicke encephalopathy and thus give thiamine 100 mg IV prior to giving glucose
Drug overdose	Obtain urine and blood toxicology screens; for suspected narcotic overdose, give naloxone IV (see text for details); use of other specific antidotes depends on history, clinical examination, and results of toxin screens
Increased intracranial pressure	Worsening level of coma, focal abnormalities, change in respiratory pattern, pupillary dilatation; intubation, hyperventilation, and mannitol or hypertonic saline infusion; possible intracranial pressure monitoring and assessing the need for neurosurgical intervention
Infection	Ceftriaxone and vancomycin for bacterial meningitis; acyclovir for herpes simplex encephalitis
Seizures	Correct any underlying metabolic or systemic problem; treat status epilepticus with lorazepam or diazepam; loading dose of phenytoin or fosphenytoin IV for long-term anticonvulsant effect; if seizures not controlled, consider barbiturates, valproate, levetiracetam; midazolam or propofol for refractory status epilepticus (see Chapter 25 for doses)
Post-cardiac arrest	If global ischemia from cardiac arrest, immediately institute therapeutic hypothermia
General medical and nursing care	Fluids and acid–base balance, electrolytes, observation of metabolic status; watch and treat changes in temperature (hyperthermia or hypothermia), agitation, and infections; prevent corneal abrasions and decubiti; correct any underlying metabolic or systemic problem

Modified from Weiner WJ, Shulman LM, eds. *Emergent and Urgent Neurology*. 2nd ed. Philadelphia: Lippincott Williams & Wilkins; 1999.

subarachnoid hemorrhages sufficient to cause coma. A CT scan should be obtained prior to the lumbar puncture to rule out a focal mass lesion or increased intracranial pressure.

The EEG may be helpful in the diagnosis of an overdose from sedatives (excessive fast activity), hepatic or uremic encephalopathy (triphasic waves), or psychogenic unresponsiveness (normal EEG). It is especially important in assessing for subclinical seizure activity (nonconvulsive status epilepticus) as a cause for prolonged, unexplained coma. An EEG with no evidence of cerebral activity can be reversibly noted secondary to barbiturate intoxication (and occasionally other drugs) and also with hypothermia.

PROGNOSIS

Overall prognosis for survival and functional cerebral recovery is dependent upon the etiology of the coma as well as the depth and duration of the insult and the patient's clinical course. For example, coma related to metabolic problems typically carries a better prognosis than that due to structural lesions.

Several studies that have dealt with postanoxic coma have revealed that the prognosis is generally better for the patient with spontaneous motor movements or appropriate movements in response to noxious stimuli and those with intact pupillary reactions and oculocephalic or oculovestibular responses. Patients studied after cardiopulmonary arrest reveal that depth and duration of postarrest coma correlated significantly with poor neurologic outcome. Motor unresponsiveness, lack of pupillary responses, and lack of oculocephalic and oculovestibular responses were associated with a poor prognosis for neurologic functional recovery. In addition, the prediction of survival and outcome could be based on a loss of consciousness alone within 3 days after cardiopulmonary arrest. Those patients not awakening within 72 hours had the worst prognosis.

Overall, however, it appears that the most specific findings on examination for poor prognosis are absent or extensor (decerebrate) motor responses and absent pupillary or corneal responses on day 3. Myoclonic status epilepticus also appears to signify a similar poor prognosis. Elevated blood levels of neuron-specific enolase (NSE) and the absence of somatosensory evoked potentials also have been found to suggest very poor outcomes.

Recent studies show that early induced hypothermia following cardiac arrest improves survival and function at 6 months.

Prognosis for patients with metabolic encephalopathies or drug overdose cannot be based solely on the level of consciousness. For example, patients with barbiturate overdose in deep coma may have no spontaneous respiration, absent oculovestibular responses, and absent cerebral activity on the EEG, yet have a complete neurologic recovery.

WHEN TO REFER THE PATIENT TO A NEUROLOGIST

A neurologist should be consulted for almost all comatose patients, especially when the etiology of the coma is uncertain. The neurologist will aid in arriving at a diagnosis, localize the abnormalities, and assist in the treatment of the underlying cause of coma. In addition, the neurologist will be able to help assess prognosis for survival and functional recovery (e.g., ability to function independently). This information also will enable the family and all treating physicians to make important further decisions regarding the patient's medical care.

Always Remember

- Coma occurs due to bilateral, diffuse cerebral hemisphere dysfunction, upper brainstem dysfunction, or a combination of the two.
- The goal of the neurologic examination is to determine the presence, location, and nature of the underlying process creating the decreased level of consciousness and also to aid in prognostication.
- Every patient who appears to be in coma should be assessed for the possibility of the locked-in syndrome.
- Overall prognosis for survival and functional cerebral recovery is dependent upon the etiology of the coma, the severity and duration of the insult, and the patient's clinical course.

QUESTIONS AND DISCUSSION

1. A 24-year-old man is brought to the emergency room with a decreased level of consciousness that developed over several hours. On arrival, he is intubated for diminished respirations. Examination reveals no response to verbal command, including the command to blink his eyes. He has small, reactive pupils (2 mm), intact horizontal oculocephalic reflexes, and no motor response to painful stimuli. Which of the following is the most likely etiology of this patient's condition?
   A. Left middle cerebral artery infarct
   B. Metabolic encephalopathy
   C. Pontine hemorrhage
   D. Pontine infarction
   E. Right hemispheric intracerebral hemorrhage

The correct answer is B. Metabolic encephalopathies can cause profound coma with preserved pupillary responses. The gradual onset of coma is also consistent with a metabolic process but is not specific for this cause. A pontine lesion could also cause small reactive pupils but would typically be associated with impaired horizontal eye movements. In addition to the profound coma with preserved pupillary reflexes, the lack of other lateralizing findings makes other structural lesions unlikely.

2. Which of the following findings is most likely to be seen in a patient with a right hemispheral destructive lesion?
   A. Lack of caloric responses, eyes conjugately deviated to the left, and left hemiplegia
   B. Right eye deviated to the right, left eye midline, and left hemiplegia
   C. Eyes conjugately deviated to the right, left hemiplegia, and intact caloric responses
   D. Ocular bobbing and left hemiplegia
   E. Present caloric responses, eyes conjugately deviated to the left, and left hemiplegia

The correct answer is C. Eyes "look toward" a destructive hemispheral lesion. Caloric responses are preserved because the pathway for the oculovestibular responses does not involve hemispheral connections. Eyes "look away" from the side of a destructive pontine lesion.

3. A 64-year-old man suffers a 10-minute out-of-hospital cardiac arrest. Examination 2 days after the event shows that he is comatose, with no response to commands. He has roving horizontal eye movements, intact pupillary responses, and bilateral decorticate posturing to noxious stimuli. Which of the following is the most likely localization of his neurologic dysfunction?
   A. Bilateral cerebral hemispheres
   B. Medulla
   C. Midbrain
   D. Pons
   E. Right cerebral hemisphere

The correct answer is A. This patient's examination is consistent with intact brainstem function but severely impaired bilateral hemispheric dysfunction, typical of patients after severe anoxic–ischemic encephalopathies due to cardiac arrest.

4. A 76-year-old woman develops the sudden onset of unresponsiveness while eating dinner with her family. Examination in the emergency department shows small reactive pupils, brisk spontaneous downward movements of her eyes, absent oculocephalic reflexes, and bilateral decerebrate (extensor) posturing. She appears to blink her eyes to command. Which of the following is the most likely etiology of her condition?
   A. Diffuse cerebral anoxia
   B. Hypoglycemia
   C. Left middle cerebral artery infarct
   D. Pontine infarct
   E. Right basal ganglia hemorrhage

The correct answer is D. This patient's signs and symptoms are most compatible with the "locked-in" syndrome due to a high pontine lesion (typically an infarct) causing quadriplegia and impaired lateral eye movements; these patients are actually awake and alert but can communicate only with vertical eye movements and blinking. This patient's finding of ocular bobbing is also commonly seen in this condition.

SUGGESTED READING

Bates D. Predicting recovery from medical coma. *Br J Hosp Med*. 1985;33:276.

Bernard SA, Gray TW, Buist MD, et al. Treatment of comatose survivors of out-of-hospital cardiac arrest with induced hypothermia. *N Engl J Med*. 2002;346:557.

Buettner WW, Zee DS. Vestibular testing in comatose patients. *Arch Neurol*. 1989;46:561.

Fisher CM. The neurological examination of the comatose patient. *Acta Neurol Scand*. 1969;45(suppl 36):1.

Hamel MB, Goldman L, Teno J, et al. Identification of comatose patients at high risk for death or severe disability. *JAMA*. 1995;273:1842.

Hoesch RE, Geocadin RG. Therapeutic hypothermia for global and focal ischemic brain injury—a cool way to improve neurologic outcomes. *Neurologist*. 2007;13:331.

Hoffman RS, Goldfrank LR. The poisoned patient with altered consciousness: controversies in the use of a "coma cocktail." *JAMA*. 1995;274:562.

Jennett B, Teasdale G, Braakman R, et al. Prognosis of patients with severe head injury. *Neurosurgery*. 1979;4:283.

Levy DE, Caronna JJ, Singer BH, et al. Predicting outcome from hypoxic-ischemic coma. *JAMA*. 1985;253:1420.

Lewis SL, Topel JL. Coma. In: Weiner WJ, Shulman LM, eds. *Emergent and Urgent Neurology*. 2nd ed. Philadelphia: Lippincott Williams & Wilkins; 1999.

Posner JB, Saper CB, Schiff ND, et al. *Plum and Posner's Diagnosis of Stupor and Coma*. 4th ed. New York: Oxford University Press; 2007.

Rabinstein AA, Atkinson JL, Wijdicks EF. Emergency craniotomy in patients worsening due to expanded cerebral hematoma: to what purpose? *Neurology*. 2002;58(9):1367.

Wijdicks EFM, Bamlet WR, Maramattom BV, et al. Validation of a new coma scale: the FOUR score. *Ann Neurol*. 2005;58:585.

Wijdicks EFM, Hijdra A, Young GB, et al. Practice parameter: prediction of outcome in comatose survivors after cardiopulmonary resuscitation (an evidence-based review): report of the Quality Standards Subcommittee of the American Academy of Neurology. *Neurology*. 2006;67:203.

Wijdicks EFM, Parisi JE, Sharbrough FW. Prognostic value of myoclonus status in comatose survivors of cardiac arrest. *Ann Neurol*. 1994;35:239.

Young GB, Ropper AH, Bolton CF. *Coma and Impaired Consciousness*. New York: McGraw-Hill; 1998.

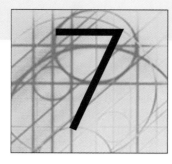

7

Cerebrovascular Disease

ROGER E. KELLEY AND ALIREZA MINAGAR

key points

- Stroke is easily recognized in the older patient with risk factor who presents with sudden onset of a focal neurologic deficit.

- Stroke prevention remains the most effective management since interventional therapy in acute ischemic stroke (the most common type) remains limited.

- Recent antiplatelet trials advanced an evidence-based approach toward secondary stroke prevention.

- Anticoagulant therapy is primarily utilized for deep venous thrombosis prophylaxis in patients with acute ischemic stroke.

- Anticoagulant therapy has a potential role in ischemic stroke prevention if there is a documented cardioembolic source, in hypercoagulable conditions, in cerebral sinovenous thrombosis, and perhaps in cerebrovascular dissection.

- There is a growing literature on interventional therapy in acute ischemic stroke, but intravenous recombinant tissue plasminogen activator, initiated within 3 hours of presentation, remains the only FDA-approved medication.

- Endovascular techniques are becoming increasingly utilized for cerebrovascular anomalies such as aneurysms and arteriovenous malformations.

Cerebrovascular disease includes both primary ischemic stroke (large artery thrombotic, e.g., lacunar-type, embolic, and hemodynamic, small artery thrombotic, e.g., watershed-type, vasculitis-induced infarction, vascular dissection-induced infarction, and sinovenous thrombotic infarction) and hemorrhagic stroke (primary intracerebral hemorrhage [ICH] and subarachnoid hemorrhage [SAH]). In addition, one can see hemorrhagic

TABLE 7.1	Major Etiologies of Stroke

Primary Ischemic	Primary Hemorrhagic
Thrombotic	Hypertensive hemorrhage
Large artery	Aneurysmal rupture
Small artery (lacunar)	Bleeding from an AVM
Sinovenous thrombosis	Bleeding diathesis
Vascular dissection	Bleeding related to neoplasm
Mechanical obstruction, e.g., surgical complication	Cerebral amyloid angiopathy
Hemodynamic, e.g., hypotension	Iatrogenic, i.e., related to antithrombotic therapy
Embolic	Septic aneurysm
Cardiogenic	
Aortic arch atheromata	
Artery-to-artery	
Arteritis	

transformation of an initially ischemic stroke and this is one of the major concerns with the use of either recombinant tissue plasminogen activator (rt-PA) or anticoagulant therapy in acute ischemic stroke. Stroke, which is a generic term for damage to the central nervous system (CNS) on a vascular basis, is a common presentation in the emergency department. Most strokes are readily diagnosed on the basis of a sudden constellation of neurologic deficits in a patient with well-recognized risk factors for cerebrovascular disease.

It is estimated that there are roughly 750,000 first or recurrent strokes in the United States per year. This translates to approximately 250 stroke patients per 100,000 per year. The frequency of stroke type varies depending on the patient population. For example, a retirement community is more likely to have patients of advanced age with a relatively high incidence of atherosclerotic disease seen in tandem with hypertension, diabetes mellitus, hyperlipidemia, and coronary artery disease. A hospital in a community of young and middle-aged people will tend to see more esoteric causes of stroke, such as lupus vasculitis, hypercoagulable states, sinovenous occlusive disease as a complication of pregnancy, stroke related to oral contraceptive use, paradoxical cerebral

embolism related to an atrial septal defect, and vascular dissection (which often has trauma as an initiating factor).

Roughly 80% to 85% of all stroke is primary ischemic and 15% to 20% is primary hemorrhagic. Of the ischemic strokes, approximately 50% to 60% are large artery thrombotic; 20% are small artery thrombotic (lacunar-type); 15% to 20% are cardiogenic or artery-to-artery emboli; and 5% to 10% are less common etiologies such as vasculitis, dissection, septic or nonseptic emboli, or sinovenous occlusive disease. Approximately 5% to 6% of all strokes are SAH, usually related to rupture of a cerebral aneurysm or bleeding from an arteriovenous malformation (AVM), whereas 10% to 15 % are primary ICH. The major stroke etiologies are listed in Table 7.1.

■ SPECIAL CLINICAL POINT: Determination of stroke mechanism is important since it has a direct impact on management.

IDENTIFICATION OF THE STROKE-PRONE INDIVIDUAL

It has become increasingly important to identify patients with risk factors for stroke (Table 7.2) because there is an increasing armamentarium of

TABLE 7.2

Risk Factors for Stroke

Major Risk Factors	Minor Risk Factors
Age	Hypercholesterolemia
Sex	Oral contraceptives
Race	Migraine
Genetic predisposition	Obesity
TIA/prior stroke	Physical inactivity
Hypertension	Mitral valve prolapse
Acute myocardial infarction	Patent foramen ovale
with thrombus	Bacterial endocarditis
Diabetes mellitus	Marantic endocarditis
Cigarette smoking	Sick sinus syndrome
Valvular heart disease	Aortic arch atheromatia
Atrial fibrillation	Polycythemia
Dilated cardiomyopathy	Bleeding diathesis
Peripheral vascular disease	Sympathomimetic agents including cocaine
Sickle cell anemia	Hyperhomocysteinemia
Hypercoagulable state	Thrombocytosis

potential therapies to reduce stroke risk. Conversely, the interventional therapies for acute stroke remain quite limited. Transient ischemic attack (TIA) is a warning of ischemic stroke, and it can precede up to 15% of all stroke. It represents an opportunity to identify a patient who is at particular risk for ischemic stroke in an effort to institute effective prevention. Prior stroke and TIA are major identifiers of stroke-prone individuals. In a study of patients with TIA presenting to the emergency room (ER), 10.5% of patients returned to the ER within 90 days with a stroke and half of these events occurred within 2 days of the TIA. The risk of recurrent stroke is very much reflective of the stroke mechanism and how aggressively risk factors are managed. The risk of recurrent stroke is 10% to 12% per year, but this can be impacted by optimal blood pressure management, aggressive control of hyperlipidemia, smoking cessation, and an effective diet and exercise programs.

■ **SPECIAL CLINICAL POINT: A transient ischemic attack (TIA), when properly recognized, represents an important opportunity to effectively intervene before the stroke occurs.**

The risk of stroke increases exponentially with age, and the risk is higher for males. African Americans appear to be more susceptible to stroke than Caucasians. For example, intracranial stenosis, which can account for up to 10% of all ischemic stroke, tends to be more prevalent in African Americans, Hispanics, and Orientals. In contrast to African Americans, Caucasians appear to be more susceptible to symptomatic extracranial carotid stenosis. Naturally, the presence of contributing factors to atherosclerosis, such as hypertension, hyperlipidemia, diabetes mellitus, familial predisposition, and smoking consumption impact on stroke type and frequency. In addition, cumulative cardiac factors can play a major role in predisposition to cardioembolic stroke. An example of this is atrial fibrillation. Lone atrial fibrillation (AF) in a person under 60 years of age is not a significant risk factor for stroke. However, the coexistence of AF with such factors as valvular heart disease, ischemic cardiomyopathy, hypertension, or prior embolic events translates into a much greater risk of cardioembolic stroke.

■ **SPECIAL CLINICAL POINT:** So-called "lone atrial fibrillation" (atrial fibrillation in a patient less than 60 years of age with a structurally normal heart and no risk factors for stroke) is associated with a stroke risk that is essentially that of an age-matched individual without atrial fibrillation.

CLINICAL EVALUATION

The history is obviously a vital aspect of the diagnostic assessment of patients presenting with stroke-like symptoms. The most common presentation for stroke is the sudden onset of focal neurologic deficit(s) in a patient with risk factors for stroke, with increasing age being a particularly important indicator. The term "stroke in the young" promotes recognition of patients 45 years of age or younger who do not have a readily identifiable predisposing factor. In such circumstances, more esoteric explanations for the stroke should be sought such as lupus vasculitis, primary CNS vasculitis, drug-induced vascular compromise, moyamoya disease, sickle cell disease, paradoxical cerebral embolus, meningovascular syphilis, and sinovenous thrombosis and hypercoagulable conditions.

Proper recognition of stroke has become even more important with the advent of thrombolytic therapy, specifically rt-PA, which must be administered intravenously within 3 hours of symptom onset. This is the only agent presently available for acute ischemic stroke. To be eligible for rt-PA, patients need to be assessed, have certain blood tests performed, and have a noncontrast computed tomography (CT) brain scan performed within the 3-hour time window before the agent can be infused (Fig. 7.1). The initial history must place emphasis on determination of the exact time that the symptoms began and pertinent past medical factors such as prior bleeding, recent surgery, or trauma that might enhance the bleeding complication rate with rt-PA. It is important to note that patients who wake up with their deficits have to have the onset assigned to the time that they were last neurolog-

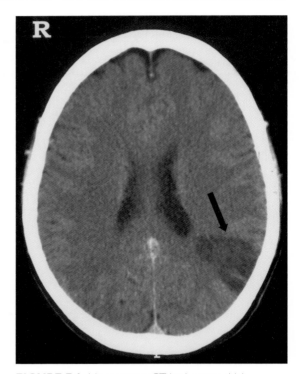

FIGURE 7.1 Noncontrast CT brain scan which demonstrates an infarct *(arrow)* that has already evolved. This would mitigate against the use of recombinant tissue plasminogen activator (rt-PA) in such a circumstance, as there is already hypodensity implying already infarcted tissue and the onset would be presumably well beyond 3 hours based on this scan. The distribution of the infarct is the left watershed region between the middle cerebral artery and posterior cerebral artery that can imply a hemodynamic mechanism.

ically unaffected. For example, if they woke up with a stroke at 6 AM and were last awake at 11 PM the evening before, then it has to be assumed that the stroke occurred just after 11 PM. However, if the patient had gone to the bathroom at 5 AM, and they were perfectly fine, and then went back to bed and awakened at 6 AM with the stroke, it can be assumed that the stroke occurred just after 5 AM. This would translate into a 2-hour window of opportunity for treatment with rt-PA (i.e., 6 to 8 AM).

The use of rt-PA mandates a more standardized approach to the neurologic evaluation for a patient with acute stroke, and this, fortunately, has been extended to most stroke patients even if they are not candidates for the medication. For example, it is important to obtain a CT brain scan at the time of presentation to readily distinguish a primary ischemic stroke from a primary hemorrhagic stroke. Generally, contrast is not necessary unless there are clinical concerns that the patient might have a tumor or abscess instead of a stroke. It is important to recognize that the CT brain scan has a sensitivity of 90% to 95% for the detection of SAH. Therefore, clinical suspicion for SAH, even with a negative CT brain scan, mandates the performance of a lumbar puncture unless there are contraindications. In addition to the CT brain scan, routine immediate blood work includes a complete blood count (CBC), platelet count, metabolic profile, prothrombin time (PT)/international normalization ratio (INR), and partial thromboplastin time (PTT).

Furthermore, a more standardized approach to the neurologic examination has been adopted to quantitate the degree of deficit in a more objective and reproducible pattern. This is especially pertinent for patients who are potentially eligible for rt-PA. The National Institutes of Health (NIH) Stroke Scale is used to provide such standardization. This is in recognition that rt-PA should only be considered for patients with a significant neurologic deficit at the time of presentation; rt-PA should not be used if the patient is rapidly improving. There are potentially greater risks of complications of rt-PA and a reduced chance of benefit from therapy when the patient has a high score on their NIH Stroke Scale. This scale correlates with severity of neurologic deficit.

■ **SPECIAL CLINICAL POINT: The greater the time from the onset of stroke, the greater the evolution of an infarction pattern by CT brain scan, the greater the degree of neurologic deficit, the poorer the control of blood pressure, the higher the admission blood glucose, as well as possibly the greater the age of the patient, the greater the likelihood of hemorrhagic transformation with rt-PA.**

There are certain presentation characteristics that help identify the stroke mechanism (Table 7.3). For example, cerebral embolus, as opposed to thrombosis, tends to occur with maximum neurologic deficit at onset. There can be syncope and/or seizure at the time of presentation due to the sudden cessation of the circulation. Involvement of different vascular territories and a documented source of cardiogenic embolus

TABLE 7.3 Features of Thrombotic Versus Embolic Stroke	
Thrombotic	**Embolic**
Stepwise progression	Sudden onset of maximal deficit
Premonitory TIA	Source of cardiogenic embolus
Atherosclerotic disease	Multiple vascular territory involvement
Carotid distribution infarct	Association with syncope at onset
Middle cerebral artery	Association with seizure at onset
Anterior cerebral artery	Hemorrhagic transformation of the infarct
Penetrating artery distribution, i.e., lacunar-type	Branch occlusion pattern on brain scan or angiography
Other evidence of large vessel disease	Embolic involvement of other organs
	Severe deficit at onset followed by rapid resolution

are other features strongly supportive of an embolic mechanism. Conversely, thrombotic stroke tends to occur in a stepwise fashion, is reported to be more commonly associated with premonitory TIA, and is associated with risk factors for atherosclerosis or lipohyalinosis. Embolic events tend to result in cerebral artery branch occlusions.

DIAGNOSTIC EVALUATION

Table 7.4 outlines the first-, second-, and third-tier diagnostic studies that are part of the stroke evaluation. The first tier represents the routine studies that are performed on any patient presenting with symptoms of TIA or stroke. Obviously the clinical picture will affect the choice and speed with which the study is performed. For example, a patient presenting with new-onset TIA should undergo immediate evaluation of the potential ischemic mechanism in an effort to intervene before a stroke occurs.

The same is true for relatively minor stroke associated with resolution of signs and symptoms within days to weeks. However, there is usually little to offer the patient who is moribund from a stroke.

■ **SPECIAL CLINICAL POINT: It is important to determine whether or not particular testing will impact management. This will help avoid unnecessary costs as well as testing that may be associated with risks that are best avoided.**

The CT brain scan is often the only neuroimaging study that is necessary for acute stroke evaluation. Contrast is usually not necessary, and this represents a practical and cost-effective approach for most patients. However, there are certain patients in whom a magnetic resonance imaging (MRI) brain scan may provide worthwhile information that may affect patient management—for example, in the patient with an atypical or fluctuating clinical picture with evidence of brainstem or cerebellar involvement an MRI typically provides a much better image

TABLE 7.4		
Hierarchy of Studies in Acute Ischemic Stroke		

First tier	**Third tier (if clinically indicated)**
Noncontrast CT brain scan	Cardiac stress test
CBC, platelet count, PT, INR, and PTT	Transesophageal echocardiogram
Serum chemistry profile EKG	Cerebral arteriography
Fasting lipid profile	HIV test
	Syphilis testing
Second tier (if clinically indicated)	Sickle cell prep
Contrast-enhanced CT brain scan	Bleeding time
MRI brain scan	Platelet function studies
Carotid/vertebral duplex scan	Special clotting studies
Transcranial Doppler ultrasonography	Fasting homocysteine level
Transthoracic echocardiogram	C-reactive protein
Holter monitor	Proteins C and S levels
Magnetic resonance angiography and/or	Proteins C and S levels
venography vs. CT angiography	Antiphospholipid antibodies
Blood cultures	Genetic testing for MELAS (mitochondrial myopathy,
ESR	lactic acidosis, and stroke-like episodes), Fabry
Lumbar puncture	disease, CADASIL (cerebral autosomal-dominant
Urine drug screen	arteriopathy with subcortical strokes and
	leukoencephalopathy), etc.

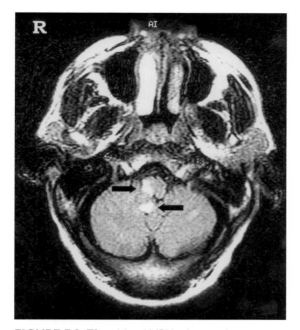

Diffusion-weighted imaging (DWI) as a component of the MRI brain scan in acute ischemic stroke allows detection of cellular injury and cytotoxic edema (Fig. 7.3). MR perfusion imaging can identify brain tissue that is susceptible to infarction but that is in a potentially salvageable state. Thus, a so-called "perfusion–diffusion mismatch" might be of value in identifying acute ischemic stroke patients who are most likely to respond to rt-PA. However, such an approach requires ready availability of these MRI techniques and immediate reading of images. Any delay associated with obtaining these studies further prolongs the initiation of rt-PA, which limits the usefulness of perfusion–diffusion images. In situations in which there is some difficulty in distinguishing an ischemic stroke from another process, the finding of hypointensity on the

FIGURE 7.2 T2-weighted MRI brain scan that demonstrates signal hyperintensity with the anterior arrow pointing to a right brainstem infarct and the posterior arrow showing infarction within the cerebellum.

of this area and can help to confirm the clinical impression (Fig. 7.2). Other potential advantages of MRI include the greater safety of using contrast-enhanced MRI, as opposed to contrast-enhanced CT scan. In addition, magnetic resonance angiography (MRA) and venography (MRV) have the ability to provide a reasonably accurate view of the extracranial and intracranial circulation, which often provides information complementary to the MRI. CT angiography (CTA) appears to have better definition than MRA in most circumstances. However, CTA requires intravenous infusion of iodine-based contrast. These less-invasive studies vary in quality between institutions and do not yet have the accuracy of the "gold standard" for the evaluation of the cerebral circulation, which remains intra-arterial cerebral arteriography.

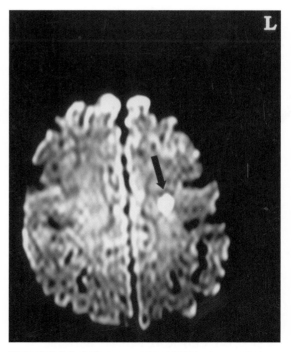

FIGURE 7.3 Diffusion-weighted MRI brain scan that demonstrates an acute left hemispheric superficial cortical infarct (arrow).

apparent diffusion coefficient (ADC) image that correlates with hyperintensity on the DWI, in the same region, supports acute ischemia (see Chapter 4, Fundamentals of Neuroradiology).

Cardiac evaluation is of value in the assessment of potential cardiogenic sources of embolism. This can include imaging of the aortic arch where atheromata have the potential to break off and enter the brain circulation. However, one must factor in the costs versus benefits of extensive cardiac evaluation unless the results are going to definitely affect management of the patient. Specifically, transesophageal echocardiography (TEE) and long-term cardiac monitoring are reserved for patients with a reasonable chance of having a potential cardiogenic source of embolism and who should be considered for anticoagulant therapy. The potential coexistence of coronary artery disease in patients with ischemic stroke must be considered because this association is not uncommon. Cardiac stress testing might be appropriate in some patients with cerebral events.

■ **SPECIAL CLINICAL POINT: There is clearly an indication for cardiac evaluation in stroke since it can impact management and has the distinct potential to prevent recurrent stroke.**

Cryptogenic stroke might require assessment with longer term cardiac telemetry in an effort to identify paroxysmal AF. TEE usually is restricted to patients who have unexplained stroke (i.e., with no risk factors for stroke). TEE is useful when there is concern about a possible patent foramen ovale in a patient with the possibility of paradoxical cerebral embolus. TEE is useful to assess the left atrium and left atrial appendage and to more effectively assess the aortic arch for atheromata. Vegetations, either septic or nonseptic, as well as thrombus formation tend to be better detected with TEE. Concern about possible bacterial endocarditis mandates blood cultures.

■ **SPECIAL CLINICAL POINT: Bacterial endocarditis is in the differential diagnosis of stroke especially in patients who are at increased risk and for stroke patients with a fever and/or newly detected heart murmur.**

An erythrocyte sedimentation rate can be useful for the detection of endocarditis, atrial myxoma, or a vasculitic process. Syphilis serology and human immunodeficiency virus testing also can be important in susceptible individuals presenting with stroke-like symptoms.

Evaluation for a hypercoagulable state is predicated on the clinical picture of prior thromboembolic events, a positive family history, a history of spontaneous abortions, and unexplained ischemic stroke in a young person. Antiphospholipid antibody titers are particularly important when there is a well-documented hypercoagulable state or in patients with systemic lupus erythematosus in association with ischemic stroke. Protein C, protein S, and antithrombin III deficiencies are evaluated in young patients with unexplained stroke, but the yield tends to be quite low unless there is a history of thromboembolic events and/or a positive family history. Thrombocythemia, with a platelet count greater than 1,000,000/μL, polycythemia, and sickle cell disease are additional hematologic factors associated with ischemic stroke. Conversely, a low platelet count or factor deficiency can result in a bleeding diathesis with secondary ICH.

Noninvasive vascular imaging includes carotid and vertebral duplex ultrasound, which combines the anatomic information of B-mode scanning with the physiologic information of Doppler and transcranial Doppler ultrasonography (TCD), which allows assessment of the flow velocities of the intracranial major arteries, as well as MRA and CTA. However, routine intra-arterial cerebral arteriography remains the "gold standard" for the most accurate information about the extracranial and intracranial circulation. This is useful for the detection of intracranial or extracranial vascular stenosis, possible vasculitis, vascular dissection, the presence of an aneurysm, or the presence of an AVM. Moyamoya disease, with progressive occlusion of the intracranial vasculature, is another entity that requires assessment with angiography.

Second- and third-tier studies are performed in an effort to prevent a subsequent event. The plasma homocysteine level and C-reactive protein (CRP) level also can help to identify individuals with an enhanced risk of ischemic stroke. Both elevated levels of homocysteine and CRP have been implicated. The finding of a relationship between CRP levels and stroke risk raises the possibility that inflammation is a potential mechanism for ischemic events.

CLINICAL ASPECTS OF ISCHEMIC STROKE AND TIA

Presentation and Localization

Of particular importance is the distinction between carotid distribution versus vertebrobasilar distribution ischemia. Carotid endarterectomy is of value for stroke prevention in symptomatic patients when carotid stenosis ipsilateral to the involved cerebral hemisphere is demonstrated. However, it is not expected that prophylactic carotid endarterectomy would be of any value for a patient presenting with vertebrobasilar distribution symptoms who also was found to have moderate or severe carotid stenosis. The features that help to distinguish carotid distribution symptoms of stroke or TIA from vertebrobasilar distribution are outlined in Table 7.5.

Middle cerebral artery (MCA) infarction typically results in contralateral weakness with greater involvement of the face and arm than the leg. Involvement of the dominant hemisphere is often associated with aphasia. Expressive aphasia (Broca) is related to involvement of the foot of the inferior frontal gyrus of the dominant hemisphere, which abuts the motor strip. Expressive aphasia is usually associated with significant contralateral hemiparesis. On the other hand, receptive aphasia (Wernicke) is related to involvement of the posterior aspect of the superior temporal gyrus of the dominant hemisphere. It is uncommon to have contralateral weakness with involvement of this vascular territory and the patient will present with impaired comprehension and with speech output that can have a "word salad" quality. Involvement of the superior and inferior division of the MCA, usually seen with MCA stem involvement, will typically result in a global or so-called "mixed" aphasia with pronounced contralateral hemiparesis and hemisensory deficit. Involvement of the anterior cerebral artery typically causes contralateral hemiparesis with the leg more involved than the arm or face. Involvement of the posterior cerebral artery territory results in contralateral homonymous hemianopsia often with little, if any, associated motor or sensory findings.

TABLE 7.5 — Carotid Versus Vertebrobasilar Distribution of Stroke/TIA Symptoms

Carotid Distribution	Vertebrobasilar Distribution
Aphasia	Bilateral visual loss
Transient monocular blindness (amaurosis fugax)	Ataxia
	Quadriparesis
Hemiparesis	Perioral numbness
Hemiparesis	"Crossed" sensory or motor deficits
Hemisensory deficit	Two or more of the following:
Homonymous hemianopsia in combination with motor or sensory deficit	Vertigo, syncope, diplopia, nausea, dysarthria, and dysphagia
	Drop attack especially when seen in association with a sensory or motor deficit

Vertebrobasilar arterial involvement can be recognized by so-called "crossed" findings such as involvement of one side of the face and the other side of the body. Isolated symptoms such as vertigo or diplopia rarely represent vertebrobasilar stroke, but a constellation of findings such as dysarthria, ataxia, and gaze paresis are typical findings of vertebrobasilar insufficiency in susceptible individuals.

Small vessel thrombotic (lacunar-type) stroke (Fig. 7.4) can have a number of presentations. However, the most common include five so-called "classic" lacunar presentations: pure motor stroke, pure sensory stroke, hemiparesis–hemiataxia, clumsy-hand dysarthria, and sensorimotor. The hallmark is lack of cortical involvement, and there are characteristic locations such as the posterior limb of the internal capsule for pure motor stroke and the thalamus or the centrum semiovale for pure

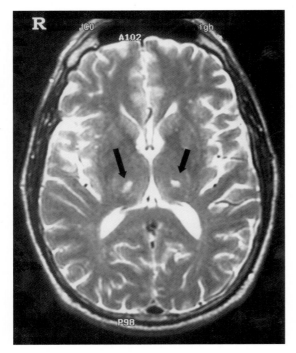

FIGURE 7.4 T2-weighted MRI brain scan that demonstrates bilateral thalamic lacunar-type infarcts (*arrows*).

sensory stroke. A clue to pure motor stroke related to lacunar-type infarction of the posterior limb of the internal carotid artery is a contralateral symmetrical pure motor involvement with relatively equal involvement of the face, arm, trunk, and leg.

■ **SPECIAL CLINICAL POINT: Lacunar-type stroke accounts for up to 20% of stroke and is primarily an in situ thrombotic process that does not necessarily require an extensive evaluation of a cardiogenic source of embolus or evaluation for carotid surgery.**

OPTIMIZATION OF ISCHEMIC STROKE PREVENTION

Atherosclerosis is a primary factor in the pathogenesis of ischemic stroke. It has been clearly established that the formation of atherosclerotic plaque correlates with stroke risk. Measures that interfere with the deposition of plaque material are the most effective means for reducing the incidence of stroke and TIA. Lipohyalinosis of the small penetrating arteries, with secondary occlusion, is the most common mechanism of lacunar-type stroke. Effective blood pressure control is of particular importance for both primary and secondary stroke prevention. Two agents identified for their potential in preventing secondary stroke are ramipril and perindopril plus a diuretic.

Statins are established for the primary prevention of stroke in certain high-risk patients. Statins, and other lipid-lowering agents, have been associated with a 25% relative risk reduction in fatal and nonfatal stroke. However, there has been an increase in the risk of primary hemorrhagic stroke with lipid lowering associated with statin therapy. Smoking cessation is of utmost importance.

Antithrombotic agents can be of benefit in stroke prevention, as well as in acute ischemic stroke treatment, but one must weigh risk versus benefit in terms of choice of therapy. For example, aspirin was not found to be of benefit in the primary prevention of stroke in middle-aged healthy men. However, some benefit was observed in women for primary stroke prevention. Warfarin is recognized as the agent of choice in the primary prevention of stroke in patients with a documented source of cardioembolic source such as higher risk AF. Warfarin also has a place in the management of certain conditions associated with a hypercoagulable state.

Aspirin is the first line of antiplatelet therapy for protection against ischemic stroke in patients with symptoms of stroke who do not have a cardiogenic source of embolism or a hypercoagulable state. For patients who are symptomatic on aspirin (aspirin failures), alternative antiplatelet agents should be considered. The choices may include combination of low-dose aspirin–high-dose dipyridamole (25/200 mg twice a day) or clopidogrel at 75 mg/day. The decision about substituting an antiplatelet agent, and which agent to use, often is based on several factors including cost, purported efficacy, and risk of side effects. In a recent study, there was no evidence of superiority of low-dose aspirin–long-acting higher-dose dipyridamole over clopidogrel in prevention against recurrent ischemic stroke. In terms of clopidogrel, which has marginal superiority over aspirin, at best, for ischemic stroke prevention, two studies of the combination of aspirin and clopidogrel revealed no benefit for stroke prevention and an enhanced risk of bleeding complications. Table 7.6 outlines the potential prophylactic medications available.

Carotid endarterectomy is the most effective means of preventing stroke in patients with symptomatic high-grade carotid stenosis. There is possibly some potential benefit for patients with 50% to 69% symptomatic stenosis, but the greatest benefit is in those with 70% to 99% stenosis. Careful patient selection and risk versus benefit analysis is required. Carotid angioplasty is an option for patients who have unacceptable surgical risk but who clearly may benefit from correction of their stenosis. This is an evolving procedure, but it may be particularly attractive for certain patients with asymptomatic carotid stenosis where the potential

TABLE 7.6 Pharmacologic Treatment Approaches for Stroke Prevention

Antihypertensives
 Ramipril
 Perindopril with diuretic
 Alternative antihypertensives
Antiplatelet agents
 Aspirin 81 mg to 325 mg/day
 Clopidogrel 75 mg/day
 Ticlopidine 250 mg with meals b.i.d.
 Aspirin/dipyridamole 25/200 mg b.i.d.
Anticoagulant therapy
 Warfarin
Lipid-lowering agents
 Statins
 Cholestyramine
 Ezetimibe
 Fenofibrate
 Chlofibrate
 Niacin
 Gemfibizol
 Fenofibrate
 Colesvelam
 Colestipol
Smoking cessation agents
 Buproprion
 Varenicline
 Nicotine administration devices

benefits of endarterectomy do not justify the risks.

ACUTE ISCHEMIC STROKE INTERVENTION

rt-PA is approved for acute ischemic stroke in patients who fulfill the criteria for its use (Table 7.7). It is associated with a 30% increased chance of full neurologic recovery at 3 and 12 months compared to placebo. It is most effective when given early, and the more normal the CT brain scan, the more likelihood of benefit. Conversely, the greater the evolution of the infarct by CT brain scan, the less likelihood of a good response and the greater the chance of ICH as a complication. This is seen

TABLE 7.7

Indications and Contraindications to the Use of Recombinant Tissue Plasminogen Activator for Acute Ischemic Stroke

Indications	Contraindications
Evaluation and management within 3 hours	Hemorrhage on CT brain scan
Persistent significant neurologic deficit on exam	Uncontrolled hypertension with persistent systolic
Absence of severe anemia, severely abnormal blood	BP >185 and diastolic BP >110 mm Hg
glucose, or other severe metabolic disturbance	History of prior intracranial hemorrhage
History of bleeding diathesis	Platelet count <100,000 mL
Patient or caregiver amenable to treatment with	Active anticoagulant therapy
rt-PA which may include informed consent	Active internal bleeding
No associated seizure activity at onset	Recent serious head trauma
No recent arterial or lumbar puncture	Recent ischemic stroke
	Recent intracranial surgery
	Clinical suspicion for subarachnoid hemorrhage
	Recent myocardial infarction

in approximately 6.4% of patients treated with rt-PA for acute ischemic stroke. The percentage might be higher in older individuals, but benefit can still be seen (Flow Chart 7.1).

Aspirin at a dose of 160 to 300 mg/day appears indicated in acute ischemic stroke as long as there is no medical contraindication. The primary benefit is to reduce the risk of early recurrent stroke. Of note, neither aspirin nor anticoagulant therapy should be given within 24 hours of the use of rt-PA to help protect against the 6.4% risk

of hemorrhagic transformation of the initially ischemic infarct (Fig. 7.5). The primary indication for anticoagulant therapy in acute ischemic stroke is for deep venous thrombosis prevention related to immobility from the stroke.

■ **SPECIAL CLINICAL POINT: The use of 160 to 320 mg/day of aspirin is recognized as having the potential to positively impact outcome.**

There are certain standard measures for acute stroke management (Table 7.8). These include

FLOW CHART 7.1. APPROACH TO USE OF RECOMBINANT TISSUE PLASMINOGEN ACTIVATOR IN ACUTE ISCHEMIC STROKE.

Presentation → Initial assessment → Review of potential → Dosing
                                    contraindications

Within 3 hours

Noncontrast CT brain scan, CBC, platelet count, PT/INR, PTT, and EKG

No bleed by CT scan, No bleeding diathesis, No recent MI or stroke, No prior intracerebral hemorrhage, No severe hyper- or hypoglycemia, No recent surgical intervention, No seizure at onset

0.9 mg/kg up to 90 mg IV with 10% over 1 minute and the rest over 1 hour, no antiplatelets or anticoagulants for 24 hours

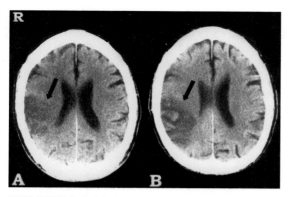

FIGURE 7.5 A: Noncontrast CT brain scan that reveals an acute right middle cerebral artery distribution infarct *(arrow)*. **B:** Follow-up of noncontrast CT brain scan several days later that reveals hemorrhagic transformation of the infarct (area) with increased density now observed reflecting blood.

protection of the airway with aspiration precautions, careful monitoring of the vital signs, and early mobilization if at all possible. In acute ischemic stroke, it is important not to be overly aggressive with blood pressure control, and

TABLE 7.8	Guidelines for the General Management of the Patient with Acute Stroke

1. Stability of vital signs
2. Avoidance of aggressive blood pressure control in acute ischemic stroke
3. Avoidance of glucose- or dextrose-containing intravenous fluids in acute ischemic stroke
4. Initiation of aspirin therapy in acute ischemic stroke if no contraindication
5. Protection of airway with aspiration precautions
6. Assessment of swallowing capacity
7. Early mobilization as clinically indicated
8. Bowel program
9. Prevention of pressure sores
10. Antiembolus measures
11. Rehabilitation therapy evaluation as indicated by the deficit
12. Social service evaluation
13. Assessment for evidence of poststroke depression
14. Long-term management of risk factors for stroke

systolic blood pressures of 160 ± 20 mm Hg and diastolic blood pressure of 100 ± 10 mm Hg are not usually treated in the first several days to weeks of the acute event. This is in recognition of the potential for sudden drops in blood pressure to reduce cerebral perfusion and cause extension of the infarction related to disruption of cerebral autoregulation in acute stroke. It is also well recognized that elevated blood glucose can have a deleterious effect on stroke outcome and enhances the risk of complications with rt-PA.

■ **SPECIAL CLINICAL POINT: It is important to avoid aggressive blood pressure control in acute ischemic stroke as this can promote cerebral hypoperfusion with extension of the infarction.**

INTRACEREBRAL HEMORRHAGE

Clinical Approach

The most common causes of ICH are listed in Table 7.9. Hypertensive ICH most commonly affects the basal ganglionic–thalamic region; pontine hemorrhage and cerebellar hemorrhage are other common locations. The patient typically presents with maximal deficit at

TABLE 7.9	Causes of Spontaneous Intracerebral Hemorrhage

1. Hypertension
2. Intracranial aneurysm
3. Arteriovenous malformation
4. Bleeding diathesis
5. Complication of anticoagulant therapy
6. Illicit drug use (e.g., cocaine)
7. Mycotic aneurysm
8. Hemorrhagic metastasis
9. Bleeding into a primary brain tumor
10. Bleeding into a brain abscess
11. Arteritis (primary, connective tissue disorder, syphilitic, etc.)
12. Amyloid angiopathy
13. Hemorrhagic leukoencephalopathy

onset, and a patient who complains of sudden severe headache followed by obtundation and focal neurologic deficit, in association with a markedly elevated blood pressure, usually is found to have ICH rather than ischemic stroke. However, small hematomas can present with minor deficit; this is why it is important to obtain a CT brain scan immediately at presentation because this distinguishes an intracerebral hematoma from an evolving infarct. It is important to recognize that acute bleeding is visible immediately on CT brain scan, whereas it takes 3 to 6 hours or longer for an acute ischemic stroke to evolve on the CT brain scan.

Lobar hematomas are less likely associated with a hypertensive mechanism; other etiologies need to be considered. Roughly one half of all lobar hematomas are not attributable to hypertension. Alternative explanations include cerebral amyloid angiopathy. This is typically seen in patients older than 60 and/or is characterized by lobar hematoma, dementia, and congophilic (amyloid) angiopathy on pathologic specimen. This entity is important to recognize clinically because surgical evacuation should be avoided. The involved vessels tend to be quite friable, and this can be associated with an unexpected challenge in terms of control of bleeding. Vascular anomalies such as AVMs and aneurysms are also in the differential diagnosis of lobar hemorrhage.

A platelet count below 30,000/μL can be associated with brain hemorrhage as can factors VIII and IX deficiency, with the latter two entities being familial in nature. Routine PT, PTT, and bleeding time obtained in patients with ICH can be useful to assess platelet dysfunction. Hypofibrinogenemia is another potential hematologic explanation for ICH. In addition, the presence of fibrinogen degradation products with fragmented erythrocytes suggests disseminated intravascular coagulation. Acquired immune deficiency syndrome can have a multitude of effects that can promote ICH; one of them is severe thrombocytopenia. Meningovascular syphilis also remains in the differential diagnosis of ICH.

Certain drugs including cocaine and amphetamines promote ICH. Such agents, with a sympathomimetic effect, can cause a sudden increase in blood pressure that can "unmask" a preexisting cerebrovascular anomaly such as an AVM or aneurysm. There also can be a vasculitic effect with so-called "beading" of the cerebral blood vessels similar to what one can see with a connective tissue disorder such as systemic lupus erythematosus and polyarteritis nodosa. Phenylpropanolamine, a sympathomimetic agent, which, until recently, was commonly found in cough and cold over-the-counter preparations and in appetite suppressants, has been implicated as a factor in ICH.

■ **SPECIAL CLINICAL POINT: The urine drug screen (UDS) is an important part of the evaluation of unexplained stroke and can help to explain an intracerebral hemorrhage.**

Bleeding into a primary CNS neoplasm or metastatic disease can occur. The most likely metastatic lesions associated with ICH include lung, breast, thyroid, renal cell, and melanoma. Bleeding related to septic embolism from bacterial endocarditis as well as nonseptic embolism from marantic endocarditis is possible. It is also possible to have bleeding into a brain abscess.

Treatment

In hypertensive ICH, bleeding can persist for 6 hours, which can produce major deleterious outcomes. There has been controversy about what degree of blood pressure control is desirable in the acute setting. There has been concern that aggressive reduction of a markedly elevated blood pressure can lead to secondary hypoperfusion of brain tissue surrounding the hematoma and lead to worsening of the outcome. However, this has not been demonstrated. It is recognized that expansion of the hematoma to a critical level, related to persistent intracranial bleeding, can accurately identify those patients with no hope for meaningful recovery. It appears that aggressive blood pressure management, with

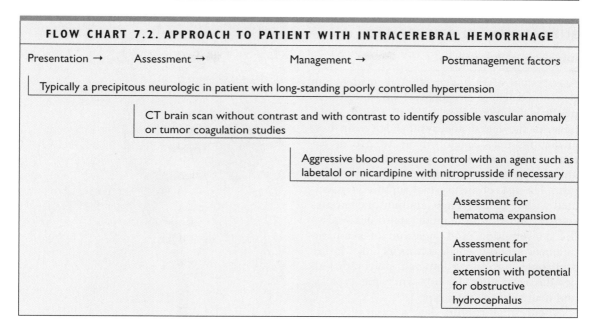

FLOW CHART 7.2. APPROACH TO PATIENT WITH INTRACEREBRAL HEMORRHAGE

Presentation →   Assessment →   Management →   Postmanagement factors

Typically a precipitous neurologic in patient with long-standing poorly controlled hypertension

CT brain scan without contrast and with contrast to identify possible vascular anomaly or tumor coagulation studies

Aggressive blood pressure control with an agent such as labetalol or nicardipine with nitroprusside if necessary

Assessment for hematoma expansion

Assessment for intraventricular extension with potential for obstructive hydrocephalus

agents such as nicardipine or labetalol, can reduce expansion of the hematoma, and limit end organ damage to other areas such as the heart and kidneys (Flow Chart 7.2). ICH associated with severely elevated blood pressure can be treated with sodium nitroprusside because of its effectiveness in rapidly lowering the blood pressure. However, this agent can increase cerebral blood flow and promote increased intracranial pressure.

■ **SPECIAL CLINICAL POINT: The consensus is for effective management of acute blood pressure for hypertensive intracerebral hemorrhage, although the degree of control remains controversial.**

Surgical evacuation of primary ICH remains controversial especially for those involving the basal ganglia or thalamus. However, there is clearly a benefit for surgical removal of a cerebellar hematoma that is associated with any evidence of pressure effect on the brainstem. In addition, cerebral lobar hematoma resulting in significant mass effect with resultant worsening of the neurologic condition is probably best managed with surgical evacuation as long as a

critical area of the brain, such as the speech area, is not going to be severely compromised by the intervention. Acute obstructive hydrocephalus related to intraventricular extension of the hematoma may respond effectively to placement of an intraventricular drain and a ventricular shunt may become necessary. However, the risks versus the benefits of such a procedure, in such a clinical setting, remain controversial. Recent reports suggest that the prognosis for recovery is improved with thrombolytic therapy through the ventricular drain to help clear clot formation and restore normal CSF flow pathways.

■ **SPECIAL CLINICAL POINT: Surgical intervention may be indicated in cerebellar hematoma, particularly with evidence of pressure on the brainstem.**

ICH related to the use of unfractionated heparin requires immediate discontinuation of the heparin infusion and infusion of protamine sulfate. Warfarin-related ICH is managed most effectively with fresh frozen plasma. It can take vitamin K up to 8 to 24 hours to correct a prolonged prothrombin time, which is far too long in such an emergency setting.

SUBARACHNOID HEMORRHAGE

Intracranial Aneurysm

Aneurysmal SAH has an annual incidence in the United States of roughly 1 in 10,000 people. It is estimated that 0.5% to 1% of adults have an incidental aneurysm. Each year, new aneurysms may develop in up to 2% of patients with previously ruptured aneurysms, and the rupture rate is up to 6 per 10,000 per year. The risk of aneurysmal rupture is associated with female sex, age, amount of cigarettes smoked, hypertension, moderate-to-heavy alcohol consumption, and ingestion of sympathomimetic agents. Genetic factors include Marfan syndrome, autosomal-dominant polycystic kidney disease, Ehlers–Danlos syndrome Type IV, and neurofibromatosis type 1.

Aneurysmal rupture has a mortality rate that approaches 50%. It is extremely important to recognize that a "warning leak" can precede a major rupture in up to 25% of patients and that recognition of this premonitory syndrome can be life saving. Patients presenting with an atypical or particularly severe headache, especially when there is clinical evidence of meningeal irritation, are most worrisome. The CT brain scan has a sensitivity of roughly 90% to 95% during the initial 24 hours of the bleed, whereas the lumbar puncture has essentially 100% sensitivity. Thus, the lumbar puncture is indicated even if the CT brain scan appears to be completely negative, but there is clinical suspicion for an aneurysmal bleed.

■ **SPECIAL CLINICAL POINT: It is important to recognize the potential of a "warning leak" in patients presenting with atypical or severe "thunderclap"-type headache even if the CT brain scan does not clearly demonstrate evidence of subarachnoid blood.**

Cerebral arteriography remains the definitive study for documentation of an aneurysm or aneurysms because they can be in multiple

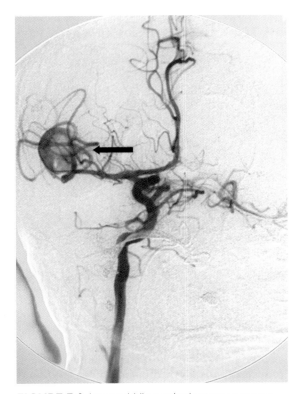

FIGURE 7.6 Large middle cerebral artery aneurysm *(arrow)* demonstrated on an intra-arterial cerebral arteriogram.

locations, and they typically are seen at branching points of the major cerebral arteries (Fig. 7.6). MRA and spiral CTA have value for noninvasive "screening" purposes. Roughly 80% to 85% of cerebral aneurysms are seen in the anterior circulation, with the most common locations at the junction of the internal carotid artery and the posterior communicating artery, in the region of the anterior communicating artery, and at the trifurcation of the MCA. Posterior circulation aneurysms most commonly are found at the tip of the basilar artery or at the junction of a vertebral artery with the posterior inferior cerebellar artery.

The clinical manifestations of a ruptured cerebral aneurysm typically reflect its location. Most patients have a severe headache with clinical evidence of meningeal irritation (i.e., neck stiffness and pain), which is aggravated by neck motion. Some patients have syncope as the primary manifestation, with headache as a more minor component of the presentation. Subhyaloid hemorrhage on funduscopic examination can be an important clue. So-called "classic" presentations include the patient stating they are experiencing the "worst headache" of their life with no localizing neurologic features or having a severe headache with a third cranial nerve palsy. The third nerve palsy identifies the location of the aneurysm at the junction of the internal carotid artery with the posterior communicating artery in the vicinity where the third cranial nerve is traversing from the midbrain toward the eye.

The major therapeutic approach is to have early surgical clipping, or endovascular coiling, of the ruptured aneurysm as soon as possible in an effort to prevent further bleeding. There are a number of potential complications of the initial rupture (Table 7.10), and rebleeding is the most worrisome. Up to 10% to 20% of patients will suffer rebleeding if early intervention, within the first 48 to 72 hours of presentation, cannot be performed. The International Subarachnoid Aneurysm Trial (ISAT) found that endovascular coiling of an aneurysm that has bled, when accessible to such a coiling procedure, was just as efficacious as and safer than surgical clipping. In this procedure, the placement of endovascular coils within the aneurysm induces electrothrombosis, and obliteration, of the aneurysmal sac. A recent follow-up to this study demonstrated similar benefits to surgical clipping over 10 years of follow-up.

■ **SPECIAL CLINICAL POINT: There is increasing use of endovascular intervention with aneurysmal subarachnoid hemorrhage. However, potential risks versus benefits, including the expertise of the particular interventionalist versus the neurosurgeon performing clipping of the aneurysm, must be factored into the decision-making process.**

Another complication is vasospasm. This tends to correlate with the amount of subarachnoid blood present, and it is most commonly seen 3 to 15 days after the initial rupture. Nimodipine, a calcium channel blocker, is available to help prevent aneurysmal rupture-induced vasospasm. Some centers now are using endovascular balloon angioplasty or intravascular infusion of vasodilating agents, such as verapamil, in an effort to protect against hypoperfusion, with secondary cerebral infarction, that can be seen as a consequence of vasospasm. In an effort to serially monitor for potential vasospasm in a noninvasive fashion, transcranial Doppler is often used to detect elevation of the mean flow velocity, which reflects narrowing of the intracranial vessel diameter. This can be useful for guidance in terms of more aggressive approaches toward evolving vasospasm.

TABLE 7.10	Complications of Aneurysmal Rupture

1. Rebleeding
2. Vasospasm with secondary ischemia
3. Hydrocephalus
   a. Obstructive
   b. Communicating
4. Diffuse cerebral edema
5. Chemical meningitis
6. Subdural hematoma
7. Intracerebral hematoma

Arteriovenous Malformation

An AVM is an anomaly of embryonal development in which there is a conglomeration of arteries and veins with no intervening capillaries. The prevalence of AVM in the general population is estimated at 0.14%, and most remain clinically silent throughout life. They are reported to be twice as common in men as in women. Although present at birth, they tend to become clinically evident most commonly between the ages of 10 and 40 years.

Approximately 50% of people who become symptomatic from an AVM present with either ICH, SAH, or both. It is the second most common cause of spontaneous SAH after aneurysmal rupture. Approximately 30% of patients with AVM present with seizures; the remaining 20% present with headache, focal neurologic deficit, or cognitive impairment. Roughly 25% of patients with ICH secondary to AVM suffer serious morbidity or death. Overall, the first bleed is fatal in 4.6% of patients. In a population-based long-term follow-up study, the risk of first hemorrhage is lifelong and increases with age. The recurrence rate for brain hemorrhage is roughly 7% for the first year following the initial bleed. Of the patients with AVM who present with seizure, 1% will suffer ICH within 1 year. The headache that is associated with AVM can be very difficult to distinguish from migraine, and there is always the possibility that the two coexist.

Fortunately, the risk of rebleeding from an AVM is not similar to that of aneurysmal rupture. The most effective course is to surgically remove the AVM, if feasible. However, not all AVMs can be resected because of the extent of the vascular supply, the location, or both. AVMs located within the deep brain structures or those involving vital brain function areas are the most challenging from a surgical approach. In an effort to reduce the vascular supply of the AVM, endovascular occlusion has been used. With the use of superselective vascular catheterization, one can insert a permanent balloon, sclerosing drugs, quick-acting glues, or thrombosing coils to interrupt the vascular supply. In certain instances, these endovascular procedures can obliterate the AVM. However, the usual purpose is to allow the AVM to be more effectively, and safely, managed from a surgical standpoint. This is in recognition of the proposed surgical risk of extirpation based on size of the lesion, type of venous drainage, and location.

Radiotherapy is an alternative to more invasive approaches. It can involve the use of gamma knife, proton beam, or linear accelerator. The purpose is to focus the radiotherapy at the vascular supply of the AVM in an effort to promote occlusive vascular injury, over multiple courses of therapy, in an effort to thrombose the involved vessels. Theoretically, radiotherapy, also known as radiosurgery, can obliterate the AVM in a best-case scenario and remove its risk of ever bleeding or rebleeding. It is important to point out that both radiotherapy and endovascular occlusion are in the developmental stages, and it is expected that outcome will improve as these techniques are perfected.

WHEN TO REFER TO A NEUROLOGIST

The edict "time is brain" is particularly important in patients with acute ischemic stroke who present within the timeframe for rt-PA. Expertise in the use of rt-PA enhances outcome. Neurologic expertise is also of value in patients who require a more sophisticated opinion in reference to recurrent symptoms of stroke or TIA. This can include optimal choice of antiplatelet therapy versus anticoagulant therapy. In terms of symptomatic carotid stenosis, the neurologist can provide expertise and experience in terms of risks versus benefits of procedures such as carotid endarterectomy versus carotid angioplasty with stenting. They can also provide a perspective on optimal choice of imaging such as carotid ultrasound versus MRA versus CTA versus routine intra-arterial cerebral angiography. One can also obtain informed opinions about the evaluation and management of the patient with unexplained ICH as well as the optimal approach to the patient with aneurysmal rupture and the patient with an AVM.

SPECIAL CHALLENGES FOR HOSPITALIZED PATIENTS

It is important to recognize that patients presenting with acute stroke or new-onset TIA require immediate evaluation and management. The sooner the mechanism of the ischemia is determined, the better to make an informed choice in terms of optimal management. Patients who are neurologically unstable should be admitted to an intensive care unit. This is particularly important for monitoring after having received rt-PA. Noninvasive vascular imaging (MRA and CTA) has become quite good. However, there continue to be challenges in terms of the accuracy of less-invasive imaging studies, including carotid and vertebral ultrasound and transcranial Doppler, compared to routine cerebral angiography. Outside of a routine electrocardiogram (EKG) on admission, along with transthoracic echocardiography when appropriate, cardiac monitoring can be especially important for patients who are at significant risk for cardiac arrhythmia as an explanation for their symptoms. TEE might also be useful, but it might also cloud the picture when there is the not uncommon finding of a patent foramen ovale or mitral valve prolapse. Many medical centers now have stroke units available, which allow a multidisciplinary approach toward the various special needs of the patient with acute stroke. These include nursing staff with special expertise in neurologic monitoring of patients with stroke; supervision by neurologists with special expertise in stroke; and a dedicated stroke rehabilitative staff to address communication disorders secondary to stroke, cognitive dysfunction, psychologic sequelae including depression, swallowing, and/or respiratory impairment. The staff also can assess and treat motor dysfunction, incoordination, and gait impairment.

QUESTIONS AND DISCUSSION

1. A 67-year-old right-handed male presents to your ER complaining of aphasia, right homonymous hemianopsia, and right hemiparesis. He noted the symptoms upon awakening at 7 AM, and it is now 9 AM. Which of the following would be a contraindication to administration of rt-PA in this case?

Always Remember

- Transient ischemic attack is a medical emergency that requires expeditious evaluation and management.
- Time is of the essence in the evaluation of the patient with acute ischemic stroke who is a potential candidate for tissue plasminogen activator.
- It is best to avoid aggressive blood pressure treatment in patients with acute ischemic stroke, as this can promote extension of the infarct.
- Most evidence suggests that more aggressive blood pressure control is indicated for patients presenting with intracerebral hemorrhage.
- The primary indication for anticoagulant therapy in the acute ischemic stroke period is for deep venous thrombosis prophylaxis.
- Aspirin tends to improve outcome in acute ischemic stroke with the recommended dose of 160 to 325 mg/day as long as there is no contraindication to the use of aspirin.
- The CT brain scan is not 100% sensitive for the detection of minor bleeding that can occur with rupture of an intracranial aneurysm. A lumbar puncture is indicated if there is any clinical support for this diagnostic possibility.

A. A CT brain scan that reveals no evidence of intracerebral hemorrhage
B. Routine blood work that reveals no significant metabolic disturbance such as severe hypoglycemia or hyperglycemia
C. A CT brain scan that reveals a hyperdense middle cerebral artery reflective of a clot within the involved middle cerebral artery
D. An INR of 1.1
E. An inability to pinpoint the time of symptom onset

The correct answer is E. This patient would be a potential candidate for rt-PA if he presents with an ischemic stroke within 3 hours of onset and with enough time to exclude contraindications to the use of this drug. A CT brain scan is mandatory to exclude intracerebral hemorrhage or evolution of the infarct to the point that there is already significant tissue damage present, which would raise serious questions about the exact onset of the ischemic insult and would increase the likelihood of hemorrhagic transformation as a complication of the therapy. Patients also must have enough of a deficit to warrant the use of this agent, and they should not be demonstrating significant spontaneous resolution of their signs and symptoms during the evaluation period because this contraindicates the need for this potentially dangerous agent. One must exclude a severe metabolic derangement, such as a very low or very high blood glucose, which can produce focal neurologic deficit. It is also important to exclude focal seizure activity as part of the presentation because this can contribute to the neurologic deficit. Contraindications include a clinically significant bleeding diathesis or anticoagulant therapy that is in a therapeutic range. In this specific case, the time that the patient was last asymptomatic (presumably when he went to sleep) must be determined.

2. A 73-year-old right-handed woman presented to the local hospital ER several weeks ago with an episode of left-sided numbness and weakness that lasted for 5 to 10 minutes before resolving completely. She has minor bilateral stenosis by carotid ultrasound, a normal MRI brain scan, a normal EKG, and a normal routine blood work. She is placed on aspirin 81 mg/day and comes to your office for follow-up 1 month later and reports having five identical episodes since the initial presentation. Which of the following would be most appropriate at this time?
A. Add clopidogrel to the aspirin

B. Evaluate for possible intracranial occlusive disease with conventional 4-vessel cerebral arteriography
C. Order a transesophageal ECHO (TEE) to rule out a cardiac source of embolism
D. EEG to evaluate for possible focal seizure activity
E. Substitution of low-dose aspirin–high-dose long-acting dipyridamole for the present aspirin dose

The correct answer is D. Two recent studies showed absolutely no benefit from the combination of aspirin and clopidogrel for ischemic stroke protection with an increased risk of bleeding complications. This patient might have significant intracranial artery stenosis as an explanation for her recurrent symptoms, despite aspirin, and guidance for alternative therapy might be aided by such documentation with noninvasive imaging (e.g., transcranial Doppler study, MRA, or CTA) before risking conventional angiography. Although it is possible that she has a transient cardiac arrhythmia, such as atrial fibrillation, or valvular disease as an explanation for her recurrent symptoms, cardioembolism is unlikely to result in six identical transient ischemic attacks. On the other hand, focal seizure activity is frequently stereotyped and can mimic TIA. It is currently not clear that substitution of low-dose aspirin–high-dose long-acting dipyridamole is superior to aspirin for stroke prophylaxis.

3. A 35-year-old right-handed woman presents to your ER with a several hour history of progressive aphasia and right hemiparesis. She has no history of hypertension, diabetes, or hypercholesterolemia. The CT brain scan reveals an evolving left middle cerebral artery distribution infarct. She has been on an oral contraceptive for the past 6 months but is on no other medications. She does not smoke and has no family history of vascular disease. Review of systems is significant for occasional dull

headaches without associate symptoms, but she reports that she recently returned from a business trip to Thailand. Which of the following is most likely to have caused her stroke?

A. Use of oral contraception
B. Complicated migraine
C. Parasitic infection
D. Paradoxical embolus associated with the presence of a patent foramen ovale
E. Giant cell arteritis

The correct answer is E. The risk of stroke related to oral contraceptives is low, but it is enhanced in older patients, those who smoke, those with other risk factors for vascular disease as well as those with a strong family history of early vascular disease. Migrainous infarction is felt to be a not uncommon cause of "stroke in the young." This small, but real, risk can be potentially enhanced by oral contraceptive use as a contributing factor, as oral contraceptives have the potential to exacerbate migraine, as well as increase the risk of stroke, and this combination might be a particularly important factor in migraine with aura. In this case, however, the patient's history does not suggest migraine, and she does not have significant vascular risk factors. Although the patient reports travel overseas, a parasitic infection is unlikely as an explanation for her stroke. But it is now well recognized that prolonged air travel can promote deep venous thrombosis of the legs. This, in association with the not uncommon finding of a patent foramen ovale, can lead to what has been termed "paradoxical cerebral embolism." The patient is not likely to have giant cell arteritis, a disease of the elderly.

4. A 38-year-old right-handed woman presents to your ER with severe headache and is found to have some pain on motion of her neck. She experienced a similar, but milder, headache 1 week earlier. She was evaluated at a different ER, had a negative CT brain scan, and was sent home with a diagnosis of "migraine." However, she has no history of significant headache prior to these two episodes. She is afebrile with normal vital signs. Her neurologic exam is normal. You elect to obtain a noncontrast CT brain scan, and it is officially read as normal. Which diagnostic test should be performed before she is sent home?

A. An MRI brain scan
B. An EEG
C. A serum protein electrophoresis
D. A lumbar puncture
E. An ESR

The correct answer is D. A patient presenting to the ER with a severe headache is always a cause for concern, especially if it is called "the worst headache of my life." Atypical headaches also should raise particular concern so that one does not miss the so-called "warning leak" of subarachnoid hemorrhage or an early meningitis or encephalitis. The CT brain scan has sensitivity of the order of 90% to 95% within the first day of an aneurysmal subarachnoid hemorrhage, and, thus, it does not fully exclude the possibility of such a life-threatening bleed. The MRI brain scan is not clearly superior to CT brain scan in the acute setting for the detection of blood. To completely exclude this possibility, when there is any clinical suspicion, one must perform a lumbar puncture. An ESR is an important test for the older patient presenting with headache to help in the evaluation for possible temporal arteritis. In this particular patient, it is important to keep in mind that migraine often presents itself by the time patients reach the age of 35.

SUGGESTED READING

Adams HP Jr. Secondary prevention of atherothrombotic events after ischemic stroke. *Mayo Clin Proc.* 2009;84:43.

Berrouschot J, Rother J, Glahn J, et al. Outcome and severe hemorrhagic complications of intravenous thrombolysis with tissue plasminogen activator in very old (≥80 years) stroke patients. *Stroke.* 2005;36:2421.

Friedlander RM. Arteriovenous malformations of the brain. *New Engl J Med.* 2007;356:270.

Sacco RL, Diener HC, Yusuf S, et al, for the PRoFESS Study Group. Aspirin and extended-release dipyridamole versus clopidogrel for recurrent stroke. *N Engl J Med.* 2008;359:1238.

Suarez JI, Tarr RW, Selman WR. Aneurysmal subarachnoid hemorrhage. *N Engl J Med.* 2006;354:387.

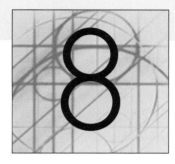

Headache Disorders

AMY WILCOX VOIGT AND JOEL R. SAPER

key points

- Primary headache disorders reflect intrinsic, possibly genetically determined vulnerability to recurring headaches.

- Secondary headaches can mimic the primary disorders, thus justifying aggressive diagnostic pursuit for patients with frequent or changing headache patterns or those with neurologic symptoms or findings.

- Progression from intermittent migraine to daily or almost daily chronic migraine results from a variety of factors, such as genetic, hormonal, psychological, and metabolic, including obesity.

- Acute medication overuse exceeding 3 days a week, week after week, and month after month is a major cause of progression from intermittent headache to more frequent headache referred to as *medication overuse headache*.

- Effective headache treatment requires individualized programs, using abortive (acute) and preventive medications and occasionally, if appropriate, behavioral therapy. Intractable cases must be referred to advanced systems of care, including specialists and comprehensive headache programs.

- Chronic administration of opioids for frequent headaches is discouraged.

INTRODUCTION

Primary headache disorders are highly prevalent conditions affecting tens of millions of U.S. citizens and hundreds of millions of individuals worldwide. The lifetime prevalence of common headache disorders can be more than 78%, with migraine prevalence greater than 20% in adult females. The economic and quality-of-life burden of migraine alone is substantial, with the most disabled half of migraine sufferers accounting for more than 90% of migraine-related work loss. Barriers to successful care include failure to diagnose properly, underestimation by both the professional and public domains of the morbidity of these conditions, and denied access to appropriate treatment.

PRIMARY AND SECONDARY HEADACHES

Primary headaches include those in which intrinsic dysfunction of the nervous system, often genetic in origin, predisposes to increased vulnerability to headache attacks. Examples include cluster headache and migraine. Secondary headaches are those in which the headache is secondary to an organic or physiologic process, intracranially or extracranially.

Table 8.1 is a short overview version of the International Headache Society's (IHS) classification of primary headaches. Table 8.2 lists some of the more frequently occurring categories of illnesses that produce secondary headaches.

MIGRAINE

■ **SPECIAL CLINICAL POINT: Migraine is a complex neurophysiologic disorder characterized by episodic and progressive forms of head pain in association with numerous neurologic and nonneurologic (autonomic, psychophysiologic)**

TABLE 8.1	Abbreviated International Headache Society Classification for Primary Headache Disorders

Episodic migraine
  With aura (including basilar [brainstem] migraine)
  Without aura
Chronic migraine (new IHS criteria)
Cluster headache (episodic/chronic)
Tension-type headache (episodic/chronic)

IHS, International Headache Society.

TABLE 8.2	Secondary Headache Conditions

More than 300 conditions can produce secondary headaches. Among the conditions are the following:
  Cerebrovascular/cardiovascular ischemia
  Metabolic disorders
  Intracranial mass lesions
  CSF hypotension/hypertension
  Infectious disorders (systemic, intracranial)
  Endocrine dysfunction
  Cervical (neck) disorders
  Temporomandibular/dental disorders

CSF, cerebrospinal fluid.

accompaniments. These can precede, accompany, or follow the headache itself.

Migraine is classified into three major subtypes:

1. Migraine with aura—characterized by heralding neurologic events lasting 30 minutes to 1 hour and preceding the head pain attacks (only 15–20% of migraine attacks). A migraine aura should last longer than 5 minutes and less than 60 minutes. If an aura is consistently less than 5 minutes in duration, then a "secondary aura" should be suspected (arteriovenous malformation, epileptic aura). If an aura lasts longer than 60 minutes in duration, it is termed a "prolonged aura," and an underlying coagulopathy or other cerebral pathology should be ruled out.

2. Migraine without aura—in which attacks of migraine and accompaniments occur without clear-cut preheadache neurologic symptomatology. This is the most common form of migraine (80% to 85%). A *prodrome* is a period of time, up to 24 hours or so, prior to the aura or headache phase in which mental or physiologic events herald the next phases of migraine. The prodrome may consist of subtle or less than subtle phenomena, such as excessive yawning, food cravings, and mental changes, such as excitability, anxiety, elation, or even depression. Many

have misinterpreted the prodrome as a "trigger" phenomenon for the headache, but in actuality the prodrome represents the earliest phases of the ensuing attack.

3. Chronic or transformed migraine—frequently a progressive form of migraine in which intermittent attacks occur at increasing frequency, eventually reaching 15 or more days per month. By definition, chronic migraine occurs on a backdrop of episodic migraine without aura, often accompanied by comorbid neuropsychiatric phenomena. Chronic migraine frequently is associated with medication overuse and "rebound."

■ **SPECIAL CLINICAL POINT:** Comorbid conditions associated with migraine, particularly chronic migraine, include depression, anxiety and panic disorders, bipolar disorder, obsessive–compulsive disorder, character disorders, and perhaps fibromyalgia.

Migraine—Clinical Symptoms

Between 80% and 90% of patients with migraine have a family history. In childhood, there is a ratio of 1:1, males to females, but in adulthood a 3:1 female-to-male gender ratio occurs. This is primarily thought to result from the adverse influence on the headache mechanism by estrogen. At older ages, the gender ratio again declines to almost 1:1, further suggesting that estrogen is likely to be influential.

Each attack generally lasts between 4 and 72 hours and can be accompanied by a wide range of autonomic and cognitive symptoms. In complex cases, particularly in chronic migraine, a likely association with several neuropsychiatric comorbid disorders, including depression, panic/anxiety syndromes, sleep disturbance, obsessive–compulsive disorder, and others, occurs. Predisposed individuals are particularly vulnerable to provocation (triggering) by certain extrinsic and intrinsic events, including hormonal fluctuation, weather changes, certain foods, delayed meals and fasting, extra sleeping time, stress, and others.

TABLE 8.3 | **Key Concepts in Migraine Pathogenesis**

Trigeminal-mediated perivascular (neurogenic) inflammation resulting in painful vascular and meningeal tissue

The perivascular release of vasoactive neuropeptides, particularly calcitonin gene-related peptide (CGRP)

The development of allodynia and central sensitization as attacks progress

The presence of an active "modulator zone" in the dorsal raphe nucleus of the midbrain during migraine attacks

Activation and threshold reduction of neurons in the descending trigeminal system and dorsal horn of upper spinal cord (C2–C3)

The deposition of nonheme iron in the brainstem, roughly correlated to increasingly frequent attacks

A yet-to-be-defined relationship with nitrous oxide

Pathophysiology of Migraine

■ **SPECIAL CLINICAL POINT:** Migraine is a brain disorder that renders the brain "hypersensitive" and overresponsive to a variety of internal and external stimuli. Trigeminal/cervical connections and cervical activation may be important phenomena in the clinical manifestations, pathogenesis, and treatment. The key features of current pathophysiologic understanding are identified in Table 8.3.

TENSION-TYPE HEADACHE

This controversial disorder is classified into both episodic and chronic forms. Episodic forms have certain features that overlap with migraine without aura, although there is a general absence of throbbing pain and autonomic accompaniments. Chronic tension-type headache overlaps in clinical features with chronic migraine. Both forms of tension-type headache may be present in patients who have otherwise typical migraine headaches. Some authorities believe that these disorders are variant forms of migraine.

CHRONIC DAILY HEADACHE

Chronic daily headache is a frequency-based descriptive term that embodies four overlapping clinical subtypes. These include the following:

1. Chronic/transformed migraine, with or without medication overuse (see below).
2. Chronic tension-type headache, with or without medication overuse.
3. New daily persistent headache—sudden onset followed by persistent head pain without the progressive features of chronic migraine but that often is associated with comorbid and medication misuse features. New daily persistent headache, while considered by some to be a primary headache disorder, may actually be a secondary headache entity, the etiology of which is uncertain at this time.
4. Hemicrania continua—unilateral, generally persistent hemicranial discomfort with some features of migraine and cluster headache and that in 20% of cases appears to arise as a consequence of head trauma. This entity also may actually represent a secondary headache disorder.

MEDICATION OVERUSE HEADACHE (FORMERLY CALLED REBOUND HEADACHE)

■ **SPECIAL CLINICAL POINT:** Medication overuse headache (MOH), formerly referred to as rebound headache, is a self-sustaining headache condition characterized by persisting and recurring headache (usually migraine forms) against a background of chronic, regular use of centrally acting analgesics, ergotamine tartrate, or triptans. The descriptive features of this condition are noted in Table 8.4. Table 8.5 reflects the current IHS criteria for MOH.

Among the most important clinical concerns is that MOH can be a progressive disorder, perhaps prompting the conversion of intermittent

TABLE 8.4 | Features of MOH

- Weeks to months of excessive use of abortive agents, with usage exceeding 2–3 days/week
- Insidious increase of headache frequency
- Dependable and predictable headache, corresponding to an irresistible escalating use of offending agents at regular, predictable intervals
- Evidence of psychological and/or physiologic dependency
- Failure of alternate acute or preventive medications to control headache attacks
- Reliable onset of headache within hours to days following the last dose of symptomatic treatment

MOH, medication overuse headache.

headache to daily headache, and ultimately has toxic and perhaps fatal implications because of the compulsive and often physiologically dependent features that reflect this medication/headache cycle. Also, MOH imposes a refractoriness to otherwise appropriate treatment, thereby forcing the discontinuation of these drugs before more appropriate medication treatment will be effective. The authors of this chapter believe that there are certain behavioral underpinnings to the development of MOH in some, but not all, patients. Addressing these, if present, is essential in order

TABLE 8.5 | New International Headache Society Criteria for Headache Attributed to Medication Overuse

A. Headache present on >15 days/month
B. Regular overuse of one or more acute/symptomatic treatment drugs
   1. Ergotamine, triptans, opioids, or combination analgesic medications ≥10 days/month on a regular basis for >3 months
   2. Simple analgesics or any combination of ergotamine, triptans, or analgesic opioids on >15 days/month on a regular basis for >3 months without overuse of any single class alone
C. Headache has developed or markedly worsened during medication overuse

to remedy the acute problem and maintain prevention in the long run.

CLUSTER HEADACHE AND ITS VARIANTS

Cluster headache is a relatively rare disorder that affects more men than women in a ratio of 3:1. Current concepts of pathophysiology suggest disturbances within the hypothalamus with relevant involvement of autonomic systems and alterations in melatonin function. Melatonin "fine-tunes" endogenous cerebral rhythms and homeostasis.

The clinical features of cluster headache include the presence of headache cycles or bouts (clusters) lasting weeks to months and occurring one or more times per year or less. During these periods, repetitive attacks of short- lasting headache occur daily. Individual attacks of headache last 1 to 3 hours (averaging 45 minutes). The attacks are associated with focal orbital or temporal pain, which is always unilateral, is of extremely severe intensity, and is accompanied by lacrimation, nasal drainage, pupillary changes, and conjunctival injection. Attacks of headache commonly occur during sleeping times or napping and can be provoked by ingestion of alcohol or nitroglycerin. It is interesting that a high likelihood of blue or hazel-colored eyes; ruddy, rugged, lionized facial features; and a long history of smoking and excessive alcohol intake characterize the majority of men with cluster headache. Table 8.6 lists the clinical distinctions between cluster headache and migraine.

Cluster headache may occur in its episodic form (bouts or cycles of recurring headaches followed by a period of no headache [remission], lasting weeks to years) or in a chronic form without an interim period, with headache attacks daily for years without interruption. Treatment differences may exist.

TABLE 8.6 | **Clinical Features Distinguishing between Cluster and Migraine Headaches**

Feature	Cluster	Migraine
Location of pain	Always unilateral, periorbital; sometimes occipital referral	Unilateral and bilateral
Age at onset (typical)	Onset 20 years or older	10–50 years (can be younger or older)
Gender difference	Majority male	Majority female in adulthood
Time of day	Frequently at night, often same time each day	Any time
Frequency of attacks	1–6 per day	1–10 per month in episodic form
Duration of pain	30–120 minutes	4–72 hours
Prodromes	None	Often present
Nausea and vomiting	20%	85%
Blurring of vision	Infrequent	Frequent
Lacrimation	Frequent	Infrequent
Nasal congestion/drainage	70%	Uncommon
Ptosis	30%	1%–2%
Polyuria	2%	40%
Family history of similar headaches	7%	90%
Miosis	50%	Absent
Behavior during attack	Pacing, manic, and agitation	Resting in quiet, dark room

TABLE 8.7	Trigeminal Autonomic Cephalgias

Cluster headache
Chronic and episodic paroxysmal hemicrania
SUNCT (short-lasting unilateral neuralgiform headaches with conjunctival injection and tearing) syndrome
Cluster-tic syndrome (the association of cluster headache with trigeminal neuralgia symptomatology)

TABLE 8.8	Therapeutic Categories of Treatment for Primary Headache

- Nonpharmacologic treatment, including behavioral therapy
- Pharmacologic treatment (acute and preventive)
- Interventional procedures, including:
  - Neuroblockade (nerve, facet, epidural space)
  - Neurotoxin treatment (botulinum toxin)
  - Radiofrequency and cryolysis procedures
  - Neurostimulation
  - Hospital/rehabilitational programs

In addition to cluster headache, several short-lasting headache entities are recognized and currently are classified with cluster headache in a category referred to as the *trigeminal autonomic cephalgias*. These disorders are characterized primarily by the presence of short-lasting headaches of variable duration—seconds (short-lasting unilateral neuralgiform headaches with conjunctival injection and tearing [SUNCT]) to 3 hours (cluster headache). The attacks are associated with autonomic features. Table 8.7 lists the current members of the trigeminal autonomic cephalgia group.

TREATMENT OF PRIMARY HEADACHES AND RELATED PHENOMENA

The following represents the key principles in the approach to treatment of primary headaches and related phenomena. These key treatment principles include the following:

- Diagnosing the specific primary headache entity
- Determining attack frequency and severity
- Establishing the presence or absence of comorbid illnesses (e.g., psychiatric, neurologic, medical)
- Identifying confounding factors, including external or internal phenomena, such as the following:
  - MOH
  - Psychological and behavioral illness and medication factors (e.g., estrogen replacement, nitroglycerin, etc.)

- Hormonal disturbances
- Use of or exposure to toxic substances
- Others
- Identifying previous treatment successes and failures

Treatment Modalities

Numerous treatment modalities are available (Table 8.8). Nonpharmacologic treatments can be very helpful, particularly when combined with pharmacologic therapy. Behavioral modification, biofeedback, exercise, and dietary manipulation add a dimension of help beyond the administration of medications and also provide patients a method of helping themselves. Pharmacologic therapy provides the essential treatment for the majority of patients with primary headache. Increasing attention has focused on the important contribution that interventional treatment may provide patients with primary headache. Occipital nerve blocks, although not reversing the primary problem, can be particularly useful for symptomatic treatment.

Nonpharmacologic Treatments for Primary Headaches

A variety of factors related to health, habits, and education can assist patients with headache. Education on headache triggers and eliminating headache-producing behaviors can be essential. Reduction of medication use and the treatment of rebound provide a fundamental and critical element to the treatment of patients with chronic headache when medication overuse phenomena exist. Discontinuing smoking, establishing regular eating and sleeping patterns, and getting regular exercise are reported as helpful by many patients with headache. Biofeedback and behavioral treatment, together with cognitive behavioral therapy, may be of value in many cases and essential in some.

Treatment of MOH

MOH requires treatment because continued use of the medication renders patients refractory to effective treatment. Outpatient and inpatient strategies are available, depending on the intensity of medication usage and the characteristics of the case. Table 8.9 identifies important general principles in the treatment of rebound or medication misuse headache.

■ **SPECIAL CLINICAL POINT: MOH, which most likely results from chronic changes to receptors, must be distinguished from headaches resulting from toxic substances or other exposure to agents or drugs.**

These have a direct provocative influence. The discontinuation of offending medication is often a challenging process. During the period

of "detoxification" headache, emotional events escalate and patients often become desperate in their search for calming agents and the treatment of pain. Many cases can be treated in an outpatient setting or in an infusion center, where IV therapies can be administered during the day. More severe and complex cases require hospitalization during which 24-hour fluid replacement, IV protocols to treat the pain, and supportive measures can be provided in an acute care setting with 24-hour nursing supervision and monitoring. Hospitalization is generally required in patients with behavioral and/or psychological confounding factors or when complex drug regimens, including opioids and others, add additional layers of complexity to the case. Emotional support as well as behavioral treatment are necessary both on an inpatient and on an outpatient level of care.

Table 8.10 identifies some of the IV medications that are used in intravenously administered treatment protocols to address acute headache and treat medication overuse during the withdrawal phases. Patients are also provided both preventive and other orally or parenterally administered acute treatments. Among those acute treatments that will not cause MOH when given more than 3 days/week (which is often necessary in the acute phases of treatment

---

TABLE 8.9 | General Principles in the Treatment of MOH

Discontinuation of offending agent (taper if contain opioid or barbiturate)

Aggressive treatment of resulting severe "withdrawal" headache

Hydration, including intravenous fluids and support in severe cases (treat nausea)

The development of pharmacologic prophylaxis

Implementation of behavioral therapies

Use of outpatient infusion or hospitalization techniques for advanced and severe conditions

MOH, medication overuse headache.

TABLE 8.10 | Parenteral Regimens to Treat Intractable Headaches

- Dihydroergotamine (0.25–1 mg IV or IM, t.i.d.)
- Diphenhydramine (25–50 mg IV or IM, t.i.d.) (Swidan et al., 2005)
- Various neuroleptics (i.e., chlorpromazine 2.5–10 mg IV, t.i.d.; droperidol 0.325–2.5 mg IV, t.i.d.)
- Ketorolac (10 mg IV, t.i.d.; 30 mg IM, t.i.d.)
- Valproic acid (250–750 mg IV, t.i.d.)
- Magnesium sulfate (1 g IV, b.i.d.)
- Hydrocortisone (100 mg t.i.d. for 3 days)
- Sumatriptan (4–6 mg s.c., cannot use more than 2 days/week)

IV, intravenous; IM, intramuscular; t.i.d., three times a day; b.i.d., two times a day; s.c., subcutaneous.

of MOH) are hydroxyzine, nonsteroidal anti-inflammatory agents, baclofen, neuroleptics, and others. Steroids might also be used for short-term intervention.

Pharmacologic Treatment of Migraine

The pharmacologic treatment of headache involves the use of abortive (acute) and preventive medications. Abortive treatments are used to terminate evolving or existing attacks. Preventive treatment is implemented to reduce the frequency of attacks and prevent overuse of acute medications. Most patients require combination treatment. Preemptive treatment is a short-term preventive course of therapy used in anticipation of a predictable event, such as a menstrual period, or vacation-related headache. There is a wide variety of pharmacologic agents used in headache management. Table 8.11 lists various routes of delivery that can be utilized in the treatment of headache.

Acute Treatment of Migraine

There are numerous agents used for the acute treatment of migraine. Some agents, such as analgesics, are of general value for pain, whereas others, such as the ergots and triptan medications, are specific and influence receptor and transmitter systems thought to be relevant

TABLE 8.11	Routes of Delivery of Medications

- Oral
- Nasal spray (sumatriptan/zolmitriptan/DHE)
- Rectal (neuroleptics, indomethacin)
- Transdermal (lidocaine)
- Parenteral
  Subcutaneous (sumatriptan/DHE)
  Intramuscular (DHE, ketorolac, diphenhydramine, hydroxyzine, neuroleptics, etc.)
  Intravenous (DHE, ketorolac, valproic acid, steroids, magnesium sulfate, neuroleptics)

DHE, dihydroergotamine.

TABLE 8.12	Categories of Medications Used in the Acute Treatment of Migraine

Simple and combined analgesics (acetaminophen, excedrin, nonsteroidal anti-inflammatory drugs, and others)
Mixed analgesics (barbiturate and simple analgesics, such as aspirin ± acetaminophen ± caffeine)—often avoided because of the likelihood of dependency and misuse
Ergot derivatives, including dihydroergotamine
Triptan medications, including the following:
  Sumatriptan
  Naratriptan
  Almotriptan
  Rizatriptan
  Zolmitriptan
  Frovatriptan
  Eletriptan

to migraine pathogenesis. Table 8.12 lists the various categories of abortive agents.

The triptans represent narrow-spectrum, receptor-specific (serotonin [5-HT$_1$]) agonists that stimulate the 5-HT$_1$ receptors to reduce neurogenic inflammation. The ergot derivatives are broader spectrum agents affecting the serotoninergic receptors and also alpha-adrenergic and dopamine receptors (and others).

■ **SPECIAL CLINICAL POINT: Whereas many patients respond well to the triptans, others appear to require the additional use of ergot derivatives.**

Experienced clinicians are adept at administering several of the triptans as well as the ergots. Short-acting, rapidly effective triptans include almotriptan, sumatriptan, rizatriptan, zolmitriptan, and eletriptan, whereas naratriptan and frovatriptan have the longest half-lives. Several delivery formulations are available in addition to tablets: injection (sumatriptan), nasal spray (sumatriptan and zolmitriptan), and rapidly dissolving forms (zolmitriptan and rizatriptan).

Patients who have not responded to less potent medications require triptans or ergots for maximum benefit. It is imperative that the trip-tans, and probably the ergot derivatives as well, be administered to patients in the early phases of an ensuing headache attack, at the first sign of a migraine aura or at the onset of headache pain, to bring about maximum benefit and re-duce the possibility of recurrence (the return of headache within the same 24-hour period). Acute medications are used in conjunction with antinauseants and in combination with each other for maximum efficiency (do not combine ergots and triptans). Clinicians must be familiar with important contraindications and safety warnings of each of these medication groups as well as adverse effects and influence on hepatic metabolism, particularly when these drugs are used in combination with others.

Finally, for reasons that are not fully under-stood but perhaps related to the cervical/trigem-inal connections, occipital nerve blocks may relieve acute migraine attacks in some individu-als. This method has been used historically by anesthesiologists but is increasingly used by neurologists and others treating headache. Long-term value is rare, but short-term relief frequently is seen, and an adjunctive value is widely appreciated.

Preventive Treatment of Migraine

Many agents are available for the prevention of migraine. However, the clinician must deter-mine when preventive pharmacotherapy should be introduced. Table 8.13 lists certain clinical guidelines that can be used to make this determination.

The categories of medications useful in pre-vention are listed in Table 8.14. A wide range of therapies is available, and increasingly useful are those that appear to work on specific neuro-transmitter systems. The reader will note that several of these categories do not relate to vascu-lature or blood flow, suggesting that the primary pathogenesis of migraine seems more likely to involve neuronal rather than vascular dynamics.

Tricyclic antidepressants and beta blockers are well-established, first-line medications for

---

TABLE 8.13 | **Guidelines for Determining the Need for Preventive Treatment**

1. Disability from migraine headaches (loss of time at work or at home)
2. Migraine headaches occurring 2 or more days per week
3. Patient is overusing acute medication (analgesic-rebound headache)
4. Risk of persistent neurologic dysfunction because of the headache condition (hemiplegic migraine, migraine with prolonged aura)
5. Acute medications are contraindicated or ineffective
6. Patient preference, provided clinical justification exists

---

preventive treatment of migraine in those pa-tients who do not have contraindications or restrictions to either medication. Calcium chan-nel blockers are generally not as effective. The anticonvulsants have considerable value and are particularly useful in the presence of neuropsy-chiatric comorbidities or other conditions, such

---

TABLE 8.14 | **Categories of Preventive Medications**

Tricyclic antidepressants (particularly amitriptyline, nortriptyline, and doxepin)

Beta-adrenergic blockers (particularly propranolol and nadolol)

Calcium channel blockers (verapamil)

Anticonvulsants (valproic acid, gabapentin, topiramate)

Ergot derivatives (methylergonovine and methysergide)[a]

Monoamine oxidase inhibitors (for refractory cases)

Others
  Selective serotonin reuptake inhibitors
  Neuroleptics
  Tizanidine
  Botulinum toxin
  Riboflavin

[a]After 4 to 6 months of daily use of ergot derivatives, diagnostic pursuit of evidence of cardiac, pulmonary, or retroperitoneal fibrosis must be undertaken.

as seizures or bipolar disorders, which might accompany migraine.

The selective serotonin reuptake inhibitors (SSRIs) and serotonin norepinephrine reuptake inhibitors (SNRIs) are helpful for neuropsychiatric comorbidities, such as depression and panic and anxiety disorders, but generally do not have a strong antimigraine influence, although venlafaxine (an SNRI) and fluoxetine (an SSRI) do have supportive data in episodic migraine and/or chronic migraine. Some patients with migraine-related headaches benefit from the antidopaminergic influence of the new neuroleptics, although the potential for adverse effects limits their widespread use. Tizanidine, an alpha-adrenergic agonist, has been shown effective in an adjunctive, preventive role. Botulinum toxin increasingly is administered for the prevention of chronic migraine, but not intermittent migraine. Numerous uncontrolled studies support efficacy, but there is a paucity of controlled data at this time, although supportive data may be available shortly. If botulinum toxin is shown to work for chronic migraine, it is likely to work through a central mechanism and not through a primary muscular influence.

The treatment of chronic migraine is similar to that of episodic migraine. Treatment is directed at both the daily or almost daily pain and periodic attacks. Because of the likely presence of a progressive course, medication overuse, and neuropsychiatric comorbidities in this population, a more comprehensive approach beyond medications alone is required. This includes cognitive behavioral therapy and other forms of psychotherapy and family therapy. Organic illness must be ruled out with appropriate testing in patients with frequent or daily headache and in those with neurologic findings (see later).

Treatment of Cluster Headache

Cluster headache responds and is treated differently than migraine. Because cluster headache attacks generally occur numerous times daily

TABLE 8.15	Acute Treatment of Cluster Headache

Oxygen inhalation (8–10 L/min 100% oxygen via non-rebreather face mask)
Triptans/dihydroergotamine (limit 1–2 dosages/day, 2–3 days/week)
Occipital nerve blocks

(one to eight), the use of abortive medications is limited to only a few agents that are safe for such frequent use. Unlike migraine, preventive therapy is necessary for cluster headache unless the typical cluster cycle is 2 weeks in duration or less.

Table 8.15 lists the agents useful in the acute management of cluster headache, which is limited by the need to use medications up to several times a day when effective preventive is not available or has not yet become effective. Many clinicians have found that occipital nerve blocks, with or without steroids, may not only terminate an acute cluster attack but may prevent subsequent attacks, at least for a day or longer.

Table 8.16 lists the available preventive agents for the treatment of cluster headache. The most reliable agents for prevention are the steroids, but because of their inherent risks with long-term usage, they are inappropriate except in transitional regimens. Steroids can be used, for example, at the onset of treatment while other preventive agents are being titrated upward; during particularly vulnerable times, such as when traveling; or when other medications

TABLE 8.16	Preventive Agents for Cluster Headache

Steroids
Lithium carbonate
Verapamil
Valproic acid
Topiramate
Baclofen
Melatonin
Indomethacin

TABLE 8.17	Recommended 7-Day Prednisone Program		
Day	Breakfast (mg)	Lunch (mg)	Dinner (mg)
1	20 (4 pills)	20	20
2	20	20	20
3	20	15 (3 pills)	15
4	15	15	10 (2 pills)
5	10	10	10
6	10	5 (1 pill)	5
7	5	5	

Available as 5 mg tablets; 60 tablets should be dispensed.

are in transition. Table 8.17 lists a recommended prednisone protocol.

For intractable cases, hospitalization is recommended. In some cases surgical intervention is required, but surgical treatment is limited because of the likelihood of postsurgical painful sequelae. Occipital nerve injection is effective in treating some acute attacks, and subcutaneous occipital stimulation has been reported as anecdotally effective. Recently hypothalamic stimulation has been shown effective in desperate clinical circumstances.

Treatment of Other Primary Headache Disorders

Chronic paroxysmal hemicrania (CPH) and episodic paroxysmal hemicrania (EPH), as well as hemicrania continua, are characteristically sensitive to treatment with indomethacin at a dose of 25 to 50 mg three times a day. SUNCT syndrome may respond to lamotrigine, topiramate, or gabapentin.

DIAGNOSTIC TESTING AND SECONDARY HEADACHE DISORDERS

More than 300 entities may produce symptoms of headache, many of which mimic the primary headache disorders. The clinician has the burden of ruling in and ruling out potentially relevant

conditions in patients with recurring or persistent headache. Diagnostic testing includes a wide range of studies, including the investigation of metabolic, endocrinologic, toxic, dental, traumatic, cervical, and infectious disorders and space-occupying lesions. Disturbances of cerebrospinal fluid (CSF) pressure, ischemic disease, and allergic conditions must be considered. Table 8.18 lists diagnostic tests that are among those that should be considered in intractable or variant cases.

Important specific conditions to consider include those of the temporomandibular or dental structures, sphenoid sinuses (must specifically image and evaluate for sphenoid sinus disease), carotid and vertebral dissection syndromes, and cerebral venous occlusion. Table 8.19 lists some of the disease categories that must be considered. Because of the relevance of the cervical spine to the descending trigeminal system and headache physiology (trigeminal cervical connection), disturbances at the level of the upper cervical spine and its nerves and joints have become

TABLE 8.18	Diagnostic Tests to Consider in Refractory Cases
Physical examination	
Metabolic evaluation	
Hematologic	
ESR/CRP	
Endocrinologic	
Chemistry	
Toxicology (drug screens)	
Standard x-rays	
Neuroimaging	
MRI/MRA/MRV	
CT/CTA/CTV	
Arteriography	
Dental and otologic examination	
Lumbar puncture	
Diagnostic blockades	
ESR	
CRP	

ESR, erythrocyte sedimentation rate; CRP, C-reactive protein.

TABLE 8.19	Secondary Headache Disorders

- Traumatic disease (cryptic or obvious)
- Carotid/vertebral dissection syndromes
- CSF disturbances (CSF leak syndromes, intracranial hypertension)
- Toxic or environmental exposure syndromes
- Nasal/dental/temporomandibular conditions
- Ocular disturbances
- Metabolic/hormonal disturbances
- Alterations of sleep–wake cycle
- Intracranial pathology
  - Vascular/ischemic/hemorrhage/vasculitis
  - Tumor, mass lesions, AV malformations
  - Infectious (encephalitis, meningitis)
- Obstructive/structural disorders (Arnold–Chiari malformation)
- Connective tissue disorders
- Disorders of the upper cervical spine

CSF, cerebrospinal fluid; AV, arteriovenous.

TABLE 8.20	Possible Reasons for Intractability

- "Rebound" (medication overuse headache) or excessive medication overuse, toxicity, etc.
- Wrong diagnosis (wrong primary or undetected secondary causes) or nondiagnosis
- Medication selection not proper/dosages not adequate
- Psychological barriers
- More aggressive treatment required: hospitalization
- Current or previous use of opioids
- Requires interventional therapy
- Beyond current pathophysiologic understanding

important targets for the treatment of otherwise pharmacologically resistant headaches. Premature or excessive use of interventional procedures is unwarranted, but when selective and expertly administered, they clearly have a role in the overall spectrum of diagnosis and treatment for headache conditions. Treatments such as implantable stimulators are on the horizon.

REFERRAL AND HOSPITALIZATION

There are indeed patients who are intractable to standard primary and secondary level care. Table 8.20 lists some possible reasons for intractability. It is advisable to refer patients with intractable headache to specialists, specialized clinics, and tertiary centers.

■ **SPECIAL CLINICAL POINT: Hospitalization is required for many complex patients whose medication misuse or the presence of intractable pain and behavioral/ neuropsychiatric** symptomatology have reached an intensity and complexity that make outpatient therapy no longer appropriate.

Hospitalization

Many patients with intractable headache can and do respond to the more aggressive therapeutic environment and milieu in specialty inpatient programs when outpatient therapy has failed to establish efficacy. Recently Lake and Saper (2009) have published outcome data on 276 consecutive patients admitted to the Michigan Head Pain & Neurological Institute, demonstrating that 75% of these intractable patients reported moderate to significant headache reduction at the time of discharge. Inpatient programming provides for the ability to address pain, toxic, physiologic, and behavioral issues, while at the same time observing various patient pain patterns and patient behaviors, which can be very informative and influential in treatment strategies. Table 8.21 lists the criteria that can be used when hospitalization is considered.

Hospitalization for acute and prolonged headache is a complex undertaking because it must address not only the refractoriness of the symptoms, the often-present confounding influence of MOH (rebound), but also the

TABLE 8.21	Criteria for Hospitalization

1. Moderate to severe intractable headache, failing to respond to appropriate and aggressive outpatient or emergency department services and requiring repetitive, sustained, parenteral treatment
2. The presence of continuing nausea, vomiting, and diarrhea
3. The need to detoxify and treat toxicity, dependency, or rebound phenomena and require monitoring services against withdrawal symptoms, including seizures
4. The presence of dehydration, electrolyte imbalance, and prostration, requiring monitoring and intravenous fluids for the presence of unstable vital signs
5. The presence of repeated previous emergency department treatments
6. The presence of serious concurrent disease (e.g., SAH, intracranial infection, cerebral ischemia, severe hypertension or hypotension, etc.)
7. To simultaneously develop an effective pharmacologic prophylaxis in order to sustain improvement achieved by parenteral therapy
8. To acutely address other comorbid conditions contributing or accompanying the headache, including medical or psychological illness
9. Concurrent medical and/or psychological illness requiring careful monitoring in high-risk situations (i.e., severe hypotension, coronary artery disease, etc.)

SAH, subarachnoid hemorrhage.

behavioral and psychological factors that often influence these dilemmas. Discontinuation of medication and the weaning process bring with them a predictable escalation of headache and the emotional factors that are characteristic to that patient. The principles of hospitalization are listed in Table 8.22.

Hospitalization length of stay varies, depending on the intensity and type of medication that is overused and that requires discontinuation, the amount of pain and its duration during this weaning process, the behavioral issues that emerge, and the confounding factors that often are present in patients with these symptoms. Developing a preventive treatment during this time is difficult because it takes time for medications to work and because generally patients are in a refractory period that may last up to weeks to months after discontinuation of the offending agents.

TABLE 8.22	Principles of Inpatient Care

Interrupt daily/intractable headache with parenteral protocols
Discontinue offending analgesic medications if rebound is present
Implement preventive pharmacotherapy
Identify effective abortive therapy
Treat behavioral and neuropsychiatric comorbidities
Use interventional modalities when indicated
Educate
Discharge and outpatient planning along with case management

When and When Not to Administer Opioids

■ **SPECIAL CLINICAL POINT: Experience and evidence support the avoidance of sustained opioid administration in the chronic headache population.**

Administration of opioids in acute situations when other treatments are contraindicated or established to be ineffective remains appropriate in selected cases, but dose and amounts of prescriptions should be limited and monitored carefully to avoid misuse. Sustained opioid administration should be extremely limited and considered only in the following selected circumstances:

> When all else fails, following a full range of advanced services, including detoxification
>
> When standard agents are contraindicated
>
> In the elderly or during pregnancy

Saper et al. (2008) provide detailed criteria for the administration of sustained opioid therapy in the headache population.

Experience suggests that, although some patients with difficult headache problems initially respond to sustained opioid therapy, there is significant risk for untoward reactions and confounding of the already complex problem. Sustained opioid therapy for intractable headache should not be started on a primary care level, and patients who do not respond to standard treatment should be referred to specialists and/or centers where more complex regimens of treatment can be offered, where rebound and the underlying behavior can be treated, and where psychological influences on headache refractoriness can be most effectively addressed.

■ **SPECIAL CLINICAL POINT: Use of opioids in the treatment of headache should be severely restricted, and if used, must be carefully monitored by those who administer the medication. If opioids are prescribed, measures must be in place to ensure that multiple doctors are not writing prescriptions for these drugs.**

Those who choose to administer chronic opioids must be prepared to calculate appropriate dosages, see patients frequently, perform appropriate urine drug screens, and monitor usage carefully through collaboration with other treating physicians and collateral sources, such as spouses. Unfortunately, this is not always the case, and many of the problems associated with opioid use have resulted from failure to carefully select appropriate patients and effectively monitor those prescribed these medications.

Always Remember

- Primary headaches, particularly migraine, are considered potentially life-long disorders and require not only aggressive treatment but maintenance therapy that changes over the course of a patient's life.
- In patients with migraine and cluster headache, headaches due to secondary causes can emerge, and therefore the clinician must be alert to the possibility that there is a superimposed condition, thus justifying vigilance and appropriate testing whenever patterns change, new symptoms develop, or unexplained phenomena occur.
- A range of treatments is available from medications to behavioral therapy to rehabilitative approaches. Patients with intractable symptoms should be referred to advanced programs for comprehensive treatment approaches.
- Opioids are generally discouraged in the treatment of chronic headaches. Chronic administration for maintenance treatment has shown to both be counterproductive and contribute to the progression of headache conditions.

QUESTIONS AND DISCUSSION

1. A 36-year-old woman develops onset of severe right-sided orbital pain lasting 2 to 3 hours. The attacks may occur three times a day, and each attack is associated with conjunctival injection, tearing, and nasal drainage. During each attack, the patient paces and at times pounds her fists in pain. Alcohol is reliably able to provoke an attack.

   Which of the following is the likely diagnosis?

   A. Cluster headache
   B. Migraine with aura
   C. Migraine without aura
   D. Chronic paroxysmal hemicrania
   E. Tension-type headache

Which is likely to apply to this condition?

A. The patient is a cigarette smoker.

B. Menstrual periods affect the attack.

C. The patient would feel better if she sought a quiet, cool, dark room.

D. Physical therapy would be of benefit.

E. Antidepressants are likely to be helpful.

The answer to the first part of the question is A and the answer to the second part of the question is also A. Cluster headache is the diagnosis, and the case description is quite characteristic of a cluster attack.

Alcohol can be provocative in both disorders, but the distinct combination of conjunctival injection, tearing, nasal drainage, pacing, and duration of attacks is much more likely in cluster headache than in migraine. By definition migraine lasts at least 4 hours.

Paroxysmal hemicrania lasts no more than an hour and usually less and is not associated with major autonomic disturbances. Tension-type headache is not associated with any of these characteristics.

Cluster headache patients are frequently heavy smokers, whereas that is much less likely for the other conditions. Cluster headache patients are not influenced by menstrual periods, do not generally pace, rarely if ever benefit from physical therapy, and are generally not helped by antidepressants, except that lithium can be helpful and does have an antidepressant value.

2. When comparing migraine with cluster headache, which of the following is true?

A. Both are influenced by estrogenic fluctuation

B. Both predominantly affect females

C. Both have attacks averaging 4 to 12 hours in duration

D. Both are associated with autonomic disturbances

E. Both usually have first onset in adolescence

The correct answer is D. Both are associated with autonomic disturbances. Both migraine and cluster headache are characterized by parasympathetic disturbances, including eye tearing, nasal drainage, and other autonomic symptoms, although in cluster headache these are more reliable and diagnostic in their presentation. In migraine they may not occur in dramatic form.

Estrogen is influential in migraine but not in cluster headache, a predominantly male illness. Migraine is more common in females, but cluster headache is much more common in males. Migraine averages 4 to 72 hours, whereas cluster headache lasts no more than 3 hours. Migraine often has its onset in adolescence, whereas cluster headache generally starts later in life.

REFERENCES

Lake AE, Saper JR, Hamel RL. Comprehensive inpatient treatment of refractory chronic daily headache. *Headache*. 2009;49:555–562.

Saper JR, Lake AE III. Continuous opioid therapy (COT) is rarely advisable for refractory chronic daily headache: limited efficacy, risks, and proposed guidelines. *Headache*. 2008;48:838–849.

Swidan SZ, Lake AE III, Saper JR. Efficacy of intravenous diphenhydramine versus intravenous DHE-45 in the treatment of severe migraine headache. *Curr Pain Headache Rep*. 2005;9(1):65–70.

SUGGESTED READING

Argoff CE. A focused review of the use of botulinum toxins for neuropathic pain. *Clin J Pain*. 2002;18:S177–S181.

Bartsch T, Goadsby PJ. Stimulation of the greater occipital nerve (GON) enhances responses of dural responsive convergent neurons in the trigeminal cervical complex in the rat. *Cephalalgia*. 2001;21:401–402.

Boes CJ, Dodick DW. Refining the clinical spectrum of chronic paroxysmal hemicrania: a review of 74 patients. *Headache*. 2002;42:699–708.

Burstein RH, Cutrer FM, Yarnitsky D. The development of cutaneous allodynia during a migraine attack. *Brain*. 2000;123:1703–1709.

Ferrari MD, Roon KL, Lipton RB, et al. Oral triptans (serotonin 5-HT1b/1d agonist) in acute migraine treatment: a meta-analysis of 53 trials. *Lancet*. 2001;358:1668–1675.

Freitag FG, Lake AE III, Lipton R, et al. Inpatient treatment of headache: an evidence-based assessment. *Headache*. 2004;44(4):342–360.

Goadsby PJ. Short-lasting primary headaches: focus on trigeminal autonomic cephalgias and indomethacin-sensitive headaches. *Curr Opin Neurol*. 1999; 12:273–277.

Goadsby PJ, Lipton RB, Ferrari MD. Migraine—current understanding and treatment. *N Engl J Med*. 2002;246:257–270.

Holroyd KA, O'Donnell FJ, Stensland M, et al. Chronic tension-type headaches are characterized by near daily headaches and are often difficult to manage in primary practice. *JAMA*. 2001;285:2208–2215.

Jakubowski M, Levy D, Goor-Aryeh, et al. Terminating migraine with allodynia and ongoing central sensitization using parenteral administration of cox1/cox2 inhibitors. *Headache*. 2005;45:850–861.

Limmroth V, Katsarav AZ, Fritsche G, et al. Features in medication overuse headache following overuse of different acute headache drugs. *Neurology*. 2002;59:1011–1014.

Mao J. Opioid-induced abnormal pain sensitivity: implications in clinical opioid therapy. *Pain*. 2002;100: 213–217.

Meng ID, Porreca F. Headache currents. Basic science: mechanisms of medication overuse. *Headache*. 2004;1:47–54.

Mokri B. Low cerebrospinal fluid pressure syndromes. *Neurol Clin*. 2004;22(1):55–74.

Nixdorf DR, Heo G, Major PW. Randomized control trial of botulinum toxin A for chronic myogenous orofacial pain. *Pain*. 2002;99:465–473.

Olesen J. Classification and diagnostic criteria for headache disorders, cranial neuralgias, and facial pain. *Cephalalgia*. 1988;8(suppl 7):1–96.

Olesen J, Tfelt-Hansen P, Welch KMA, eds. *The Headaches*. 2nd ed. Philadelphia: Lippincott Williams & Wilkins;2000.

Ozyalcin SN, Talu GK, Kizitan E, et al. The efficacy and safety of venlafaxine in the prophylaxis of migraine. *Headache*. 2005;45:144–152.

Peres MF, Rozen TD. Melatonin in the preventive treatment of chronic cluster headache. *Cephalalgia*. 2001;21:993–995.

Saper JR. What matters is not the differences between triptans, but the differences between patients. *Arch Neurol*. 2001;58(9):1481–1482.

Saper JR. Chronic daily headache: a clinician's perspective. *Headache*. 2002;42:538.

Saper JR. Approach to the intractable headache case: identifying treatable barriers to improvement. Continuum: lifelong learning in neurology. *Neurology*. 2006;12:259–284.

Saper JR, Hamel RL, Lake AE III. Medication overuse headache (MOH) is a biobehavioral disorder. *Cephalalgia*. 2005;25:545.

Saper JR, Lake AE III. Borderline personality disorder and the chronic headache patient: review and management recommendations. *Headache*. 2002; 42:663–674.

Saper JR, Lake AE III, Hamel RL, et al. Long-term scheduled opioid treatment for intractable headache: 3-year outcome report. *Cephalalgia*. 2000;20:380.

Saper JR, Lake AE III, Madden SF, et al. Comprehensive/tertiary care for headache: a 6-month outcome study. *Headache*. 1999;39:249–263.

Saper JR, Silberstein SD, et al. *Handbook of Headache Management*. 2nd ed. Philadelphia: Lippincott Williams & Wilkins;1999.

Silberstein SD. Practice parameter: evidence-based guidelines for migraine headache (an evidence-based review): Report of the Quality Standards Subcommittee of the American Academy of Neurology. *Neurol*. 2000;55:754–762.

Silberstein SD, Lipton RB, Dalessio DJ, eds. *Wolff's Headache and Other Head Pain*. 7th ed. New York: Oxford University Press;2001.

Silberstein SD, Lipton RB, Dodick DW, eds. *Wolff's Headache and Other Pain*. 8th ed.. New York: Oxford University Press;2008.

Silverman SB. Cervicogenic headache: interventional, anesthetic, and ablative treatment. *Curr Pain Headache* Rep. 2002;6:308–314.

Weiller CA, May A, Limmroth V, et al. Brainstem activation and spontaneous human migraine attacks. *Nat Med*. 1995;1:658–660.

Weiner RL, Reed KL. Peripheral neurostimulation for control of intractable occipital neuralgia. *Neuromodulation*. 1999;2:217–221.

Welch KM, Welch KM, Nagesh V, et al. Periaqueductal gray matter dysfunction in migraine: cause or the burden of illness. *Headache*. 2001;41:629–637.

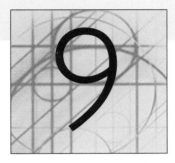

Epilepsy

DONNA C. BERGEN

key points
- Seizures are diagnosed by taking a careful history from the patient and/or a witness of the attacks.
- A single electroencephalogram may be normal in patients with epilepsy.
- Onset of epilepsy is most common in children and in the elderly, but may occur at any age.

A tonic–clonic seizure may occur acutely at any time of life as a result of trauma, metabolic disturbances, stroke, alcohol withdrawal, substance abuse, or other causes. Approximately 6% of the population has an afebrile seizure at some point in their lives. The recurring seizures of the chronic disorder called epilepsy also may begin at any time of life and include various other types of seizures. The prevalence of epilepsy in the United States is about 0.5%, making it one of the most common neurologic disorders. Incidence across the lifespan is a U-shaped curve, with the first year of life and old age being times of highest risk.

Epilepsy is a disorder primarily of the cerebral cortex, with seizures occurring when populations of neurons discharge in abnormal patterns. The pathophysiology of epileptic disorders is not well understood, and varies depending on seizure type and epilepsy syndrome (see Types of Seizures). Many of the genetically determined epilepsies, for example, have been shown to be the result of channelopathies or inborn structural abnormalities of neurotransmitter receptors. The many animal models of focal epilepsies, however, suggest that glial proliferation, loss of inhibitory neuronal activity, cortical remodeling, excessive excitatory activity, and other chronic cortical changes all may play a part in producing an acquired epileptogenic focus.

TYPES OF SEIZURES

The diagnosis of epilepsy is made on the basis of the clinical history of the seizures taken from the patient and often from a witness. The prototypical seizure, the tonic–clonic seizure (previously called *grand mal* seizure), often starts with sudden loss of consciousness, with the patient falling stiffly (the tonic phase); this is followed by rhythmic jerking of the limbs and torso (the clonic phase), which slows and then stops abruptly. Such seizures usually last only 60 to 90 seconds. The patient awakens after a period of postictal stupor, which usually lasts less than 15 minutes, but confusion may persist considerably longer. Such seizures coincide with very rapid, abnormal cortical and subcortical neuronal activity, which is recruited so rapidly that it appears synchronously in all brain areas when recorded on an electroencephalogram (EEG).

The physiologic abnormalities that may accompany these attacks include apnea, hypoxemia, acidosis, and autonomic disruptions such as cardiac arrhythmias and hypertension. Pulmonary edema can occur and may play a role in the syndrome of sudden death that occurs occasionally even in young, otherwise healthy patients with epilepsy. Other physical complications may include dislocation of the shoulder, vertebral collapse, and aspiration pneumonia.

Focal or partial seizures begin in a localized cortical area, with the clinical ictal phenomena being determined by the brain region involved. For example, seizures beginning with abnormal neuronal activity in primary motor cortex may cause initial twitching of the face or limb, depending on the exact site of onset. The patient with an occipital ictal focus may report flashing lights or globes, often in the visual field contralateral to the focus. Foci in the temporal lobes often produce autonomic symptoms such as nausea or complex psychic experiences such as intense feelings of familiarity (*déjà vu*) or feelings of strangeness. Such recalled seizure onsets commonly are called auras; although commonly construed as warnings of seizures they actually reflect the beginnings of the seizures themselves. The duration of focal seizures is generally 30 to 60 seconds.

Focal seizures that end without impairment of consciousness are termed *simple* partial seizures. Whether they begin with an aura or with sudden loss of awareness, focal seizures that at some time impair consciousness are called *complex* partial seizures. A witness typically reports that the patient stares and becomes unreactive, and that the patient may carry out simple motor activities such as picking at the clothes, walking about, or most typically smacking the lips. Complex partial seizures also last about a minute and may or may not be followed by postictal confusion. Both simple and partial seizures may spread throughout the brain, developing into a typical tonic–clonic seizure.

■ **SPECIAL CLINICAL POINT: An aura represents the beginning of a seizure, and its nature is determined by the site of onset in the cerebral cortex.**

There are also less dramatic seizure types, many occurring more commonly in children than in adults. An *absence* seizure (previously called petit mal seizure) refers to a brief episode of loss of awareness, occuring without warning, lasting for a few seconds, and ending with immediate resumption of consciousness. The patient usually stops what she is doing; the eyes remain open or may blink rapidly, but the patient does not fall. Absences may occur many times per day. Patients often are unaware of them, and they commonly are noted first by family members or teachers.

Another brief seizure type is the *myoclonic* seizure, which consists of sudden, brief single or repetitive jerks of the limbs without warning. Myoclonic seizures occur without warning and generally last only a few seconds. Consciousness sometimes is impaired, but like the absence seizure, the myoclonic seizure is followed by immediate return to full awareness without a postictal state.

Less common are the brief *atonic* or *akinetic* seizures, which consist of sudden falls without warning, usually but not always with loss of consciousness. Although brief, these seizures can be very dangerous, with patients often suffering injuries to the face or skull.

EPILEPSY SYNDROMES

The *primary generalized epilepsies* are a group of disorders which usually present in childhood, respond well to treatment, and may have high rates of remission. They generally are considered genetic in origin, most having nonspecific inheritance patterns but definite family clustering. The seizure types seen in these syndromes vary and may include generalized tonic–clonic seizures, absence seizures, and myoclonic seizures.

Patients with primary generalized epilepsies usually have normal neurologic examinations, are of normal intelligence, and give no history suggesting preexisting brain pathology. The EEG shows normal background activity, often interrupted by bursts of generalized spike-and-wave discharges. Primary generalized epilepsies make up 30% to 40% of childhood epilepsies.

Virtually all of the primary generalized epilepsies are age related, beginning and often remitting at specific times of life. The most common syndrome is that of *febrile seizures*, which occur in nearly 5% of children, generally between the ages of 1 and 3 years. Uncomplicated febrile seizures stop by the age of 5 years and are not associated with an increased risk of seizures in later life. On the contrary, when the seizures are prolonged (30 minutes or more), repeated, or followed by postictal hemiparesis (Todd's paralysis), children do have an increased risk of developing a chronic seizure disorder, which sometimes appears years later in the form of complex partial or other seizure types. Such syndromes are called complicated febrile seizures.

Childhood absence epilepsy usually begins between the ages of 4 and 10 years with the appearance of absence seizures. In 30% to 40% of cases, tonic–clonic seizures appear around the time of puberty. Seizures usually respond easily to medical treatment, and the remission rate by young adulthood may reach 80% to 90%. Before treatment, the EEG usually shows normally developed background activity interrupted by hyperventilation-induced three per second spike-and-wave activity (see Diagnosing Epilepsy), which is characteristic and helpful for diagnosis.

Juvenile myoclonic epilepsy is one of the most common genetically based epilepsies, with onset between the ages of 10 and 20 years. Patients usually present with a tonic–clonic seizure occurring without warning, often in the early morning. If specifically asked, they also give a history of recent involuntary jerks of the limbs or dropping of objects from the hands. These myoclonic seizures also occur most commonly in the morning and often immediately precede the "big" seizure that usually brings them to medical attention. Sleep deprivation or alcohol use commonly triggers seizures. The EEG shows characteristic polyspike-and-wave discharges elicited by strobe lights. The seizures themselves, however, are not sensitive to flashing lights. This type of epilepsy persists for decades or may even be lifelong.

■ **SPECIAL CLINICAL POINT:** **Juvenile myoclonic epilepsy is one of the most common types of epilepsy, and though generally responsive to treatment, may require lifelong therapy.**

In contrast to the previously mentioned seizure types, almost all adult epilepsies, as well as the majority beginning in childhood, are focal or *localization-related epilepsies*, with focal or partial seizures. The occurrence of focal seizures implies the existence of focal brain pathology. An almost unlimited variety of clinical seizure phenomena may occur, depending on the site of brain injury.

In the diagnosis of all forms of epilepsy, taking a meticulous history from the patient as well as from witnesses to the seizures is essential. The precise sequence of events making up the attacks reveals the site of seizure onset in the brain and the route and extent of seizure propagation through the brain. For example, a patient with a meningioma growing over the right cerebral hemisphere may present with focal motor seizures of the left leg resulting from irritation of nearby cerebral motor cortex by the tumor. Such an attack may spread down along the precentral (motor) gyrus, sequentially involving the cortex controlling the left arm. If the patient remains conscious throughout the seizure, the episode is called a simple partial seizure. Commonly, however, intrinsic cerebral inhibitory mechanisms fail to keep the seizure localized, and the electrical discharge may spread suddenly into thalamic and other brain structures with strong, widespread cortical projections. In this case, a generalized tonic–clonic seizure ensues. Unless the clinician obtains the history of focal onset of such an attack, a mistaken diagnosis of primary generalized epilepsy may be made, and a search for localized brain disease may be left undone.

A completely different symptom complex may be reported by the patient with temporal lobe injury, such as that following encephalitis, anoxia, or complicated febrile convulsions. A complex partial seizure often begins with a subjective experience such as a sudden feeling of strangeness or an abrupt sensation of nausea moving upward from the epigastrium. If the seizure discharges remain confined to a small area of the temporal lobe, the attack may not proceed further and may end in 30 to 60 seconds. If, however, the seizure spreads throughout both sides of the limbic system, consciousness may be altered or lost. The patient may stare vacantly or may appear to look about, becoming unresponsive and often making simple movements (automatisms) such as lip smacking, grimacing, or hand wringing. He may stand or sit still or may walk about aimlessly. Because of the intimate relationship between limbic cortical structures and the hypothalamus, autonomic signs and symptoms such as piloerection, change in skin color, borborygmus, or an urge to urinate are common in complex partial seizures. If the seizure stops at this point, the altered behavior also stops abruptly, but the patient may remain confused for several minutes or longer. If the seizure has started in the speech-dominant hemisphere, language function may be temporarily impaired postictally. If the ictal activity spreads further, however, a full-fledged tonic–clonic seizure occurs. Patients may be able to describe vividly the onset or aura of such attacks, but many subjects with temporal lobe seizures have no recall of events before loss of consciousness, and the physician must rely on witnesses for a full description of the episodes.

Focal epilepsy, with or without secondary generalization of the attacks, is by far the most common form of seizure disorder seen by the primary care physician and by most neurologists. Within this category, complex partial seizures are the most prevalent type. Many patients with partial seizures find complete relief from attacks with medication, but about 30% continue to have some seizures even with competent medical advice and optimal therapy.

The clinical picture becomes even more complex in the patient with multifocal or diffuse brain injury. Such a person may be subject to two or sometimes three seizure types. Generalized motor convulsions, focal seizures of any type, or absence attacks all may occur chronically. Additional patterns also may be present, often as fragments (tonic seizures) or distinctive types of episodes such as sudden losses of muscle tone with falling (akinetic seizures). Patients with these multiple seizure types nearly always bear other stigmata of serious cerebral injury such as mental retardation or cerebral palsy. In such cases, seizures are often difficult if not impossible to control with drugs, are almost always lifelong, and are best handled with the help of a neurologist or epileptologist.

Epilepsy takes a heavy toll on many aspects of patients' lives. Although prejudicial attitudes are softening gradually, epilepsy is still a condition often hidden from those outside the family. Social stigmatization is still surprisingly high, often affecting employment, insurability, and self-esteem. When the condition is poorly controlled, it can dominate and define relationships between parents, children, spouses, and siblings. Children may be sheltered excessively by parents and teachers, which may cause social maturation to be delayed or prevented. Depression and anxiety are very common and underdiagnosed in those with epilepsy, and suicide rates are above average. Learning difficulties in children with epilepsy are common and sometimes overlooked.

■ **SPECIAL CLINICAL POINT: Mood disorders occur in many patients with epilepsy and are often missed unless sought for by physicians.**

Details of state regulations vary, but usually the patient with epilepsy who cannot demonstrate complete, long-term control of the attacks is prohibited from driving. Public transportation and car pools are often inadequate solutions for day-to-day autonomy. Because a diagnosis of epilepsy has far-reaching implications for the life of the patient, it is essential that the diagnosis be neither missed nor misapplied.

DIAGNOSING EPILEPSY

Epilepsy is diagnosed through the patient's history—not by head scans, EEGs, or the neurologic examination. In cases when a seizure disorder is suspected, the physician must spend adequate time with the patient and often with witnesses to the attacks to make a reliable diagnosis.

In most cases, asking the patient for a detailed account of the last episode, or of the last one the patient recalls well, often evokes precise details and a coherent impression. Physicians should ask what the patient was doing when the attack began. They should inquire about the first thing that occurred when the attack started and what happened next. They also should ask how the patient felt after the episode ended and if any focal weakness or speech difficulty was present, details that might reveal the focal nature of the seizure.

The stereotypy of the attacks is an important diagnostic point, because for the individual patient, seizures are highly consistent events. Even when there is more than one seizure type, each type has its own stereotypy. Significant variation in the pattern of attacks argues against epilepsy.

The duration of seizures is generally invariant. Except for brief absence or myoclonic seizures, which generally last 5 to 15 seconds, most focal or tonic–clonic seizures last 30 to 90 seconds. The postictal recovery period depends on the type of seizure, but actual seizure-like episodes that last many minutes to hours are usually not epileptic.

Finally, a brief history from a witness is often crucial. What does the witness see and how does the attack begin? Patients with complex partial seizures sometimes recall the aura that begins the seizure, but are unaware of the subsequent loss of awareness. A witness may provide the crucial description of the blank stare and unresponsiveness typical of this type of seizure. The details of such seizures are crucial in discussing safety issues such as driving.

Discriminating between absence and complex partial seizures sometimes may be a diagnostic hurdle. The latter is much more common than the former, especially in adults. Making the correct diagnosis is important because only complex partial seizures imply the presence of focal brain disease and the therapies for the two types vary somewhat. If a reliable witness can be found, the two seizure types can be distinguished accurately by the duration of the attack. Almost all absence seizures last less than 15 seconds, and many are shorter. However, most complex partial seizures continue for more than 30 seconds, with many lasting 1 to 1.5 minutes. Auras, automatisms, and postictal confusion are common with complex partial seizures but are not characteristic of absence seizures. Postictal language difficulty or other focal neurologic signs may be reported after a complex partial seizure.

An EEG almost always demonstrates abnormal, repetitive neuronal discharges (spikes) during a seizure. In the far more usual case, when seizures are not occurring, interictal EEGs often show single spikes that often are reported as "epileptiform discharges" on EEG reports. Such discharges may be focal or diffuse ("generalized"), depending on the type of epilepsy. Some are so characteristic of specific epilepsy syndromes that an expert electroencephalographer may be able to corroborate the likely clinical diagnosis very specifically, given an adequate history. This rule is particularly true in patients with childhood absence epilepsy where the EEG shows characteristic three per second discharges and in subjects with complex partial seizures associated with focal spikes over the temporal lobe.

Epilepsy, however, cannot be diagnosed by the EEG alone. Although the typical abnormality is seen in more than 80% of untreated patients with absence seizures, there is a dismaying 50% false-negative rate in a single EEG in patients with focal seizures. In addition, the EEG may be falsely positive in up to 5% to 10% of children, that is, epileptiform discharges are seen although the child does not have nor will develop epilepsy. This is seen especially in those with a family history of epilepsy. Focal epileptiform discharges in adults are much more specific, however, occurring in fewer than 2% to 3% of those without active epilepsy or a history of epilepsy.

When a diagnosis of epilepsy is made, and even after a single first seizure, magnetic resonance scanning of the head with infusion is indicated, unless a specific genetically determined, nonfocal epilepsy syndrome is identified with some assurance. Most patients, even those with focal epilepsy, have normal scans, but up to 30% demonstrate focal pathology such as cortical migrational abnormalities, mesial temporal sclerosis, vascular malformations, infarctions, or neoplasms.

DIFFERENTIAL DIAGNOSIS

Neurocardiogenic (vasovagal) syncope is generally easily diagnosed, because the typical prodrome almost always is remembered vividly by the patient. Giddiness, weakness, sweating, nausea, and fading or graying-out of vision are highly suggestive of true syncope. Urinary incontinence is not rare in syncope; tongue biting, however, is rare and usually implies a convulsion.

Witnesses report the victim of syncope as crumpling or sliding to the ground, whereas the patient with convulsions usually falls stiffly. Consciousness is regained very quickly after syncope, whereas confusion or somnolence is common after seizures. The diagnosis of neurocardiogenic syncope may be made more difficult by the occurrence of a few myoclonic jerks during the syncope, which may be reported by witnesses as seizure activity (so-called "convulsive syncope"). A history of the typical prodrome and syncopal triggers (dehydration, overheating, prolonged standing, micturition) will prevent confusion.

■ **SPECIAL CLINICAL POINT: Syncope is easily diagnosed because of the typical prodrome or trigger and often includes brief myoclonic jerking.**

Cardiogenic or Stokes–Adams attacks also must be differentiated from seizures. Most patients with this syndrome are late middle aged or elderly. The patient usually loses consciousness without warning or after brief palpitations. The patient usually falls suddenly and limply to the ground. Syncope from cardiac arrhythmias rarely causes incontinence or tongue biting. The attacks are usually short, and consciousness is regained quickly and completely.

Panic attacks sometimes are mistaken for seizures, particularly if they include an element of dissociation reported as altered consciousness. The typical symptom complex of fear, chest pain, dyspnea, numbness (especially in the fingertips and lips as a result of hyperventilation), and weakness is not typical of seizures.

Pseudoseizures or psychogenic seizures usually present as seizure-like attacks that do not respond to antiepileptic drug (AED) treatment. Like true seizures, pseudoseizures vary from convulsive-like episodes to transient alterations in consciousness or sensation, but the astute clinician may note incongruous or atypical elements in the history. For example, the person with pseudoseizures resembling tonic–clonic seizures may report continuing awareness of surroundings even during the throes of an attack. Symptoms may vary from episode to episode. Urinary incontinence and even bodily injury occur with surprising frequency in pseudoseizures and do not rule out the diagnosis. A firm diagnosis can be made only with the help of the EEG (see Management of Epilepsy). Pseudoseizures and true epileptic seizures occasionally occur in the same patient, making diagnosis and treatment particularly difficult.

MANAGEMENT OF EPILEPSY

Medical therapy is begun once a diagnosis of epilepsy has been firmly established, that is, after at least two unprovoked seizures (Flow

Chart). The goal of treatment should be complete control of seizures, and the ideal therapy is a single drug without side effects. This goal is initially achievable in 70% of patients. Eventually, a substantial minority of patients (10% to 30%) will demonstrate refractoriness to drug therapy, however (see Surgical Therapies).

Epilepsy is a fearsome diagnosis for most patients or parents, so the physician should be prepared to spend some time dispensing information about the disorder, its prognosis, expectations of therapy, problems relating to pregnancy, and safety measures. Informational pamphlets can be acquired from a local or regional Epilepsy Foundation office; the phone number for the national office is 800-332-1000, and the Web site is www.epilepsyfoundation.org.

The choice of initial treatment depends on an accurate diagnosis of seizure type(s). Absences and myoclonic seizures, for example, respond to valproate, lamotrigine, zonisamide, levetiracetam, and topiramate, and these drugs also prevent tonic–clonic and focal seizures. Ethosuximide, however, will stop absence seizures but not other seizure types. Most other AEDs are effective against the most common seizure types (i.e., focal seizures and tonic-clonic seizures) (Table 9.1). Treatment of the patient with mental retardation, cerebral palsy,

TABLE 9.1 | Treatment of Common Seizure Types

Partial (focal) seizures
Phenytoin (Dilantin, Phenytek)
Carbamazepine (Tegretol, Carbatrol)
Valproate (Depakote)
Primidone (Mysoline)
Phenobarbital
Gabapentin (Neurontin)
Lamotrigine (Lamotrigine)
Topiramate (Topamax)
Tiagabine (Gabitril)
Oxcarbazepine (Trileptal)
Zonisamide (Zonegran)
Levetiracetam (Keppra)
Pregabalin (Lyrica)
Lacosamide (Vimpat)

Absence seizures
Ethosuximide (Zarontin)
Valproate
Lamotrigine
Zonisamide
Levetiracetam

Myoclonic seizures
Valproate
Lamotrigine
Zonisamide
Levetiracetam

Drugs are listed in order of FDA approval, not necessarily by preference.

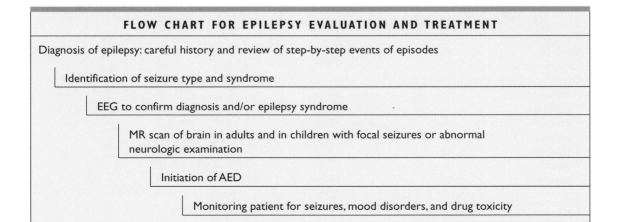

FLOW CHART FOR EPILEPSY EVALUATION AND TREATMENT

Diagnosis of epilepsy: careful history and review of step-by-step events of episodes

Identification of seizure type and syndrome

EEG to confirm diagnosis and/or epilepsy syndrome

MR scan of brain in adults and in children with focal seizures or abnormal neurologic examination

Initiation of AED

Monitoring patient for seizures, mood disorders, and drug toxicity or structural cerebral pathology who has multiple seizure types or akinetic seizures is particularly challenging and usually requires the assistance of a neurologist or epileptologist.

Because many AEDs cause side effects if introduced too quickly, standard practice is to start the chosen AED strictly according to instructions on the package insert, or even slower. This practice involves starting with a low dosage and building to a recommended effective dose or serum level. An exception is phenytoin, which generally is started at a full, usually well-tolerated, adult daily dosage of 300 mg/day. In emergency situations such as initial multiple seizures, intravenous loads with phenytoin, valproate, or levetiracetam are all well tolerated.

The effective dose of many AEDs is often very close to the dose that causes side effects, and interactions among AEDs themselves and between some AEDs and other drugs are common. Careful attention to the pharmacokinetics of the AED is essential, and the physician managing epilepsy must be aware of all drugs that the patient chronically or intermittently ingests (Table 9.2).

SERUM ANTIEPILEPTIC DRUG LEVELS

Recommended "therapeutic" serum levels of AEDs are values below which patients have been observed to be at risk for seizures, and above which many patients complain of dose-related side effects. It is prudent to titrate doses of carbamazepine, phenytoin, valproate, and the barbiturates to within the usual therapeutic levels. Optimal therapeutic levels for the other AEDs have not been well established, although clinical laboratories provide estimates, and these AEDs usually are increased to a therapeutic *dosage* (Table 9.2). If seizures or side effects occur, an AED dosage may be increased or decreased carefully within or even sometimes outside normal levels or dosages. If the first AED fails to control the seizures, a second drug may be added; when the dosage is stable, the first, ineffective drug can then be withdrawn slowly.

Serum AED levels also can aid decision making when a patient taking more than one drug becomes toxic. Drug levels may be helpful if patient adherence is questionable. When drawn at the same time of day, and without interference from other medications or illness (e.g.,

TABLE 9.2 Properties of AEDs			
AED	**Plasma Half-Life**	**% Protein Bound**	**Target Levels (μg/mL)**
Ethosuximide	30–60	<10	40–100
Gabapentin	5–9	0	4–16
Lamotrigine	15–24[a]	55[a]	2–20
Levetiracetam	7	<10	20–60
Oxcarbazepine	10–15	40	5–50
Phenobarbital	65–110	45	10–30
Phenytoin	10–24	90	10–20
Primidone	8–15	<20	4–8
Tiagabine	2–9	96	5–70
Topiramate	12–30	15	2–25
Valproate	5–15	70–90	50–150
Zonisamide	50–70	55	10–40

[a]60 hours when used with valproate.
AED, antiepileptic drug.

gastrointestinal upsets), AED levels are usually remarkably stable from sample to sample.

SOME INDIVIDUAL ANTIEPILEPTIC DRUGS

Although some general principles govern their use, individual AEDs vary enough in their metabolism, side effects, and interactions with other drugs to require separate comment. *Carbamazepine*, especially in one of its long-acting forms, is an older AED still used commonly for focal or tonic–clonic seizures. A readily reversible rash occurs in about 3% to 5% of patients, but serious hypersensitivity reactions are rare. Early, mild leucopenia may be seen but is generally reversible and is only rarely a significant problem. Predictable, reversible, dose-related side effects are blurred vision, diplopia, and nausea. Chronic side effects may include macrocytosis, low-normal serum levels of folate, and hyponatremia.

Despite common long-term side effects, phenytoin is still often prescribed. It is available in a parenteral form, a loading dose is well tolerated, and most adults achieve a therapeutic blood level on a "standard" 300 mg/day dosage. Dose-related toxicity typically includes nystagmus, tremor, and ataxia. Elevated serum alkaline phosphatase, macrocytosis, and low serum T_4 (but normal thyroid-stimulating hormone) are common and require no action. The metabolism of phenytoin is saturable, so that small increases in dosage within the therapeutic range may cause disproportionately large increases in serum levels. Therefore, changes in daily doses should be no more than 25 to 50 mg at one time. The common long-term cosmetic effects of phenytoin, which include acne, hirsutism, gingival hyperplasia, and possibly coarsening of facial features may be significant, especially in children.

Both carbamazepine and phenytoin, along with the now little used phenobarbital and primidone, are powerful inducers of certain P450 hepatic enzymes, and phenytoin is strongly protein bound, so physicians prescribing these drugs must always be aware of possibly significant pharmacologic interactions with other drugs (e.g., warfarin [Coumadin], certain antimicrobials). These drugs reduce the serum levels of valproate, lamotrigine, topiramate, tiagabine, zonisamide, oxcarbazepine, and each other.

Valproate is generally tolerated well, but side effects such as weight gain and tremor are common, and alopecia can present a problem. Fatal toxic hepatitis has been reported, mainly in young children on polytherapy during the first 6 months of use; the drug is not recommended for children younger than 2 years of age. Blood levels tend to vary more than they do with other anticonvulsants, so they are less useful. Drug interactions with valproate may be significant: it is an inhibitor of certain liver metabolic pathways, and the drug dramatically raises the serum level of lamotrigine. Valproate's metabolism may be enhanced by enzyme-inducing medications including phenytoin and carbamazepine.

Since 1993 many new AEDs, most of them pharmacologically unrelated to older AEDs, have become available for treatment of seizure disorders (i.e., lamotrigine, topiramate, gabapentin, tiagabine, zonisamide, oxcarbamazepine, levetiracetam, pregabalin, and lacosamide). All are U.S. Food and Drug Administration-approved as treatment of focal (partial) and tonic–clonic seizures. All but gabapentin, pregabalin, tiagabine, and lacosamide have been successfully used for treatment of absence and myoclonic seizures as well. The "therapeutic" blood levels of these AEDs show much wider variation than those of the older drugs and may not be as clinically useful. Many of these drugs offer some advantages in terms of fewer drug interactions. All are considerably more costly than the older AEDs, but most are available as generic preparations.

Gabapentin and *pregabalin* are derivatives of gamma-aminobutyric acid (GABA), the main inhibitory neurotransmitter of the brain. They demonstrate no interactions with other drugs and are therefore very useful in the elderly, who are often taking a variety of other pharmaceuticals. The most common dose-related side effect is drowsiness. Patients should be warned that weight gain is common with chronic use.

Lamotrigine must be introduced very slowly to reduce the incidence of skin rash to a tolerable 3% to 4%. Titration and doses must be moderated, when valproate also is used, because of pharmacokinetic interactions. It is generally well tolerated, although insomnia may limit its use. Dose-limiting side effects include diplopia, nausea, and dizziness.

Levetiracetam can be introduced at a therapeutically effective dose of 1000 mg/day. It is generally well tolerated, although high doses can be associated with changes in mood or even cognition.

Oxcarbazepine is a derivative of carbamazepine, with the advantage of fewer drug interactions and with a similar side effect profile. Hyponatremia may be a problem, especially in the elderly or in those with already low serum sodium.

Topiramate and *zonisamide* are sulfonamide derivatives, with topiramate especially requiring slow dose titration to minimize cognitive and behavioral side effects. Weight loss with chronic use may be considerable. The concomitant use of hepatic enzyme-inducing drugs such as phenytoin or carbamazepine significantly lowers the blood level of these drugs. Nephrolithiasis has been reported.

Tiagabine is another GABA agonist, whose metabolism is briskly enhanced by enzyme-inducing drugs, and its dose must be managed accordingly. Twice-a-day dosing has been shown to be effective.

COMPLICATIONS OF EPILEPSY AND ANTIEPILEPTIC DRUGS

The psychosocial complications of epilepsy may be significant, even in the absence of other obvious cerebral pathology. The prevalence of major depression and anxiety is high; the incidence of suicide is about double that in the general population. Complaints of significant memory deficits for recent events are almost universal in those with focal limbic system epilepsy and can worsen if uncontrolled seizures persist. Atten-

tion deficit disorder is a frequent accompaniment in children, and learning disorders are common and generally underdiagnosed.

Long-term use of the enzyme-inducing AEDs has convincingly been shown to increase the risk of bone thinning and folate deficiency. Relatively higher serum cholesterol levels, and low levels of folate, have consistently been observed as well. The metabolism of some B vitamins may also be increased. Similar adverse effects on bone metabolism have been shown with valproate. For these reasons, patients on enzyme-inducing AEDs or valproate should be given supplemental calcium with vitamin D (e.g., 500 mg twice a day), and those on enzyme inducers should take a daily multivitamin. Early bone density scans for both men and women are increasingly recommended.

■ **SPECIAL CLINICAL POINT: Standard practice is to add a multivitamin and supplemental calcium with vitamin D when patients take valproate or an enzyme-inducing AED.**

For "rescue" therapy in patients with clusters of seizures, prepackaged syringes of *diazepam* gel for rectal use are safe for home use and are very effective. Oral lorazepam (usually 1–2 mg for adults) can also be used, but takes longer to be effective.

SURGICAL THERAPIES

A novel treatment for drug-resistant epilepsy is vagus nerve stimulation, shown to be effective in treating partial and tonic–clonic seizures. This pacemaker-like device is implanted subcutaneously, and it operates both by programmed, intermittent stimulation and by being switched on when a seizure is felt or seen to begin. Although about 30% of patients improve with vagus nerve stimulation, it is always used with concomitant AEDs, and complete cessation of seizures is unusual.

If three appropriate AEDs at therapeutic dosages fail to control epilepsy in adults or children, the possibility of surgical therapy should be considered because continued drug resistance to multiple therapies is likely. The most common procedure is temporal lobectomy, which has a low morbidity and a high probability of complete cessation of seizures, particularly in patients with mesial temporal sclerosis.

STOPPING ANTIEPILEPTIC DRUGS

Many epilepsies, particularly those beginning in childhood, eventually go into remission. The point at which AEDs may be safely stopped in well-controlled patients is debatable. A seizure-free period of 2 years in children and 3 years in adults is considered a reasonable time at which to consider a trial without drugs. Permanent remission rates in children with absence epilepsy reach 80% to 90%, but relapse is the rule in juvenile myoclonic epilepsy. Drug withdrawal fails in the more common adult focal epilepsies in 30% to 50% of cases.

DIETARY AND ALTERNATIVE OR REHABILITATIVE TREATMENTS

The ketogenic diet and its variants are high-fat, low-protein/carbohydrate diets sometimes used for short periods in children with intractable epilepsy. It customarily is initiated and supervised by a pediatric neurologist, usually with the assistance of a dietitian experienced in its use. No other dietary changes, herbs, or supplements have been found to help in the treatment of epilepsy.

Hypnosis has been successful in isolated cases but is not customarily used. In the absence of complications, no specific physical or occupational rehabilitation is necessary in treating epilepsy.

WOMEN AND EPILEPSY

Phenytoin, carbamazepine, the barbiturates, and topiramate all enhance the metabolism of oral contraceptive hormones; high-dose preparations with 50 g of estradiol are recommended. Folate metabolism also is enhanced by phenytoin, carbamazepine, and the barbiturates. Because inadequate maternal folate has been associated with spinal bifida, supplemental folic acid should be given to all women of reproductive capacity taking these drugs.

All of the AEDs that have been studied have been shown to increase the rate of fetal malformations by about a factor of 2, and all AEDs are category C or D drugs in pregnancy. Valproate has been associated with a significant increased risk of midline neural tube defects. Because of the serious risks of seizures during pregnancy, however, most women with epilepsy continue to use an AED when pregnant. Stopping or changing an AED after pregnancy is discovered generally is not advised. Serum AED levels characteristically fall during pregnancy and need careful monitoring.

SPECIAL CHALLENGES FOR MANAGING HOSPITALIZED PATIENTS

Patients with epilepsy who are admitted to hospital for other conditions should have their routine AEDs continued. Currently, the only chronically used AEDs available in parenteral form are phenytoin, valproate, levetiracetam, phenobarbital, and lacosamide. If patients cannot take their usual AED by mouth for

---

Always Remember

- Epilepsy is diagnosed by taking a careful history.
- Almost all adult onset epilepsies are focal in nature, so MR scanning of the brain is essential.
- Complete cessation of seizures using a single AED without side effects is the goal of therapy for all patients.
- Failure of two AEDs suggests that the diagnosis may be incorrect or that the patient has intractable epilepsy requiring referral to a neurologist.

more than 24 hours, a parenteral AED should be used, preferably with the help of a neurologist. Many surgical procedures will interrupt oral AED therapy by less than a day, and the usual drug simply may be resumed as soon as the patient is able to take it.

WHEN TO REFER THE PATIENT TO A NEUROLOGIST

Although most patients with epilepsy are helped to achieve substantial control of seizures, at least 10% to 30% of patients on optimal drug therapy continue to have seizures serious or frequent enough to cause major disruptions to life. If seizures have not been completely controlled after 2 years, or if the patient has failed to respond to two AEDs, such patients should be referred to a neurologist or epilepsy center. Some of these patients turn out to have disorders other than epilepsy; some have types of seizures responsive to more appropriate AEDs; others are appropriate for surgical therapy.

QUESTIONS AND DISCUSSION

1. Patients with primary generalized epilepsy may have which of the following types of seizures?
   A. Absence
   B. Myoclonic
   C. Grand mal
   D. All of the above
   E. None of the above

The correct answer is D. Patients may have any combination of these seizures. Sometimes grand mal attacks are preceded or led into by clusters of absence or myoclonic spells.

2. The physiologic substrate of clinical seizure activity is:
   A. Abnormal neuronal discharge
   B. Hyperactive glial potentials
   C. Repeated disturbances in cerebral blood flow
   D. Excessive gabaergic activity

The correct answer is A. In focal epilepsy, groups of hyperirritable neurons, perhaps affected by loss of inhibitory input, excessive excitatory activity, and anatomic distortions, overact and are able to hypersynchronize the activity of other neuronal populations. This activity spreads and causes focal or even generalized seizures.

3. High blood levels of phenytoin usually are accompanied by:
   A. Somnolence
   B. Hair loss
   C. Ataxia
   D. Pulmonary edema
   E. Weakness

The correct answer is C. Ataxia is much more common than somnolence. Sedation is caused by phenytoin only at extremely high levels, as would be caused by deliberate overdosing. Hair loss may occur with valproate but not with phenytoin. Neither pulmonary edema nor muscle weakness is typical of phenytoin effect. Ataxia is seen in most patients with blood levels higher than 30 mg/dL.

4. The true statement about vagal nerve stimulation for epilepsy control is:
   A. Approximately 30% of patients undergoing this procedure improve.
   B. The aim of vagal nerve stimulation is to eliminate AEDs.
   C. The treatment is not useful to treat partial and tonic–clonic seizures.
   D. The stimulator is limited because patients cannot turn on the stimulator at the time of their seizure onset, even if they have a well-defined aura.

The correct answer is A. A novel treatment for drug-resistant epilepsy is vagus nerve stimulation, shown to be effective in treating partial and tonic–clonic seizures. This pacemaker-like device is implanted subcutaneously, and it operates both by programmed, intermittent stimulation and by being switched on when a seizure is felt or seen to begin. Although about 30% of patients improve with vagus nerve stimulation, it is always used with concomitant AEDs, and complete cessation of seizures is unusual.

SUGGESTED READING

Amar AP. Vagus nerve stimulation for the treatment of intractable epilepsy. *Expert Rev Neurother*. 2007;7: 1763–1773.

Arif H, Hirsch LJ. Treatment of status epilepticus. *Semin Neurol*. 2008;28:342–354.

Brodie MJ, French JA. Management of epilepsy in adolescents and adults. *Lancet*. 2000;356:323–329.

Cross JH, Jayakar P, Nordli D, et al.; International League against Epilepsy, Subcommission for Paediatric Epilepsy Surgery; Commissions of Neurosurgery and Paediatrics. Proposed criteria for referral and evaluation of children for epilepsy surgery: recommendations of the Subcommission for pediatric epilepsy surgery. *Epilepsia*. 2006;47(6):952–959.

Duncan JS, Sander JW, Sisodiya SM, et al. Adult epilepsy. *Lancet*. 2006;367:1087–1100.

French JA, Pedley TA. Initial management of epilepsy. *N Engl J Med*. 2008;359:155–176.

Haut SR, Shinnar S. Considerations in the treatment of a first unprovoked seizure. *Semin Neurol*. 2008;28: 289–296.

LaFrance WC Jr, Kanner AM, Hermann B. Psychiatric co-morbidities in epilepsy. *Int Rev Neurobiol*. 2008;83: 347–383.

Sirven JI. Acute and chronic seizures in patients older than 60 years. *Mayo Clin Proc*. 2001;76:175–183.

Tomson T, Hiilesmaa V. Epilepsy in pregnancy. *Brit Med J*. 2007;335:769–773.

Wyllie E, Gupta A, Lachhwani DK. *The Treatment of Epilepsy: Principles and Practice*. 4th ed. Philadelphia: Lippincott Williams & Wilkins; 2005.

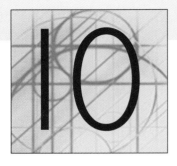

Sleep Disorders

RUŽICA KOVAČEVIĆ-RISTANOVIĆ
AND TOMASZ J. KUŹNIAR

key points

- Insufficient sleep time and sleep apnea are the two most common causes of excessive daytime sleepiness.

- Obstructive sleep apnea is suspected on the basis of snoring and excessive daytime sleepiness.

- Obstructive sleep apnea may be associated with significant morbidity related to sleepiness and morbidity/mortality related to its cardiovascular effects.

- Taking a good sleep history is a key to diagnosis and the first step to successful treatment of insomnia.

- Narcolepsy typically presents in an adolescent/young adult with excessive sleepiness, sleep attacks, and cataplexy.

leep is a subject that has fascinated physicians and the public since antiquity. A search for a "sleep center" in the brain has demonstrated the complexity of the sleep process, the multiplicity of structures involved in sleep, and the reciprocal interactions necessary for the initiation and maintenance of this behavior.

The structures found to facilitate sleep are the basal forebrain (i.e., the preoptic area of the hypothalamus, specifically the ventrolateral preoptic nucleus [VLPO], promoting sleep via gamma-aminobutyric acid [GABA]/galanin activity), the area surrounding the solitary tract in the medulla, and the midline thalamus. It has been proposed that the sleep-promoting role of the anterior hypothalamus results from its inhibitory action on the posterior hypothalamic awakening neurons nuclei (mainly tuberomammillary histaminergic

neurons [TMN] projecting widely to the cortex). Structures found to facilitate waking are wake-promoting hypocretin (orexin) system and the ascending reticular-activating system of the pons and midbrain and posterior hypothalamus. The role of the hypothalamus has been revised recently since the discoveries of sleep-promoting GABA/galanin activity in the VLPO and wake-promoting hypocretin (orexin) system activity in the dorsolateral hypothalamus around the perifornical nucleus. Although no direct interaction between the VLPO and hypocretin systems is reported, both systems innervate the main components of ascending arousal systems such as adrenergic locus coeruleus (LC), serotonergic dorsal raphe (DR), dopaminergic ventrotegmental area (VTA), and histaminergic TMN. The VLPO (GABA/galanin) system inhibits and the dorsolateral hypothalamic (hypocretin [orexin]) system activates these "arousal" systems.

Destruction of the VLPO system results in insomnia, whereas destruction of the hypocretin system results in narcolepsy (hypersomnolence/sleep attacks and cataplexy). The control of alternating sleep stages (NREM [nonrapid eye movement]/REM [rapid eye movement] cycling) is attributed to interaction between antagonistic aminergic and cholinergic systems in the brainstem. The aminergic and cholinergic systems also are involved in the process of cortical activation of arousal. In addition to the previously mentioned systems, the dopaminergic system is involved in control of alertness as well, especially the ventral tegmental area (A10). Dopaminergic neurons of the VTA but not substantia nigra (SN) are excited by hypocretins, and there is a greater hypocretin innervation of the VTA than SN. Dopaminergic neurons in the ventral periaqueductal gray (PAG) also are activated during wakefulness. The dopaminergic system, including the descending A11 projection, may be particularly important for sleep disorders accompanied by anomalies of sleep-related motor control (cataplexy and periodic limb movement [PLM] disorder). Circadian sleep rhythm is modulated by the hypothalamic suprachiasmatic nucleus (SCN). The SCN sets the body clock period to approximately 25 hours, with the light and schedule cues (*zeitgebers*, "time givers") entraining it to 24 hours. The retinohypothalamic tract conveys light stimuli to the SCN that directly influences its activity. Melatonin has been implicated as a modulator of light entrainment because it is secreted maximally during the night by the pineal gland (hormone of darkness). Thus, the anterior hypothalamus may serve as a center for "sleep switch" under the influence of the circadian clock.

Understanding the neurochemistry of sleep is important for practical reasons. The discovery of the involvement of different neurotransmitters and neuromodulators in control of arousal and sleep has raised the possibility of more specific treatments of sleep disorders (e.g., hypocretin agonists and/or GABA/galanin antagonists for treatment of excessive sleepiness).

Most current treatments for sleep disorders do not relate to the known neurochemical substrates for sleep. Even more important, the myriad effects of currently used medications on sleep (those used to alter sleep and those used for an unrelated purpose) should be understood.

The important clinical, diagnostic, and therapeutic features of some sleep disorders are described in this chapter. Useful guidelines for diagnosis and therapy also are presented, although there are few universally accepted treatments for common sleep complaints.

SLEEP ARCHITECTURE

Because the workup of many patients with sleep disorders involves the use of a sleep laboratory, it is important to understand the tests available and the parameters measured. A portion of the sleep recording, referred to as a polysomnogram (PSMG) of a normal subject, is shown in Figure 10.1. Three basic parameters are needed to define the stage of sleep: an electroencephalogram (EEG), an electro-oculogram (EOG), and an electromyogram (EMG). The normal EEG of an alert, resting subject with closed eyes shows an 8- to 12-Hz posterior activity known as alpha. Two major sleep stages are distinguished: NREM and REM sleep; the nomenclature of NREM sleep has recently changed. Electroencephalographically NREM sleep has three stages. Stage N1 sleep is the stage of NREM sleep that directly follows the awake state. An EEG shows a low-voltage tracing of mixed frequencies predominantly in the theta band with alpha activity less than 50%, vertex sharp activity, and slow eye movements. Stage N2 sleep is the stage of NREM sleep that is characterized by the presence of sleep spindles (12 to 14 Hz) and K-complexes against a relatively low-voltage, mixed-frequency background. High-voltage delta waves may constitute up to 20% of N2 sleep. In the new diagnostic description of stage N3 of NREM sleep, at least 20% of the period consists of EEG waves less than 2 Hz; this stage is commonly referred to as slow wave sleep. Stage N3

ROC/LOC

C₄/A₂

EMG

O₂ SAT.

N/OT

TSG

TACH.

ECG

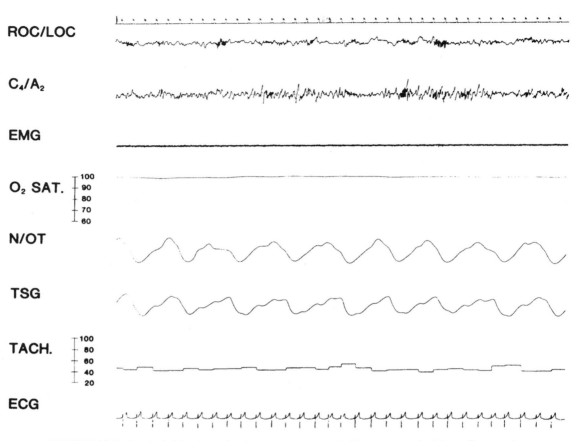

FIGURE 10.1 A typical eight-channel polysomnogram recorded from a normal adult man in stage 2 of nonrapid eye movement sleep. Electro-oculogram (ROC/LOC) recorded from right outer canthus referred to left outer canthus; electroencephalogram (EEG) (C4/A2) recorded from the right central lead referred to the right mastoid; electromyogram (EMG) recorded from the submental musculature; arterial oxygen saturation (O2SAT) transduced by an ear oximeter; nasal and oral airflow (N/OT) recorded by a thermocouple mounted in a plastic respiratory mask; thoracic movement (TSG) recorded by a strain gauge; heart rate recorded by a cardiotachometer; electrocardiogram (ECG) recorded from V5 referred to the left mastoid.

sleep occurs predominantly in the first third of the sleep period (Fig. 10.2).

REM sleep alternates with the NREM sleep at about 90-minute intervals in adults and 60-minute intervals in infants. The EEG pattern during REM sleep resembles stage 1 sleep but is accompanied by REMs. In addition, EMG activity is low. There is a general activation of the autonomic system, with a higher average respiratory rate, heart rate, and blood pressure, and, more importantly, much more pronounced variability throughout the REM period. In about 80% of awakenings from REM sleep, people recall vivid dreams, compared to only 5% of awakenings from NREM sleep. However, in about 60% to 80% of awakenings from NREM sleep, people may recall thought-like fragments. Population studies have shown

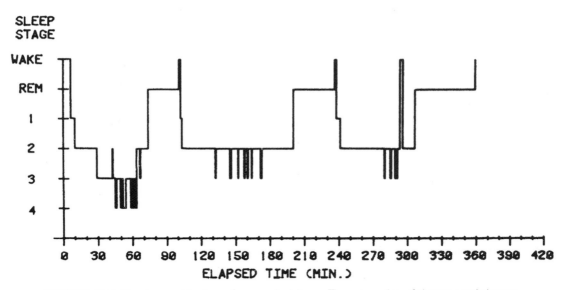

SLEEP
STAGE

FIGURE 10.2 The sleep architecture of a normal adult man. The progression of electroencephalogram (EEG) stages of sleep demonstrates a concentration of stages 3 and 4 within the first half of the sleep period. Episodes of rapid eye movement (REM) sleep occur at approximately 90-minutes intervals, and the majority of REM appears within the latter half of the sleep period. Waking arousals are few.

that the percentage of time spent in each stage varies with age and sex. Figures 10.1 and 10.2 represent a sleep PSMG and architecture plot from a normal adult.

CLASSIFICATION OF SLEEP ABNORMALITIES

The recently updated international classification of sleep disorders (International Classification of Sleep Disorders-2, ICSD-2) divides sleep disorders into (a) insomnias, (b) sleep-disordered breathing, (c) hypersomnias of central origin, (d) circadian rhythm disorders, (e) sleep-related movement disorders, and (f) parasomnias. The most common clinical correlates of these disorders are insomnia and excessive daytime sleepiness, although some sleep disorders do not cause any daytime symptoms. Future advances in the understanding of the pathophysiology of sleep disorders

will result in improved classification along the lines of pathology.

SLEEP DISORDERS ASSOCIATED WITH INSOMNIA

Insomnia is a perception of inadequate, disturbed, insufficient, or nonrestorative sleep despite an adequate opportunity to sleep, accompanied by daytime consequences of inadequate sleep. A Gallup phone survey found that 36% of Americans suffer from some type of sleep disorders. Occasional insomnia was reported by 27% of respondents, and chronic insomnia was reported by 9%.

Among the intrinsic sleep disorders are psychophysiologic insomnia, sleep-state misperception (paradoxical insomnia), restless legs syndrome and idiopathic insomnia, all of which produce the complaint of insomnia. Similarly, many extrinsic sleep disorders such as inadequate sleep hygiene, environmental sleep disorder, altitude insomnia, adjustment sleep disorder, limit-setting sleep disorder, food allergy insomnia, hypnotic-dependent sleep disorder, alcohol-dependent sleep disorder, and sleep-disordered breathing are likely to be accompanied by insomnia. Among circadian rhythm sleep disorders, delayed sleep-phase syndrome is associated with a complaint of sleep-onset delay, whereas advanced sleep-phase syndrome is accompanied by a complaint of early awakening. In general, the pattern of insomnia may be primarily (a) difficulty falling asleep (sleep-onset delay, sleep-onset insomnia), (b) early morning arousal (premature awakening, terminal insomnia), or (c) premature awakening(s), sleep fragmentation with inability to fall asleep again (sleep-maintenance insomnia).

Insomnias can be transient or acute (lasting less than 3 to 4 weeks) or chronic (lasting longer than that). Multiple factors can trigger transient insomnia, including life stress, brief illness, rapid change of time zones, drug withdrawal, use of central nervous system (CNS) stimulants, and pain. Transient insomnia is experienced by everyone, and recovery usually is rapid.

Chronic insomnia may be lifelong. It usually is related to chronic psychophysiologic arousal, psychiatric disorders, use of drugs and alcohol, and other medical, toxic, and environmental conditions. However, it also may represent a primary sleep disorder in the form of sleep apnea syndrome, alveolar hypoventilation syndrome, PLMs of sleep, and RLS.

SLEEP-ONSET DELAY

Sleep-onset delay is a common problem and probably accounts for most patients who present with a complaint of insomnia. It usually has psychogenic causes. Sleeplessness may develop from a continued association with stimulating practices and objects at bedtime. Such patients sleep better away from their bedrooms and usual routines, for example, while on vacation.

A conditioned internal factor also may develop in the form of apprehension about unsuccessful and excessive efforts to sleep. Conscious efforts to fall asleep result in CNS arousal. These patients consider themselves "light sleepers." They often have multiple somatic complaints such as back pains, headaches, and palpitations that lead to occasional abuse of alcohol, barbiturates, minor tranquilizers, and hypnotics. The sleep of such patients in the sleep laboratory is usually better than at home because the conditioning factors that are active at home are reduced in the laboratory. Multiple specific psychiatric illnesses associated with anxiety, such as personality disorders (e.g., anxiety and panic disorders, hypochondriasis, obsessive–compulsive disorders), and schizophrenia, also can be associated with sleep-onset difficulty.

Drugs also can compromise the initiation of sleep. When obtaining a history, the physician should inquire specifically about possible precipitants of drug-induced insomnia. In addition to steroids and dopaminergic agents, xanthine derivatives (e.g., caffeine and theophylline) may cause sleep disruption. A frequently overlooked class of agents is the beta-adrenergic agonists, such as terbutaline and phenylethylamine derivatives (used as stimulants, appetite suppressants, and decongestants). If such medications are taken late in the day, and in increasing amounts because of the development of tolerance, they easily can cause sleep-onset delay as well as sleep fragmentation and "lightening" of sleep. Such inadequate sleep provokes daytime symptoms such as sleepiness, which is responsible for a further increase of ingestion of the drug to promote alertness.

In addition to the psychologic and drug-induced causes of sleep-onset delay, patients who have a disturbed circadian rhythm may have the same sleep complaint. In delayed sleep-phase syndrome, patients naturally fall asleep at 2 or 3 AM or later. They cannot fall asleep if they go to bed at conventional times. If they must get up for a job or school at 6 AM, they will be sleepy in the morning. However, they have no trouble going to sleep and getting full rest if they can go to bed late and sleep until midday. This pattern is characteristic (and probably physiological) in late adolescence and early adulthood. A change in lifestyle and a course of chronotherapy at a sleep disorder center can correct this problem. Delayed sleep-phase syndrome may also be treated with a morning session of bright light, which may be combined with an early evening dose of melatonin. Similarly, evening exposure to bright light and light restriction in the morning (wearing dark goggles) may be useful in treatment of advanced sleep-phase disorder. Chronotherapy, an individually designed sleep schedule consisting of a gradual sleep-onset time delay until a desired time is reached, may also help patients with irregular sleep–wake patterns, who sleep for short and variable periods throughout the 24 hours. These people have difficulty falling asleep at conventional times because they have napped recently. Shift workers and those who travel frequently across time zones often experience sleep-onset delay (in addition to jet lag) and may also benefit from a combined bright light–melatonin treatment.

Similar delay in sleep onset may result from misalignment between the natural body's circadian rhythm and work schedule (shift work disorder). Other conditions that may induce similar clinical presentation of troubles falling asleep and/or sleepiness include jet lag disorder, and irregular circadian rhythm sleep disorders, related to either lack of sleep hygiene. Infrequent free-running circadian sleep rhythm disorder is most frequently seen in blind persons; lack of entrainment of the circadian rhythm results in non-24-hour rhythm.

Treatment

The treatment of chronic insomnia is a significant challenge. It is highly individualized, and no uniform approach can be recommended. The physician should first identify any underlying conditions, which may include psychiatric disorders such as depression, alcohol or substance abuse, chronic medical disorders, sleep apnea, aging, and alteration in the circadian rhythm. Treatment then should be based on concurrent problems, age, and hepatic and renal function. The mainstay of treatment is the exploration and correction of maladaptive nighttime behaviors. This behavioral therapy, typically involving a series of meetings with the managing physician or therapist can be supplemented with carefully chosen, typically short-term, pharmacological therapy. Specific interventions that are typically used in this setting are discussed below.

■ **SPECIAL CLINICAL POINT: In treating sleep-onset delay, pharmacologic treatment should be used judiciously and should be combined with nonpharmacologic treatments.**

Counseling plays an important role in the therapy of sleep disorders. If the physician spends time talking with these patients, he or she may find that they actually are attempting to discuss problems that they find difficult to raise, such as impotence, marital discord, or alcoholism in a family member. The complaint may be resolved if attention is given to these problems, regardless of whether sleep behavior actually is altered.

Sleep hygiene includes setting a fixed hour for retiring each night, eliminating daytime naps, avoiding drinking caffeine-containing beverages and engaging in anxiety-producing activities at night, and ensuring that the bedroom is quiet, dark, and comfortable. Because patients may not think of over-the-counter preparations as drugs, mentioning the need to avoid sympathomimetic substances may prove fruitful. Physical exercise is advised, if taken at least a few hours before bedtime.

Only a few practical points concerning *behavioral therapies* need to be reviewed here. Techniques that attempt to increase relaxation, either through biofeedback or more conventional learning paradigms, may be valuable if they are aimed at a specific physiologic disturbance. For example, a patient whose PSMG indicates a large amount of muscle activity prior to falling asleep might benefit from EMG biofeedback. These techniques generally will require the facilities of a sleep laboratory. Attempts at operant and classic conditioning as aids in treating insomnia also have had some limited success. A widely accepted behavioral modification technique—stimulus control—is especially useful in correcting maladaptive association of arousal with bedtime routine. Other techniques aimed at reducing tension include progressive muscular relaxation and autogenic training.

Sleep restriction relies on restricting time spent in bed to the estimated sleep time the patient accumulates during the night, as documented by sleep logs, and then gradually increasing it until an optimal sleep time is achieved. This treatment is based on the observation that insomniacs spend too much time in bed in an attempt to obtain more sleep. Reduction of time spent in bed leads to a state of mild sleep deprivation, which is likely to result in faster sleep onset, improved sleep continuity, and deeper sleep. Stimulus control therapy is a formal set of behavioral advices and entails going to bed only if sleepy, getting out of bed when unable to sleep, using the bed and bedroom for sleep only, arising at the same time every morning, and avoiding naps.

Cognitive therapy focuses on maladaptive thoughts that produce an emotional arousal, such as unrealistic expectations about sleep requirements, negative consequences of insomnia, and misattributions of daytime difficulties to poor sleep.

Pharmacologic treatment can be used in the management of insomnia; however, the use of medications must be considered carefully. These medications are most helpful when their use is self-limited, such as during acute hospitalization or as part of a more comprehensive program of sleep hygiene. In the latter case, they may allow the physician time to explore the roots of the sleep disturbance more thoroughly and implement behavioral treatments.

The choice of a sedative agent is dictated primarily by the duration of clinical sedation; ideally, the hypnosedative effect should cease by the time the patient arises. An effective hypnotic drug should decrease sleep latency and increase the total sleep time. The value of a hypnotic depends on the balance of its efficacy and side effects. The efficacy is defined by its ability to induce and maintain sleep, and it directly depends on the drug's dose, absorption, and duration of action. Thus, an efficacious hypnotic is absorbed rapidly and has duration of action consistent with the sleep period (usually around 8 hours). Ideally, such a hypnotic has no adverse effects. However, hypnotics with duration of action that exceeds the sleep period usually lead to residual sedation during daytime. In contrast, use of short-acting hypnotics in doses higher than required often is associated with major adverse effects such as rebound insomnia and anterograde amnesia. Dependence is also an undesirable possibility with the use of hypnotics. This possibility can be minimized by the intermittent use of low doses, together with limited duration of drug intake and gradual withdrawal if treatment has been continuous for more than a month. The available drugs have a surprisingly heterogeneous set of effects on sleep architecture.

Although almost all agents used as hypnosedatives will suppress REM sleep when given in sufficiently large quantities, two patterns of effects are seen at lower doses. Barbiturates, chloral hydrate, anticholinergics, tricyclics, and ethanol demonstrate REM suppression, whereas most benzodiazepines decrease stage N3 sleep. They all appear to decrease sleep latency and reduce the number of spontaneous awakenings. Although the drugs that have the least effect on sleep architecture may offer a theoretic advantage in the therapy of insomnia, there is no clear demonstration that they induce "better" sleep. Data on commonly used sleep-promoting medications and some miscellaneous agents are summarized in Table 10.1.

Sleep latency usually is decreased with these agents, and there is seldom a reason to use more than a single agent in the treatment of insomnia. A failure to obtain an adequate response on the first night does not imply a need to increase the dosage immediately; a trial of at least two

TABLE 10.1 | **Commonly Used Sleep-Promoting Medications**

Drug Name	Initial Dose (mg)	Maintenance Dose (mg)	Drug Interactions
Temazepam[a]	7.5–15	15–30	Combination contraceptives may stimulate glucuronide conjugation of temazepam
Estazolam[a]	1	1–2	Ketoconazole inhibits CYP 450 3A and 2C family of enzymes
Triazolam[a]	0.125	Usually 0.25	Drugs inhibiting cytochrome P450 CYP 3A such as ketoconazole, itraconazole and nefazodone, and erythromycin
Lorazepam[a]	1	1–2	Combination contraceptives may increase glucuronidation; quetiapine reduces the clearance
Alprazolam	0.25	0.5	Drugs that inhibit alprazolam's metabolism via CYP 450 3A including fluoxetine, propoxyphene, diltiazem, isoniazid, and macrolide antibiotics
Clonazepam	0.5–1	1–2	Cytochrome P450 inducers such as phenytoin, carbamazepine, and phenobarbital cause a 30% decrease in plasma clonazepam levels; inhibitors of P450 family of enzymes, such as oral antifungal agents, should be used cautiously
Chlodiazepoxide[a]	5–10	10–25	Antacids slow absorption; disulfiram inhibits its hepatic metabolism (hydroxylation and dealkylation); ketoconazole reduces its clearance
Zolpidem	5–10 (6.25)[b]	10–20 (12.5)[b]	Potent inducers of CYP 450 3A4 (carbamazepine, phenytoin, rifampicin) reduce its hypnotic effect; ketoconazole causes increased plasma concentrations, SSRIs and zolpidem may lead to delirium
Zaleplon	5–10	10–20	Drugs that are potent CYP 450 3A4 inducers (rifampin, phenytoin, carbamazepine, phenobarbital) may cause its ineffectiveness.
Eszopiclone	1–2	3	Drugs that are potent CYP 450 3A4 inducers (rifampin, phenytoin, carbamazepine, phenobarbital) may cause its ineffectiveness
Amitriptyline[c]	10–25	50	Other antidepressants: SSRIs, type 1C antiarrhythmics
Desipramine[c]	25	50	Anticholinergic and sympathomimetic drugs
Imipramine[c]	25	50	Anticholinergic drugs (excessive anticholinergic effects); MAO inhibitors contraindicated
Nortriptyline[c]	25	25–75	Baclofen—short-term memory loss; barbiturates can increase metabolism of TCAs; TCAs may inhibit the uptake of bethanidine into NE neuron and reduce anti-HTN effect; concurrent administration with drugs capable of prolonging QT interval is contraindicated; belladonna potentiation of anticholinergic activity
Doxepin[c]	25	25–50	MAO inhibitors, alcohol, tolazamide (hypoglycemia)

(continued)

TABLE 10.1

Commonly Used Sleep-Promoting Medications *(continued)*

Drug Name	Initial Dose (mg)	Maintenance Dose (mg)	Drug Interactions
Chloral hydrate[a]	500	500–1000	Increased free levels of phenytoin, initial enhancement of anticoagulation by coumarins because of increased free levels; furosemide
Diphenhydramine	25–50	50–100	Enhanced risk for adynamic ileus, urinary retention, chronic glaucoma with tricyclics and other antihistamines

CYP, cytochrome P enzyme; SSRI, selective serotonin reuptake inhibitor; MAO, monoamine oxidase; NE, norepinephrine; TCA, tricyclic antidepressant; HTN, hypertension.
[a]Additive effect of other central nervous system depressants and centrally acting muscle relaxants.
[b]Extended release formulation.
[c]Drugs that inhibit cytochrome P450 2D6 (quinidine, phenothiazines, and bupropion) may inhibit metabolism of TCAs via inhibition of CYP 450 2D6.
Other antidepressants: SSRIs, anticholinergic, and sympathomimetic drugs; some TCAs may increase half-life and bioavailability of oral anticoagulants, with amphetamine-like agents-enhanced amphetamine effects; amprenavir may increase serum concentration of TCAs and lead to arrhythmias, due to inhibition of CYP 450 3A4 isoenzyme.

or three nights is indicated. Sleep induction is related to the rate of drug absorption. Sleep maintenance is related to dosage and half-life. The timing of the intake of the medications is, therefore, important. Hypnotics with longer half-lives (lasting more than 24 hours) show increased efficacy with two or three nights of administration, but they also show increased residual daytime effects. Some benzodiazepines, such as flurazepam, produce persistent long-acting metabolites and cause definite impairment in alertness, motor performance, and cognitive function in the morning. Because of the intrinsic "tapering" effect of compounds with long half-lives, rebound and/or withdrawal phenomena appear to be unlikely; when they do occur, such effects are delayed in onset and are relatively mild. However, there is a much higher likelihood of rebound or withdrawal effect after abrupt discontinuation of short-half-life hypnotics, for which dose tapering is appropriate. When the initial therapy is unsuccessful, changing classes of medications may be useful.

In the last two decades, sleep medicine has seen an almost complete replacement of barbiturates by benzodiazepines, followed by an introduction of nonbenzodiazepine hypnotics in place of benzodiazepines. Only five benzodiazepines are currently marketed for hypnotic purposes in the United States: triazolam, temazepam, quazepam, flurazepam, and estazolam. Various benzodiazepine anxiolytics (e.g., diazepam, alprazolam, lorazepam, or oxazepam) also are prescribed for insomnia associated with anxiety disorders. Unfortunately, there is limited evidence to support their efficacy for these disorders. The drug of choice for sleep-onset insomnia differs from that for sleep-maintenance insomnia (i.e., triazolam for the former, and temazepam for the latter).

Onset of action after an oral dose depends on rapidity of absorption from the gastrointestinal tract. Duration of action of a single dose of a benzodiazepine hypnotic depends on its distribution (e.g., it may concentrate in sites such as adipose tissue, where it exerts no pharmacologic activity) and on elimination and clearance. With repeated administration at a fixed dosing rate, a drug will accumulate in plasma and brain until a steady state is reached. Time necessary to reach a steady-state condition depends only on the drug's elimination half-life. For a drug such as triazolam with a very short elimination half-life, accumulation will be complete within 1 day;

that is, the mean plasma concentration will be no higher after multiple days of therapy than after the first day. At the other extreme is a drug such as flurazepam, with its principal active metabolite desalkylflurazepam. This compound has a very long elimination half-life; 2 weeks or more of long-term treatment will be necessary for a steady state to be attained. The rate of drug disappearance following discontinuation after long-term treatment will mirror the rate of accumulation (i.e., the longer the elimination half-life, the more time will be needed for the drug to disappear). A potential benefit of accumulating a benzodiazepine is that persistence of drug at the receptor sites throughout each 24-hour dosing interval increases the likelihood of a daytime anxiolytic effect, a potential benefit for patients with both anxiety and insomnia. For short half-life hypnotics such as triazolam, however, increased daytime anxiety has been reported in some studies, possibly attributable to wide fluctuations in plasma and receptor-site concentrations between doses. Estazolam, a relatively new benzodiazepine, remains effective as a hypnotic for at least 6 weeks of continuous administration at a dosage of 2 mg at bedtime, with no evidence of clinically significant tolerance. It improves sleep latency and total sleep time, reduces the number of nocturnal awakenings, and improves both depth of sleep and sleep quality in adults with chronic insomnia.

■ **SPECIAL CLINICAL POINT: In the last decade, several nonbenzodiazepine hypnotics have become the most commonly prescribed medications for insomnia. Their main advantage compared to the benzodiazepines is their favorable side effect profile, less potential for residual daytime effects, and less potential for abuse.**

Zolpidem, and its slow-release formulation, is a benzodiazepine receptor ligand structurally unrelated to benzodiazepines (an omega 1-selective nonbenzodiazepine hypnotic). It has an elimination half-life of 3.5 to 5.1 hours (mean, 4 hours). In young adults, zolpidem leads to a marked increase in slow wave sleep, with reduction of N2

and no change in REM sleep. In middle-aged patients, there is a reduction of wakefulness after sleep onset (WASO) time and increase of N2 sleep, without changes in REM sleep.

Zaleplon is a nonbenzodiazepine hypnotic from the pyrazolopyrimidine class. It interacts with the GABA–BZ receptor complex, selectively on omega-1 receptor on the alpha subunit of the GABA A receptor complex. In controlled trials it shortened sleep latency. It is metabolized by aldehyde oxidase and to a lesser degree by CYP 450 3A4. Inhibitors of these enzymes may decrease its clearance and enhance sedative/hypnotic effect. Due to its short half-life of only 30 minutes, it may be used for initial as well as maintenance insomnia.

Eszopiclone is a cyclopyrrolone compound, a nonbenzodiazepine hypnotic that has been approved by the U.S. Food and Drug Administration (FDA) for treatment of insomnia. It has an onset of action of 1 hour and half-life of about 6 hours. Eszopiclone has been shown to decrease sleep latency and improve measures of sleep continuity. It has not been associated with the development of tolerance over 6 months of use.

A structurally new compound with a distinct mechanism of action was recently introduced in treatment of insomnia. Ramelteon is a nonsedating melatonin receptor agonist that is rapidly absorbed from the GI tract, gives a peak concentration at 0.5 to 1.5 hours and has the half-life of 1 to 2.5 hours. It then undergoes extensive liver metabolism, yielding weak, active metabolites that have an elimination half-life of 2 to 5 hours. Ramelteon produces modest shortening of sleep latency.

Precautions

Patients who are pregnant, who are alcoholic, or who have sleep apnea should not be given hypnotics, except in low doses and only in special circumstances. Preference for nonbenzodiazepines over benzodiazepines is based on the former's lower toxicity and potential for abuse. The prescribing of hypnotics to children is not recommended, except for rare use in the treatment of night terrors or severe somnambulism. Benzodiazepine metabolism varies and is largely age dependent. The elimination half-life of diazepam in healthy men may increase threefold to fourfold from 20 years of age to 80 years of age. The elimination of hypnotics is decreased in elderly people who might have a low renal glomerular filtration rate, a reduced hepatic blood flow, and a decreased activity of hepatic drug-metabolizing enzymes. The choice of hypnosedatives for elderly patients with sleep-onset delay, especially when they are acutely hospitalized, is complicated by the risk of a paradoxical excitation at nighttime (sun-downing), which may be precipitated or exacerbated by medication. Although diphenhydramine has been useful in many of these patients, there is a risk of increasing their confusion because of its anticholinergic effect. These problems can be minimized by adjunctive measures, such as leaving a light on in the patient's room, and by frequently reorienting the patient to the unfamiliar surroundings. A family member occasionally may be required to stay with the patient.

Because of the intrinsic "tapering" effect of long-half-life compounds, rebound and withdrawal phenomena appear to be unlikely; when they do occur, such effects are delayed in onset and are relatively mild. However, there is a much higher likelihood of rebound or withdrawal effect after abrupt discontinuation of short-half-life hypnotics, so dose tapering is appropriate.

Although many of these drugs, especially the benzodiazepines, have been marketed with emphasis on their short duration of action, many have long-acting active metabolites. This is often a problem in the patient who experiences a decrement in liver function. Sedative effects are additive and may convert what would have been a mild metabolic encephalopathy into a coma days after the initiation of treatment.

Non-benzodiazepine hypnotics are generally better tolerated and associated with fewer side effects. Dizziness, hypersomnolence, and headache are the most common side effects of zolpidem, zaleplon, and eszopiclone. Zolpidem has been associated with complex behaviors in sleep, including sleep eating. Patients taking eszopiclone may report an unpleasant taste in the mouth.

Alternative Therapies

The most popular and well-studied herbal treatment of depression is St. John's wort (*Hypericum perforatum*), a remedy used for wound healing, sedation, and pain relief. Its use as a hypnotic has not been studied systematically, but it may promote "deep sleep" and prolong REM latency.

Valerian root (*Valeriana officinalis*) has been used widely for its hypnotic properties. A limited number of human studies suggest that valerian could be used as a mild hypnotic with minimal side effects. It seems to affect GABA metabolism and reuptake, mainly GABA A receptors, 5HT-1a, and adenosine receptors. Numerous herbs are used in combinations by traditional Chinese medicine. However, there are no well-designed studies to document their effectiveness and safety.

Anxiety disorders often are linked to insomnia. Anxiety may respond to kava kava (*Piper methysticum*). Its mechanism of action is thought to involve GABA A receptors.

Melatonin is used to reset the circadian clock and help proper positioning of the sleep cycle within a 24-hour period, but it also has a mild direct sedative–hypnotic effect (the most common doses are 2–10 mg 30 minutes to 2 hours before bedtime). Caution should be exercised in patients with known cardiovascular disease because melatonin reportedly causes vasoconstriction in coronary and cerebral arteries of rats. Other possible side effects are inhibition of fertility, increased depression or induced depression, suppression of male libido, retinal damage, and hypothermia. Melatonin's interactions with other drugs are not fully understood, which is of particular concern in the elderly population. As with other dietary supplements, there is a concern about purity of the product. Catnip (*Nepeta cataria*) is used as a "tonic" for sleep, as is chamomile (*Marticaria recutita*). Several other herbs are used as sleep aids because of their reported sedative effects: gotu cola (*Centella asiatica*), hops (*Humulus lupulus*), lavender (*Lavandula angustifolia* and others), passionflower (*Passiflora incarnata*), and scullcap (*Scutellaria lateriflora*). Hepatoxicity was described for scullcap when used in combination with valerian root, but this may have resulted from substitution of a particular herb with species of germander (*Teucrium*).

The FDA recalled all products of L-tryptophan in the United States, but it still is manufactured worldwide. It has resurfaced in the form of 5-hydroxytryptamine. It was found that the new product contains the same impurities previously found in L-tryptophan responsible for eosinophilia–myalgia syndrome. L-tryptophan also is found in some protein supplements.

RESTLESS LEGS SYNDROME

Insomnia characterized by marked sleep-onset delay may result from RLS because of increasing severity of unpleasant sensations in the limbs when at rest at night. The patient experiences disagreeable deep sensations of creeping inside the calves whenever at rest (sitting or lying down). These dysesthesias cause an almost irresistible urge to move the limbs and thus interfere with the sleep onset. Movements bring a relief of the sensation, but it typically lasts only an instant. Although majority of patients with RLS also have sleep-related PLMs, coincident PLMs are not required for the diagnosis of RLS.

■ **SPECIAL CLINICAL POINT: The diagnosis of RLS relies entirely on the patient's symptoms, and no laboratory testing is necessary to make it.**

Revised criteria emphasize the onset of symptoms with rest and a clear circadian pattern to the symptoms. The four essential criteria for the diagnosis have been published and widely accepted:

1. A sensation of an urge to move the limbs (usually legs)
2. Motor restlessness to reduce sensations
3. Onset or worsening of the symptoms when at rest
4. Marked circadian variation in occurrence or severity of symptoms, with worsening or sole presence of symptoms in the evening.

Once asleep, approximately 85% of patients with RLS experience PLMs causing numerous arousals and poor quality of sleep. Many patients with RLS experience PLMs while awake (PLMs of wakefulness, PLMW), especially in sedentary situations. Although total sleep time may be markedly reduced and sleep efficiency is very low, patients with RLS generally do not report sleepiness and/or sleep attacks, but they usually complain of tiredness and not feeling fully alert.

Prevalence of RLS is 5% to 10% and it increases with age. In the majority of studies, RLS is more prevalent in women. The large majority of patients afflicted by RLS appear to represent idiopathic cases, unrelated to any other medical condition as a possible cause.

Several secondary causes of RLS have been well documented: pregnancy, iron deficiency, and end-stage renal disease. Neuropathies and radiculopathies have been accepted as possible secondary causes of RLS, specifically neuropathy associated with rheumatoid arthritis and diabetes mellitus. Some studies suggest other causes of secondary RLS, including peripheral vascular disease, chronic obstructive pulmonary disease, asthma, and fibromyalgia.

The exact pathophysiology of RLS is unknown. However, several studies suggest subcortical dopamine system's dysfunction, which results in reduction of the spinal and possibly cortical inhibition that may be state dependent. The positron emission tomography and single-photon emission computed tomography studies showed small decreases in dopaminergic function in the striatum of patients with RLS compared to control subjects. All the clinical conditions (end-stage renal disease, iron deficiency, pregnancy) associated with iron deficiency also are associated with RLS. Low brain iron may lead to dopaminergic dysfunction, as documented by decreased D2R, decreased dopamine transporter, and increased extracellular dopamine in rats deprived of iron in early life. In some cases, restless legs and PLMs are caused or exacerbated by dietary substances (e.g., caffeine) or medications (e.g., neuroleptics and tricyclic antidepressants).

Drug Treatment

Accepted and fairly successful treatments for restless legs and PLMs include dopaminergic drugs, opioids, and some miscellaneous drugs. Treatment choices are the same for primary and secondary RLS.

■ **SPECIAL CLINICAL POINT: Given the prevalence of iron deficiency in RLS, assessing iron and ferritin levels is essential. If iron deficiency is noted, iron supplementation is usually needed for adequate control of RLS symptoms, along with an investigation of the reasons of iron deficiency. Typically, achieving the ferritin level of 50 mg/L or more is the goal. Oral iron supplementation is more effective if it is taken on an empty stomach and 60 minutes before a meal.**

Among pharmacological agents used for RLS, dopaminergic medications are now considered first-line agents (Table 10.2). The dopaminergic agent carbidopa/levodopa (Sinemet) improves all of the features of both RLS and PLM disorder, including discomfort in the legs, involuntary movements during the waking state (dyskinesias while awake), PLMs during sleep, and sleep fragmentation, but its use has been decreasing, because of the augmentation that develops with its continued use. Side effects include gastrointestinal discomfort, nausea, and vomiting. Augmentation consists of increasing intensity of the symptoms, earlier onset of the symptoms in the day, reduced time at rest before symptoms start, and in some cases, more widespread dysesthesias and restlessness. Rebound is a phenomenon of reappearance of

RLS symptoms in the morning, after the effects of a dose of levodopa wears off. Carbidopa/levodopa, especially its sublingual formulation (Parcopa), may be still useful in control of episodic, intermittent RLS symptoms, especially during long periods of inactivity (air flights etc.).

Bromocriptine is another dopaminergic agonist that has been used successfully, but is no longer commonly used, because of common side effects, including nasal stuffiness, gastrointestinal discomfort, especially hypotension, and ergot-related fibrosis. Another ergot-based dopamine agonist, pergolide has been withdrawn from the market.

Non-ergot, direct dopamine agonists are very effective therapeutic agents in the treatment of RLS. Pramipexole (Mirapex) and ropinirole (Requip) are currently used as a treatment of choice. They are typically introduced at lowest doses, and titrated up every few days until they control evening and nocturnal symptoms. At doses used to treat RLS, the side effects of these medications are typically minor, and involve dizziness, lightheadedness, and insomnia. At higher doses, the dopamine agonists may produce sleep attacks—a sudden sensation of overwhelming sleepiness.

Gabapentin is now considered an alternative treatment of mild RLS, especially if coinciding with neuropathy, chronic pain, or neurodegenerative diseases, such as Parkinson disease and dementia. Typical side effects of gabapentin include gait unsteadiness and somnolence.

Numerous opioids have been used, such as codeine, propoxyphene (Darvon), oxycodone (Percodan), pentazocine (Talwin), levorphanol (Levo-Dromoran), and methadone. Their effectiveness has been tested formally by only a few studies. Although widely prescribed for the treatment of PLMs, clonazepam was not shown to reduce symptoms of RLS, and even reduction of PLMs seems to be small.

Alternative Treatments

The behavioral manipulations of avoidance of smoking, certain drugs, and alcohol are almost

TABLE 10.2 | **Medications for Treatment of Restless Legs Syndrome**

Drug Name	Initial Dose (mg)	Maintenance Dose (mg)	Drug Interactions
Levodopa[a]	25/100	Up to 300 mg maximum	MAOI, tricyclics especially in elderly with cardiac disease (reduced L-dopa response, arrhythmias, hypertension); isoniazid; phenytoin (reduced effectiveness)
Bromocriptine[a]	2.5	2.5–20	With cyclosporine bromocriptine inhibits CYP450 3A and increases cyclosporine levels; macrolide antibiotics, clarithromycin, erythromycin inhibit bromocriptine metabolism; droperidol reduces its therapeutic efficacy
Pramipexole	0.125	0.25–3	Kava may decrease the effectiveness of pramipexole
Ropinirole	0.25	0.5–6	Ropinirole is a substrate for CYP 450 1A2, any inhibitor (ciprofloxacin) or inducer of this enzyme may require dose adjustment; estrogens also reduce its oral clearance; dopamine antagonists may reduce its effect
Codeine[b]	15	15–60	Quinidine inhibits CYP 450 2D6 (stops production of morphine); rifampin induces CYP 450 isoenzymes and reduces its effectiveness
Hydrocodone[b]	5–10	Up to 30	Same as codeine
Hydromorphone[b]	2	3–4	Rifampin reduces its effectiveness because of CYP 450 isoenzymes' induction
Morphine[b]	10–30	Up to 60	Somatostatin (antagonizes analgesic effect); Yohimbine enhances analgesic effect; metformin (increased risk for lactic acidosis); MAOIs contraindicated
Oxycodone[b]	10	Up to 30	Same as codeine
Methadone[b]	5–10	Up to 20–40	Phenytoin, carbamazepine, rifampin (inducers of CYP 450 3A4 isoenzyme) reduce their levels and even cause withdrawal symptoms; nonnucleoside reverse transcriptase inhibitors (inhibit or induce CYP 450 isoenzymes); fluconazole, fluvoxamine (inhibitors of CYP 3A4 isoenzyme
Propoxyphene	65	130	Carbamazepine (CBZ), propxyphene reduces CBZ's hepatic metabolism, CBZ toxicity metoprolol, propanolol levels rise (inhibition of hepatic metabolism); ritonavir (inhibits propxyphene's metabolism)
Iron (Fe sulfate, Fe gluconate) with vitamin C	150	150–300	Aluminum-, calcium-, or magnesium-containing products may reduce iron absorption; cholestyramine (reduced iron absorption because it binds to iron); cirpofloxacin, levofloxacin (reduced absorption due to chelation); generally decreased bioavailability of quinolone antibiotics due to chelation; levothyroxine (reduced absorption); decreased levodopa absorption

MAOI, monoamine oxidase inhibitor; CYP, cytochrome P enzyme; AUC, area under the curve.

[a]Dopamine antagonists (neuroleptics) are likely to diminish their effectiveness.

[b]Other CNS depressants and centrally acting muscle relaxants; opioid agonist/antagonists (withdrawal symptoms); inducers of CYP 450 isoenzymes may reduce their effectiveness.

routinely recommended to patients complaining of insomnia. Avoidance of over-the-counter stimulants such as decongestants with pseudoephedrine, phenylephrine, and appetite suppressants such as phenylpropanolamine is advised, especially at bedtime.

Moderate exercise prior to bedtime, vigorous enough to cause release of beta-endorphin, is suggested, preferably before 7 PM. Light calisthenics or stretching for 5 to 10 minutes at bedtime supplements the exercise regimen. Stress reduction (meditation, yoga, and relaxation response) combined with sleep hygiene complements other behavioral techniques.

Distraction or counterstimulation of the legs is another approach. It includes hot foot socks or ice packs; rubbing feet, pounding thighs, or wearing socks to bed. Massage, electrical stimulation, acupuncture, hypnosis, and cognitive therapy add to the repertoire of these approaches. Sclerotherapy, once thought to represent a promising option in patients with varicose veins, is unlikely to alleviate the symptoms. Magnesium is noted to improve PLMs and RLS. In addition to iron, a supplementation of vitamin E, B_{12}, folate, and B_6 is useful, especially in cases with documented deficiencies. Valerian root and kava kava may be helpful as mild hypnotic–sedative agents.

EARLY MORNING AWAKENING

Early morning awakening can be seen in numerous clinical settings, including depression, use of some drugs, and advanced sleep-phase syndrome. Endogenous depression is characterized by a typical premature awakening and an inability to fall asleep again, with variable sleep-onset disturbance depending on the individual's component of agitation. A key polysomnographic finding is shortened REM sleep latency, which is considered by some experts to be a biologic marker of depression, in addition to an increased intensity of REM sleep. Deep (delta) NREM sleep also is reduced; this is a relatively nonspecific feature.

In contrast, bipolar depression frequently is associated with hypersomnia; however, this state again is accompanied by a shortened REM latency and reduced stage N3 sleep. The onset of sleep is delayed and sleep is short in mania and hypomania. Insomnia may precede all other symptoms of depression, and restoration of sleep may be the first sign of recovery.

In patients with early morning awakening, sedative therapy usually is accompanied by an unacceptable degree of morning sedation. Antidepressants appear to offer the best results and should be the initial form of therapy. Tricyclic antidepressants with sedative properties, such as amitriptyline (Elavil) and trimipramine (Surmontil), reduce sleep latency and improve sleep continuity. Trazodone, a nontricyclic, also is used widely for treatment of insomnia in patients who are depressed. Although an improvement in sleep often precedes an improvement in mood, changes of affect should determine the endpoint in therapy.

Drug-induced early morning awakening may occur with the use of some short-acting benzodiazepines, such as oxazepam or lorazepam. They are almost completely inactivated by a conjugation in the liver, and they have few residual morning aftereffects. Patients who drink alcoholic beverages prior to sleep may develop early morning awakening, apparently related to an increase in REM sleep (REM rebound) after the alcohol is metabolized. An underlying psychiatric problem should be considered, as in any patient with an alcohol-related problem. Therapy involves a slow withdrawal of the causative agent.

Advanced-sleep-phase syndrome may mimic a pattern of early morning awakening typical of depression. It is seen most frequently in elderly people. There are no established treatments for this condition, although reverse chronotherapy or exposure to light in the evening accompanied by light deprivation in the morning may be helpful. Either treatment requires the skills of experts in sleep disorders centers.

SLEEP FRAGMENTATION

A major complaint of frequent awakenings at night often signals the presence of a primary sleep disorder, specifically sleep apnea or PLMs. Multiple medical conditions also can interfere with sleep maintenance, whereas psychiatric etiology is a less likely explanation.

In sleep apnea, sleep disruption is caused by cessation of breathing during apneic periods and subsequent short awakenings. While these events may be very frequent, they are usually not realized by the patient, and only reported by his or her bed partner. Occasionally, patients with sleep apnea do realize that they wake up frequently at night; this presentation is more frequent in central rather than obstructive sleep apnea, and in women.

PLM disorder is a condition in which insomnia is associated with the occurrence of periodic episodes of repetitive and highly stereotypical leg jerks during sleep. These are followed consistently by a partial arousal. Patients are often unaware of the movements at night; rather, they report frequent nocturnal awakenings and unrefreshing sleep. A bed partner usually can provide an accurate description of the movements.

Medical conditions that sometimes lead to insomnia include alveolar hypoventilation, which in adults could be secondary to massive obesity; chronic obstructive pulmonary disease; myopathy; cordotomy; or lesions involving structures that control sleep and breathing, including stroke. Primary alveolar hypoventilation (previously termed "Ondine curse") typically presents in infants and is associated with a further worsening of hypercapnia and hypoxemia in sleep. Gastroesophageal reflux with regurgitation, heartburn, and dyspepsia; nocturnal angina; sleep-related asthma; nightmares; and cluster headaches all may cause a serious insomnia as a result of severe sleep fragmentation. Other medical and neurologic conditions can be associated with this form of insomnia, including CNS infections, head traumas, nocturnal epilepsy, fibromyalgia,

chronic pain, and endocrine diseases such as hyperthyroidism and Addison disease. In these patients, treatment of the underlying disorder can be expected to alleviate the sleep disturbance and thus obviate the need for hypnotics. Of note, hypercortisolism (especially iatrogenic) should be considered if sleep fragmentation is prominent. Parkinsonian patients receiving therapy with levodopa also are subject to this complaint. These patients frequently report daytime napping and their response to hypnosedatives and tricyclics is unpredictable. Not taking dopaminergic drugs after eating supper is helpful for many patients. Another cause of sleep fragmentation is bruxism (teeth grinding).

WHEN TO REFER THE INSOMNIAC TO A SLEEP SPECIALIST

Primary care physicians and other nonspecialists may attempt to treat an acute insomnia, especially if the trigger or the etiology is easily identifiable. The treatments include a short course of hypnotics or simple behavioral interventions (sleep hygiene). When patients present with chronic (more than 6 months) insomnia, it is advisable to refer the patient to the sleep specialist for formal evaluation and a trial of behavioral and/or medical therapy.

SPECIAL CHALLENGES FOR HOSPITALIZED PATIENTS

Anesthesiologists have to be aware of the reactions some of the patients with RLS may develop if given antidopaminergics. The reaction can be severe and look as a "forme fruste" neuroleptic malignant syndrome (crampy stiffness without fever). This is especially likely to occur when patients awaken after they were given droperidol (a potent, long-acting dopamine antagonist) while withdrawing from fentanyl (a potent, short-acting μ-opiate agonist). The timing of this emergency coincides with circadian enhancement of RLS (late afternoon). Recommended substitutes for nausea include on-dansetron (5HT-3 blocker) and domperidone (large molecule dopamine antagonist, which does not penetrate the blood–brain barrier, but area postrema has none). Domperidone is not available in the United States.

Patients with RLS may tolerate the following antipsychotic medications: quetiapine and clozapine. Although many patients have trouble sleeping in the hospital, during hospitalization special attention must be given to subjects with RLS.

SLEEP DISORDERS ASSOCIATED WITH HYPERSOMNOLENCE

Included in this category of sleep disorders associated with hypersomnolence are intrinsic and extrinsic sleep disorders as well as parasomnias and disorders associated with medical/psychiatric disorders. The chief symptoms include an inappropriate and undesirable sleepiness during waking hours, decreased cognitive and motor performance, an excessive tendency to sleep, unavoidable napping, an increase in total sleep over 24 hours ("true" hypersomnia), and a difficulty in achieving full arousal on awakening. The term *hypersomnolence* in a strict sense should be reserved for patients who have a demonstrable tendency to fall asleep in the waking state when sedentary or who have sleep "attacks." There also may be diminished alertness in the waking state, described by the term *subwakefulness*. In all patients presenting with these symptoms, it is important to separate excessive daytime somnolence from less specific symptoms of tiredness, fatigue, malaise, or depression.

■ **SPECIAL CLINICAL POINT: Insufficient sleep time is the most prevalent reason for daytime sleepiness; responding to the demands of everyday life many people wake up to an alarm clock every day, curtailing their natural sleep. Prolonging sleep time, with an aim of spontaneous arousals on most days, is frequently the first advice to a sleepy patient.**

Other major causes of excessive daytime sleepiness include sleep apnea syndrome and narcolepsy.

SLEEP APNEA

A potentially lethal condition, sleep apnea is an abnormal breathing pattern during sleep defined as a cessation of airflow at the level of the nostrils and the mouth, lasting for at least 10 seconds. Depending on the criteria employed, the estimated prevalence of sleep apnea syndrome ranges from 2% to 10% of the adult population. It is the most frequent diagnosis in sleep disorder centers and the most frequent cause of excessive daytime sleepiness. Apneas are subdivided by type: obstructive apnea secondary to a sleep-induced obstruction of the airway (Fig. 10.3); central apnea secondary to decreased respiratory muscle activity; and mixed apnea combining both phenomena. Mixed apnea usually starts as a central apnea (with no respiratory effort) and develops into an obstruction later. Obstructive apneas are much more common than central apneas; typically either obstructive or central apnea predominates in each patient.

Obstructive sleep apnea (OSA) is caused by pharyngeal collapse during inspiration and not by an active musculature contraction. Contributing factors may include abnormal anatomic relationships among the muscular or bony structures of the nasopharynx, oropharynx, or hypopharynx (e.g., a short thick neck, macroglossia, micrognathia, retrognathia, a relatively small and low-positioned hyoid bone, or a narrow pharynx). Alternatively, inappropriate involuntary respiratory control of the pharyngeal (genioglossus) and diaphragmatic muscle tone may be responsible. Occasionally patients demonstrate increased compliance of their pharyngeal walls, especially when they have fatty or redundant pharyngeal and submucosal folds, or, less frequently, enlarged tonsils. As an end-result, patients with OSA have an imbalance between the forces that tend to collapse the upper airway

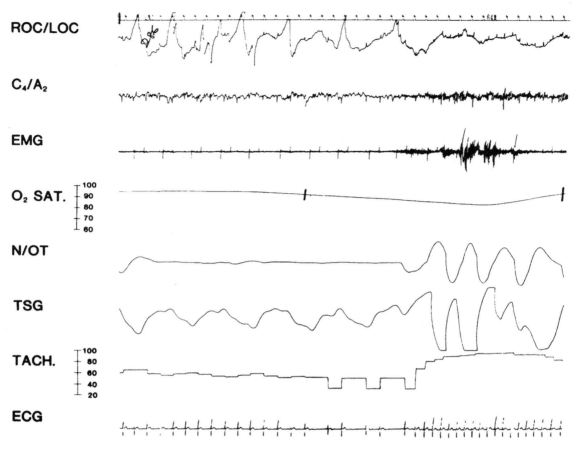

FIGURE 10.3 Obstructive apnea. During the of rapid eye movement (REM) stage, airflow ceases for 21 seconds while unsuccessful respiratory effort continues, indicating obstruction of the upper airway. Oxygen saturation falls to 81%. Immediately prior to the resumption of ventilation, the electrocardiogram (ECG) demonstrates second-degree atrioventricular block. When ventilation occurs, sinus rhythm appears in the electroencephalogram (EEG) and tachycardia is evident in the ECG.

and forces that keep it open. Although many patients with OSA are moderately overweight, morbid obesity is present only in a minority.

■ **SPECIAL CLINICAL POINT: Sleep apnea should be suspected in an individual with snoring, witnessed pauses in breathing at night, and excessive daytime sleepiness. Obesity and elevated blood pressure are frequently present.**

Obstructive sleep apneas are more prevalent with increasing age and worsen after alcohol or sedative drug intake. Important features in the clinical history are often best confirmed by interviewing the bed partner are loud snoring and witnessed respiratory pauses, frequently alarming to the bed partner. Awakenings due to choking sensation or loud sounds produced by snoring (snort arousals) are sometimes reported. Sensation of excessive sweating at night, related to sympathetic activation produced by apneas, is frequently present. Finally, patients with OSA frequently report dryness in the mouth/throat upon awakening, and, less commonly, morning headaches that are present upon awakening and disappear quickly during the day. Suspicion of OSA is frequently raised by excessive daytime sleepiness, and restless sleep with frequent awakenings. On examination, a large neck circumference (≥17 inches in males and ≥16 inches in females), micrognathia and retrognathia and excessive oropharyngeal soft tissue should suggest the diagnosis of OSA. Objective confirmation of the diagnosis is made with an attended or unattended sleep study that typically records EEG, electrocardiogram, oximetry, breathing effort, and airflow.

■ **SPECIAL CLINICAL POINT: In sleep apnea, the patient is usually unaware of nocturnal symptoms and may be resistant to undergoing an evaluation of sleep; presence of a bed partner during history intake may greatly facilitate the evaluation.**

Waking respiratory functions are usually within normal limits. Hypertension has been reported in >50% of patients with OSA. Alveolar hypoventilation, associated with an elevated waking $PaCO_2$, occasionally accompanies OSA. Increased $PaCO_2$ of 45 mmHg or higher has been reported in 23% of obese patients with OSA, and may be due to hypoventilation, or a coexistence of OSA and chronic obstructive pulmonary disease, COPD (*overlap syndrome*).

Sleep apneas substantially affect the cardiovascular system, and association between several cardiovascular diseases and OSA is now well documented. Marked cyclic sinus arrhythmia appears during sleep and apnea. This rhythm pattern is characterized by progressive sinus bradycardia during apnea (heart rates of less than 40 beats/min are not uncommon) with an abrupt reversal and sinus acceleration at the arousal and onset of ventilation, caused by a sudden sympathetic output. Second-degree atrioventricular block, prolonged sinus pauses, nonsustained ventricular tachycardia, and paroxysmal atrial tachycardia episodes also occur. Furthermore, systemic and pulmonary artery pressures increase in association with obstructive apneas. There is an independent

association of hypertension and OSA, and sleep apnea has been detected in 22% to 30% of patients with systemic hypertension. Sleep apnea increases the risk of ischemic heart disease, cardiovascular death, congestive heart failure (CHF), and atrial fibrillation. Finally, recent reports link OSA with the development or worsening of insulin resistance and type 2 diabetes.

Central sleep apnea is not a single disease entity but results from any one of a number of processes that produce instability of respiratory control. In contrast to patients with OSA, these patients are older; they complain mainly of sleep fragmentation; they are not overweight; and they have less pronounced oxygen desaturation and a more moderate hemodynamic impact. There is no definite sex distribution. Central sleep apnea may be present in a sizeable proportion of patients with CHF. In this group, central apneas are due to increased sensitivity of the respiratory center to pCO_2, producing relative hypocapnia, and prolonged circulation time; in patients with CHF, central apneas frequently alternate with periods of hyperpnea, to cause periodic breathing pattern.

Complex sleep apnea, a recently recognized entity, combines the presence of OSA with central apneas that become apparent when treatment of obstructive events is attempted. These patients typically present with a phenotype close to a patient with OSA and their condition is only revealed during sleep testing and trial of therapy of OSA.

Upper airway patency does not need to be fully compromised for symptoms of daytime sleepiness to develop. The upper airway resistance syndrome (UARS) is accompanied by subjective and objective evidence of pathologic sleepiness. In some individuals, even a minor reduction of airway patency with sleep onset may lead to a modest increase in upper airway resistance and a slight decrease of tidal volume without hypoxemia. In response to increased resistance, inspiratory muscles increase their effort to maintain normal tidal volume. This compensatory increase in respiratory effort usually triggers a brief alpha EEG arousal (3 to 14 seconds in duration), interrupting further development of obstruction before oxygen desaturation occurs. If the alpha EEG arousals are frequent, clinically significant daytime sleepiness may arise. Snoring is noted in most, but not all, of these individuals.

Both central and OSA can be a complication of another medical or neurologic disorder, including brainstem infarction, lateral medullary syndrome, bulbar poliomyelitis, medullary neoplasms, syringomyelia and syringobulbia, olivopontocerebellar atrophy, Alzheimer disease, encephalitides, Creutzfeldt–Jakob disease, postencephalitic parkinsonism, cervical cordotomy, neuromuscular disorders affecting intercostal muscles and the diaphragm (such as myasthenia gravis), higher cervical spinal poliomyelitis, Guillain–Barré syndrome, limb–girdle dystrophies, and especially myotonic dystrophy. Hypoventilation and daytime drowsiness are prominent in all of these disorders. Enlarged tonsils (an especially important factor in the etiology of sleep apnea and snoring in children), myxedema, micrognathia and other facial and mandibular abnormalities, platybasia, neck infiltration secondary to Hodgkin disease, lymphoma, or radiation therapy to the neck, acromegaly, and familial or acquired dysautonomia (usually mixed central and OSA) may all cause OSA.

Of special interest is the development of postpolio syndrome years after the acute stage of poliomyelitis. It starts with fatigue, new muscular weakness, musculoskeletal pain, and dysphagia. During sleep, patients experience central and obstructive sleep apnea, which is worse during REM sleep because of the combined REM sleep–induced atonia and abnormal motor (phrenic) output caused by medullary dysfunction. Poliomyelitis also can cause atrophy of respiratory accessory muscles and thoracoabdominal muscles, leading to severe chest deformity such as kyphoscoliosis. Furthermore, impairment of cranial motor nerves (hypoglossal, facial, and trigeminal) may adversely affect tongue and other upper airway muscles. As a

consequence, all types of apneas may occur. These patients are vulnerable to develop respiratory failure with acute respiratory infection and may require assisted ventilation in intensive care units until the infection is controlled.

EVALUATION OF SUSPECTED SLEEP APNEA

The evaluation of patients suspected of having sleep apnea syndrome includes a full daytime and sleep history obtained not only from them but also (and most importantly) from their bed partner. A physical examination should concentrate on blood pressure, evidence of right heart failure, and abnormal skeletal and muscle configurations of the face and neck. The ear, nose, and throat examination is of primary importance. Chest radiographs and electrocardiograms are useful for evaluating pulmonary hypertension, determining the status of the right and left ventricles, and establishing possible coexistence of other cardiopulmonary disorders. A complete blood count may document the presence of polycythemia in chronic hypoxemia or right-sided heart failure. Pulmonary function studies with arterial blood gas sampling may be necessary to determine airway obstruction, or investigate for primary hypoventilation during the waking state and document hypo- and hypercapnia. The primary test that establishes the diagnosis of OSA is a polysomnographic study (PSMG), which is essential in an estimation of the severity of sleep-disordered breathing, sleep fragmentation, and oxihemoglobin desaturations. The severity of sleep apnea, defined by the so-called "apnea-hypopnea index," AHI (i.e., the number of episodes per hour of sleep), the degree of oxygen desaturation, sleep fragmentation and the presence of significant arrhythmias will be derived from sleep study and will guide future treatment (Fig. 10.4). Availability of sleep centers has been one of the major factors limiting the frequency of diagnosis of OSA. Recently, the use of home devices that give a limited number of physiological variables in

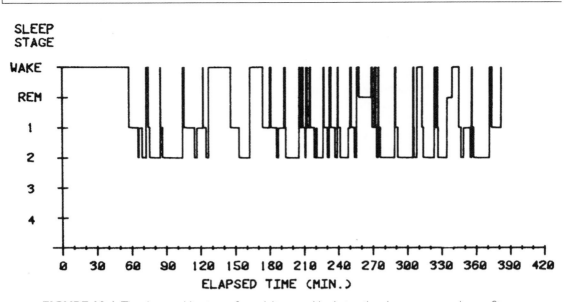

FIGURE 10.4 The sleep architecture of an adult man with obstructive sleep apnea syndrome. Stages 3 and 4 are lacking; frequent arousals occur, which fragment the sleep cycle; rapid eye movement (REM) sleep is much reduced as a proportion of the sleep period; and REM periodicity is abolished. The majority of the sleep period consists of nonrapid eye movement (NREM) stages 1 and 2.

sleep has been approved as a means to diagnose OSA.

Treatment of Sleep Apnea

The treatment of sleep apnea syndromes depends on its cause (Table 10.3). An important general treatment is weight loss, provided the loss of weight is not only achieved but also maintained. Similarly, abstinence from alcohol and avoidance of hypnosedative drugs are advocated.

Pharmacologic approaches including acetazolamide, theophylline, naloxone, medroxyprogesterone, and clomipramine have not been studied systematically on large numbers of subjects. The only widely used drug is protriptyline, which may exert a beneficial effect in an occasional patient with OSA. Its effect may be the result of a reported direct action on the muscle tone of the upper airway. A recent crossover unblinded trial of protriptyline and fluoxetine suggests equal effectiveness of either

drug, with about 30% to 50% of patients showing improved oxygenation during sleep. Similar results have been recently reported with mirtazapine.

A number of studies suggest that the administration of oxygen may be a useful method of treating central sleep apnea, although the mechanism by which it reduces central apneic events has not been established. It is hypothesized that the potential destabilizing influence of the hypoxic ventilatory response on respiratory control may be counteracted by the administration of oxygen. However, in some cases, hypercapnia and the frequency of OSA may increase.

Due to the effect of gravity on the airway, OSA is typically worse in the supine than in nonsupine position of sleep. In some situations, sleep apnea is only present in the supine position, while the lateral sleep is normal. If this is a case, restriction of sleep position may be used to control apnea. Several devices that make supine sleep uncomfortable by placing a bulky

TABLE 10.3 | **Treatment Options for Sleep Apnea**

Behavioral interventions
  Weight loss
  Avoidance of alcohol and sedatives
  Avoidance of supine sleep position
  Discontinuation of smoking
Continuous positive airway pressure treatments
  Nasal or oral positive airway pressure (NCPAP or OPAP)
  Bilevel positive airway pressure (BPAP)
  Auto-adjusting positive airway pressure (Auto-PAP)
Oral appliances
Surgical procedures
  Bypass surgery
    Tracheostomy
Upper airway reconstructions
  Soft-tissue modifications (Uvulopalatopharyngoplasty [UPPP], laser-assisted UPPP [LAUP], somnoplasty,
    radiofrequency volumetric reduction of the tongue, laser lingual resection—lingualplasty, tongue base
    suspension, tonsillectomy)
Skeletal modifications
  Mandibular osteotomy with genioglossal advancement and hyoid suspension, maxillomandibular osteotomy and
    advancement, hyoid myotomy and suspension to mandible, hyoid myotomy and suspension to thyroid cartilage,
    anterior hyoid advancement, transpalatal advancement pharyngoplasty, nasal surgery
Pharmacologic agents
  Medroxyprogesterone, decongestants, nasal steroids, antihistamines, protryptiline, and serotonergic agents:
    fluoxetine and other selective serotonin reuptake inhibitors, L-tryptophane

object on patient's back, such as a tennis ball t-shirt, are used to this effect.

The most widely used treatment of OSA is nasal continuous positive airway pressure (CPAP), which acts by establishing a "pneumatic splint" to the upper airway. CPAP is produced by a blower unit, which then pressurizes, via a conducting hose, a tight fitting nasal, oronasal, or oral mask. Pressurized air then causes elevation of the pressure in the oropharynx, thus reversing the transmural pressure gradient across the oropharyngeal airway, which results in airway opening. Poor compliance is a major obstacle limiting this otherwise successful treatment.

■ **SPECIAL CLINICAL POINT: Many patients with sleep apnea resist the use of CPAP. The main reasons for poor compliance are discomfort from the mask, poor mask fit resulting in air leakage, and trouble breathing against the incoming air. Early intensive support with phone calls and follow-up visits improve long-term compliance with CPAP.**

Newer devices are now equipped with systems that lower the pressure during an early expiration, improving comfort of breathing. Additionally, some patients do not use their CPAP due to social or cosmetic reasons and due to nasal obstruction.

Some patients whose apneas are eliminated with CPAP continue to have non-apneic desaturations, especially during REM sleep. These patients may have chronic obstructive pulmonary disease in addition to sleep apnea (overlap syndrome). In such situations, supplemental oxygen may be beneficial. The benefits derived from oxygen treatment should be verified either by a polysomnography or an overnight oximetry.

Bilevel positive airway pressure in a spontaneous mode (BPAP-S) offers an effective alternative for patients who are uncomfortable while expiring against the high pressures delivered by CPAP. This device allows independent titration of expiratory (EPAP) and inspiratory (IPAP) airway pressure. The difference between the EPAP and IPAP reflects the pressure support delivered by the device. BPAP is typically used in cases of comorbid obesity, intrinsic lung disease, and chest deformity, conditions associated with hypoventilation.

A bilevel device can also be used to provide spontaneous ventilation with a pressure support, with a minimal back-up rate (non-invasive mechanical ventilation, NIMV or bilevel positive airway pressure in spontaneous-timed mode, BPAP-ST). This mode of therapy is typically used in central sleep apnea and in conditions associated with hypoventilation. A variation of this treatment modality, an adapt-servo ventilator has been recently introduced to specifically address central apneas, especially in a form of periodic breathing pattern. The device detects the patient-generated flow and supplements it, breath by breath, with a variable, rather than constant pressure support. This modality has been shown to resolve a large proportion of idiopathic and opioid-related central sleep apnea, Cheyne–Stokes breathing, and complex sleep apnea.

Several surgical techniques have been used in treatment of OSA. Sometimes, correction of nasal obstruction can result in significant reduction of sleep apneas. Similarly, in cases of airway obstruction due to excess lymphoid tissue (most common etiology of OSA in children, less common in adults), an adenoidectomy or tonsillectomy can be curative. Attempts to promote uvulopalatopharyngoplasty (UPPP) as an alternative surgical treatment of sleep apnea have not been successful. Multiple studies indicate at best a success rate of 33% to 70%. The success rate may improve somewhat, provided selection of patients is based on the determination of the level of obstruction prior to the surgery. More encouraging are results of UPPP in the treatment of snoring. A 75% to 100% success rate for the elimination of snoring has been reported; this is not unexpected as structures generating the sounds of snoring are surgically removed. This may be misinterpreted as a sign of apnea cure, but the apneas may persist despite the disappearance of snoring. Laser-assisted uvulopalatoplasty, involving partial resection of the uvula and soft palate using a laser, is a simple surgical procedure that can be done on an outpatient basis in two to seven sessions without general anesthesia. It seems highly effective in eliminating habitual snoring, with success rates from 70% to 84%. Similarly, placement of implants within the soft palate reduces snoring but is unlikely to resolve apnea. Finally, surgical correction of the maxillofacial anomalies (maxillary advancement, mandibular advancement, surgery involving the attachment of the genioglossus to the mandible, hyoid bone suspension) has been used to correct sleep apnea in patients with craniofacial abnormalities.

There are at least 35 oral appliances that have been developed to help with snoring and sleep apnea. They all focus on the nasopharyngeal inlet and position of the base of the tongue. They either attach to the tongue and pull it forward directly or advance the mandible, and hence, the attachment of the genioglossus muscle, thus opening the retrolingual space in the throat. Typically the oral appliances are used in patients with mild to moderate sleep apnea who prefer oral appliances to CPAP, do not respond to CPAP, or are not candidates for CPAP therapy. Based on a recent pooled analysis of several trials, oral appliances are able to reduce the apnea-hypopnea index to <10 in about 50% of treated patients. Use of oral appliances has also been associated with improved daytime sleepiness. Compliance of patients with oral appliances is comparable to that of CPAP and side effects (salivation and teeth discomfort) are generally mild, though frequent.

In summary, although significant progress in evaluation and treatment of sleep-disordered breathing has been made, the exact etiology and pathophysiologic mechanism(s) currently are unknown. Sleep-disordered breathing has a profound effect on health. The range of sequelae varies from sudden death or cor pulmonale to failure to thrive or to perform at work and school. If unrecognized, lifelong problems may arise.

NARCOLEPSY

Narcolepsy is a syndrome consisting of excessive daytime sleepiness and abnormal manifestations of REM sleep. The latter includes frequent sleep-onset REM periods, which may be subjectively appreciated as hypnagogic (sleep-onset) or hypnopompic (sleep-offset) hallucinations, and dissociated REM sleep-inhibitory processes (i.e., cataplexy and sleep paralysis). The appearance of REM sleep within 10 minutes of sleep onset is considered evidence for narcolepsy. In narcolepsy, the patient falls asleep in the midst of activities, although most people will stay awake during animated conversation, walking, eating, or coitus.

The cardinal symptoms of narcolepsy are excessive daytime sleepiness, sleep attacks, and cataplexy. Although sleep attacks are characteristic of this disease, excessive sleepiness is equally disturbing (i.e., a permanent, sometimes profound, impairment of vigilance or wakefulness between attacks). Sleep attacks usually last about 15 minutes. The patient awakens refreshed, and there is a definite refractory period of 1 to 5 hours before the next attack. Cataplexy is a sudden decrease in, or abrupt loss of, muscle tone that either is generalized or limited to particular muscle groups. Cataplexy ranges from weakness in the muscles supporting the jaw, or a sense of weakness in the knees, to a complete muscular weakness causing the patient to slump to the floor, unable to move. Cataplectic attacks characteristically are initiated by laughter, surprise, outbursts of anger, or a feeling of exaltation. These attacks generally last for only a few seconds or for as long as 30 minutes.

An auxiliary symptom of narcolepsy includes sleep paralysis, which occurs while the patient is falling asleep or waking from sleep. Consciousness is preserved, and it is accompanied by an intense feeling of fear. Hallucinations also occur at the onset of sleep or on awakening, and they are usually frightening. Automatic behavior, sometimes reported as a "blackout," is a reflection of severe sleepiness. Nocturnal sleep also is disturbed with frequent awakenings, frequent sleep-onset REM periods, and vivid dreams. The combination of excessive daytime sleepiness and cataplexy is pathognomonic for narcolepsy.

The diagnosis of narcolepsy is based on the presence of excessive daytime sleepiness, sleep attacks, cataplexy, and other auxiliary symptoms. Typically the diagnosis is made by ruling out other causes of sleepiness (insufficient sleep time, presence of sleep apnea or PLM disorder, or use of medications or substances of abuse), and confirming the pathologic sleepiness by the Multiple Sleep Latency test (MSLT), showing a mean sleep latency of 5 minutes or less, with two or more sleep-onset REM periods. Presence of shortened nocturnal REM latency (<20 minutes) may support the diagnosis.

■ **SPECIAL CLINICAL POINT: It is advised that prior to MSLT testing all medications that might affect the central nervous system (anxiolytics, sedatives, stimulants, antidepressants) be stopped for 2–4 weeks. Further, sufficient sleep time 2 weeks prior to testing should be documented with actigraphy or a sleep log. In all instances, a polysomnogram is recorded on the night prior to the MSLT.**

More than 85% of all narcoleptics with definite cataplexy share a specific human leukocyte antigen (HLA) allele, HLA DQB1-0602 (most often in combination with HLA DR2), compared to 12% to 38% of the general population in various ethnic groups. DQB1-0602 may represent a genetic marker for the disorder, indicating the presence of the possible narcolepsy-susceptibility gene on chromosome 6. A negative test for DQB1-0602 does not rule out diagnosis of narcolepsy because a rare narcoleptic patient with cataplexy may be DQB1-0602 negative. Only 8% to 10% of narcoleptics are aware of another member of the family with narcolepsy/cataplexy. Prevalence studies have shown that the risk for a first-degree relative of a patient having narcolepsy with cataplexy is 1% to 2%. Usually, patients with narcolepsy can be reassured that the illness will not develop in their relatives. However, a 1% to 2% risk is 10 to 40 times higher than the prevalence observed in the general population, suggesting the existence of genetic predisposing factors. Twin studies demonstrated only a 25% to 31% concordance rate for narcolepsy in monozygotic twins. Genetic factors are defining susceptibility, but other (environmental) may trigger the onset of the disease. Although almost all diseases associated with the specific HLA allele are autoimmune in nature, an extensive search for known general markers (cerebrospinal fluid [CSF] oligoclonal bands, serum immunoglobulin levels, lymphocyte subset ratios) of autoimmune activation was negative.

However, as postulated by Mignot in 1995, the possibility of autoimmune cell destruction in a small part of the brain has become more likely in light of the discovery of the hypocretin system and its crucial role in the development of narcolepsy.

Genetic canine narcolepsy has been shown to be caused by mutations in the hypocretin-2 receptor gene. Almost simultaneously another group reported on the phenotype of the preprohypocretin (the precursor to two peptides: hypocretin-1 and hypocretin-2) knockout mice. The homozygous mice were observed to have numerous periods of "behavioral arrests." Twenty-four-hour EEG recordings revealed an increased amount of sleep during the dark period, reduced REM latency, and sleep-onset REM periods. Thus, a mouse model of narcolepsy with cataplexy was discovered.

Both discoveries prompted intense research in humans. Hypocretin-containing neurons are localized in the dorsolateral hypothalamus around the perifornical nucleus. In humans, the number of hypocretin-containing neurons is estimated to range from 15,000 to 20,000 to 50,000 to 80,000. These cells project widely to the entire brain: cerebral cortex, basal forebrain structures, such as the diagonal band of Broca; the amygdala; and the brainstem areas such as reticular formation, raphe nuclei, and LC. The role of hypocretin transmission in human narcolepsy has been confirmed by finding of low hypocretin levels in CSF in narcoleptics, compared to controls, and absence of hypocretic-containing neurons in the brains of patients with narcolepsy.

Treatment of Narcolepsy

Treatment of narcolepsy comprises treatment of the two most disabling symptoms of narcolepsy: excessive daytime sleepiness/sleep attacks and cataplexy (Tables 10.4 and 10.5).

In the rare patient, successful treatment involves only improved sleep hygiene, as previously described. Most patients, however, will need stimulants, primarily dextroamphetamine or methylphenidate. Stimulants enhance the release and inhibit the reuptake of catecholamines and, to a lesser extent, serotonin in the CNS. Stimulants are likely to reduce but not eliminate excessive daytime sleepiness and performance deficits. Methamphetamine in doses higher than those recommended for treatment of obesity was found to normalize sleepiness and performance in eight subjects studied, but it rarely is used because of concerns about abuse and related adverse behaviors.

Side effects often limit the use of stimulants. The dose-related clinically significant side effects include irritability, agitation, headache, tachycardia, hypertension, and peripheral sympathetic stimulation. Stimulants may be associated with dependence. A novel wake-promoting agent, modafinil usually is grouped

TABLE 10.4

Wake-Promoting Drugs for Treatment of Excessive Daytime Sleepiness

Drug Name	Initial Dose (mg)	Maintenance Dose (mg)	Drug Interactions
Dextroamphetamine	5	5–60	Because it is an indirect-acting sympathomimetic, may precipitate HTN crisis if taken with MAOI; with beta blockers may produce severe HTN, arrhythmias with tricyclics; may diminish the effectiveness of the anti-HTN drugs; may delay absorption of phenobarbital, ethosuximide, phenytoin
Methylphenidate	5–10	10–60	May decrease hypotensive effect of guamethidine; may inhibit metabolism of coumarin anticoagulants, some anticonvulsants, phenylbuthazone, and tricyclic drugs; safe use with clonidine and other alpha-2-agonists has not been systematically evaluated
Methamphetamine	10	10–50	MAOIs contraindicated; may decrease hypotensive effect of guanethidine; insulin requirement may be changed; phenothiazines antagonize stimulant effect of the amphetamines
Modafinil	100–200	200–400	Coadministration of potent CYP 450 3A4 inducers (carbamazepine, phenobarbital, rifampin) or inhibitors of CYP 450 3A4 inhibitors (ketoconazole, itraconazole) could alter modafinil's levels; it is a very modest CYP 3A4 inducer (cyclosporine, steroidal contraceptive clearance may increase). Because it is reversible inhibitor of CYP 2C19 (used for alternative metabolism of tricyclics) in patients deficient in CYP 2D6 the levels may rise
Selegiline	10	10–40	Stupor, muscle rigidity, hyperpyrexia with meperidine, and MAOIs (severe agitation, hallucinations, and death); severe toxicity with tricyclics and SSRIs
Sodium oxybate	3 g in two doses	3–9 g in two doses	Other CNS depressants and centrally acting muscle relaxants (benzodiazepines, opioids, barbiturates, ethanol, etc.)

HTN, hypertension; MAOI, monoamine oxidase inhibitor; CYP, cytochrome P enzyme; SSRIs, selective serotonin reuptake inhibitors.

with stimulants but seems to have a different mechanism of action that is not fully understood at present time. Modafinil increases the levels of dopamine and noradrenaline in several parts of the CNS. It activates glutamate-dependent pathways and reduces GABA-ergic transmission. The advantage of modafinil over other stimulants is lower frequency and severity of side effects, especially less irritability and agitation; however, if it is titrated rapidly, headache may emerge. Selegiline (monoamine oxidase [MAO] B inhibitor), combined with a low tyramine diet, also improves daytime sleepiness. Sodium oxybate was recently approved by the FDA for treatment of cataplexy and excessive daytime sleepiness in patients with narcolepsy.

TABLE 10.5

Anticataplectic Medications

Drug Name	Initial Dose (mg)	Maintenance Dose (mg)	Drug Interactions
Imipramine	10	10–100	See Table 10.1
Nortriptyline	25	25–75	See Table 10.1
Protriptyline	5	5–40	See Table 10.1
Clomipramine	25	50–150	Interactions same as for other TCAs; combination with tranylcypromine is particularly hazardous and the serotonin syndrome developed with concurrent use of moclobemide
Fluoxetine	20	20–80	It inhibits CYP 450 2D6 isoenzyme; this may require reduction of the dose of concomitant medication; thioridazine is contraindicated because of potential fatal arrhythmias; elevations of carbamazepine, phenytoin, tricyclics, clozapine levels were observed; also some benzodiazepine levels rose; sumatripan—weakness, incoordination, hyperreflexia; other tightly protein-bound drugs (warfarin, digitoxin)
Paroxetine	20	20–60	Weakness and hyperreflexia if used with almotripan; inhibition of TCA metabolism in some people—it is an inhibitor of CYP 450 2D6 and may inhibit other P450 isoenzymes including CYP 3A4; its metabolism can be inhibited by bupropion; cimetidine may increase serum concentrations of paroxetine via inhibition of CYP 450 metabolism of paroxetine; serotonin syndrome with MAOI—concurrent use contraindicated; increased serum concentration of clozapine with SSRIs; cyproheptadine reduces its effectiveness by antagonizing postsynaptic serotonin
Sertaline	25	50–100	Combination with other CNS drugs was not studied systematically; potential interaction with other drugs tightly bound to proteins (warfarin, digoxin) may result in increased levels; cimetidine led to significant increases in AUC and prolonged half-life
Citalopram	20	20–60	Substrate for CYP 450 3A4 and 2C19, is expected to interact with potent inhibitors of CYP 450 3A4 (ketoconazole, itraconazole, and macrolide antibiotics), and potent inhibitors of CYP P450 2C19 (omeprazole), but no clinically significant interactions observed; increased metoprolol levels; sumatripan in combination resulted in weakness, hyperreflexia, and incoordination
Sodium oxybate	3 g in two divided doses	3–9 g in two divided doses	See Table 10.4

TCA, tricyclic antidepressant; CYP, cytochrome P enzyme; MAOI, monoamine oxidase inhibitor; SSRIs, selective serotonin reuptake inhibitors; AUC, area under the curve.

Tricyclic antidepressants have been traditionally used in treatment of narcolepsy (as a REM suppressant) and cataplexy. Cataplectic attacks respond to imipramine, nortriptyline, and protriptyline. One of the most effective drugs for treatment of cataplexy is clomipramine, a triglyceric with a potent serotonin-uptake inhibitor. Side effects, mainly resulting from their anticholinergic properties, may limit the use of tricyclics. The most frequently reported side effects are dry mouth, increased sweating, sexual dysfunction (impotence, delayed orgasm, erection, and ejaculation dysfunction) weight gain, tachycardia, constipation, blurred vision, and urinary retention and xerostomia. Sudden discontinuation of tricyclics is likely to result in severe worsening of cataplexy and even status cataplecticus. Newer antidepressants with more exclusive inhibition of serotonin uptake (e.g., fluoxetine, paroxetine, and sertraline) are useful alternatives in the management of cataplexy, with fewer anticholinergic side effects. The anticataplectic effects of these drugs are most likely related to their desmethyl metabolites, which are potent adrenergic uptake inhibitors.

An FDA-approved drug for treatment of cataplexy is sodium oxybate. Sodium oxybate is a salt of a CNS depressant, gamma-hydroxybutyric acid. Published and reported data indicate its powerful effect in control of cataplexy, improvement of sleep quality, with increase in slow wave sleep, and reduction of daytime sleepiness. Side effects are mild (nausea, vomiting, dizziness, enuresis, dream abnormality, headache), and the drug is generally well tolerated. Given the high potential for misuse, the drug is strictly regulated.

Improvements observed with the use of L-tyrosine, codeine, or propranolol have not been documented in controlled trials. When sleep fragmentation is a major complaint, judicious use of short-acting hypnotics once or twice per week may be helpful. Significant improvement of nocturnal sleep with sodium oxybate was reported in double-blind, placebo-controlled trials.

Pharmacologic approaches are generally not entirely satisfactory, and many patients benefit from social support provided by Narcolepsy Network and other similar organizations.

Alternative Wake-Promoting Agents

Caffeine is a mild stimulant derived from the seeds, leaves, or fruits of 60 plant species. These plants are sources of caffeine for beverages such as coffee (*Coffea arabica*, *Coffea canephora*) or black or green tea (*Camellia sinensis*). Kola (*Kola acuminata*), guarana (*Paullinia cupana*), and mate (*Ilex paraguariensis*) are sources of caffeine for cola and other citrus beverages.

Herbal medicinal products containing caffeine include herbal teas, antioxidant green tea preparations, and weight loss formulations. Weight loss preparations often combine caffeine with ephedrine-containing products. Caffeine enhances alertness presumably via antagonism of the adenosine receptors. Ephedra is the source of ephedrine, an over-the-counter compound used for treatment of asthma. Ephedrine also is used and abused for energy, weight loss, and body building. Lesser known sources of ephedrine or related compounds are Indian sida (*Sida cordifolia*) and bitter orange (*Citrus aurantium*), sometimes found in energy or weight loss preparations. Ginseng (*Panax ginseng*—Korean ginseng) is a substance used to counteract fatigue (mild stimulant) or enhance performance. Siberian ginseng (*Eleutherococcus senticosus*) is used to enhance physical endurance and work capacity. There is no known herbal treatment for cataplexy.

INSUFFICIENT SLEEP

Insufficient sleep is the most frequent cause of daytime somnolence. The individual is voluntarily, but often unwittingly, chronically sleep deprived. Although this relationship may seem self-evident, most patients are unaware that their chronic sleep deprivation is responsible for their continuous excessive sleepiness. When these individuals obtain adequate sleep, their complaint of somnolence during the day disappears. In the most typical scenario, the sleep debt is built over weekdays and is partially relieved by prolonged sleep time on weekends.

Various other medical and medicinal causes of excessive daytime somnolence deserve mention. Hypnosedatives, anticonvulsants, antihypertensives, antihistamines, and antidepressants are common causes. A withdrawal from stimulants also may give rise to severe sleepiness. Multiple medical and toxic conditions may be associated with drowsiness: hyperglycemia (prior to ketoacidosis or nonketotic coma), hypocortisolism, hypoglycemia, hypothyroidism, panhypopituitarism, hepatic encephalopathy, hypercalcemia, renal insufficiency, vitamin B_{12} deficiency, chronic subdural hematoma, encephalitis, intracranial neoplasm (primary or secondary), meningitis, or the aftereffects of trauma. Hypersomnolence is a misnomer in many of these conditions because more often a state of obtundation occurs. There are also two rare periodic disorders of excessive sleepiness: (a) Kleine–Levin syndrome, characterized by recurrent periods of extended sleep, megaphagia, sexual disinhibitions, and social withdrawal if awake, and (b) menstruation-associated hypersomnia, a period of sleepiness during a patient's menstrual period (without observed changes in behavior).

When to Refer the Patient with Hypersomnia to the Sleep Specialist

Excessive daytime sleepiness is most frequently the result of sleep deprivation, poor sleep hygiene, prescribed or nonprescribed drugs, or sleep apnea. However, it is often a life-threatening symptom in situations requiring full vigilance (driving, operating machinery, combat, etc.). Primary care physicians are advised to use short (one-page) screening questionnaires in their outpatient offices because the patients often do not volunteer the information. If the screening is positive, the patient should be referred for the evaluation and workup in a sleep center. Of particular importance is quick and proper diagnosis and treatment of the sleep disorders accompanied by severe sleepiness (OSA, narcolepsy) in professional drivers.

Special Challenges for Hospitalized Patients

Of all types of hypersomnolence, sleep apnea poses prominent challenges to hospital personnel who may not be familiar with patients carrying this diagnosis. For a patient with diagnosed sleep apnea, useful guidelines include optimizing all associated medical conditions before elective surgery and using local or required anesthesia without sedation or narcotic use whenever possible. Full general anesthesia with adequate control of the airway is preferred to deep sedation. Patients should be extubated only after they fully wake up, and preferably in a nonsupine position. CPAP should be used postoperatively as soon as it is feasible in all patients who had used CPAP prior to surgery. Continuous, rather than intermittent oximetry monitoring is indicated in postoperative patients with sleep apnea; it can take place in the intensive care unit, stepdown, telemetry, or general ward setting. Patients with the following are especially at risk and require extreme vigilance: heavy narcotic requirement, severe sleep apnea (based on sleep study/clinical suspicion), and severe systemic manifestations. These patients should be observed in the intensive care unit.

PARASOMNIAS

Parasomnias, which include a heterogeneous group of behavioral disturbances that occur only during sleep or are exacerbated by sleep, do not have a common pathophysiologic mechanism. They represent disorders of arousal, partial arousal, and sleep-stage transitions.

Disorders of arousal (confusional arousals, sleep walking, and sleep terrors) all arise from NREM sleep, usually delta sleep; can be triggered by forced arousal from delta sleep; and are prevalent in childhood. Arousals from delta sleep are characterized by confusion, disorientation in time and space, and slow speech and mentation. These confusional arousals usually occur in children and may progress into sleepwalking (somnambulism) or sleep terror (*pavor nocturnus, incubus*). Typically there is very little if any recall for the event the following morning and minimal if any recall of dreamlike mentation. Most somnambulistic episodes last a few seconds to a few minutes. A sleep terror is an arousal from NREM sleep accompanied by a piercing scream or cry and behavioral manifestations of intense anxiety indicating autonomic arousal. Autonomic manifestations include mydriasis, perspiration, piloerection, rapid breathing, and tachycardia. Morning amnesia for the episode is the rule. Several groups of factors contribute to the occurrence of disorders of arousal. They include predisposing factors (genetic factors), factors causing increased amount of delta sleep or difficulty awakening (age, recovery from prior sleep deprivation, fever, CNS depressant drugs, etc.), and factors causing sleep fragmentation (pain, environmental stimuli, stimulants, stress, sleep apnea, PLMs, etc.).

There is often a concurrence of more than one of these disorders in the same child, and a hereditary predisposition to parasomnias has been noted. Somnambulism in children is not considered to be caused by psychologic factors, although its persistence into adulthood may represent a serious problem and occasionally may be associated with diverse forms of personality disturbance and psychopathology. Most children grow out of this condition between the ages of 7 and 14 years. It is important to protect patients against injury by, for example, installing safety rails at the head of stairways and placing locks on windows. If predisposing and triggering factors are identified, every effort should be made to minimize or avoid them. Many patients respond to benzodiazepines: triazolam, clonazepam (0.5–2.0 mg), and diazepam (5–10 mg) in the usual evening doses. Tricyclic drugs, such as imipramine, desipramine, and clomipramine in the doses of 10 to 50 mg, also may be effective.

REM sleep behavior disorder, recurrent isolated sleep paralysis and nightmare disorder are all classified as parasomnias usually associated with REM sleep. A nightmare is an arousal from REM sleep with the recall of a disturbing dream, accompanied by anxiety and much less prominent autonomic arousal. The awakened patient instantly is oriented and alert. Vocalization, fear, and motor activity are less intense than in sleep terrors. Nightmares are more likely to occur in the second half of the night, when more prolonged REM episodes are likely to occur. Withdrawal from alcohol, amphetamines, or hypnotics may lead to REM sleep rebound and cause nightmares.

REM sleep behavior disorder (RBD) is a parasomnia characterized by vigorous motor activity, instead of atonia, in response to dream content, often resulting in an injury. Manifestations of acting out dreams include laughing, talking, chanting, singing, yelling, swearing, gesturing, reaching, grabbing, arm flailing, punching, kicking, sitting up, jumping out of bed, crawling, and running movements.

■ **SPECIAL CLINICAL POINT: A high percentage of patients with RBD have a demonstrable underlying neurologic disorder, typically a synucleinopathy (Parkinson disease, dementia with Lewy bodies, multiple system atrophy or pure autonomic failure); RBD may predate the onset of other neurological symptoms by years.**

A minority of cases are idiopathic and tend to occur in the elderly. Transient RBD has been seen in association with acute drug intoxications and withdrawal states.

Making the bedroom environment safe for the patient by moving the furniture away from the bed, placing a mattress on the floor next to the bed, and keeping any weapons out of the bedroom are mainstays of management of RBD. Clonazepam (initial dose 0.5–1.0 mg) is the drug of choice for treatment of RBD. Anecdotal reports suggest effectiveness of clozapine, quetiapine, and melatonin.

Sleep-related enuresis is involuntary micturition beginning usually during deep NREM sleep in an individual who has or should have voluntary waking control of the bladder. In contrast to this idiopathic nocturnal enuresis, symptomatic enuresis is the result of urogenital or other diseases and is generally less benign. Idiopathic enuresis and somnambulism tend to disappear by late childhood or adolescence, probably representing a phenomenon of delayed maturation. At 5 years of age, 15% of boys and 10% of girls are still enuretic. Recommended treatment includes tricyclic antidepressants (e.g., imipramine, 25–75 mg at bedtime [approximately 1.0–1.5 mg/kg/day]) and daytime bladder exercises aimed at increasing bladder capacity. Oxybutynin chloride has been used with variable success. Intranasal desamino-D-arginine vasopressin (DDAVP) at low doses has been shown to have a definite effect, especially in children older than age 9 years and adults. Conditioning with a buzzer and pad is the most successful treatment for enuresis, but success may depend on continued use of the buzzer.

Parasomnias also include a cluster headache and the related (but more chronic) condition of paroxysmal hemicrania. Cluster headaches occur in REM sleep and may be related to an increased cerebral blood flow during REM sleep. About 45% of patients with seizure disorders have seizures mainly during sleep. Generalized seizures are markedly activated by NREM sleep; specifically, generalized tonic–clonic seizures are most common during stages 1 and 2 NREM sleep. Partial seizures may occur during NREM and REM sleep. Prolonged EEG monitoring may be necessary in some difficult cases when a diagnosis of epileptic (as opposed to non-epileptic) episodic behavior is needed.

Sleep-related eating disorder may occur in association with OSA, somnambulism, daytime eating disorders, medication abuse; it may occur in isolation. A sleep-related eating disorder is characterized by almost nightly eating and weight gain that patients attribute to the nocturnal eating. Most patients are only partially conscious during the eating episode. Two thirds of patients with this condition are women who generally are concerned about the weight gain. Daytime binge eating or obsessive–compulsive disorder is absent. Treatments include clonazepam, carbidopa/levodopa, and fluoxetine and topiramate. Cases of sleep-related eating disorder due to zolpidem have been described.

Other parasomnias that may occur in childhood as well as in adulthood include bruxism, head banging (*jactatio capitis nocturna*), abnormal swallowing, and painful penile erections. Whether these conditions require a polysomnographic evaluation and treatment depends entirely on the persistence of the symptoms and the degree of the patient's disability. Nocturnal groaning (catathrenia) is a parasomnia characterized by groaning or monotonous vocalization and is predominantly seen in REM sleep.

Alternative Treatments

There are no alternative treatments, other than anecdotal reports of alarms triggered by assumption of an erect posture, presumably accomplishing an awakening. If fully awake, the patient is less likely to be exposed to injury, consume undesirable food, or the like.

When to Refer the Patient with Parasomnia to the Sleep Specialist

Age, frequency, and the type of parasomnia should guide the nonspecialist to refer the patient. In childhood usually the parents are initiating the referral because the events could be dramatic and the parents are concerned about the safety of their child.

Always Remember

- In a patient with psychophysiological *insomnia*, behavioral therapy typically results in more sustained benefit than pharmacologic therapy alone.
- The diagnosis of *restless legs syndrome* is made on purely clinical grounds and does not require any testing in the sleep laboratory unless some other sleep pathology is suspected.
- *Insufficient sleep time* is the most common reason for hypersomnolence. Extending sleep time with a goal of spontaneous, rather than alarm-triggered awakenings is typically one of the first steps in evaluating a person with hypersomnolence.
- Patients with *obstructive sleep apnea* are frequently not aware of the severity of their nocturnal and diurnal symptoms and may resist formal evaluation. Involving their bed partner in this evaluation during the history taking may facilitate it.
- Most problems with continuous positive airway pressure (CPAP) compliance by patients with *obstructive sleep apnea* are due to mask problems. Early intensive support— follow-up visits and phone calls improve long-term compliance with CPAP.
- In most patients with suspected *narcolepsy*, all CNS-active medications (anxiolytics, sedatives, antidepressants, and stimulants) should be stopped 2 to 4 weeks prior to sleep evaluation.
- Appearance of *REM behavior disorder* with dream enactment may be an early sign of neurodegenerative disease.

QUESTIONS AND DISCUSSION

1. A 23-year-old man presents with a chief complaint of "narcolepsy." His history indicates the presence of sleep attacks, cataplexy, sleep paralysis, and hypnagogic hallucinations for the last 4 years. He states he has never been treated for the disorder and recognized his problem from reading about narcolepsy in a magazine. The neurologic examination is normal. The physical examination reveals a nervous man with a heart rate of 102 beats/min, but otherwise normal vital signs. The remainder of the physical examination is normal. A routine complete blood count, general chemistry screen, electrocardiogram (ECG), and chest x-ray film are normal. A thyroid battery is within normal limits. Which of the following is the most appropriate management of this patient?
    A. Prescription of D-amphetamine, 5 mg three times daily
    B. Administration of D-amphetamine in combination with a tricyclic antidepressant
    C. Routine all-night PSMG
    D. Urine screening for amphetamine metabolites
    E. Scheduling for a series of daytime naps in the sleep laboratory

The correct answer is D. The usual practice is to screen the urine for amphetamine metabolites before doing a more involved study. It is usually a bad sign to have a patient who knows the classic symptoms of narcolepsy and maintains he has never been diagnosed or treated. In most cases of narcolepsy, excessive daytime sleepiness and sleep attacks are initial symptoms of the disease, whereas associated symptoms develop later. A patient with all components of the syndrome early in the course of the disorder is subject to suspicion. Once urine samples are known to be "clean," all-night PSG and MSLT are useful to establish the diagnosis. If a patient is suspected of covert stimulant use, a prolonged period of abstinence should be documented before assuming that an REM-onset sleep episode is narcolepsy (because the same pattern may appear as part of stimulant withdrawal). Empiric therapy with stimulants is a practice that should be avoided.

2. A 36-year-old schoolteacher is referred for an evaluation of excessive somnolence. The patient states that he feels extremely drowsy unless he is actively involved in a novel behavior. The problem has been present for at least 3 years but seems to be getting worse. He has fallen asleep at the wheel of his car twice in the last 6 months. He denies a significant history of alcohol ingestion and is not taking medications. The physical examination reveals a large (160-cm, 82-kg) individual with normal vital signs. The physical and neurologic examinations are normal. After leaving the room to answer a call, you return to find the patient sleeping. A routine blood count reveals hemoglobin of 17 g/dL, with normal indices and normal white blood cell count. Biochemical screening is normal. A routine ECG is normal. Thyroid hormone levels and cortisol determinations are unremarkable. A urine screen for sedatives is unrevealing. Which of the following studies is most appropriate at this time?
   A. EEG
   B. CT of the head
   C. MRI of the brain
   D. All-night PSMG study, with respiratory and cardiac monitoring and if negative, followed by a series of daytime naps in the sleep laboratory

The correct answer is D. This is a fairly typical history in a sleep clinic—the diagnostic possibilities include narcolepsy, sleep apnea, and idiopathic hypersomnia. The history given, however, lacks the important details that would help clarify these diagnostic possibilities such as a history of snoring, cataplectic episodes or episodes of sleep paralysis, episodic amnesia, morning headache, or a family history of a similar problem. Any of the possibilities could be entertained from this history. The patient's weight and sex make sleep apnea statistically more likely, but

sedative drug abuse is too frequently a cause of this symptom to overlook it as a possibility. Our usual approach is to screen for sedatives, then to proceed with an all-night PSMG, with respiratory and cardiac monitoring. If the results are negative, daytime naps are studied with an MSLT the following day to exclude narcolepsy. The studies in answers A, B, and C are rarely of any value in evaluating these patients. In this particular case, an all-night PSMG documented the presence of a severe OSA with associated cardiac arrhythmias. The elevated red blood cell count appeared to be a secondary complication of nocturnal apnea.

3. You are consulted by a 23-year-old man who described episodes of "amnesia." On several occasions, he has found himself at various locations with no recollection of having traveled to them. He recollects being at another location hours before; his memory for previous events is good, and he denies any other symptoms preceding the attack. Observers have seen him during an episode, and he appeared distracted but carried on social conversations appropriately and on one occasion drove a car without incident. He appears relatively stable, and attacks occur in situations that seem devoid of any emotional importance. The patient does not drink alcohol. The neurologic examination is normal. A sleep-deprived EEG without sedation is read as normal, although it is noted that drowsiness is followed quickly by the onset of low-voltage fast activity. Biochemical studies including a 6-hour glucose tolerance test are all normal. An MRI of the brain is normal. Empiric therapy with phenytoin (100 mg three times daily) leads to worsening of the symptoms. Which of the following disorders is most compatible with this history?
   A. Pseudoseizure or hypoglycemia
   B. Narcolepsy–cataplexy syndrome or sleep apnea syndrome
   C. Somnambulism

D. Transient global amnesia or amnestic migraine

E. Complex partial seizure

The correct answers is B. The episodes described are typical of "automatic behavior" syndrome. This behavioral abnormality is associated with the appearance of "microsleep" episodes, which electroencephalographically are stage N1 sleep. Sleep apnea and narcolepsy are associated with this disorder. Although the diagnosis of complex partial seizures is difficult to rule out on the basis of a normal EEG, the adverse response to empiric anticonvulsants is more typical of an "automatic behavior" syndrome. Transient global amnesia presents a similar clinical picture but is an entity restricted to late middle life; frequent recurrences are unusual in this syndrome. Somnambulism is a similar phenomenon but is more frequent in childhood and arises from a period of normal sleep; it is usually a stage N3 sleep event.

Amnestic migraine may produce recurrent amnestic episodes but usually does so in the presence of more typical migrainous episodes. There is some question of whether this is a sui generis disorder or this represents the coexistence of two phenomena in a single individual.

Pseudoseizures rarely are characterized by amnesia and are usually situationally related. Hypoglycemia may present as transient decrease in consciousness, but is usually associated with signs of sympathetic stimulation; history of apparent normal behavior during the episode makes it less likely.

Appropriate management in this case would include an all-night PSMG and if negative followed by the Multiple Sleep Latency test the next day as well as a routine 16-channel EEG. A careful history-taking directed specifically toward cataplexy, daytime napping, nocturnal apnea, and snoring would help in a differentiation of the underlying condition. Hypnosedatives, anticonvulsants, and diazepam usually cause worsening of the symptoms. In patients with sleep apnea of any cause, proper medical or surgical management has been reported to alleviate this symptom complex.

4. A 43-year-old accountant is referred for sleep evaluation for snoring and bizarre nighttime behaviors. For the past several years, his sleep has been very active; a bed partner reports snoring, snorting, vocalizations, frequent position changes, and repeated leg movements. On several occasions he has been noted to wake up and not knowing where he was, he also could not recognize his bed partner for a brief period of time. There were single episodes of sleep paralysis and sleep hallucinations, but no cataplexy. His daytime functioning is impaired by his stressful job, his obesity, and significant sleepiness that tend to develop in the afternoons. In the evening he tends to fall asleep in front of TV, but denies any leg discomfort or urge to move the legs. He moved and changed his job 3 years prior to this evaluation, and gained 50 lbs since. He is otherwise healthy, has not had any neurological problems in the past, and does not take any medications.

On examination, he is obese with the body mass index (BMI) of 44.5 kg/m^2, has a large tongue with side indentations, short thick neck, bilaterally decreased breath sounds, and minimal peripheral edema.

Which of the following diagnoses is the most likely?

A. Narcolepsy without cataplexy

B. Confusional arousals

C. Restless legs syndrome

D. Obstructive sleep apnea

E. Nocturnal epilepsy

The correct answer is D. Obstructive sleep apnea is the most likely explanation of this variety of symptoms presented by the patient. Obstructive sleep apnea typically presents with snoring and excessive daytime sleepiness; obesity is a known risk factor. OSA may produce, via sleep fragmentation related to apnea-related arousals, whole number of nighttime symptoms ranging from frequent position changes, leg movements, vocalizations, confusional arousals, to apparent REM-intrusion phenomena such as sleep paralysis and sleep hallucinations.

Narcolepsy typically presents in adolescents and young adults; late presentation in a middle-aged adult is uncommon, but delayed diagnosis is frequent. Also, the sleep of a patient with narcolepsy is highly fragmented, but typically devoid of parasomnias. The patient does not report daytime symptoms characteristic of RLS. Confusional arousals with or without more complex behaviors, is a parasomnia typical for children; the multitude of other nocturnal symptoms make it unlikely in this patient. Nocturnal epilepsy may present as bizarre behavior at night, but these are usually stereotyped in nature. Presence of daytime sleepiness and physical examination findings typical of OSA make this diagnosis more likely.

SUGGESTED READING

American Academy of Sleep Medicine. *The International Classification of Sleep Disorders*. 2nd ed. Westchester: American Academy of Sleep Medicine; 2005.

Ancoli-Israel S, Roth T. Characteristics of insomnia in the United States: results of the 1991 National Sleep Foundation survey. I. *Sleep*. 1999;22 (suppl 2): S347–S353.

Benarroch EE. Suprachiasmatic nucleus and melatonin: reciprocal interactions and clinical correlations. *Neurology*. 2008;71(8):594–598.

Boeve BF, Silber MH, Saper CB, et al. Pathophysiology of REM sleep behaviour disorder and relevance to neurodegenerative disease. *Brain*. 2007;130(pt 11): 2770–2788.

Caples SM, Garcia-Touchard A, Somers VK. Sleep-disordered breathing and cardiovascular risk. *Sleep*. 2007;30(3):291–303.

Chemelli RM, Willie JT, Sinton CM, et al. Narcolepsy in orexin knockout mice: molecular genetics of sleep regulation. *Cell*. 1999;98:437–451.

Fahey CD, Zee PC. Circadian rhythm sleep disorders and phototherapy. *Psychiatr Clin North Am*. 2006;29(4): 989–1007; abstract ix.

Gay P, Weaver T, Loube D, et al. Evaluation of positive airway pressure treatment for sleep related breathing disorders in adults. *Sleep*. 2006;29(3):381–401.

Gross JB, Bachenberg KL, Benumof JL, et al. Practice guidelines for the perioperative management of patients with obstructive sleep apnea: a report by the American Society of Anesthesiologists Task Force on Perioperative Management of patients with obstructive sleep apnea. *Anesthesiology*. 2006;104(5):1081–1093; quiz 1117–1118.

Guilleminault C, Chowdhuri S. Upper airway resistance syndrome is a distinct syndrome. *Am J Respir Crit Care Med*. 2000;161(5):1412–1413.

Hauri P, Linde S. *No More Sleepless Nights*. New York: Wiley; 1996.

Kushida CA, Littner MR, Hirshkowitz M, et al. Practice parameters for the use of continuous and bilevel positive airway pressure devices to treat adult patients with sleep-related breathing disorders. *Sleep*. 2006;29(3):375–380.

Lin HC, Friedman M, Chang HW, et al. The efficacy of multilevel surgery of the upper airway in adults with obstructive sleep apnea/hypopnea syndrome. *Laryngoscope*. 2008;118(5):902–908.

Lin L, Faraco J, Li R, et al. The sleep disorder canine narcolepsy is caused by a mutation in the hypocretin (orexin) receptor 2 gene. *Cell*. 1999;98:365–376.

Littner MR, Kushida C, Anderson WM, et al. Practice parameters for the dopaminergic treatment of restless legs syndrome and periodic limb movement disorder. *Sleep*. 2004;27(3):557–559.

Mahowald MW, Schenck CH. Non-rapid eye movement sleep parasomnias. *Neurol Clin*. 2005;23(4):1077–1106, vii.

Montplaisir J, Boucher S, Poirier G, et al. Clinical, polysomnographic, and genetic characteristics of restless legs syndrome: a study of 133 patients diagnosed with new standard criteria. *Mov Disord*. 1997;12:61–65.

Morgenthaler T, Kramer M, Alessi C, et al. Practice parameters for the psychological and behavioral treatment of insomnia: an update. An American Academy of Sleep Medicine report. *Sleep*. 2006;29(11):1415–1419.

Morin CM. *Insomnia: Psychological Assessment and Management*. New York: Guilford Press; 1993.

Morin CM, Bootzin RR, Buysse DJ, et al. Psychological and behavioral treatment of insomnia: update of the recent evidence (1998–2004). *Sleep*. 2006;29(11): 1398–1414.

Morin CM, Hauri PJ, Espie CA, et al. Nonpharmacologic treatment of chronic insomnia. An American Academy of Sleep Medicine review. *Sleep*. 1999;22: 1134–1156.

Parish JM, Somers VK. Obstructive sleep apnea and cardiovascular disease. *Mayo Clin Proc.* 2004;79(8): 1036–1046.

Phillips B, Ancoli-Israel S. Sleep disorders in the elderly. Review. *Sleep Med.* 2001;2:99–114.

Powell NB, Riley RW, Robinson A. Surgical management of obstructive sleep apnea syndrome. *Clin Chest Med.* 1998;19:77–86.

Schenck CH, Mahowald MW. Rapid eye movement sleep parasomnias. *Neurol Clin.* 2005;23(4):1107–1126.

Sherin JE, Shiromani PJ, McCarley RW, et al. Activation of ventrolateral preoptic neurons during sleep. *Science.* 1996;271:216–219.

Silber MH. Clinical practice. Chronic insomnia. *N Engl J Med.* 2005;353(8):803–810.

Taheri S, Zeitzer JM, Mignot E. The role of hypocretins (orexins) in sleep regulation and narcolepsy. *Annu Rev Neurosci.* 2002;25:283–313.

Wing YK. Herbal treatment of insomnia. *HKMJ.* 2001;7: 392–402.

Winkelman JW. Clinical and polysomnographic features of sleep-related eating disorder. *J Clin Psychiatry.* 1998;59:14–19.

Young T, Palta M, Dempsey J, et al. The occurrence of sleep-disordered breathing among middle-aged adults. *N Engl J Med.* 1993;328(17):1230–1235.

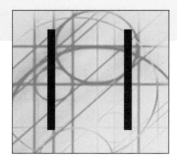

Multiple Sclerosis

PETER A. CALABRESI AND SCOTT D. NEWSOME

> **key points**
> - Multiple sclerosis (MS) is an immune-mediated, multiphasic, mutifocal disease of the central nervous system.
> - The primary etiology of MS is unknown; however, the disease has features of inflammation, demyelination, axonal injury, and neurodegeneration.
> - Visual dysfunction, sensory disturbances, and gait impairment are very common presenting symptoms.
> - MRI is the single most useful test in confirming the diagnosis of MS.
> - Early and accurate diagnosis is paramount.
> - Initiating early disease-modifying treatment can influence the clinical course.
> - Symptomatic therapy can greatly improve MS patients' quality of life.

ultiple sclerosis (MS) is a neurodegenerative disease with early intense inflammation of the central nervous system (CNS). The primary etiology of MS remains unknown and is likely multifactorial. The disease is characterized pathologically by inflammatory infiltrates and demyelination, followed by varying degrees of secondary axonal degeneration.

■ SPECIAL CLINICAL POINT: Multiple sclerosis is the most common nontraumatic cause of neurologic disability in young adults and affects approximately 400,000 people in the United States. An estimated 200 people per week are newly diagnosed.

MS affects women two to three times more commonly than men. Most patients start with a period of unpredictable relapses and remissions, which in the majority is followed by an accumulation of neurologic dysfunction and a chronic progressive course. The life expectancy has been shown to be only 6 to 7 years less than that for a control population without MS, but the emotional and economic cost to society as a result of the disability is enormous.

HISTORY

The earliest account of a disease that appears likely to have been MS is found in writings from the 14th century, describing the illness of a Dutch nun, "Blessed Lidwina of Schiedam." The earliest pathologic descriptions by Carswell and Cruveilhier date to between 1838 and

1845. Charcot is generally credited with the first comprehensive account of the clinical and pathologic features of MS, which was published in 1868.

EPIDEMIOLOGY

Epidemiologic studies have shown that MS has an unequal geographic distribution, with large regional and ethnic variations in the prevalence of disease (Fig. 11.1). MS is rare in the tropics and increases in frequency at higher latitudes north and south of the equator. The prevalence in the United States is reported at 57.8 per 100,000 and is almost twice as common in the Northern as compared to the Southern United States. The prevalence rate has been increasing, probably because of better recognition of MS and improved treatment of complications with a correspondingly increased longevity of those affected. Prevalence rates of less than 5 per 100,000 are found in Asia, Africa (except English-speaking whites in South Africa), and northern South America. MS is also said to be much less common among Eskimos, Gypsies, and African Americans. However, these patterns may be changing with increased travel; cases of MS have been reported in native Africans who have not traveled out of the country, and the prevalence of African Americans with MS has not been reexamined adequately in the magnetic resonance imaging (MRI) era of diagnosis.

Migration studies suggest that the risk of acquiring MS is related to the location in which one has lived before puberty. Individuals migrating from high- to low-risk areas decreased their expected risk of developing MS, as determined from their area of birth. Conversely, migration from low- to high-risk areas increased the risk of acquiring MS. The reliability of migration studies has been questioned, and no definite conclusions can be made from these data.

Numerous instances of MS clusters have been reported. Several clusters have been related to exposure to heavy metals and canine distemper virus, but no conclusive link has been established. Genetic studies strongly suggest that the disease is polygenic and that genetic factors may have a stronger influence in determining susceptibility to MS than environmental factors.

PATHOLOGY OF MULTIPLE SCLEROSIS

Classic descriptions of the MS lesion as predominantly demyelinating with relative sparing of axons still hold true today. Modern tools

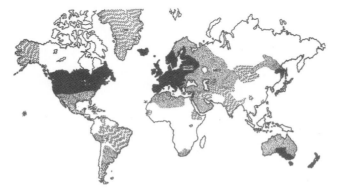

FIGURE 11.1 Map of the world depicting areas of high prevalence (30+/100,000, *solid*), medium prevalence (5–29/100,000, *dotted*), and low prevalence (0–4/100,000, *dashed*). White areas are regions without data or people. (From Kurtzke JF, Wallin MT. Epidemiology. In: Burks JS, Johnson KP, eds. Multiple sclerosis: diagnosis, medical management, and rehabilitation. New York: Demos Medical Publishing; 2000. Reproduced with permission from Demos Medical Publishing.)

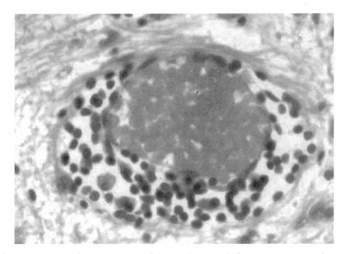

FIGURE 11.2 Perivenular infiltrate typical of the early acute inflammatory event in an active lesion.

have afforded more detailed descriptions of the immunologic and structural events occurring within lesions and have reemphasized the secondary axonal degenerative stage of the lesion. Major advances in the classification of MS pathology have been made from biopsy and rapid autopsy material. Clinicopathologic correlations using MRI and spectroscopy provide hope that advances in our understanding of the pathologic state will allow guided therapeutic interventions.

The MS plaque appears to begin with the migration of lymphocytes and macrophages across the blood–brain barrier into the perivenular space (Fig. 11.2). This is followed by diffuse parenchymal infiltration by inflammatory cells, edema, and active stripping of myelin from axons by macrophages, leading to multifocal areas of demyelination (Fig. 11.3). Subsequently, astrocytic hyperplasia and the accumulation of lipid-laden macrophages ensue. As plaques enlarge and coalesce, the initial perivenular

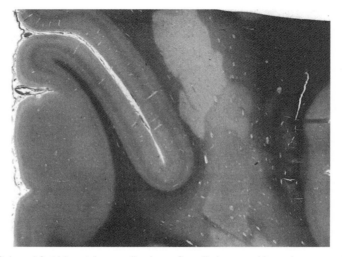

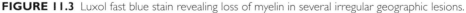

FIGURE 11.3 Luxol fast blue stain revealing loss of myelin in several irregular geographic lesions.

distribution of the lesions becomes less apparent. The inflammatory reaction is usually less pronounced in grey matter, probably because of the smaller amount of myelin in these areas. The extent of axonal loss in the demyelinated areas is highly variable. The sparing of axons is relative, and some axonal loss occurs in almost all lesions and can become substantial in severe cases. Axonal loss can also occur very early and even be present during the first clinical attack.

Plaquelike areas of pale myelin staining are called shadow plaques and are generally regarded as evidence of partial remyelination. Several studies have confirmed a remarkable potential for oligodendrocyte proliferation and partial remyelination, which seems to be impeded by as-yet-unknown local factors.

Myelin and Nerve Conduction

Proteolipid protein (PLP), myelin basic protein (MBP), and their isoforms make up 80% to 90% of the myelin sheath with 2',3'-cyclic nucleotide 3'-phosphohydrolase (CNPase), myelin-associated glycoprotein (MAG), myelin oligodendrocyte protein (MOG), and other minor proteins making up the rest. Both PLP and CNPase are restricted to CNS myelin, whereas MBP constitutes about 10% of the protein in PNS myelin. Lipids constitute 80% of the dry weight of myelin. Cultured oligodendroglial cells contain a family of gangliosides of which GM_3 and GM_1 are the principal components.

One oligodendrocyte usually forms internodal segments of myelin on several different nerve fibers. This differs from the peripheral nervous system, where one Schwann cell contributes myelin to only one internodal segment. This difference may account, in part, for the much greater efficiency of regeneration in peripheral myelin. The nodes of Ranvier have a high concentration of sodium channels concentrated in the nodal membrane, which are required for saltatory conduction. During an episode of inflammatory demyelination, conduction may be transiently impaired as a result of edema, loss of myelin, and some degree of metabolic dysfunction of the nerve axon. Conduction can recover acutely on resolution of edema, subacutely with redistribution of sodium channels along the internodal membrane, or chronically after partial remyelination.

Pathologic Correlations with Magnetic Resonance Imaging

■ **SPECIAL CLINICAL POINT: The profound impact of modern imaging technologies, particularly MRI, is evident from its expanding role in the diagnosis and prognosis of MS.**

High signal (bright) T2-weighted lesions correlate well with the presence of lesions on gross pathology. However, T2 lesions lack specificity for microscopic tissue pathology and seem to represent a composite of factors including edema, demyelination, remyelination, gliosis, and axonal loss. Therefore, the T2-lesion burden does not correlate strongly with clinical disability even in clinically eloquent areas of the CNS (brainstem and spinal cord) because not all T2 lesions purport the destructive axonal pathology. Indeed, this is exactly what the T2-weighted lesion volume studies show—a weak but significant correlation with clinical disability (Expanded Disability Status Scale, or EDSS, and cognitive impairment). Because of the imprecise specificity of T2 images, more emphasis is being placed on T1-weighted images in which persistent low signal (black holes) seems to correlate better with axonal dropout and clinical disability. However, one must be cautious because during the acute enhancing phase of a lesion, and perhaps for several months thereafter, low signal T1 lesions may represent extracellular edema that can resolve.

Another misunderstood aspect of imaging is that there is a temporal sequence of lesion pathology such that acute contrast-enhanced lesions correlate well with the perivenular infiltrate and the likelihood of a clinical exacerbation but also predict future formation of black holes and brain atrophy. Indeed in a clinical trial of interferon beta (IFNβ), the drug suppressed inflammation on the MRI in the first year of treatment but did not slow brain atrophy until the second year. This suggests that those axons that were already demyelinated prior to treatment may follow an inexorable course of degeneration during the first year of treatment, but the axons that were salvaged from demyelination by suppression of the inflammatory attack in the first year are spared degeneration in the second year. This also would explain why in two recent short-term trials of potent immunosuppressive drugs used for 12 months or one dose, contrast-enhancing lesions were reduced, but there was no effect on progression of disability or brain atrophy. Newer methods such as magnetization transfer imaging, diffusion tensor imaging, and proton magnetic resonance spectroscopy (^{1}H-MRS) may be more sensitive measures of underlying structural pathology.

ETIOLOGY AND IMMUNOPATHOGENESIS

Although the cause of MS remains uncertain, our understanding of the underlying mechanisms and pathology has grown enormously.

■ **SPECIAL CLINICAL POINT: The best formulation of the pathogenesis of MS is that the disease is an autoimmune process that occurs in a genetically susceptible individual after an environmental exposure.**

This hypothesis is supported by an extensive and diverse literature but is based on three seminal discoveries. The recognition by Rivers that the acute paralytic encephalitis that occasionally followed rabies and small pox vaccination was an autoimmune reaction to contaminating self-proteins led him to the discovery of experimental allergic encephalomyelitis (EAE), which has since been studied extensively as an animal model for MS. The discoveries that genes influence disease susceptibility and specifically that the human leukocyte antigen class II region on the short arm of chromosome 6 is associated with the risk of developing MS have led to a multitude of studies suggesting that polygenetic influences predispose certain individuals to acquiring MS. Finally, the observations made regarding latitudinal gradient, migration, and disease clustering have strongly suggested an environmental role in the disease. Although no specific microbial agent has stood the test of time, modern molecular immunology has provided numerous potential mechanisms through which numerous infections could mediate autoimmunity.

Genetics

Genetic susceptibility to MS has long been suspected, based on widely differing prevalence in different ethnic populations. Family studies have found that first-degree relatives of patients are at 20-fold increased risk of developing MS. Furthermore, monozygotic twins are more likely to be concordant for MS (20% to 40%) than dizygotic twins (3% to 4%). Nonbiologic first-degree (adopted) relatives are no more likely to develop MS than the population at large, which further supports the notion that familial clustering for MS is largely genetic in origin. However, unless one invokes incomplete penetrance of genes, the twin studies also suggest a strong environmental component because no more than 40% of monozygotic twins are concordant for MS. Widely different MS prevalence among similar high-susceptibility genetic groups that inhabit different environments (such as Anglo-Saxons in England versus in South Africa) presumably must be tied to this second, environmental element of disease etiology. Studies of candidate genes and whole-genome screens suggest that multiple weakly acting genes interact epistatically to determine risk toward MS, as suspected from epidemiologic studies. Recently, various single-nucleotide polymorphisms (SNPs) associated with a higher risk of developing MS were identified on the interleukin-2 receptor α gene, interleukin-7 receptor α gene, and confirmed in the HLA-DRA locus.

Immunology of Multiple Sclerosis

The inflammatory reaction in MS is of unknown origin. Although no infectious agent has been proved to be the cause of MS, it is hypothesized that many common viruses can trigger autoimmune-mediated demyelination in susceptible individuals through molecular mimicry (cross-reactivity between microbial proteins and myelin). In addition, there is evidence that quiescent autoreactive T cells that are present in healthy individuals may be activated through bystander activation by cytokine or polyclonal T-cell activation mediated by bacteria or viruses.

■ **SPECIAL CLINICAL POINT: It remains uncertain how tissue injury (to myelin, oligodendroglia, axons, and neurons) occurs in MS, but the inflammatory events surrounding the vast majority of acute MS lesions seem to suggest a direct immune-mediated pathology.**

The MS lesion resembles a delayed-type hypersensitivity (DTH) reaction, containing activated T cells, B cells, numerous mononuclear phagocytes, inflammatory cytokines, and adhesion molecules. Electron microscopy studies suggest the macrophage may play a major role in the direct stripping of myelin from axons, although this could be a secondary phagocytic response

to excitotoxic injury of oligodendrocytes or neurons. There has been more emphasis recently on the role of innate immune cells in MS, specifically, dendritic cells and microglia. These cells seem to help facilitate the proinflammatory immune response in MS and direct autoreactive T-cell function within the CNS through antigen presentation. Therapies directed toward these cells could prove to be very beneficial.

DISEASE COURSE AND CLINICAL PATTERNS

The clinical course of MS is divided into categories according to neurologic symptoms as they develop over time. A new classification for MS categories was developed by consensus among MS experts (Table 11.1).

Relapsing–Remitting Multiple Sclerosis

Relapsing–remitting MS (RR-MS) is the most common form in patients younger than age 40 years. Patients may develop focal neurologic symptoms and signs acutely or over a few days.

TABLE 11.1 | **Multiple Sclerosis Clinical Categories**

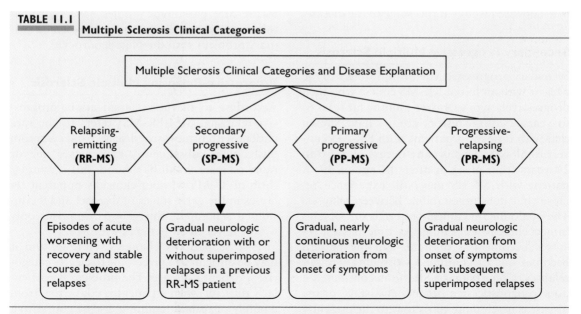

Lublin FD, Reingold SC. Defining the clinical course of multiple sclerosis: results of an international survey. *Neurology.* 1996;46:907–911.

These exacerbations or attacks are remarkably unpredictable and heterogeneous in character, probably because they result from varying degrees of inflammation that can occur in any part of the brain or spinal cord.

■ **SPECIAL CLINICAL POINT: Common presentations of multiple sclerosis include blurred or double vision, sensory symptoms (numbness, tingling, or pain), weakness, vertigo, or impaired balance.**

A new symptom will commonly present over 24 to 72 hours, stabilize for a few days or weeks, and then improve spontaneously over 4 to 12 weeks. Subsequent new focal symptoms or signs typically follow the initial attack months or years later and again remit partially or completely. It is very common for old symptoms to persist or reoccur, especially in response to periods of stress such as infections or prolonged elevations of core body temperature. Over time, it becomes difficult to determine whether the symptom flare represents a new exacerbation or worsening symptoms referable to past disease. Recovery from relapses is often incomplete, and permanent disability can accumulate in a stepwise fashion at this stage of the disease.

Secondary Progressive Multiple Sclerosis

Secondary progressive MS (SP-MS) refers to the patient with an initial RR-MS course who then progressively worsens over months (at least 6) to years. Natural history studies have shown that with time most patients with RR-MS convert to SP-MS. This usually occurs after 10 to 20 years from onset or after the age of 40. A patient with SP-MS may still experience relapses but does not stabilize between relapses. The predominant clinical pattern is one of continued clinical worsening. As time passes, relapses become less discrete, and the pattern becomes one of continued worsening without relapses. Conversion to SP-MS is considered a poor prognostic sign because this stage of the disease is much more refractory to the presently available immunomodulatory therapies. Some

patients with SP-MS spontaneously stabilize for considerable periods, although they only rarely recover after deficits have persisted for 6 months. The pathogenic mechanisms underlying conversion from RR-MS to SP-MS may relate to failure of remyelination and progressive axonal injury.

Primary Progressive Multiple Sclerosis

Primary progressive MS (PP-MS) accounts for approximately 10% to 15% of patients and is characterized by progressive worsening from the onset of symptoms without interposed relapses. Patients with PP-MS are more likely to be men and older than 40 years of age at symptom onset. This form of the disease often presents with progressive gait disorder as a result of leg weakness, spasticity, and impaired coordination. In cases of progressive neurologic dysfunction, it is extremely important to rule out structural pathology, infections, and hereditary and other neurodegenerative diseases. Patients with PP-MS have fewer gadolinium-enhancing brain lesions on MRI, less tissue inflammation on histopathologic assessment, and less cerebrospinal fluid (CSF) inflammation than typical for SP-MS; pathologic studies have suggested this form of the disease may represent a primary problem with the oligodendrocyte.

Progressive-Relapsing Multiple Sclerosis

According to the new classification, progressive-relapsing MS (PR-MS) refers to the rare patient with progressive disease from symptom onset, who subsequently experiences one or more relapses. In all likelihood, this is another form of SP-MS without clinically apparent relapses in the early stages of disease, and if considered separately, this group comprises only 6% or fewer of all patients with MS.

Disease patterns change over time, and it may be difficult at a given time to clearly categorize a patient's disease. The problem is particularly difficult when a patient is converting from a purely relapsing–remitting disease course to a purely progressive disease course. This has been termed "relapsing progressive MS" by some and "transitional MS" by others, but these disease categories cannot be defined precisely by current methods. Observation for as long as 1 year may be required to categorize such a patient with confidence.

Clinically Isolated Syndromes and Prognosis

■ **SPECIAL CLINICAL POINT: In the era of partially effective prophylactic MS therapies, there has been increased emphasis on making a diagnosis early in the course of the disease to initiate appropriate preventative treatment.**

The use of MRI as a diagnostic tool is discussed later. T2-lesion burden at the time of first MS symptoms (optic neuritis, transverse myelitis, etc.) not only determines the likelihood of converting to clinically definite MS but is also predictive of future disability. For example, a patient with a single episode of optic neuritis and an abnormal brain MRI has a 50% to 80% risk of subsequently being diagnosed with MS in 5 to 10 years. The frequency of gadolinium-enhancing lesions correlates with the likelihood of having a clinical exacerbation and predicts future brain atrophy. However, because T2-weighted lesions lack specificity for tissue pathology and gadolinium enhancement is transient (2 to 8 weeks), T1 hypointense lesions (black holes) and brain atrophy may be a better measure of axonal loss and have been shown to correlate more strongly with both present and future disability. The presence of mild atrophy or persistent T1 black holes early in the course of MS should alert the physician to a potentially aggressive form of the disease.

OTHER VARIANTS OF MULTIPLE SCLEROSIS AND IMPORTANT MIMICKERS

Several other variants of MS have been described and are important to recognize.

Marburg Disease

An acute rapidly progressive form of MS, often called Marburg disease, is characterized by a person who develops acute or subacute progressive neurologic deterioration, leading to severe disability within days to months. The disease may progress steadily to a quadriplegic obtunded state with death as a result of intercurrent infection, aspiration, or respiratory failure from brainstem involvement. Postmortem studies have documented inflammation in the optic nerves, optic chiasm, cerebral hemispheres, and spinal cord. The pathology reveals a pronounced mononuclear cell infiltrate with severe axonal damage and tissue necrosis.

Neuromyelitis Optica

Neuromyelitis optica (NMO) or Devic disease refers to the patient who presents with both optic neuritis and transverse myelitis, occurring either simultaneously or separated by a few months to years. Several features differentiate this disease from classical MS, including older age of onset, higher female to male incidence (9:1), limited white matter lesions on a brain MRI, multilevel contiguous typically central spinal cord lesions (three or more vertebral levels), and severe disability and death as a result of respiratory failure in one third of all patients. NMO also seems to be more common than MS in non-Caucasians. Pathologically, the syndrome is variable with some lesions characterized by inflammation and demyelination, but it is invariable with severe necrosis and many patients having cavitary lesions in the spinal cord. Those patients who survive the acute attack commonly follow a course with features indistinguishable from RR-MS but have a worse prognosis. An NMO serum biomarker (NMO-IgG) has recently become commercially available, which can help differentiate this disease from MS. This distinction is of utmost importance since the therapeutic interventions are different for NMO and MS. While the NMO-IgG blood test is highly specific and the majority of clinically diagnosed NMO patients will be NMO-IgG positive, a negative blood test does not exclude the diagnosis.

Acute Disseminated Encephalomyelitis

Acute disseminated encephalomyelitis (ADEM) and its hyperacute form, acute necrotizing hemorrhagic encephalopathy (ANHE), are thought to be forms of immune-mediated inflammatory demyelination. They differ from MS in that they are typically monophasic, whereas MS is by definition multiphasic or chronically progressive. Patients with ADEM or ANHE usually present with fever, headache, meningeal signs, and altered consciousness, which are exceedingly rare in MS. Multiple reports of clinical and pathologic overlap have been published. Some authors have suggested that the MRI can be used to differentiate MS from ADEM, but no reliable clinical criteria to differentiate the two processes exist.

PRECIPITATING FACTORS

Exposure to viruses and bacteria has been associated with precipitating disease exacerbations. The risk of an exacerbation decreases during pregnancy, with the rate being decreased by approximately two thirds in the third trimester. The risk of an acute attack in the first 3 months postpartum is increased and has been estimated that 20% to 40% of postpartum patients with MS will have an exacerbation. The decreased relapse rate during pregnancy is probably related to a family of immunosuppressive hormones and Th2. Overall, pregnancy probably has little overall effect on the course of the disease, and therefore remains a realistic possibility for woman with MS. There is increasing evidence that vitamin D deficiency may play an important role in MS. Recent studies have suggested that higher serum vitamin D levels correspond to a decreased risk of developing MS. It is well established that vitamin D receptors are present within immune cells and may promote immune regulation. The anti-inflammatory cytokine, transforming growth factor-β_1 (TGF-β_1), is typically decreased in MS and increases upon vitamin D supplementation. This association further supports the contributions of environmental factors, especially since sunlight exposure provides a major source for vitamin D. This could also explain the unusual geographical distribution of MS.

SYMPTOMS AND SIGNS

See Tables 11.2 and 11.3.

Optic Neuritis

Multiple sclerosis commonly affects the optic nerves and chiasm, and approximately 30% of patients present with visual symptoms. In acute optic neuritis, the patient experiences monocular loss of central vision and often has eye or brow pain, which worsens on lateral eye movement. The symptoms may present over a few hours to 7 days, with a few cases progressing over several weeks. Loss of visual acuity and color perception are often considerable. Most patients will recover significantly after 2 to 3 months, although continued improvement

TABLE 11.2	Initial Symptoms in Patients with Multiple Sclerosis
Symptom	**Percentage**
Sensory disturbance in one or more limbs	33
Disturbance of balance and gait	18
Vision loss in one eye	17
Diplopia	13
Progressive weakness	10
Acute myelitis	6
Lhermitte's symptom	3
Sensory disturbance in face	3
Pain	2

Paty DW, Poser CM. Clinical symptoms and signs of multiple sclerosis. In: Poser CM, ed. *The Diagnosis of Multiple Sclerosis.* New York: Thieme & Stratton; 1984:27.

TABLE 11.3 | **Common Symptoms and Signs in Patients with Multiple Sclerosis**

Symptom	Sign	Comment
Visual blurring (central)	Diminished acuity (central)	Syndrome of optic neuritis seen usually early in disease
Vision loss/eye pain	Scotoma/deafferented pupil	
Diplopia	Internuclear ophthalmoplegia	May be associated with nausea, vertigo, or other brainstem signs
Oscillopsia	Rarely other oculomotor weakness, flutter, or dysmetria	
Loss of dexterity	Upper motor neuron signs often affecting legs early and arms later	Develops in many MS patients over time
Weakness		
Tightness and pain		
Shaking	Intention tremor, dysmetria, dysarthria, truncal or head titubation	Occurs in 30% of patients; may be the predominant manifestations in some patients
Imbalance		
Paresthesias	Decreased vibration and position sense in legs > hands	Sensory symptoms are often painful and distressing
Loss of sensation	Decreased fine sensation in hands	
Bandlike disturbance	Sensory level	
Falls	Wide-based gait	Gait disturbances are common in MS and can cause severe disability
Lack of coordination	Ataxic and unsteady gait	
Inability to concentrate or learn	Diminished concentration, processing speed, or verbal learning on neuropsychologic testing	May be subtle or have severe impact on patient and family; severe dementia in <10% of patients
Easily distractible		
Emotional lability	Episodic crying or laughing	Distressing to patient; generally not related to patients' actual emotions
Depression	—	Commonly underrecognized or underestimated
Fatigue	—	Disabling in many patients with MS; does not correlate with severity of motor signs
Pain	—	Numerous etiologies (see text)
Urinary urgency, hesitancy, frequency, and incontinence	Requires urodynamic testing to fully characterize type of bladder dysfunction	Often complicated by intercurrent UTI

MS, multiple sclerosis; UTI, urinary tract infection.

can occur as long as a year later; however, some patients sustain permanent damage and can become blind. Acuity is variably diminished in the affected eye. A central or centrocecal scotoma (marked enlargement of the blind spot to involve central vision) can be documented at the bedside with an Amsler grid, and red desaturation can be demonstrated with color plates or with a red-tipped hat pin. Using the swinging flashlight test in a darkened room, one can demonstrate a defect in the afferent pathway such that pupillary constriction in the affected eye is greater with contralateral than with direct light stimulus. A positive test reveals a relative afferent pupillary defect, sometimes called a Marcus Gunn pupil. Funduscopic examination is usually normal in acute retrobulbar neuritis. When the optic nerve is affected anteriorly, the disc may be congested and swollen, thus resembling papilledema. Several months after an optic neuritis, the disc often appears pale, especially at the temporal border, and this can provide evidence of a previous attack. Occasionally, optic nerve demyelination and axonal damage can manifest silently and is noticed only in the setting of other symptoms suggestive of MS.

A novel noninvasive eye scan called optical coherence tomography (OCT) is now being used to assess MS patients. The scan provides high-resolution quantifiable images of the retinal nerve fiber layer that have been shown in recent studies to reflect optic nerve damage even in asymptomatic eyes. OCT scans may prove to be a very important biomarker for disease monitoring and therapeutic effectiveness; however, since OCT scans are not specific for MS/optic nerve pathology, they are not considered a diagnostic test to the exclusion of a thorough eye exam.

Oculomotor Syndromes

Eye movement abnormalities are also extremely common in MS and include broken (saccadic) smooth pursuits, nystagmus, ocular dysmetria (overshooting target), isolated extraocular muscle palsies, and the classical internuclear ophthalmoplegia (INO).

■ SPECIAL CLINICAL POINT: An INO results from damage to the medial longitudinal fasciculus, and its presence in a young adult, particularly when bilateral, is highly suggestive of MS.

In its complete form, one eye is unable to adduct and the other has abducting nystagmus. More commonly one observes varying degrees of adduction lag with dysconjugate nystagmus. The patient is asked to make a rapid saccade from midline to a laterally situated target, and the examiner focuses on whether the eyes move in a conjugate manner. The condition is frequently bilateral, with one eye being more involved than the other. Quantitative infrared oculography has demonstrated that the frequency of subtle INOs is probably much greater than can be clinically appreciated.

Motor Dysfunction

Weakness, spasticity, hyperreflexia, and Babinski's sign (upgoing toe) are common manifestations of damage to the pyramidal tracts (corticospinal tracts) in patients with MS. This most commonly presents in the legs (spastic paraparesis) because of the relative length that these fibers have to travel, which makes them more susceptible to numerous areas of demyelination and noticeable conduction delays. It is not uncommon for cervical lesions to manifest first in the lower extremities. Concomitant symptoms include stiffness, spasms, and pain. Extreme hyperreflexia causes clonus, which is usually described by the patient as a shaking or tremor.

Cerebellar Signs

End-point tremor (dysmetria) on finger to nose testing is most noticeable in the upper extremities, probably because of their important role in fine movement tasks. Lower extremity and midline truncal ataxia result in gait impairment, and some patients with MS are mistaken for being intoxicated. Head or truncal titubation or scanning dysarthria (impaired prosody) can become disabling aspects of the disease.

Sensory Symptoms

Approximately one third of patients with MS present initially with sensory disturbance involving the limbs, and the majority of patients will have paresthesias as the disease progresses. Symptoms are usually described as "pins and needles" and less commonly as a loss of sensation. Paresthesias can be painful burning or electrical sensations. The sensory symptoms follow a spinal cord pattern, often with an incomplete loss of sensation to either vibration (posterior columns) or pinprick (spinothalamic) pathways. It is important to distinguish the spinal pattern from peripheral or root lesions, which follow cutaneous or dermatomal patterns of sensory loss. Occasionally, patients will describe patches of numbness or symptoms in an apparently nonanatomic distribution, which presumably could relate to multifocal areas of demyelination or may be a manifestation of psychiatric disease.

Lhermitte's phenomenon refers to an electric tingling sensation that is precipitated by neck flexion, usually into the arms or down the back. Lhermitte's phenomenon suggests cervical spinal cord disease. It is very common in patients with MS with cervical spinal cord involvement but is not specific for MS.

Pain

Pain is very common in MS and may be caused directly by abnormal firing of sensory nerves, as a result of severe spasticity, or because of secondary orthopedic injuries. Trigeminal neuralgia (TN) or atypical facial pain are common causes of severe pain in MS. Younger patients who present with TN should be evaluated for MS as this pain syndrome is more common above the age of 50.

Cognitive and Memory Symptoms

■ **SPECIAL CLINICAL POINT: Approximately 50% of patients with MS exhibit significant short-term memory loss or difficulty with concentration, attention, and processing speed.**

Cortical deficits relating to language and visual spatial function are much less common. In only a minority of patients is dementia an incapacitating aspect of the disease. Correlations between the severity of cognitive impairment and the extent of MRI changes have been found.

Psychiatric Manifestations

Inappropriate laughing and weeping, often in response to minor provocation, occurs in more than 10% of patients with MS. Approximately 50% of patients with MS will have an episode of major depression during the course of their illness, and many patients will have chronic low-level depressive symptoms. MRI studies have confirmed an association with lesion load or atrophy, especially in the frontal and temporal lobes, and depression in MS. The health care provider should have a heightened awareness of the risk of suicide in patients with MS. Depression may also be part of a bipolar illness, which is more common in patients with MS than in control populations.

Fatigue

Fatigue may be the most common single complaint of patients with MS and can be disabling. Fatigue usually comes on late in the afternoon or may occur with strenuous activity or with exposure to heat. Short rest periods usually restore function. A less specific and more generalized fatigue is also seen and may take the form of overwhelming lassitude, which can be disabling. Episodic fatigue may herald clinical disease exacerbation. The mechanisms underlying MS fatigue are unknown.

Bladder, Bowel, and Sexual Dysfunction

Bladder dysfunction is common and can be divided into two categories. Patients may fail to empty urine adequately, causing urinary hesitancy, postvoid fullness or dribbling, or frank inability to initiate urination despite a feeling of fullness. Alternatively, patients may fail to properly store urine, causing urgency, urge incontinence, dysuria, frequency, and nocturia. The correlation between bladder symptoms and the underlying pathophysiology is often imperfect; therefore, objective testing by cystometrogram is often necessary to characterize the problem and to guide management.

Constipation is also common in MS and should be managed aggressively to prevent complications. Fortunately, fecal incontinence is relatively rare but when present is socially devastating.

Sexual dysfunction is reported by 50% to 75% of patients with MS and is exacerbated by a variety of problems, including fatigue, decreased sensation, decreased libido, erectile dysfunction, spasticity, impaired lubrication, body image disorder, and depression.

Other Manifestations

Paroxysmal disorders in MS include dystonic spasms, tic douloureux, episodic paresthesias, seizures, ataxia, and dysarthria. Sleep disorders and sleep-related movement disorders (restless leg syndrome) are common in MS and can contribute to daytime fatigue. Various other disease manifestations occur more rarely, including hearing loss, spasms, aphasia, homonymous hemianopsia, gait apraxia, movement disorders (myoclonus and chorea), and autonomic dysfunction (sweating, feeling hot and cold, edema, and postural hypotension).

DIAGNOSIS OF MULTIPLE SCLEROSIS

■ **SPECIAL CLINICAL POINT: MS is diagnosed clinically through the demonstration of CNS lesions disseminated in time and space and with no better explanation for the disease process.**

There is no single diagnostic test, and several other diseases can mimic MS. Therefore, diagnostic criteria based on clinical features supplemented by laboratory tests have been used. The original and recently revised McDonald criteria were developed by a panel of MS experts and were based on review of extensive supportive scientific studies focusing on the sensitivity and specificity of MRI diagnostic criteria (Table 11.4). The major change associated with the latest criteria is that a diagnosis of MS can be made early after a clinically isolated syndrome if a follow-up MRI performed 1 month later demonstrates the formation of a new T2 lesion that is of sufficient size and location (Tables 11.5 and 11.6). These criteria also define MRI lesion characteristics that increase the likelihood of MS: number (>9), abutting the ventricles, juxtacortical, infratentorial, spinal, and contrast enhancing. As with all the criteria, the clause that "there must be no better explanation" remains a critical part of the definition of MS. Critics of these criteria have complained they are too restrictive, whereas purists remain unconvinced of the utility of MRI for diagnosis. The lack of specificity for MS of white matter lesions seen on MRI must also be remembered, and overreliance on imaging to the exclusion of the clinical picture can lead to diagnostic errors. Ultimately, how one defines the clinical syndrome of MS, within the recognized spectrum of multifocal demyelination discovered at autopsy to hyperacute demyelinating syndromes, remains an ongoing debate. The revised McDonald criteria provide an important update and have been adopted for the incorporation of patients in research studies.

Important Radiologic and Laboratory Features

Magnetic Resonance Imaging

■ **SPECIAL CLINICAL POINT: MRI is the single most useful test in confirming the diagnosis of MS.**

A brain MRI performed on a high field (>1.5 Tesla) magnet is abnormal in 95% of patients

| TABLE 11.4 | McDonald Diagnostic Criteria |

Clinical Presentation	Paraclinical Tests Needed	
	Space	Time
Two attacks; two locations	No	No
Two attacks; one location	MRI abnormal or two MRI lesions + CSF	No
One attack; two locations	No	MRI criteria or second attack
One attack; one location (CIS)	MRI abnormal or two MRI lesions + CSF	MRI criteria or second attack
PP-MS (progression for 1 year)	Need two of the following: Nine MRI brain lesions or four to eight brain lesions + VEP Two MRI cord lesions Positive CSF[a]	

CSF, cerebrospinal fluid; CIS, clinically isolated syndromes; PP-MS, primary progressive multiple sclerosis; VEP, visual-evoked potential.
[a]Evidence of oligoclonal bands or increased IgG index or both.
Modified from Polman CH, Reingold SC, Edan G, et al. Diagnostic criteria for multiple sclerosis: 2005 revisions to the "McDonald Criteria." *Ann Neurol.* 2005;58:840–846.

with clinically definite MS, and the absence of high signal abnormalities in either the brain or spinal cord is strong evidence against the diagnosis of MS. MS lesions appear as areas of high signal usually in the cerebral white matter on T2-weighted images (Figs. 11.4 and 11.5). They are typically round or ovoid but may appear as fingerlike projections extending perpendicularly from the ventricular wall that is visualized best on sagittal imaging (Dawson's fingers). Typical locations include the corpus callosum, abutting the walls of the ventricles, in the juxtacortical lesions (grey–white junction), in the posterior fossa (pons and cerebellar peduncles), and in the spinal cord (cervical twice as commonly as thoracic). Fluid-attenuated inversion recovery (FLAIR) is more sensitive than conventional T2-weighted imaging for cerebral lesions but is less useful in the posterior fossa or spinal cord. Short tau inversion recovery (STIR) images have the highest sensitivity for detecting

| TABLE 11.5 | MRI Criteria for Brain Abnormality |

Three of the following[a]:
One Gd-enhancing lesion or nine T2-hyperintense lesions if there is no Gd-enhancing lesion
At least one infratentorial lesion
At least one juxtacortical lesion
At least three periventricular lesions

Gd, gadolinium.
[a]One spinal cord lesion can be substituted for one infratentorial brain lesion. An enhancing cord lesion can substitute for an enhancing brain lesion and count twice in the MRI criteria for diagnosis (one enhancing lesion and one infratentorial lesion).
Polman CH, Reingold SC, Edan G, et al. *Ann Neurol.* 2005;58:840–846.

| TABLE 11.6 | Dissemination in Time |

Two possible ways to demonstrate imaging dissemination in time:
(1) Scan 3 months after clinical event showing a Gd-positive lesion not at same site of original event
(2) New T2W lesion at least 30 days after initial clinical event scan

Gd, gadolinium; T2W, T2-weighted.
Polman CH, Reingold SC, Edan G, et al. *Ann Neurol.* 2005;58:840–846.

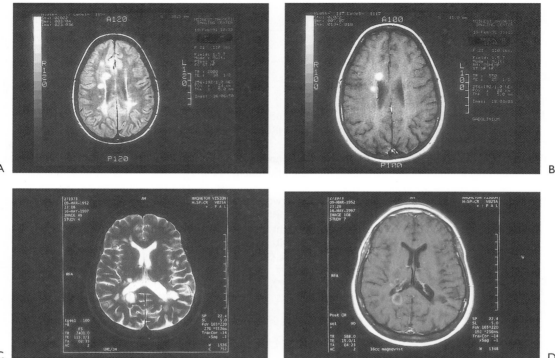

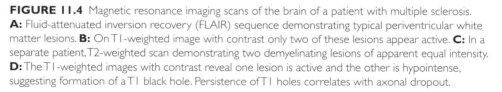

FIGURE 11.4 Magnetic resonance imaging scans of the brain of a patient with multiple sclerosis. **A:** Fluid-attenuated inversion recovery (FLAIR) sequence demonstrating typical periventricular white matter lesions. **B:** On T1-weighted image with contrast only two of these lesions appear active. **C:** In a separate patient, T2-weighted scan demonstrating two demyelinating lesions of apparent equal intensity. **D:** The T1-weighted images with contrast reveal one lesion is active and the other is hypointense, suggesting formation of a T1 black hole. Persistence of T1 holes correlates with axonal dropout.

demyelination in the spinal cord. All MRIs performed in suspected or definite patients with MS should be done before and after intravenous (IV) administration of the paramagnetic agent gadolinium diethylenetriaminepentaacetic acid (GdDTPA). Lesions that enhance after GdDTPA have been shown to represent acute inflammatory lesions and as such increase the likelihood that a lesion is related to MS as opposed to a nonspecific small-vessel disease process. Enhancing lesions are also used as a measure of disease activity in clinical trials. Enhancing lesions last only for 2 to 8 weeks and therefore can be missed easily, so FLAIR is a more reliable measure of the total burden of disease or for infrequent serial scanning. MRI is also useful for ruling out non-MS–related

structural lesions such as spinal tumors, syrinxes, Chiari malformations, and herniated disc material.

CSF Analysis

CSF studies to rule out infectious and neoplastic etiologies and to look for the presence of intrathecal immunoglobulin (Ig) synthesis are an important part of laboratory testing in cases in which the clinical picture and MRI are not diagnostic. The presence of more than 50 mononuclear cells/mm3, any neutrophils, or a CSF protein of greater than 100 mg/dL should raise concern about a diagnosis of MS. Depending on the laboratory and technique, approximately 80% to 90% of patients with clinically definite

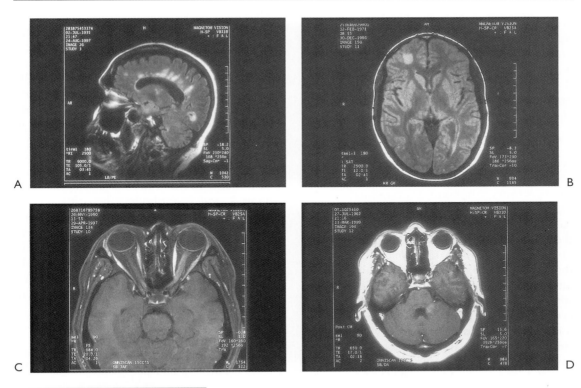

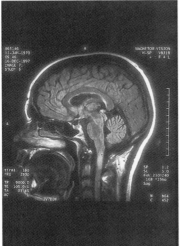

FIGURE 11.5 Magnetic resonance imaging scans of the brain of a patient with multiple sclerosis demonstrating typical lesion locations. **A:** Periventricular lesions extending perpendicularly from the ventricles (Dawson's fingers). **B:** Juxtacortical lesion. **C:** Edematous enhancing optic nerve. **D:** Enhancing lesion on the cerebellar peduncle. **E:** Lesions in the corpus callosum and high cervical cord.

MS will have two or more IgG bands present on a CSF gel electrophoresis and not in a matched serum sample (oligoclonal bands). Quantitative increases in the CSF IgG index provide similar information but do not always correlate with the presence of oligoclonal bands and should therefore also be ordered as part of CSF analysis. The sensitivity of these tests in clinically isolated syndromes is lower. In addition, oligoclonal bands are not specific for MS and have been observed in 50% of patients with infectious diseases of the nervous system and in about 15% of patients with non-inflammatory diseases such as tumors and infarctions. MBP is released after CNS tissue injury from many processes, and other than documenting an organic etiology to the clinical presentation, the test is not helpful.

Evoked Potentials

Sensory evoked potentials are used in MS to provide objective evidence to supplement subjective sensory symptoms or occasionally to reveal clinically silent lesions. This can be particularly valuable if a psychiatric basis for the symptoms is being considered or in early cases in which MRIs are inconclusive. Of the three types of evoked potentials, brainstem auditory evoked response (BAER), somatosensory evoked potential (SSEP), and visual evoked potential (VEP), the latter is the most useful because remote optic nerve disease is common and not well visualized on MRI. VEPs can also be helpful in supporting a diagnosis of PP-MS based on the McDonald criteria.

Serologic Testing

As part of excluding other disease processes, it is often prudent to obtain peripheral blood to test: vitamin B_{12}, methylmalonic acid, 25-OH vitamin D, thyroid-stimulating hormone, erythrocyte sedimentation rate, antinuclear antibodies, Lyme titer, and rapid plasma reagin. In unusual cases, more extensive testing may include antineutrophil cytoplasmic antibodies, antiphospholipid antibodies, anti-dsDNA antibodies, anti-Smith antibodies, Sjögren syndrome A and B antibodies, hepatitis profile, copper levels, ceruloplasmin, NMO-IgG, and angiotensin-converting enzyme. Rarely, human immunodeficiency virus and opportunistic infection can mimic MS. Some risk exists of obtaining false-positive tests, and some experts have questioned the cost-effectiveness of extensive serologic testing.

Errors in Diagnosing Multiple Sclerosis

Conditions commonly misdiagnosed for MS are listed in Tables 11.7 and 11.8.

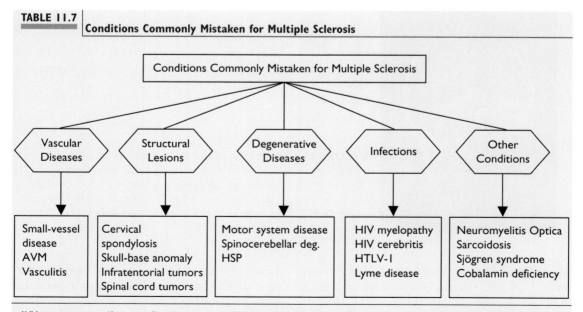

TABLE 11.7   Conditions Commonly Mistaken for Multiple Sclerosis

Vascular Diseases	Structural Lesions	Degenerative Diseases	Infections	Other Conditions
Small-vessel disease AVM Vasculitis	Cervical spondylosis Skull-base anomaly Infratentorial tumors Spinal cord tumors	Motor system disease Spinocerebellar deg. HSP	HIV myelopathy HIV cerebritis HTLV-1 Lyme disease	Neuromyelitis Optica Sarcoidosis Sjögren syndrome Cobalamin deficiency

AVM, arteriovenous malformation; Deg., degeneration; HSP, hereditary spastic paraparesis; HIV, human immunodeficiency virus; HTLV-1, human T-cell lymphotrophic virus type-1.

TABLE 11.8	Diseases That Mimic Multiple Sclerosis on MRI

ADEM	Histiocytosis
HTN/small-vessel disease	HTLV-1
CADASIL	Lyme disease
Sarcoidosis	Leukodystrophies
Vasculitis	Mitochondrial disease
Migraine	Lupus
Aging-related changes	Behçet disease
Organic aciduria	HIV

ADEM, acute disseminated encephalomyelitis; HTN, hypertension; HTLV-1, human T-cell lymphotrophic virus type-1; CADASIL, cerebral autosomal dominant arteriopathy with subcortical infarcts and leukoencephalopathy.

■ **SPECIAL CLINICAL POINT: The rules of dissemination in time and space are critical to making an accurate diagnosis of MS.**

ADEM can appear clinically and radiographically like MS but is usually a monophasic disease process. Similarly, the presence of a cervicomedullary lesion such as with a Chiari malformation can cause multiple symptoms emanating from one location in the nervous system, so careful attention to documenting a clear second location is critical. In both situations, MRI has proved extremely useful; however, T2-weighted lesions are not specific for MS, and therefore vascular, infectious, and neoplastic etiologies of multifocal disease must be considered. The extent of exclusionary testing is usually dictated by the clinical presentation. In a case of RR-MS with typical findings and confirmatory brain MRI, little other testing is necessary. In atypical presentations with unusual historical features (fever, altered level of consciousness, exposures, no relapses), strong family history, no eye findings, purely progressive disease, or very aggressive disease from onset (NMO), more extensive testing is mandatory. Finally, psychiatric disease must be considered in the patient with numerous symptoms and little objective evidence for disease. The experienced clinician, however, recognizes that early in the course of MS, objective evidence

may be lacking and comorbid psychiatric disease can be the primary symptom. The level of confidence in the diagnosis of MS increases with time, and the physician should always be alert to alternative or coexistent disease processes even in patients who carry a diagnosis of MS.

When to Refer a Patient to a Neurologist

MS is a complicated neurologic disease, and the approaches to diagnosis and treatment are changing rapidly.

■ **SPECIAL CLINICAL POINT: It is appropriate to refer any patient suspected of having MS to a neurologist with MS experience, even if the patient has had only a single clinical event.**

Symptoms that are suspicious for MS include unexplained numbness/tingling, fatigue, urinary urgency, loss of vision in one eye, or impaired coordination. Although many of these symptoms occur commonly in healthy people, it is the persistence of a symptom or multiple symptoms that should provoke further evaluation. The non-neurologist should not be dissuaded by concomitant emotionality or psychiatric disease because this can be part of the presentation of MS. A brain MRI is a good first step in screening for MS. The presence of any high signal lesions in a young person warrants neurologic consultation.

THERAPY OF MULTIPLE SCLEROSIS

Disease-Modifying Therapies

Four partially effective disease-modifying therapies (DMT) for the initial management of MS are available in the United States: IFNb-1a (Avonex), IFNb-1a (Rebif), IFNb-1b (Betaseron), and glatiramer acetate (Copaxone). Mitoxantrone (Novantrone) was approved in the United States for the treatment of worsening forms of RR-MS, PR-MS, and SP-MS. A sixth novel agent, Natalizumab (Tysabri), was reapproved for use in the United States for patients

TABLE 11.9

Pharmacologic Treatments: Immunomodulating and Acute Relapses

Drug Name	Indication	Starting Dose	Stable Dose	Comments
Avonex (Interferon beta-1a)	Relapsing MS CIS	30 mcg IM q.d.	30 mcg IM q.d.	Flulike side effects
Rebif (Interferon beta-1a)	Relapsing MS CIS	22 mcg SC t.i.w.	44 mcg t.i.w.	Flulike side effects
Betaseron (Interferon beta-1b)	Relapsing MS CIS	0.0625 mg SC q.o.d.	0.25 mg SC q.o.d.	Flulike side effects
Copaxone (Glatiramer acetate)	Relapsing MS CIS	20 mg SC q.d.	20 mg SC q.d.	Idiosyncratic chest pain/palpitations
Tysabri (Natalizumab)	Relapsing MS	300 mg IV q4 weeks	300 mg IV q4 weeks	PML and other infections reported
Mitoxantrone (Novantrone)	Worsening forms of relapsing MS and SPMS	5–12 mg/m^2 IV	5–12 mg/m^2 IV q3 months for 2–3 years	Maximum lifetime dose 140 mg/m^2 Cardiotoxicity and leukemia reported Contraindicated in avascular necrosis
Methylprednisolone	Acute relapses	1,000 mg IV q.a.m. × 3–5 days	1,000 mg IV q.a.m. × 3–5 days	

MS, multiple sclerosis; CIS, clinically isolated syndrome; IM, intramuscularly; SC, subcutaneous; IV, intravenous; SPMS, secondary progressive multiple sclerosis.

with RR-MS who have either inadequate response to first-line therapies or are intolerant to them. Table 11.9 lists these immunomodulating pharmacologic treatments.

Beta Interferons Beta interferons (IFNα) are naturally occurring cytokines with a variety of immunomodulating and antiviral activities that may account for their therapeutic utility. IFNα may act through several mechanisms including modulation of major histocompatibility complex (MHC) expression, suppressor T-cell function, adhesion molecules, and matrix metalloproteinases. All three IFNα drugs have been shown to reduce relapses by about one third in double-blind placebo-controlled trials and are recommended either as first-line therapies or for glatiramer acetate intolerant patients with RR-MS. In addition, in each of these trials, IFNβ resulted in a 50% to 80% reduction of the inflammatory lesions visualized on brain MRI. Evidence also exists

that these drugs improve quality of life and cognitive function.

The major difference between the IFNβ drugs is that Avonex is given weekly intramuscularly (IM), Rebif is given three times a week subcutaneously (SC), and Betaseron is given every other day SC. The adequacy of IFNβ-1a weekly dosing has been questioned. Studies appear to support a modest dose–response effect for IFNβ; however, one study of double dose (60 mg IM) Avonex, once a week, found no benefit over the single-dose regimen. Whether the benefit of more frequent dosing is sustained for periods longer than 2 years remains unclear, and the increased incidence of neutralizing antibodies (NAbs) with the more frequent SC dosing must also be considered.

Flulike symptoms, including fever, chills, malaise, muscle aches, and fatigue, occur in approximately 60% of patients treated with either IFNβ-1a or IFNβ-1b and usually dissipate with continued use and premedication with nonsteroidal anti-inflammatory drugs (NSAIDs). Other side effects include injection-site reactions, worsening of preexisting spasticity, depression, mild anemia, thrombocytopenia, and elevations in transaminases, which are usually not severe and rarely lead to treatment discontinuation.

Development of NAbs can occur with any of the IFNβ products. Although the results are variable, IFNβ-1a weekly IM (Avonex) is reported to have the lowest incidence. The effect of NAbs on long-term efficacy remains to be fully defined. Some experts recommend that the results of an NAb assay in patients who exhibit insufficient treatment response may guide decisions for alternative therapy.

Glatiramer Acetate Glatiramer acetate (Copaxone) is a polypeptide mixture that was originally designed to mimic MBP. The mechanism of action of glatiramer acetate is distinct from that of IFNβ; therefore, patients may respond differently to this drug. Glatiramer acetate (20 mg SC q.d.) has also been shown to reduce the frequency of relapses by approximately one third and therefore is also recommended as a first-line treatment for RR-MS or for patients who are IFNβ intolerant. Glatiramer acetate results in a one-third reduction in the inflammatory activity seen on MRI.

Glatiramer acetate is generally well tolerated and unassociated with flulike symptoms. Immediate postinjection reactions associated with administration of glatiramer acetate include a local inflammatory reaction and an uncommon idiosyncratic reaction consisting of flushing, chest tightness with palpitations, anxiety, or dyspnea, which resolves spontaneously without sequelae. Routine laboratory monitoring is not considered necessary in patients treated with glatiramer acetate, and the development of binding antibodies does not interfere with the therapeutic efficacy of glatiramer acetate.

Mitoxantrone Mitoxantrone (Novantrone) is an anthracenedione antineoplastic agent that was shown in a phase III, randomized,

placebo-controlled, multicenter trial to reduce the number of treated relapses by 67% and slowed progression on EDSS, ambulation index, and MRI measures of disease activity. It is therefore recommended for worsening forms of MS. Acute side effects of mitoxantrone include nausea and alopecia. The lifetime use of this drug is limited to 2 to 3 years (or a cumulative dose of 120 to 140 mg/m^2) because of its cumulative cardiotoxicity. Since a more rapid cardiotoxicity can occur, a new black box warning was added recommending patients to have their baseline left ventricular ejection fraction checked prior to the start of therapy and retested before each subsequent dose. There is also increasing awareness and concern about treatment-related leukemias with this drug. More cases have been identified over the last year suggesting that the risk is higher than once suspected. Mitoxantrone is a chemotherapeutic agent that should be prescribed and administered only by experienced physicians.

Natalizumab Natalizumab (Tysabri) is a novel monoclonal antibody (mAb) directed against the adhesion molecule very late antigen-4 (VLA-4) that is expressed on leukocytes (except neutrophils). This agent is the first and currently the only mAb approved for use in MS. Natalizumab prevents leukocytes from binding to the vascular endothelium, especially during inflammation and ultimately prevents their transmigration into the CNS. Natalizumab had promising results in a phase II trial and two phase III clinical trials. In the phase III trial, AFFIRM, sustained progression of disability was reduced by 42%, clinical relapse rate was reduced by 68%, and MRI activity (enhancing lesions) was reduced by 92% in the natalizumab-treated group compared to placebo. Natalizumab was removed from the market in early 2005 after two MS patients from the second phase III trial (SENTINEL) developed a rare, deadly viral infection of the brain called progressive multifocal leukoencephalopathy (PML). Both patients were on combination therapy, Avonex plus natalizumab.

One patient eventually died and the other suffered major sustained disability. Natalizumab was subsequently reintroduced to the market in 2006 with a restricted indication for use as a second-line monotherapy treatment in RR-MS. It was initially thought that PML might occur only in the setting of combination therapy; however, since reapproval, at least four more cases of PML have been confirmed. There are now a total of seven known cases of PML as of December 2008 (one case was identified postmortem in a Crohn disease clinical trial after natalizumab treatment). The absolute risk of PML associated with natalizumab use is unknown, but an estimated risk of 0.1% is quoted and based on the previous clinical trial data. Natalizumab is only available in the United States through the TOUCH program, which was implemented for careful monitoring of potential drug-related side effects (specifically PML). TYGRIS is a worldwide phase IV safety study that is monitoring the use of natalizumab abroad. Natalizumab is given intravenously every 4 weeks under the care and supervision of an experienced infusion center staff. Serious allergic reactions can occur and typically happen within 2 hours from the start of infusion. Other more common side effects include infusion-related reactions, rashes, elevated transaminases, leucopenia, reactivation of various herpetic infections, sinusitis, and bladder/bowel infections. Two cases of melanoma were recently reported after natalizumab use; however, it is unclear whether a true association exists. Close neurologic monitoring is required during natalizumab use along with frequent blood work monitoring. Natalizumab is a potent monoclonal antibody that should be prescribed and administered only by experienced physicians.

Other Drugs Used in Multiple Sclerosis Several other drugs are commonly used in MS despite the lack of U.S. Food and Drug Administration approval and definitive evidence of efficacy. Numerous small clinical trials support the modest effect of intravenous immunoglobulin G (IVIg), azathioprine, methotrexate, mycophenolate mofetil, and cyclophosphamide.

Initiation of Early Therapy

■ **SPECIAL CLINICAL POINT: Evidence is accumulating that the best time to initiate disease-modifying treatment is early in the course of the disease.**

Data indicate that irreversible axon damage may occur early in the course of RR-MS and that available therapies appear to be most effective at preventing new lesion formation but do not repair old lesions. With disease progression, the autoimmune response of MS may become more difficult to suppress. Weekly IM IFNβ-1a (Avonex) has been proved to reduce the cumulative probability of developing clinically definite MS in patients who present with a first clinical demyelinating episode and have two or more brain lesions on MRI (CHAMPS trial). High-dose interferon and glatiramer acetate therapy have further supported earlier treatment in clinical trials (ETOMS, BENEFIT, and PRECISE). Based on these data, the National Multiple Sclerosis Society (NMSS) recommends initiation of immunomodulating treatment at the time of diagnosis. The clinician must weigh these considerations against the practical concerns of young patients, for whom the prospect of starting a therapy that requires self-injection may be frightening and burdensome. There are also few long-term (more than 10 years) data regarding the safety and sustained efficacy of disease-modifying drugs. Some patients will opt to defer therapy, hoping to be among the minority of patients with benign MS, but certain MRI and clinical features should prompt the physician and patient to reconsider this approach. An MRI with contrast-enhancing lesions, large burden of white matter disease, or presence of any T1 low signal lesions (black holes) suggests a relatively poor prognosis. It may be useful to repeat the brain MRI in 6 months or 1 year to determine how quickly the disease process is evolving. The

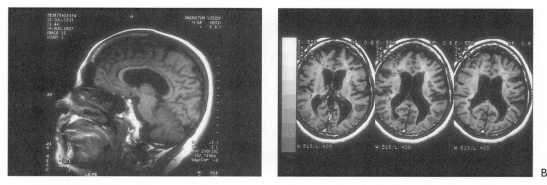

FIGURE 11.6 T1-weighted magnetic resonance imaging scans of the brain of a patient with multiple sclerosis demonstrating atrophy. **A:** Sagittal image revealing thinned corpus callosum and ventriculomegaly. **B:** Axial image with extensive ventriculomegaly and T1 black hole formation.

presence of spinal cord lesions or atrophy also suggests a poor prognosis (Figs. 11.6 and 11.7). Clinical features may be less useful for assessing prognosis, and once definite disability develops, it may be too late to treat that component of the disease.

Combination Therapy

Several trials are studying the addition of oral immunosuppressive drugs, IVIg, glatiramer acetate to IFNβ, and other agents in patients who continue to have disease activity. The rationale for this approach is based on experience with

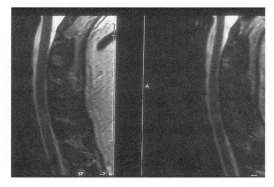

FIGURE 11.7 Magnetic resonance imaging scans of the spinal cord of a patient with multiple sclerosis revealing multiple high signal lesions best seen using the short tau inversion recovery (STIR) sequence.

other diseases, but further testing is required both to ensure its safety and to ensure that the mechanism of action of one drug does not interfere with that of the other drug. Recently, a lack of clinical efficacy was observed in the Avonex Combination Trial (Avonex and oral methotrexate) despite being well tolerated. Combination therapies may increase the risk of serious complications due to excessive immunosuppression or decreased immune surveillance, so caution is advised when considering this treatment paradigm.

Symptomatic Therapy

■ **SPECIAL CLINICAL POINT: Appropriate recognition and treatment of ongoing symptoms can greatly improve quality of life in patients with MS (Table 11.10).**

Despite the recent advances in immunomodulating therapies to decrease new disease activity, many patients continue to suffer from ongoing symptoms related to preestablished lesions.

■ **SPECIAL CLINICAL POINT: Corticosteroids are the mainstay of acute relapse treatment and are discussed as a symptomatic therapy because at this time no conclusive evidence exists that they have any effect on the natural history or long-term outcome of a disease exacerbation.**

TABLE 11.10 Pharmacologic Treatments: Symptomatic

Drug	Indication	Starting Dose	Stable Dose	Comments
Baclofen	Spasticity	5 mg t.i.d.	10–40 mg t.i.d./q.i.d.	Severe withdrawal reaction
Tizanidine	Spasticity	2 mg q.h.s.	4–8 mg t.i.d.	—
Diazepam	Spasticity, anxiety, insomnia, vertigo	2–5 mg q.h.s.	5–10 mg t.i.d.	—
Meclizine	Vertigo	12.5 mg t.i.d.	25 mg t.i.d.	—
Oxybutynin	Urinary urgency	5 mg q.d.	5–10 mg b.i.d.	Anticholinergic effects may be contraindicated with glaucoma
Tolterodine	Urinary urgency	1 mg q.d.	1–2 mg b.i.d.	Anticholinergic effects may be contraindicated with glaucoma
Sildenafil	Erectile dysfunction	50 mg 0.5–4 hours prior to intercourse	25–100 mg	Contraindicated in macular degeneration and with nitrates
Modafinil	Fatigue	200 mg q.a.m.	100–200 mg q.d./b.i.d.	Contraindicated with certain heart conditions
Amantadine	Fatigue	100 mg b.i.d.	100 mg b.i.d.	—
Gabapentin	Pain, dystonic spasms	300 mg q.h.s.	300–900 mg t.i.d./q.i.d.	—
Carbamazepine	Pain, dystonic spasms	100 mg q.d.	100–600 mg t.i.d./q.i.d.	Contraindicated in patients with preexisting cytopenias

Corticosteroids There is evidence that corticosteroids shorten the duration and severity of an exacerbation. Intravenous methylprednisolone (IVMP), 1,000 mg, is administered daily for 3 to 5 days in the office or at home by a visiting nurse. On completion of the IVMP, prednisone may be started, 60 mg orally in the morning and reduced by 10 mg every other day until tapered off. The prednisone taper is not necessary but helps reduce withdrawal symptoms in some patients. An H2 blocker or proton pump inhibitor may be coadministered in patients with a history of ulcer or heartburn. Metoclopramide may be useful in patients who develop singultus (hiccups). The effects of steroids appear to diminish with repeated usage, and many patients reach a stage of unresponsiveness to steroids. It is unclear whether that stage can be delayed or prevented by restricting the use of steroids, but this appears to be a wise approach. Patients who become refractory to a short course of IVMP may respond to higher doses (2 g/day), longer courses (10 days), or plasma exchange.

The most common side effects of treatment are irritability, difficulty sleeping, and fluid retention. Additional well-recognized risks include hypokalemia, gastrointestinal side effects, and osteoporosis. Fluid retention can be minimized by salt restriction during the therapy, and diuretic use is discouraged because of the exaggerated risk of hypokalemia. Ankle edema can be minimized by wearing elastic stockings and elevating the leg. Hypokalemia is usually not a problem in the absence of concurrent potassium wasting, such as with diuretic therapy, but in the presence of heart disease or with concurrent diuretic therapy, oral potassium replacement should be administered and electrolyte levels should be monitored during therapy. Anxiety and difficulty sleeping are usually minor problems. Patients may on rare occasions develop significant depression or mania during corticosteroid therapy.

In the Optic Neuritis Treatment Trial (ONTT), the rate of visual recovery was significantly faster in the IVMP group than in patients treated with placebo or oral prednisone, but no significant differences in visual outcome were found between groups at 6 months. Prednisone therapy alone increased the risk of new episodes of optic neuritis in either eye; however, the oral dose used was not equivalent to the IV dose. The ONTT results have led to widespread use of IVMP for patients with optic neuritis and an abnormal brain MRI, although equivalent doses of oral prednisone may be just as efficacious. Hints of a neuroprotective effect of steroids in other studies await confirmation.

Spasticity Mild spasticity may be managed by stretching and exercise programs such as aqua therapy and yoga. Drug therapy is indicated when stiffness, spasms, or clonus interfere with function or sleep. Baclofen is a good first choice for monotherapy. It exerts an antispastic effect by stimulating receptors for the inhibitory neurotransmitter, GABA. The initial dosage is 5 to 10 mg three times a day with intermittent upward dosage adjustments to achieve a therapeutic response or maximum tolerated dose, which may exceed 100 mg in some patients. Some patients may only require bedtime dosing to control nocturnal spasms. The principal limiting side effects of baclofen are confusion, sedation, or increased muscle weakness, and careful attention must be given to not overmedicate patients who are dependent on their muscle tone to ambulate. Baclofen may also unpredictably improve or worsen bladder function. Patients should never abruptly discontinue baclofen from doses greater than 30 mg/day because a withdrawal syndrome can occur consisting of confusion, seizures, or both. Tizanidine is an α-adrenergic

agonist that exerts an antispastic effect by stimulating central pathways that provide descending inhibitory input to the spinal cord. Tizanidine is best initiated very slowly, starting with 2 mg at bedtime, with gradual dosage adjustment by 2- to 4-mg increments to a maximum of 12 mg three times a day. The principal side effects are sleepiness, orthostatic hypotension, and dry mouth. Tizanidine is said to be less likely to cause motor weakness than baclofen, but its efficacy is often limited by somnolence. It can be used alone but is often successful in low doses combined with baclofen. Gabapentin and benzodiazepines also have muscle-relaxant properties. In cases of extreme spasticity, continuous intrathecal baclofen can be delivered through an implantable infusion pump placed in an abdominal subcutaneous pocket and connected to a plastic catheter that is tethered in the lumbar subarachnoid space. Occasionally, botulinum toxin injections can be used for spasticity; however, it is less effective for larger muscle groups (hamstrings) and can be technically difficult with varying success.

Pain and Spasms Patients with disagreeable paresthesias, atypical facial pain, or tic douloureux often respond to antiepileptic drugs such as carbamazepine, oxcarbamazepine, phenytoin, gabapentin, or pregabalin. Occasionally, amitriptyline can be helpful. Narcotic analgesics are rarely the solution for chronic pain in MS. For refractory TN, IV phenytoin may provide rapid relief. Baclofen, mexiletine, misoprostol, valproic acid, topiramate, and lidocaine have also been suggested but have shown variable success. Surgical procedures to relieve medically intractable pain include rhizotomy, injection of anesthetics, and gamma knife. Paroxysmal dystonic spasms can be seen in MS and respond well in most instances to low doses of some antiepileptic drugs.

Bladder, Bowel, and Sexual Dysfunction The first step in managing a neurogenic bladder is to determine whether the problem is one of failure to empty, failure to store, or a combination of both called detrusor external sphincter dyssynergia. A thorough history and urinalysis to rule out infection is appropriate. Immediate treatment of bacteriuria with antibiotics, even in the absence of typical dysuria, is necessary in MS because of the known propensity for infection to cause disease exacerbation. A postvoid residual urinary volume is the best means to determine if there is retention. Anticholinergic drugs are the initial drugs of choice for irritative bladder symptoms in the absence of infection. Oxybutynin, 5 mg, is increased gradually until symptom relief or distressing side effects, such as dry mouth, blurred vision, or worsening constipation, occur. Oxybutynin is also available in a long-acting formulation with reduced peak side effects and enhanced efficacy compared with other agents. Tolterodine, 1 to 2 mg twice a day, is a useful alternative with fewer anticholinergic side effects. Solifenacin, 5 to 10 mg daily, and Trospium, 20 mg two times a day, are newer overactive bladder agents. Propantheline bromide and hyoscyamine sulfate are older alternative anticholinergic agents. Anticholinergic drugs can be used intermittently if bladder symptoms are distressing at particular times, such as at bedtime or before a long automobile ride. The patient should be made aware of possible urinary retention with anticholinergics. Urinary residual volume should be checked after initiating therapy or should concerns arise about retention. In cases of concomitant retention and urgency, anticholinergics can be used in combination with intermittent bladder self-catheterization. Patients failing to achieve urinary continence with anticholinergic pharmacotherapy, with or without self-catheterization, need formal urologic evaluation for consideration of diversion procedures.

Drug treatment of urinary retention is usually ineffective, but some patients may benefit from attempts at decreasing bladder neck tone using α_1-adrenergic receptor antagonists such as terazosin, doxazosin, prazosin, and tamsulosin. Desmopressin, a vasopressin analogue, can be used at a dose of 20 mg by intranasal administration nightly to treat nocturnal incontinence by temporarily suppressing urine production. This approach should be used with caution in patients with hypertension or hyponatremia.

Constipation is very common in MS and should be managed aggressively to avoid long-term complications. Eating foods rich in fiber may help with mild constipation. Stool softeners and/or laxatives can be used for moderate constipation. For fecal incontinence, the addition of fiber in the form of a bulk fiber laxative (e.g., Metamucil) twice a day can provide enough bulk to the stool to allow a partially incompetent sphincter to hold in the bowel movement long enough to allow the patient to reach a bathroom. The use of anticholinergics or antidiarrheal agents may be effective for short periods to combat incontinence associated with diarrhea.

A careful sexual history to determine the problem(s) is a good first step in treating sexual dysfunction. Counseling the patient regarding avoiding the ill effects of elevated body temperature can be critical in managing problems that worsen with sexual intimacy. Erectile dysfunction (ED) in MS can be managed with sildenafil effectively initiated at 50 mg 60 minutes before intercourse (higher doses may be necessary). Sildenafil should be used with caution in older patients or in those with a history of heart disease. This agent is contraindicated in patients taking medications with nitrates in them and in patients with macular degeneration. Newer agents including vardenafil and tadalafil can also help with ED. Discontinuation of medications known to decrease libido (selective serotonin reuptake inhibitors [SSRIs]) or impotence (β-blockers) should be considered if possible.

Neurobehavioral Manifestations The most common neurobehavioral manifestation amenable to drug therapy is depression, which occurs in more than 50% of patients with MS. Moderate or severe depression should be treated with one of the SSRIs. For patients with psychomotor retardation and depression, fluoxetine, 20 to 80 mg daily, or sertraline, 50 to 200 mg daily, may be particularly effective. Paroxetine, 100 to

200 mg daily, is often useful for patients who are anxious and depressed. These drugs increase the levels of tricyclic antidepressants (TCAs), so care should be exercised in combining SSRIs with TCAs. Amitriptyline, 50 to 200 mg at bedtime, can be useful in depressed patients who are also having difficulty sleeping, headaches, or other pain. Treatment should be instituted gradually to minimize anticholinergic or CNS side effects. The patient and family should be warned of the delay between initiating therapy and observing a benefit. The pseudobulbar syndrome of pathologic laughing or weeping may respond to amitriptyline in low doses. Several newer antidepressants may be useful when the anticholinergic side effects of TCAs or the sexual side effects of SSRIs (decreased libido and orgasm) become intolerable. Bupropion, citalopram, escitalopram, and venlafaxine all may be better tolerated. Bipolar disorder is also increased in MS and commonly treated with valproic acid or lithium. SSRIs can aggravate mania complicating treatment of bipolar disorder, which may warrant psychiatric consultation.

Alprazolam, a benzodiazepine analogue, has been useful for anxiety in some patients. A dose of 0.25 to 0.50 mg two or three times a day is usually sufficient. Diazepam can be used as an alternative drug. Infrequently, antipsychotic medications are needed in MS. Atypical antipsychotic agents (risperidone, olanzapine, quetiapine) are preferred over typical agents (Haldol, Thorazine) to minimize the potential for extrapyramidal and anticholinergic side effects. As with other symptomatic therapies, the need for pharmacotherapy over time should be assessed intermittently, and the drug should be tapered if appropriate.

Fatigue Some types of MS fatigue may respond to short periods of rest, but if this is not possible, or in cases of severe fatigue, medication should be considered. Amantadine, 100 mg twice a day, may be effective in treating about one third of the cases of fatigue. Modafinil, a newer narcolepsy drug that acts as a CNS stimulant, was found to be effective in patients with MS at a dose of 200 mg in the morning. Occasionally, treatment with an SSRI (fluoxetine and sertraline) can have a positive effect on fatigue even in the absence of overt depression. 4-Aminopyridine (Fampridine or 4-AP) is an investigational voltage-gated potassium channel (Kv1.4) blocker, that may help with fatigue, endurance, and ambulation in MS by prolonging action potentials. In higher doses, this agent has been associated with seizures and confusion limiting its use. A newer sustained-release formulation of 4-AP is under intense investigation. A recent dose comparison study suggested that walking speed in some patients may improve with the sustained-release form; however, two people experienced de novo seizures at the higher dose. Future studies are planned to further assess the risk–benefit profile of this newer formulation.

Special Challenges for Hospitalized Patients Patients with MS may be hospitalized either during severe exacerbations or for other medical problems. In the case of an MS exacerbation, the patient should be screened for sources of infection and treated with antibiotics as appropriate. Rapid control of fever is also important to prevent worsening of symptoms. Exacerbations that warrant hospitalization are usually related to acute inability to ambulate or loss of self-care in the more advanced patient, and IV corticosteroids are usually instituted. Plasma exchange may be useful in steroid-unresponsive cases and requires hospitalization. Physical and occupational therapy should be initiated immediately, and a rehabilitation plan should be put in place with attention to adaptive devices for the home and orthotics or ambulation aids. For non–MS-related hospitalization, it is equally important to be vigilant about infections to prevent exacerbation. MS rarely causes respiratory compromise, and there are no absolute contraindications to anesthesia. Cosmetic surgery is discouraged, but necessary operations are usually well tolerated. Patients with MS do not have any impairment in wound healing. Postpartum exacerbations usually do not occur for several weeks after delivery and thus are not a major obstetric complication. Counseling, social work, and attention to severe depression should be considered during periods of stress such as may occur during hospitalization.

Alternative Therapies Used by Patients with Multiple Sclerosis Numerous alternative therapies have been advocated for MS but they are rarely tested in a placebo-controlled manner and, therefore, they cannot be recommended. Because MS is an unpredictable disease characterized early by relapses and spontaneous recovery, patients are very susceptible to placebo effects and misguided judgments about the efficacy of alternative therapies. Bee stings have been used for many years, and for those who are not allergic about half of patients report a temporary boost in energy perhaps related to endogenous corticosteroid release in response to cutaneous inflammation. Procarin is a patch used by some patients with MS and contains vitamin B_{12}, histamine, caffeine, and a proprietary substance. Several diets for MS, such as the Swank diet, have been popular. Acupuncture is used to relieve pain and sometimes boost energy. Low-dose naltrexone (LDN) has been used off-label for MS and other diseases. Naltrexone is an opioid receptor antagonist approved for the treatment of alcohol and opioid dependence. Its use in MS is controversial and there have been no randomized, double-blinded, placebo-controlled trials to assess LDN tolerability or efficacy. A small, open-label pilot study was done suggesting improvements in fatigue; however, the NMSS currently does not support the use of this agent until further testing is done. None of the above approaches has been tested adequately. Complementary medicine advocates recommend yoga, meditation, aqua therapy, body-cooling devices, and stress reduction, all of which are reasonable and safe approaches to dealing with MS.

Physical Therapy Physical therapy has an important role in managing MS. Regular exercise and stretching decrease MS symptoms of stiffness, weakness, and pain and improve overall well-being. Physical therapy has been shown to improve disability from MS independent of drug interventions and should be continued on a regular basis as part of a maintenance regimen.

Novel Experimental Immunomodulatory Approaches

Several treatments are being tested in preliminary trials, including antibodies to various critical immune molecules (CD25 IL-2α receptor, CD20 B-cell marker, and the CD52 leukocyte marker), phosphodiesterase inhibitors, novel NSAIDs, β-adrenergic agonists, and immunosuppressive regimens used during organ transplantation and malignancies. Of these therapies, the monoclonal antibodies (alemtuzumab, daclizumab, rituximab) and novel oral agents (fingolimod, cladribine) seem to have the most promise in MS, as shown in recent clinical trials. Despite the encouraging trial data, there have been several serious complications associated with many of these agents, which will potentially limit their future widespread use. Immunoablative protocols using extremely high doses of chemotherapies, followed by autologous stem-cell rescue, have been used in particularly aggressive forms of MS. This approach has afforded disease stabilization, both clinically and by MRI, but has an unacceptably high morbidity and mortality at present.

Remyelination and Neuroprotection

Theoretical approaches to remyelination include enhancing existing oligodendrocyte precursors or neural stem cells by using growth factors or direct transplantation of oligodendrocytes or autologous stem cells. Growth factors such as insulinlike growth factor carry the inherent risk of nonspecifically activating the immune system. Anti-LINGO antibodies appear to be a promising means of inducing endogenous remyelination by enhancing oligodendrocyte progenitor cell differentiation into myelin-forming cells in vitro and in animal models.

Always Remember

- Multiple sclerosis (MS) has features of inflammation, demyelination, axonal injury, and neurodegeneration.
- Visual dysfunction, sensory disturbances, and gait impairment are very common presenting symptoms.
- MS is diagnosed clinically through the demonstration of CNS lesions disseminated in time and space and with no better explanation for the disease process.
- MRI is the single most useful test in confirming the diagnosis of MS.
- Initiating early disease-modifying treatment can influence the clinical course.
- Symptomatic therapy can greatly improve MS patients' quality of life.
- MS is a complicated neurologic disease, and the approaches to diagnosis and treatment are changing rapidly, therefore, it is appropriate to refer any patient suspected of having MS to a neurologist with MS experience.

QUESTIONS AND DISCUSSION

1. A 24-year-old nursing school student presents to her primary care physician (PCP) with complaints of numbness and tingling in her hands for 1 month. On questioning, she responds that she has had recent fatigue and mild depression, which she attributed to stress. She denies any other past medical history and is only taking birth control pills. Her entire physical examination is normal. The next appropriate step is to:
   A. Recommend EMG/NCS to rule out carpal tunnel syndrome.
   B. Reassure her that she has no abnormal signs on examination and therefore cannot be diagnosed with multiple sclerosis at this time.
   C. Order blood tests and a brain MRI.

D. Treat her for depression and reevaluate in 3 to 6 months for improvement.

The correct answer is C. This woman could have early signs of MS, and because there is strong evidence to support early initiation of therapy, it is important to make a diagnosis. Blood testing is indicated to exclude thyroid disease, vitamin B_{12} deficiency, other inflammatory neurologic disorders, and infections. A brain MRI is the single best screening tool for MS. Depression may be a symptom of MS and should not be considered an adequate explanation for ill-defined somatic symptoms. Carpal tunnel syndrome is a common cause of hand numbness but is usually unilateral and would not explain the other reported symptoms.

2. A 36-year old woman is diagnosed with optic neuritis. Her initial brain MRI reveals several demyelinating lesions. She is referred to a neurologist, but she declines immunomodulating therapy and prefers to "wait and see." Three months later, a repeat MRI is obtained and reveals a new gadolinium-enhancing lesion. At this time:
   A. She has clinically definite MS according to McDonald criteria but treatment is not indicated because this is probably a benign case.
   B. She has clinically definite MS according to McDonald criteria and treatment with either IFNβ or glatiramer acetate would be appropriate.
   C. She has PP-MS for which unfortunately there is no treatment.
   D. In the absence of a second clinical event, she cannot be diagnosed with multiple sclerosis.

The correct answer is B. The demonstration of a new lesion on MRI more than 3 months later provides evidence for dissemination in time and now fulfills criteria for a definite diagnosis of MS. The National Multiple Sclerosis Society and many MS experts now favor early initiation of therapy. Benign MS is defined as no disability after at least 10 years and can only be diagnosed retrospectively. Progressive MS is defined as 6 months of unabated worsening without exacerbations, and 1 year of disease progression is required to make a diagnosis of PP-MS.

3. A 40-year-old woman with RR-MS presents for routine follow-up. She is being treated with IFNβ injections, and although she has had no exacerbations since being on treatment, she complains of increased stiffness in her legs, and on questioning she also admits to urinary urgency with occasional episodes of incontinence. On examination, she is more spastic and hyperreflexic in her legs than 6 months ago, but there is no clear sensory level over her spine or weakness. At this point:
   A. She should stop taking the medication as she now has secondary progressive disease.
   B. She should switch to another immunomodulating drug as she has failed IFNβ therapy.
   C. A urinalysis should be ordered to rule out a urinary tract infection.
   D. She should stop taking the medication as these are likely side effects of the IFNβ.

   The correct answer is C. Minor changes in neurologic function do not constitute progressive disease, and it is likely that the reduction in relapses suggests that the IFNβ is effective. Although exacerbation of spasticity can be a side effect of IFNβ, bladder frequency is part of underlying MS and is often a sign of urinary tract infection. Antibiotic treatment of bacteriuria often alleviates the bladder symptoms and sometimes other new symptoms as well.

4. A patient with MS presents to the office with several days of dizziness, diplopia, and trouble walking straight. There has been no obvious precipitating factor (infection, heat, stress), and she has been taking her medications on a regular basis. On examination, she is noted to have several new findings including bilateral INO,

finger to nose dysmetria, severe gait ataxia, and facial asymmetry. You recommend the following:
   A. Treatment with 2 weeks of prednisone (approximately 1 mg/kg).
   B. Strict bedrest until the symptoms resolve.
   C. A brain MRI as soon as possible to confirm an MS exacerbation.
   D. Treatment with 3 to 5 days of IV methylprednisolone (1 g/day).

   The correct answer is D. The patient is having an acute disabling exacerbation and should be treated with IV methylprednisolone. A brain MRI is a useful means of assessing disease activity (gadolinium-enhancing lesions and new T2 lesions) and determining the extent of breakthrough disease activity but is not obligatory if the clinical picture is clear.

SUGGESTED READING

Arnold DL, Matthews PM. MRI in the diagnosis and management of multiple sclerosis. *Neurology.* 2002;58:S23–S31.

Brex PA, Miszkiel KA, O'Riordan JI, et al. Assessing the risk of early multiple sclerosis in patients with clinically isolated syndromes: the role of a follow up MRI. *J Neurol Neurosurg Psychiatry.* 2001;70: 390–393.

Brex PA, Ciccarelli O, O'Riordan JI, et al. A longitudinal study of abnormalities on MRI and disability from multiple sclerosis. *N Engl J Med.* 2002;346:158–164.

Comi G. Why treat early multiple sclerosis patients? *Curr Opin Neurol.* 2000;13:235–240.

Dhib-Jalbut S. Mechanisms of action of interferons and glatiramer acetate in multiple sclerosis. *Neurology.* 2002;58:S3–S9.

Frohman EM, Zhang H, Kramer PD, et al. MRI characteristics of the MLF in MS patients with chronic internuclear ophthalmoparesis. *Neurology.* 2001;57:762–768.

Frohman EM, Racke MK, Raine CS. Multiple sclerosis—the plaque and its pathogenesis. *N Engl J Med.* 2006;354:942–955.

Grudzinski AN, Hakim Z, Cox ER, et al. The economics of multiple sclerosis: distribution of costs and relationship to disease severity. *Pharmacoeconomics.* 1999;15:229–240.

Hafler DA, Compston A, Sawcer S, et al. Risk alleles for multiple sclerosis identified by a genomewide study. *N Engl J Med*. 2007;357:851–862.

Hemmer B, Archelos JJ, Hartung HP. New concepts in the immunopathogenesis of multiple sclerosis. *Nat Rev Neurosci*. 2002;3:291–301.

Krupp LB, Rizvi SA. Symptomatic therapy for underrecognized manifestations of multiple sclerosis. *Neurology*. 2002;58:S32–S39.

Lucchinetti C, Bruck W, Parisi J, et al. Heterogeneity of multiple sclerosis lesions: implications for the pathogenesis of demyelination. *Ann Neurol*. 2000;47:707–717.

Lutterotti A, Martin R. Getting specific: monoclonal antibodies in multiple sclerosis. *Lancet Neurol*. 2008;7:538–547.

Polman CH, Reingold SC, Edan G, et al. Diagnostic criteria for multiple sclerosis: 2005 revisions to the "McDonald Criteria." *Ann Neurol*. 2005;58:840–846.

Trapp BD, Peterson J, Ransohoff RM, et al. Axonal transection in the lesions of multiple sclerosis. *N Engl J Med*. 1998;338:278–285.

Wingerchuk DM, Lennon VA, Lucchinetti CF, et al. The spectrum of neuromyelitis optica. *Lancet Neurol*. 2007;6:805–815.

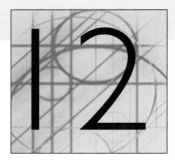

12 Parkinson Disease

BRADLEY J. ROBOTTOM, LISA M. SHULMAN,
AND WILLIAM J. WEINER

---

key points

- Parkinson disease is the second most common neurodegenerative disease worldwide.

- Parkinson disease has four major cardinal signs: resting tremor, cogwheel rigidity, bradykinesia, and postural instability.

- Resting tremor is the most common presenting symptom.

- Nonmotor symptoms such as depression, apathy, and anxiety are common and have a negative impact on quality of life.

- A variety of effective, symptomatic treatments are available.

- Antipsychotics and other dopamine blocking agents should be avoided in Parkinson disease patients.

- A careful medication history asking about exposure to dopamine blocking agents is important in making a diagnosis of Parkinson disease.

---

arkinson disease is the most common akinetic rigid syndrome and the most frequently encountered extrapyramidal movement disorder. It is a neurodegenerative disease of unknown etiology that most often begins at 58 to 60 years of age. Approximately 10% to 15% of patients will have disease onset before age 50. As the population of the United States ages, the number of people at risk for the development of Parkinson disease increases. Diagnostic and therapeutic knowledge is important not only because of the prevalence of the disorder but also because the pharmacology of Parkinson disease has led to fundamental changes in the way investigators and physicians view central nervous system neurotransmitter function.

CLINICAL FEATURES

Parkinson disease is characterized by a typical history of progressive neurologic disability and the following **four major neurologic signs: resting**

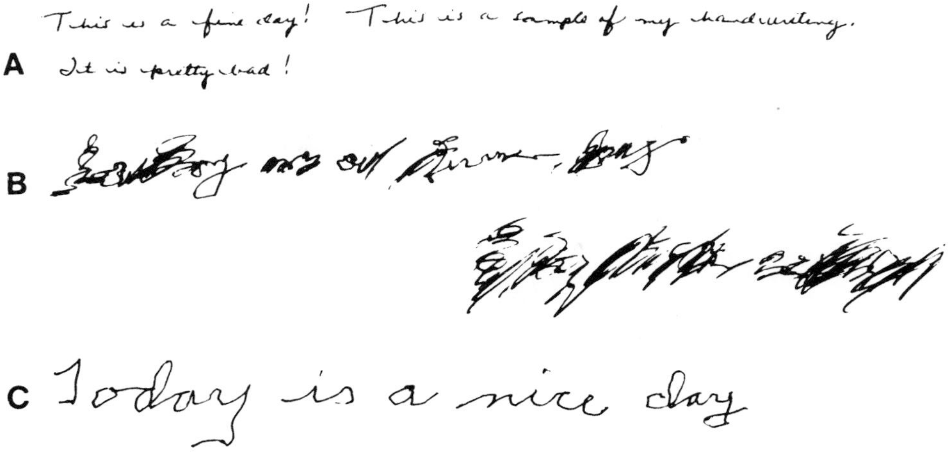

FIGURE 12.1 A: This handwriting sample from a 55-year-old patient with untreated Parkinson disease is a good example of the typical micrographic handwriting that is often characteristic of this condition. The handwriting samples shown in **(B)** and **(C)** are from a patient with essential tremor. **B:** Prior to treatment, the sample shows the typical large, sloppy script. **C:** This sample, taken from the same patient with essential tremor while being treated with propranolol (160 mg/day), shows obvious improvement. Changes in written script can provide excellent clues to the type of movement disorder that is present (see Chapter 13).

tremor, cogwheel rigidity, bradykinesia, and **impaired postural reflexes.** It is often observed that when a patient first presents to a physician for the evaluation of symptoms, the syndrome has been present for 1 to 2 years. Unilateral tremor involving a single limb is the most common presenting symptom and sign. However, careful history taking often reveals that difficulty buttoning shirts or blouses, fastening snaps, cutting food; alterations in handwriting (Fig. 12.1); a feeling of stiffness; or a feeling of overall slowness may have been noted up to 12 to 24 months earlier and that these symptoms have gradually become worse. In addition, a patient may note voice fluctuations and intermittent loss of volume. Inquiring whether the patient has difficulty rising from low, soft chairs or sofas; difficulty entering and leaving an automobile, difficulty turning in bed; or difficulty walking and maintaining balance in a crowd highlight the functional impact of bradykinesia, rigidity, gait impairment, and impaired postural reflexes. The patient may occasionally notice an inability to stop walking forward (propulsion) or backward (retropulsion). Family members may also report that the patient's facial expression has changed and that he or she does not smile as much (masked faces; Fig. 12.2), that he or she seems to stare all the time (reptilian stare), that her or his posture has become stooped and flexed (simian posture; Fig. 12.3), and that he or she has become exasperatingly slow. It may take 30 to 90 minutes to dress in the morning and even longer to disrobe in the evening.

The elucidation of this history may make the diagnosis of parkinsonism evident. Not all patients will present with all of these symptoms, and a patient will occasionally present with only a single symptom and will yet have parkinsonism. Inquiring whether the onset of symptoms was abrupt or insidious; whether there has been a gradual progression of symptoms; whether there is a family history of neurologic syndromes; and whether there is concurrent drug use, past history of encephalitis,

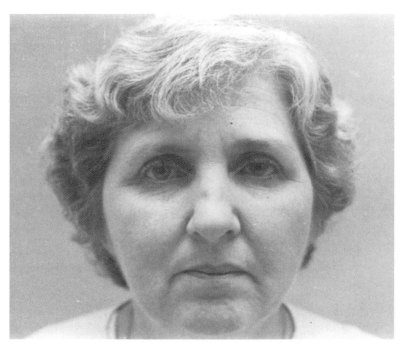

FIGURE 12.2 Typical masked faces in a patient with Parkinson disease.

or exposure to various toxins, including the use of street drugs, may help determine the etiology of the syndrome.

Resting tremor is the most frequent presenting sign in these patients. The appearance of this tremor often precipitates the patient's visit to the doctor. Parkinsonian tremor is highly characteristic and consists of a low-to-medium amplitude, with four to five cycles per second alternating movement. Tremor is defined as the involuntary rhythmic oscillatory sinusoidal movement that results from the alternating or synchronous contractions of reciprocally innervated antagonistic muscles. Resting tremor has been described as "pill rolling" because of the movement of the fingers and thumb. Its appearance resembles the activity of an "old time" pharmacist preparing a pill. The tremor, however, may begin in the hands, legs, or face and most often appears unilaterally in a single limb. It will often progress to involve the second limb of the same side before becoming bilateral. **Tremor is the initial presenting symptom in 75% of patients.** With the exception of impaired postural reflexes, the major signs of parkinsonism usually appear unilaterally. Careful observation of the tremor will reveal that it is a resting tremor that is ameliorated with purposeful movement. **A simple way of assessing whether a tremor is primarily resting, postural, or kinetic is to have the patient perform the finger-to-finger and finger-to-nose maneuver and to observe the affected limb at rest, with outstretched posture and with movement.** The patient with a resting tremor will have a marked amelioration of tremor when the arm springs into action. The patient with kinetic tremor will have no tremor at rest but will typically develop increased tremor as the hand approaches the target. When the resting limb is raised to an outstretched position, the tremor of Parkinson disease will diminish, although with maintained posture, the tremor may reappear until movement is initiated again.

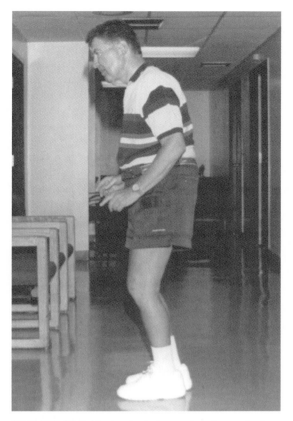

FIGURE 12.3 Moderate simian posture in a patient with Parkinson disease. Note the flexion of the upper extremities, upper trunk, and head. Facial masking is also apparent.

When the limb is totally supported and at rest, the patient with resting tremor will be seen to have the tremor, whereas those patients with kinetic tremor will not. Although resting tremor is a common early sign, tremor is rarely a source of disability.

Cogwheel rigidity is a sign that can be present either unilaterally or bilaterally, depending on the stage of illness. The patient does not complain of "cogwheeling." This sign is elicited by passive movement of the limb or neck through a full range of motion. When present, this sign is best elicited by slow flexion and extension of the wrist or neck. In addition to increased tone, a characteristic

ratchetlike sensation is appreciated by the examiner with passive movement. There are some patients in whom the initial symptomatology is cervical or low back discomfort, and the question of whether increased muscle tone is responsible for this symptom has been raised.

Bradykinesia is responsible for much of the disability associated with parkinsonism. Slowness of voluntary movement contributes to increasing difficulty with the activities of daily living such as getting in and out of a car, rising from chairs, cutting meat, preparing food, dressing, and walking. Some of these difficulties can be easily observed during an examination by watching the patient rise from a chair, walk to the examining room, and undress. Gait impairment accounts for the greatest proportion of the emerging disability, as severe gait impairment results in a loss of independence in many of these activities of daily living.

Postural reflexes refer to the ability of the patient to right himself and to keep from losing balance when sustaining postural perturbations (e.g., being jostled in a crowd). In addition, these reflexes are also important when turning around and changing direction while walking without losing balance. These reflexes can be evaluated simply and effectively by observing the patient walk 10 to 15 steps and turn around. A patient with normal postural reflexes should be able to pivot and turn without taking extra steps. In parkinsonism, one will often observe that the patient takes three to five steps to change direction. Another test of postural reflexes during the office visit is a firm backward pull on the shoulders or chest with the admonition to the patient that he should attempt to stop his backward motion in one to two steps. The examiner must be positioned behind the patient during this maneuver and prepared to stop the retropulsive movement or prevent a fall if necessary (Fig. 12.4). Impaired postural reflexes with frequent falls are a source of severe disability and injury in advanced parkinsonism (e.g., subdural hematoma, fractures of the hip or wrist). It should be noted that when postural reflex impairment is a prominent

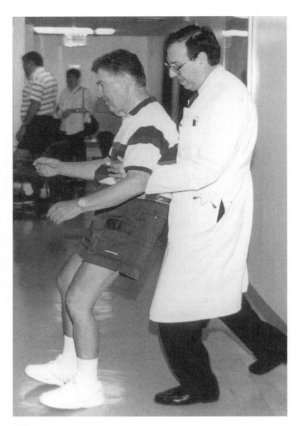

FIGURE 12.4 A loss of postural reflexes is often seen in patients with Parkinson disease. After instructing the patient to maintain his or her posture, the examiner has administered a backward thrust to the patient's chest. The postural response is quite poor: rather than maintaining a fixed postural response to the thrust or taking one or two steps backward, the patient has lost balance entirely and requires the assistance of the examiner to prevent him or her from falling to the ground.

early sign of parkinsonism, the diagnosis more often than not is not true Parkinson disease but instead one of the other neurodegenerative disorders that produces parkinsonism, such as progressive supranuclear palsy (PSP) or multiple system atrophy (MSA).

There is no single pathognomonic sign of Parkinson disease; instead, the informed and experienced clinician uses a constellation of symptoms and signs to make the diagnosis.

There is also no known biologic marker of Parkinson disease, and there is no definitive laboratory or imaging study to confirm the diagnosis. Furthermore, identifying parkinsonism by history and clinical examination does not imply that the diagnosis is Parkinson disease, which is characterized by a specific neuropathology. Patients with a minimum of two of the four cardinal symptoms (tremor, rigidity, bradykinesia, and impaired postural reflexes) in the absence of this specific neuropathology are diagnosed as having an akinetic rigid syndrome or parkinsonism, the most common cause of which is Parkinson disease. Clinical features that help distinguish Parkinson disease from other forms of parkinsonism include unilateral presentation of symptoms and signs, slow progression, resting tremor, and responsiveness to dopaminergic agents.

MECHANISMS OF DISEASE

Parkinson disease is defined pathologically by the loss of dopaminergic neurons in the substantia nigra pars compacta and the presence of intracytoplasmic Lewy bodies, which stain for α-synuclein. The idiopathic degeneration of these neurons leads to loss of dopaminergic input to the corpus striatum. The progressive failure of the nigrostriatal pathway results in the symptoms of Parkinson disease. Neuropathologic examination of the brain of a patient with a history of Parkinson disease reveals loss of the pigmented neurons in the substantia nigra and loss of dopamine in the striatum where the nigrostriatal fibers project. Olfactory dysfunction, constipation, and rapid eye movement (REM) sleep disorder may represent early nonmotor manifestations of Parkinson disease, but this remains more speculation than fact.

The etiology of Parkinson disease remains elusive. Although numerous epidemiologic studies have investigated Parkinson disease, definitive environmental factors have not been identified. Nevertheless, there are many leads, and the presence of significant environmental toxin exposure in genetically predisposed individuals remains a strong possibility. Inherited forms of Parkinson disease have been identified, the most common of which is leucine-rich repeat kinase (LRRK2) autosomal dominant Parkinson disease. LRRK2 mutations account for 10% to 40% of sporadic and inherited Parkinson disease in the Ashkenazi Jewish and North African Arab populations and lead to a typical, adult-onset Parkinson disease phenotype. Other autosomal dominant (α-synuclein) and autosomal recessive (parkin, PINK1, DJ-1) forms of Parkinson disease lead to young-onset Parkinson disease. However, surveys of large numbers of patients seen in movement disorder centers do not reveal a family history of Parkinson disease in the majority of patients with Parkinson disease. Nonetheless, identifying the α-synuclein and Parkin mutations has led to the discovery that the Lewy body is partly composed of α-synuclein and to the potential role of the proteosome in the pathogenesis of Parkinson disease. These recent genetic discoveries are very important and have opened the door to the concept that Parkinson disease may be a complex genetic disease.

The demonstration in 1967 that orally administered levodopa could produce dramatic improvement in the symptoms of Parkinson disease was a remarkable therapeutic advance. For levodopa to have a therapeutic effect, it must cross the blood–brain barrier and be decarboxylated to dopamine. The enzyme that decarboxylates dopa to dopamine is ubiquitous and also decarboxylates several other aromatic amino acids. This enzyme, termed "aromatic amino acid decarboxylase" or "dopa decarboxylase," is found in several extracerebral locations, including the gastrointestinal tract, liver, and kidney. When orally administered, levodopa is absorbed; acted on by the extracerebral decarboxylase; and converted to dopamine, which cannot cross the blood–brain barrier. If levodopa is administered alone, enormous quantities are required to overcome the peripheral decarboxylase systems and achieve a therapeutic benefit. The use of a peripheral decarboxylase inhibitor

(carbidopa) with levodopa results in a marked reduction in the dose of levodopa necessary to achieve a central effect.

Another enzyme that plays a role in determining how much levodopa circulating in the blood reaches the brain is catechol-O-methyltransferase (COMT). COMT methylates levodopa and also reduces the concentration of levodopa that is available for transport across the blood–brain barrier. Peripheral COMT inhibition is another therapeutic maneuver to enhance levodopa bioavailability in the brain to increase central dopamine activity.

An additional enzyme that affects central levodopa availability is monoamine oxidase B (MAO-B). MAO-B acts by deaminating dopamine, leading to reduced availability in the synaptic vesicles. Central MAO-B inhibition is yet another therapeutic target to ameliorate symptoms of Parkinson disease by increasing levodopa bioavailability.

Because increasing the concentration of dopamine in the striatum results in dramatic clinical improvement in patients with Parkinson disease, the neural substrate that dopamine acts on (the striatal dopamine receptors) is obviously relatively intact. The dopamine receptor sites are divided into five different subtypes, but there are two main families: the D_1 and D_5 group and the D_2, D_3, and D_4 group. Drugs acting as dopamine receptor agonists must have D_2 activity to be effective in the treatment of Parkinson disease. The dopamine receptor agonists that are available to treat Parkinson disease include ergot-derived (bromocriptine and pergolide) and non–ergot-derived (pramipexole, ropinirole, and rotigotine) compounds. Although all of the dopamine receptor agonists have D_2 activity, they have somewhat different profiles of activation for the various dopamine receptors. Although all agonists have similar efficacy and adverse event profiles, there are variations among individual patients in regard to which agonist is the most efficacious. Although the number of antiparkinsonian medications grows steadily, levodopa remains the gold standard of therapy, the most potent drug for the symptomatic treatment of Parkinson disease.

TREATMENT

All medications currently used to treat Parkinson disease only provide symptomatic relief and do not alter the underlying pathogenesis of the disorder (Table 12.1).

In other words, the natural progression of Parkinson disease continues despite current treatment. The treatment of each patient with Parkinson disease should be highly individualized to provide functional improvement. If a patient's symptoms are very mild and causing no impairment in the activities of daily living, delay of treatment may be the appropriate choice. If a patient's symptoms are mildly troublesome, with tremor as the predominant feature, low-dose anticholinergics (e.g., trihexyphenidyl, benztropine) may be all that is required. The anticholinergics, the oldest drugs available to treat Parkinson disease, remain useful because the striatum contains high levels of both dopamine and acetylcholine, and the dopamine

deficiency state in the striatum of patients with Parkinson disease results in a relatively elevated cholinergic tone. Anticholinergics exert their beneficial effect by partially correcting this relative cholinergic excess. Anticholinergics must be used with caution in older patients because they can induce memory dysfunction and confusion. In older men, anticholinergics can also lead to urinary hesitancy and retention.

Amantadine is also useful in the treatment of early Parkinson disease and can be helpful for early bradykinesia. Amantadine has anticholinergic activity, mild dopaminergic activity, and antiglutaminergic activity. Amantadine is also useful in treatment of drug-related dyskinesia in more advanced Parkinson disease. Other options for patients with early troublesome symptoms include monotherapy with the dopamine receptor agonists (pramipexole, ropinirole, or rotigotine), or low-dose carbidopa–levodopa with or without a COMT inhibitor (tolcapone or entacapone). The progression of the disease process will eventually result in the need for more powerful dopaminergic stimulation.

The use of levodopa as a precursor loading strategy to increase central dopamine and to ameliorate Parkinson disease has been one of the major therapeutic advances in neurology. However, high-dose levodopa administration without the addition of a peripheral dopa decarboxylase inhibitor, such as carbidopa, produces anorexia, nausea, and vomiting. These symptoms occur because of the high levels of circulating peripheral dopamine that are present as a result of extensive extracerebral decarboxylation and result in the stimulation of the area postrema (emesis center) of the brain. The development of peripheral dopa decarboxylase inhibitors in large part ameliorated these problems and led to the development of combination therapy with carbidopa and levodopa. This drug is available in fixed ratios of 10/100, 25/100, and 25/250, with the numerator indicating the milligram dose of carbidopa and the denominator indicating the milligram dose of levodopa. The most important advantage of this drug is the ability to administer less

TABLE 12.1	Medications Used in the Treatment of Parkinson Disease	
Dopamine Replacement	**MAO-B Inhibitors**	
Carbidopa/levodopa (Sinemet)	Rasagiline (Azilect)	
Carbidopa/levodopa/ entacapone (Stalevo)	Selegiline (Eldepryl, Zelapar)	
Dopamine Agonist	**COMT Inhibitors**	
Pramipexole (Mirapex)	Entacapone (Comtan)	
Ropinirole (Requip, Requip XL)	Tolcapone (Tasmar)	
Rotigotine (Neupro)		
Apomorphine (Apokyn)	**Anticholinergics**	
	Benztropine (Cogentin)	
NMDA Antagonist	Trihexyphenidyl	
Amantadine	(Artane)	

levodopa to obtain the same central effect with a marked reduction in nausea and vomiting. In fact, the ease of administration of carbidopa–levodopa therapy both for patient and the treating physician has resulted in it being used almost exclusively in the treatment of patients with Parkinson disease who require levodopa. Carbidopa–levodopa in a controlled-release (CR) formulation (CR 25/100, CR 50/200) provides a slower and longer-lasting effect of levodopa. CR preparations may be useful to treat motor fluctuations, nighttime bradykinesia resulting in sleep disruption, early morning painful dystonic cramps, and early morning severe bradykinesia. There is also a triple combination (levodopa/carbidopa/entacapone) tablet to treat Parkinson disease, which will allow some patients to take fewer pills daily. **Levodopa remains the most potent drug for the treatment of bradykinesia and rigidity in Parkinson disease.**

The direct-acting dopamine receptor agonists approved in the United States for the treatment of Parkinson disease include pramipexole, ropinirole, and rotigotine. Previous-generation dopamine agonists that are no longer used for Parkinson disease include bromocriptine and pergolide. Because dopamine receptor agonists exert their effect on the striatal dopamine receptors (which presumably are not involved in the substantia nigra degenerative process), it was felt that they might be an effective substitute for levodopa. Although dopamine agonists have assumed an important role in Parkinson's therapy, none of the agonists are as potent as levodopa for relief of symptoms of Parkinson disease. Clinical experience with the dopamine agonists has shown that they are effective not only in the treatment of Parkinson disease but also in ameliorating motor fluctuations in patients treated with carbidopa–levodopa. Bromocriptine, the first dopamine agonist introduced, is rarely used today both because of its cost and because the new agonists are generally more potent and effective. Pergolide, although effective, has been linked to valvular heart disease (fibrotic changes associated with

ergot-derived preparations) and withdrawn from the United States market. Pramipexole, ropinirole, and rotigotine have been approved for use in both early and late (pramipexole and ropinirole) Parkinson disease. These non-ergot dopamine agonists are effective and well tolerated in early Parkinson disease. Rotigotine is marketed as a transdermal patch, which is unique among the dopamine agonists. However, problems with the patch's medication delivery system led to its being withdrawn from the market. It is expected that rotigotine will be reintroduced at a future date. The use of these drugs instead of levodopa as initial therapy has been shown to delay the onset of drug-induced dyskinesia. They are also very helpful in managing motor fluctuations and dyskinesias in more advanced Parkinson disease.

Because there are no known neuroprotective agents that modify disease progression in Parkinson disease, treatment is directed at symptomatic improvement. **If the diagnosis of Parkinson disease is made, there is no need to start treatment with any anti-Parkinsonian medications unless the patient is experiencing functional disability in activities of daily living, on the job, or in recreational activities.**

There is continuing controversy about whether to start treatment with levodopa or a dopamine agonist when functional impairment begins. A number of clinical trials of pramipexole, ropinirole, and levodopa in early untreated patients with Parkinson disease have demonstrated that levodopa is more effective than the dopamine agonists in relieving motor symptoms and that dopamine agonists induce less motor fluctuations and dyskinesias in the early years (2 to 5) of Parkinson disease. The American Academy of Neurology issued a practice parameter examining this issue and concluded that initial symptomatic treatment of Parkinson disease could begin with either levodopa or a dopamine agonist. When choosing initial treatment, many factors including age, degree of disability, cognitive status, and cost all need to be considered.

Selegiline, an MAO-B inhibitor, also known as l-deprenyl, inhibits the catabolism of dopamine and promotes dopaminergic activity. Selegiline has been used in early Parkinson disease and has been shown to delay the need for levodopa. There has been considerable discussion as to whether this effect in early Parkinson disease is "neuroprotective" or simply symptomatic. The evidence strongly suggests that the effect of selegiline is symptomatic.

Rasagiline, another MAO-B inhibitor that is not metabolized to amphetamine byproducts, has been demonstrated to be effective in early Parkinson disease and in managing motor fluctuations in advanced Parkinson disease. Like selegiline, rasagiline has been proposed to have neuroprotective effects. A recently completed delayed-start trial of rasagiline suggested a disease-modifying effect. However, the full study results have elicited considerable controversy regarding the results. The research question is not whether the small effect size achieved is statistically significant, but is it clinically meaningful.

Entacapone and tolcapone are COMT inhibitors approved for the treatment of Parkinson disease. COMT inhibitors must be administered in combination with levodopa, resulting in increased bioavailability of levodopa to the brain. COMT inhibitors may enhance dopaminergic side effects; therefore, downward titration of carbidopa–levodopa may be required, particularly in patients who already have dyskinesia. Tolcapone and entacapone have been shown to be effective in patients experiencing motor fluctuations. Both drugs are easy to administer, and their therapeutic efficacy can be ascertained quickly. The FDA determined that hepatotoxicity associated with tolcapone necessitates stringent liver function monitoring and informed consent when prescribing this drug. Entacapone is not associated with liver toxicity. Entacapone has been combined with levodopa and carbidopa in one tablet.

It should be noted that all of the anti-Parkinson medications may be used in combination, particularly in the advanced patient with complex symptoms.

COMPLICATIONS

Although there is no question that carbidopa–levodopa is the mainstay of therapy in this disorder, numerous problems are associated with its use (Table 12.2). However, it should be recognized that several long-term follow-up studies of patients with Parkinson disease who were treated with levodopa demonstrated that at the end of 5 years of treatment, most patients' motor function was no worse than prior to treatment or, in many cases, still better than before they were treated. This finding is extraordinary because prior to levodopa therapy, the prognosis in Parkinson disease was dismal.

Several major side effects are associated with the use of carbidopa–levodopa, including drug-induced dyskinesias, drug-induced psychiatric problems, and motor fluctuations. Levodopa-induced dyskinesias are a striking long-term complication of this therapy. The dyskinesias are most often choreic. Chorea consists of irregular, unpredictable, brief, jerky movements that flit from one body part to another in a continuous random sequence. Occasionally, levodopa-induced dyskinesias are dystonic. Dystonia describes movements that are dominated by sustained muscle contraction, frequently resulting in twisting repetitive movements and abnormal postures. The dyskinesia may involve the lingual, facial, and buccal regions; the limbs; and the axial musculature. It is particularly striking to see patients with this drug-related

TABLE 12.2	Toxicity Associated with Chronic Levodopa Therapy
Central toxicity	Dyskinesias
	Motor fluctuations
	"On–Off" phenomenon
	Sleep disturbances
	Psychiatric disturbances
Peripheral toxicity	Nausea and vomiting
Mixed central and questionable peripheral toxicity	Orthostatic hypotension

movement disorder because patients with Parkinson disease were previously characterized by slowness and poverty of movement. The chorea seen in this setting may resemble the chorea seen in Huntington disease or tardive dyskinesia.

Levodopa-induced dyskinesias are common and may be seen in more than half the patients at the end of 5 years of carbidopa–levodopa treatment. However, patients with onset of dyskinesias during the first 5 years of levodopa treatment experience very mild abnormal movements that do not usually interfere with function. The severity of the chorea may increase with continued treatment, and the dose of levodopa required to elicit chorea may decrease with time. The relationship between duration of disease, levodopa treatment, and onset of dyskinesias is unclear. A reduction in levodopa dosage invariably will ameliorate this drug-induced movement disorder. Although the chorea may be severe, the parkinsonian patient often does not find the movement troubling; it is usually the family or the physician who first notices the chorea. This is probably best explained by the fact that while a patient is choreic, they are still able to move voluntarily with relative ease. Given a choice, most parkinsonian patients prefer excess movement to bradykinesia. However, severe levodopa-induced dyskinesia can be as disabling as bradykinesia.

The psychiatric side effects of long-term dopaminergic therapy include altered sleep patterns, vivid nightmares, auditory and visual hallucinations, paranoia, and psychosis. Although there may be a continuum of increasing severity of psychiatric symptomatology with increasing dopaminergic medication dose and duration, the symptoms may develop insidiously in some patients and acutely in others. These drug-related complications can be ameliorated by reduction of dopaminergic medications.

The simplest approach to drug-induced psychosis in Parkinson disease is to reduce the dosage of antiparkinsonian medications and particularly to reduce the administration of other medications that depress the nervous system, including sedatives, hypnotics, anxiolytics, anticholinergics, opiates, and muscle relaxants. When this is not sufficient to relieve hallucinations and delusions, the use of antipsychotic medications is indicated to be able to continue dopaminergic medications at a level to maintain the patient's motor function. There are several atypical neuroleptic drugs available that can reduce or abolish psychosis with less potential for extrapyramidal side effects. Clozapine is the only neuroleptic medication proven to be effective in Parkinson disease psychosis that does not produce adverse motor effects. Quetiapine is often used as a first-line treatment. Although quetiapine does not have the proven efficacy of clozapine, quetiapine also does not carry the same risk of serious adverse hematologic events. **Traditional neuroleptics should not be used for psychosis in Parkinson disease patients because of the adverse effect on motor function.** All of the atypical neuroleptics are used in much lower dosage in Parkinson disease then when indicated for schizophrenia.

Fluctuation in motor performance is an additional complication associated with both chronic dopaminergic therapy and duration of disease. After a variable period of treatment, patients note that the beneficial effects of the drug begin to wear off before they are due to take their next dose ("wearing off" or end-of-dose akinesia) and that they may be very akinetic in the morning before the first dose of medication (morning akinesia). One or more doses often do not seem to work. Later, particularly in patients on multiple overlapping doses of carbidopa–levodopa, the fluctuations from a mobile state or "on" to "off" with obvious parkinsonism may appear random with no obvious relation to dosage timing. The transition between relatively normal functions to complete reemergence of the parkinsonian state can occur in several minutes, and it can persist for up to 3 to 4 hours. Sudden, rapid, unpredictable fluctuations between these two extremes can also occur. Clinically, these fluctuations can be striking, and the dramatic nature of these transitions occasionally can be observed during an office evaluation. A patient may be seen in a severely parkinsonian state ("off") with marked cogwheel rigidity, resting tremor, and severe akinesia to the degree that the patient is unable to rise from a chair and have impaired postural reflexes to the point of falling or being unable to stand. During 5 to 6 minutes, the same patient may turn "on" and be observed to be able to stand and sit without difficulty, to have no tremor, and to be able to walk relatively normally and not look at all parkinsonian. The observer who is unfamiliar with these rapid transitions is astounded by these fluctuations, and the uninformed observer may even believe that the severe parkinsonian state, or "off," may reflect a functional or nonorganic problem.

This perplexing problem seems to be related to alterations in central dopamine receptor-site responsiveness and to fluctuating levels of available dopamine. It is a problem typically encountered only in patients with advanced Parkinson disease. There are many therapeutic maneuvers to try in a patient with motor fluctuations, including increasing the antiparkinsonian medication dose or dosing frequency, adding the controlled-release formulation of carbidopa–levodopa, adding a dopamine receptor agonist, adding a COMT inhibitor, adding a MAO-B inhibitor, or implementing a restricted-protein diet. New medications should be added one at a time. Both levodopa and the dopamine receptor agonists (pramipexole and ropinirole) must be initiated at a low dose and gradually titrated upward to the therapeutic range, whereas the COMT inhibitors (tolcapone or entacapone) and MAO-B inhibitors (selegiline and rasagiline) are initiated at an effective dose. The restricted-protein diet is mainly helpful in patients who report a significant effect of diet on their response to carbidopa–levodopa. Levodopa shares the same gastroin-testinal transport system with other aromatic amino acids, and high-protein meals result in greater competition for the uptake system, reducing the amount of levodopa available to the brain. In patients who note loss of efficacy of carbidopa–levodopa when it is administered with a protein meal, the restricted-protein diet may provide smoother motor response throughout the day. This is not a low-protein diet; it restricts daytime protein intake to enhance motor performance during the day and shifts a greater proportion of the daily protein to the evening meal.

The symptoms of Parkinson disease remain responsive to the effects of levodopa throughout the duration of the illness; however, as the disease advances, the degree of symptom relief is less dramatic as the complications of motor fluctuations, dyskinesia, and hallucinosis emerge. The administration of levodopa or a dopamine agonist should begin when the patient's ability to carry out daily functions is impaired. All of these medications are symptomatic and not disease modifying; therefore, it is important to treat a "symptom." The precise timing is individualized based on many issues including lifestyle and individual response to symptomatology. There is no benefit to withholding treatment until advanced disability ensues.

Management of advanced Parkinson disease is challenging because the clinician often confronts a double bind; the patient requires increased levodopa to improve his or her parkinsonism but needs decreased levodopa to reduce dopaminergic adverse events. The introduction of dopamine receptor agonists, MAO-B inhibitors, or COMT inhibitors can be useful for problems with motor fluctuations and drug-related dyskinesia. Dopamine receptor agonist administration provides dopaminergic stimulation of the postsynaptic striatal dopamine receptors and also often allows a reduction in carbidopa–levodopa dose. In some patients, the combination of dopamine agonist with levodopa will result in more consistent motor improvement with less dyskinesia.

SURGERY

The history of surgical treatment of Parkinson disease begins more than 60 years ago. In 1968 to 1969 when levodopa treatment became widely available, surgical procedures for Parkinson disease dropped precipitously and almost disappeared. However, in the last 15 years there has been a resurgence of interest in surgical treatment. This has developed because pharmacologic treatment has limitations, greater insight into basal ganglia function was achieved, and improved surgical techniques and technologies became available. Pallidotomy utilizing updated stereotactic techniques has been reintroduced to treat advanced Parkinson disease. In this procedure, a small lesion is made by the neurosurgeon in the globus pallidus in an attempt to disrupt the physiologic outflow of the basal ganglia and relieve the symptoms of Parkinson disease. Some centers report a 20% to 30% improvement in the motor symptoms of Parkinson disease and resolution of dyskinesia in selected patients. Neurosurgical complications include intraparenchymal hemorrhage, cerebral vascular accident, and altered mental status. Patients with severe intractable drug-related dyskinesia are generally the best candidates for this procedure.

Another surgical procedure that has largely replaced pallidotomy is deep brain stimulation (DBS). DBS is a neurosurgical stereotactic procedure in which a stimulating electrode is placed in a selected brain region (target) and wires are subcutaneously passed from the target to an electronic stimulator that is implanted in the chest wall (analogous to a cardiac pacemaker). The stimulator can be turned off and on by the patient with the use of a magnetic "wand." DBS for Parkinson's symptoms has been targeted at the Vim nucleus of the thalamus, the globus pallidus, or the subthalamic nucleus. When the target is the Vim nucleus of the thalamus, relief of tremor is most likely to be achieved; however, the other symptoms of Parkinson disease (bradykinesia, rigidity, loss of balance) are not relieved by this procedure. When the target is the globus pallidus or the subthalamic nucleus, more pervasive symptomatic relief including tremor, rigidity, bradykinesia, and dyskinesia may be achieved. Currently, the most common target for DBS is the subthalamic nucleus. DBS targeting the subthalamic nucleus provides the most robust relief of motor symptoms, but it carries a risk of cognitive or behavioral problems developing after surgery. Formal trials comparing pallidotomy to DBS procedures for Parkinson disease have not yet been reported.

There has been considerable interest in the role of fetal tissue (mesencephalon) implants in the treatment of Parkinson disease. This concept involves the transplantation of the dopamine-producing mesencephalon cells from an aborted fetal brain into the brain of the patient with Parkinson disease. Unfortunately, two well-controlled, blinded trials of human fetal tissue transplants in Parkinson disease failed to demonstrate therapeutic benefit and provoked uncontrollable dyskinesias in a number of study subjects.

Whether or not the implantation of stem cells into the basal ganglia will be beneficial to patients remains to be determined. Currently, there are many technologic problems related to the stem cells that need to be solved before clinical trials can begin.

DRUG-INDUCED PARKINSONISM

Drug-induced parkinsonism can be precipitated by any drug that reduces central dopaminergic activity (Table 12.3). Drugs that block the dopamine receptor (e.g., neuroleptics, metoclopramide) or deplete central dopamine (e.g., reserpine, tetrabenazine) often result in parkinsonian symptomatology. Parkinsonism induced by drugs can mimic all of the features seen in Parkinson disease. Akinesia and rigidity are the most common signs, and resting tremor is seen less often. Other features that may help distinguish drug-induced parkinsonism from

TABLE 12.3	Medications Causing Parkinsonism

Typical Antipsychotics	Antiemetics
Amoxapine	Chlorpromazine
Molindone	Metoclopramide
Thioridazine	Promethazine
Fluphenazine	Prochlorperazine
Loxapine	Thiethylperazine
Mesorizadine	**Neurotransmitter**
Trifluoperazine	**Depletors**
Perphenazine	Reserpine
Haloperidal	Tetrabenazine
Thiothixene	**Calcium Channel**
Pimozide	**Blockers**
Zuclopenthixol	Flunarizine
Atypical	Amlodipine
Antipsychotics	Cinnarizine
Olanzapine	**Miscellaneous**
Quetiapine	Lithium
Clozapine	Valproic acid
Risperdal	Fluoxetine
Aripiprazole	
Ziprasidone	
Paliperidone	

Parkinson disease include a clear history of exposure to a compound known to interfere with central dopamine activity, a relatively short time from onset of parkinsonian symptoms to functional impairment (about 1 to 2 months as opposed to 12 to 24 months), bilateral presentation instead of unilateral presentation of symptoms and signs, and the presence of other drug-related motor abnormalities (e.g., tardive dyskinesia; see Chapter 13).

The diagnosis of drug-induced parkinsonism requires a high index of suspicion. Once the diagnosis is made, treatment should be directed at stopping the offending drug. **In almost all patients with this syndrome, the parkinsonism will resolve over time. Resolution of drug-induced parkinsonism may take weeks to months.** If active treatment is required, anticholinergics, amantadine, and levodopa–carbidopa have been used successfully. When drug-induced parkinsonism does not resolve, Parkinson disease may have been unmasked.

FURTHER CONSIDERATIONS

Although the etiology of Parkinson disease remains unknown, there have been recent attempts to modify the natural history of this disorder and delay progression. This approach to treatment, sometimes referred to as "neuroprotective" or "disease-modifying therapy," has been based on a wide variety of theoretic and preclinical models. Attempts to modify disease progression using vitamin E (2,000 units/day) and selegiline (5 mg b.i.d.) failed. Vitamin C in doses of 1,500 to 3,000 mg/day has been proposed as an additional antioxidant treatment, but vitamin C has never been tested adequately. The results from a trial of rasagiline, which purports to show disease modification, have not yet been published. At present, there is no "neuroprotective" therapy for Parkinson disease; however, there is continued interest in disease-modifying therapies and a number of trials are in progress.

The levodopa treatment era in Parkinson disease with improved function and life expectancy led to broadening the scope of what is considered to be the central nervous system dysfunction seen in this disorder. Although James Parkinson did not originally describe cognitive dysfunction as part of the illness, it is apparent that cognitive impairment and dementia are often associated with Parkinson disease. There is evidence from the pre-levodopa era to suggest that 25% to 30% of patients with Parkinson disease eventually were institutionalized because of dementia and not because of incapacitating motor performance. However, the increased longevity and maintenance of communicative abilities in patients with Parkinson disease led to further understanding of cognitive dysfunction in Parkinson disease. Studies confirm earlier observations that as many as 25% to 50% of patients with Parkinson disease may develop dementia. Parkinson disease dementia is characterized primarily by executive dysfunction, rather than an amnestic dementia, as seen in Alzheimer disease. Trials of the acetylcholinesterase inhibitors, donepezil and rivastigmine, have both shown modest benefits on cognition in Parkinson disease dementia and may be considered for treatment.

There is considerable interest in other nonmotor symptoms of Parkinson disease including depression, apathy, fatigue, anxiety, and sleep disruption. Studies indicate that all of these nonmotor symptoms are much more frequent than previously understood, and contribute significantly to quality of life and disability in Parkinson disease.

Any drug or degenerative process that interferes with central dopaminergic activity can lead to parkinsonism. The dysfunction of the dopamine system may involve the nigral (presynaptic) neuron or the striatal dopamine receptor (postsynaptic). Drugs or degenerative processes that affect not the presynaptic nigrostriatal dopaminergic pathway but the striatal dopamine receptors may result in the same clinical signs. The latter situation is sometimes referred to as postsynaptic parkinsonism. Examples of postsynaptic parkinsonism include some drug-induced states and metabolic disturbances that result in calcification of the basal ganglia and familial striatonigral degeneration. Because the pathology in these syndromes is located primarily within the striatum and involves the dopamine receptors, it should not be surprising that carbidopa–levodopa therapy is less effective in these disorders. Other neurodegenerative disorders have elements of both presynaptic and postsynaptic dopaminergic dysfunction including the spinocerebellar ataxias (SCA), PSP, and MSA. Clinical clues to identify these syndromes include variable response to levodopa, the presence of a kinetic tremor (SCA), the failure of voluntary conjugate gaze (PSP), and the presence of severe orthostatic hypotension and other autonomic signs (MSA).

WHEN TO REFER TO A NEUROLOGIST

Parkinson disease is a common disorder, and it is believed that there may be 1 million people in the United States with this illness. Because there is no specific imaging study or biomarkers to confirm the diagnosis, Parkinson disease is a clinical diagnosis. Physicians making this diagnosis should be comfortable in determining that a patient has Parkinson disease based on the patient's history and examination. Parkinson disease is a chronic progressive illness that ultimately results in significant disability; the diagnosis is a serious one.

Although the diagnosis of Parkinson disease certainly can be made by a non-neurologist, many patients and families will ask for referral for confirmation. There is great interest in clinical research trials for neuroprotective agents for Parkinson disease, and most of these trials seek to enroll early patients. Referral of patients for possible participation in studies can be of great value for the patient because there currently are no drugs that slow the progression of Parkinson disease and it may give the patient a sense of being more proactive about dealing with this diagnosis.

The early years of symptomatic treatment are often uneventful and the patient can be cared for by the non-neurologist. If patients develop motor fluctuations, dyskinesias, or hallucinations and psychosis, referral to a neurologist is indicated for further treatment.

COMPLEMENTARY THERAPIES

Some people say that there are no alternative therapies in medicine—only therapies that work and those that do not. This applies to Parkinson disease. Few alternative therapies in Parkinson disease have been tested. High-dose vitamin E (2,000 units/day) was demonstrated to have no effect in modifying disease progression. Early studies of coenzyme Q10 were promising, but it is premature to conclude that it is "neuroprotective." Studies of coenzyme Q10 are still ongoing.

A small study of acupuncture was conducted in Parkinson disease. Acupuncture was ineffective for all motor and nonmotor symptoms with the exception of some benefit for sleep and rest.

Physical therapy is helpful for alleviating rigidity and bradykinesia in Parkinson disease. There is currently great interest on the possible interactions between exercise and cognition. Physical therapy and regular exercise may have benefits on cognition in addition to purely physical benefits. Speech therapy may also be helpful to patients with Parkinson disease. One therapy in particular (Lee Silverman Voice Treatment) is effective for hypophonia in Parkinson disease patients.

There is no special diet for most patients with Parkinson disease. In some patients with motor fluctuations that are sensitive to protein intake (after a protein meal medications may not work as well), a protein redistribution diet may be of value. A wide variety of additional treatments are marketed as possible therapeutic agents for Parkinson disease. These include over-the-counter antioxidants, food supplements, ginkgo biloba, ginseng, herbal preparations, massive doses of vitamins, spa treatments, NADH (reduced form of nicotinamide adenine dinucleotide) preparations, and chelation therapy. None of these have been shown to be effective.

SPECIAL CHALLENGES FOR HOSPITALIZED PATIENTS

When patients with Parkinson disease enter the hospital for medical or surgical conditions unrelated to Parkinson disease, special precautions are indicated. Most patients with moderate Parkinson disease have specific requirements for the timing of their medications to maintain optimum motor function. Hospital routines often do not accommodate well to complicated time-specific oral medication schedules. One way to address this problem is to have patients and families remain in control of administering the antiparkinsonian medications. The staff must remain fully informed about the medications being administered.

If hospitalized patients with Parkinson disease become agitated, with delirium or psychotic ideation, care must be taken to avoid agents that interfere with the efficacy of Parkinson disease medications. The use of traditional neuroleptics, and certain antiemetics, or gastrointestinal agents (metoclopramide) can interfere with dopamine neurotransmission and result in motor worsening.

The dramatic changes in motor function of the patient with Parkinson disease with motor fluctuations may result in confusion on the part of the hospital staff. Staff may observe a patient "on" who is able to perform all activities of daily living without assistance and later observe the same patient "off" and immobile. During "off" periods, the patient may require assistance and the staff may mistakenly believe the patient's request for assistance is not necessary. Staff education about the changeable nature of symptoms in fluctuating patients is important.

All medical and surgical services caring for patients with Parkinson disease should be proactive in instituting preventative measures to avoid deep-vein thrombosis and aspiration pneumonia in patients with Parkinson-related immobility. Fall precautions should also be taken for Parkinson disease patients with gait disturbances or impaired postural reflexes.

Always Remember

- Parkinson disease has four major cardinal signs: resting tremor, cogwheel rigidity, bradykinesia, and postural instability.
- Levodopa is the most effective medication for symptomatic treatment of Parkinson disease.
- Parkinson disease has motor, cognitive, and emotional/behavioral consequences.
- A careful history regarding exposure to dopamine blocking agents should be taken, and typical antipsychotics and metoclopramide should be avoided in Parkinson disease patients.

QUESTIONS AND DISCUSSION

1. A 62-year-old right-handed man presented to his physician with the following problems. He has noticed for the last 6 months that his handwriting has changed and that it appears small and cramped. In addition, he has the feeling that his right hand is not as strong as it used to be, and he often has to struggle to button his shirt. The week prior to his visit, his wife noticed that his right hand appeared to be shaking when he was resting quietly in an easy chair.

   The most likely diagnosis in this patient based on history alone is:
   A. Parkinson disease
   B. Wilson disease
   C. Huntington disease
   D. Dystonia

   Neurologic signs present on examination might include which of the following?
   A. Bilateral limb chorea, linguofaciobuccal dyskinesias
   B. Resting tremor of the right hand, cogwheel rigidity of the right upper extremity
   C. Fixed dystonic posturing of the right hand
   D. Kinetic tremor of the right hand
   E. Three-step retropulsion, two to three extra steps in turning maneuvers

The answer to the first part of the question is A and the answer to the second part is B. This is a typical history of Parkinson disease characterized by slow progression and a predominantly unilateral presentation of the symptoms and signs. In addition, the handwriting is described as cramped and small (micrographic). The feeling of weakness in an involved extremity is a common complaint, although there is usually no objective sign of weakness. The presence of unilateral signs of tremor and cogwheel rigidity is typical. If postural reflexes are impaired (retropulsion and increased steps on turning maneuvers) early in the presentation, the diagnosis of Parkinson disease is questionable. However, postural reflex impairment is a common sign in advanced Parkinson disease.

2. A 59-year-old right-handed woman has an 8-year history of left upper extremity resting tremor. She has been treated with carbidopa–levodopa for the last 7 years. Although she states that originally her tremor was much improved, she has been having difficulty with increasing involuntary "dancelike" gyrating, nonpurposeful movements of the left upper and lower extremities. In addition, her husband reports that occasionally his wife sees visitors in the house when they are alone. Questioning the patient reveals that she often sees people who are not really there. She speaks lucidly about this and recognizes that they are not real. The correct diagnosis in this patient would be:
   A. Dystonic posturing of the left upper extremities
   B. Tardive dyskinesia
   C. Parkinson disease with dopaminergic adverse events
   D. Wilson disease and dopaminergic adverse events

The correct answer is C. The patient's initial presenting complaint is the spontaneous appearance of a unilateral resting tremor that is relieved by dopaminergic agents. This is a characteristic early presentation of unilateral Parkinson disease, and the additional information that dopaminergic therapy ameliorated the symptoms suggests the diagnosis of Parkinson disease. The patient's present complaints are adverse events associated with chronic dopaminergic therapy, specifically levodopa-induced dyskinesias and hallucinations. Levodopa-induced dyskinesias in Parkinson disease are often choreiform and are not phenomenologically distinguishable from the chorea seen in many other choreatic states. The hallucinations reported by this patient are typical, nonthreatening visual hallucinations.

Answer A is incorrect because dystonic postures and movements are not "dancelike" and gyrating. Answer B is incorrect because there is no drug history of neuroleptic medication and tardive dyskinesia is by definition secondary to chronic dopamine receptor blockade. Answer D is incorrect because Wilson disease does not present so late in life. The average age of onset of Wilson disease presenting with neurologic symptomatology is 19 years.

The most appropriate therapy in this patient would be:
A. Raising the dose of carbidopa–levodopa
B. Adding an anticholinergic
C. Reducing the dose of carbidopa–levodopa
D. Administering a typical neuroleptic

The correct answer is C. The patient's current problems of dyskinesias and hallucinations are secondary to chronic dopaminergic stimulation, and the appropriate therapy is to reduce the dose of dopaminergic therapy if possible. These drug-induced effects will be ameliorated when dopaminergic agents are reduced. When the dose of the dopaminergic is reduced or discontinued, the patient's parkinsonian symptoms will become worse.

Typical neuroleptics should be avoided because of their high predilection for worsening motor function in patients with PD. However, if reduction in levodopa dosage results in excessive motor dysfunction with functional impairment, the addition of an atypical neuroleptic may be necessary. First, confirm that the patient is not taking other types of medications that may significantly contribute to confusion and psychotic ideation, such as sedatives, tranquilizers, and anticholinergics. If the drug regimen is simplified but the psychotic symptoms persist, choose either clozapine or quetiapine for their antipsychotic effects. Use the lowest effective dosage to avoid adverse effects. If drug-induced dyskinesia persists and is very troublesome despite maximal reduction of antiparkinsonian medications, surgical intervention may be considered.

Answer A is incorrect because this is a drug-induced syndrome and raising the dose of the drug will not ameliorate the problem—it will exacerbate it. Answer B is incorrect because anticholinergics will not improve chorea and are likely to increase the psychotic symptoms. Answer D is incorrect because typical neuroleptics lead to unacceptable motor deterioration in patients with PD.

3. A 65-year-old right-handed man presents with generalized slowing of mobility and difficulty seeing the food on his plate. His family says that his problem has been getting worse for the last 12 months and that the patient also has difficulty walking up stairs. In addition, he describes that he is having difficulty buttoning his shirt, rising from a chair, and turning over in bed. The family also reports that his facial expression has changed (he does not smile as much) and that a tremor of his left hand is occasionally noted. Examination reveals that there is a resting tremor of the left hand, cogwheel rigidity in the left upper extremity is present, and postural reflexes are mildly impaired. Additional findings include increased extensor tone in the neck and marked impairment of voluntary conjugate gaze. The patient is unable to look down voluntarily, and there is also moderate impairment of upward gaze. In addition, right and left lateral gaze are not normal. The correct diagnosis in this patient would be:
A. Wilson disease
B. Huntington disease
C. Parkinson disease
D. Progressive supranuclear palsy
E. Multiple system atrophy

The correct answer is D. PSP is an idiopathic midbrain and brainstem degenerative disorder that is characterized by parkinsonian features and progressively impaired voluntary conjugate gaze. This patient is described as having parkinsonian features (resting tremor, cogwheel rigidity, impaired postural reflexes, and mild bradykinesia) and has markedly impaired conjugate gaze. A useful office maneuver to determine whether the gaze dysfunction is supranuclear or nuclear is the doll's head procedure. In this maneuver, the head is passively flexed and extended, and in a separate maneuver, it is rotated to the right and to the left while the passive motion of the eyes is observed. In a patient with supranuclear gaze dysfunction, the eyes will move reflexly and conjugately in an appropriate direction. This maneuver and its physiology are discussed in greater detail in Chapter 20.

Answer A is incorrect because of the late onset of neurologic symptoms and the type of eye movements observed. Answer B is incorrect because of the late onset of neurologic symptoms and because the movement disorder is not that seen in adult-onset Huntington disease. Although definite parkinsonian features are present, Answer C is incorrect because of the additional findings of disturbed volitional gaze. Answer E is incorrect because of the pronounced oculomotor dysfunction.

4. The degenerative cellular pathology seen in Parkinson disease is localized primarily in the:
   A. Cerebral cortex
   B. Thalamus
   C. Cerebellum
   D. Substantia nigra
   E. Corpus striatum

The loss of cell bodies and their projection systems in the correct answer to the first part of this question results in what biochemical lesion?
   A. Loss of acetylcholine in the striatum
   B. Loss of dopamine in the striatum
   C. Loss of dopamine in the cerebral cortex
   D. Loss of acetylcholine in the cerebellum

The answer to the first part of the question is D, and the answer to the second part of the question is B. Parkinson disease is pathologically characterized by depigmentation, Lewy bodies, and cell loss in the substantia nigra. The destruction of the nigral striatal projection system results in the loss of dopamine in the striatum. Dopamine is the neurotransmitter used by this system, and the dopamine within the striatum is contained primarily within the axonal terminations of the nigral neurons.

5. A 65-year-old woman was diagnosed with Parkinson disease 9 years ago when she developed a resting tremor of the left hand. When levodopa–carbidopa treatment was started, she had a positive response and her tremor, clumsiness of the left hand, and gait improved. She is now taking levodopa–carbidopa 25/100 mg 2 tablets q.i.d., pramipexole 1 mg t.i.d., and entacapone 200 mg q.i.d. On this schedule, she experiences end-of-dose wearing off and moderate dyskinesias. She has no hallucinations or delusions, is not depressed, and is otherwise in good health. The motor fluctuations and dyskinesias have become troublesome to her.

   Management of her motor fluctuations and dyskinesia may include:
   A. Increasing levodopa–carbidopa dosage and frequency
   B. Increasing pramipexole dosage
   C. Adding an additional dopamine agonist
   D. Perform surgical procedure (DBS)

The correct answer is D. This patient has a complex problem that reflects advancing parkinsonism and drug-associated problems. Decreasing the dosage of pramipexole, entacapone, or levodopa will ameliorate her dyskinesia. However, her parkinsonism may worsen to an unacceptable degree. Another option would be to start amantadine 100 mg b.i.d. in order to reduce dyskinesia. DBS is a good therapeutic choice when medical options have been exhausted because it can alleviate both motor fluctuations and dyskinesias.

The following conditions exclude a patient from DBS surgery for Parkinson disease: unstable medical conditions, cognitive impairment, poor response to levodopa, neurobehavioral problems, and atypical parkinsonism. The DBS candidates with the best chance of a successful outcome are relatively healthy, have no cognitive impairment or significant behavioral problems (depression, anxiety), still have some good response to levodopa administration, have Parkinson disease, and understand that DBS for Parkinson disease is not a cure.

SUGGESTED READING

Cotzias GC, Van Woert MH, Schiffer LM. Aromatic amino acids and modifications of Parkinsonism. *N Engl J Med*. 1967;276:374.

Factor SA, Weiner WJ, eds. *Parkinson's Disease: Diagnosis and Clinical Management*. 2nd ed. New York: Demos Press; 2008.

Havemann J. *A Life Shaken—My Encounter with Parkinson's Disease*. Baltimore: Johns Hopkins University Press; 2002.

Jankovic J, Marsden CD. Therapeutic strategies in Parkinson's disease. In: Jankovic J, Tolosa E, eds. *Parkinson's Disease and Movement Disorders*. 3rd ed. Baltimore: Williams & Wilkins; 1998:191.

Miyasaki JM, Martin W, Suchowersky O, et al. Practice parameter: initiation of treatment for Parkinson's disease: an evidence-based review: report of the Quality Standards Subcommittee of the American Academy of Neurology. *Neurology*. 2002;58:11–17.

Miyasaki JM, Shannon K, Voon V, et al. Practice parameter: evaluation and treatment of depression, psychosis, and dementia in Parkinson disease (an evidence-based review): report of the Quality Standards Subcommittee of the American Academy of Neurology. *Neurology*. 2006;66:996–1002.

Pahwa R, Factor SA, Lyons KE, et al. Practice parameter: treatment of Parkinson disease with motor fluctuations and dyskinesia (an evidence-based review): report of the Quality Standards Subcommittee of the American Academy of Neurology. *Neurology*. 2006;66:983–995.

Shulman LM, Gruber-Baldini AL, Anderson KE, et al. The evolution of disability in Parkinson disease. *Mov Disord*. 2008;23:790–796.

Suchowersky O, Reich SG, Perlmutter J, et al. Practice parameter: diagnosis and prognosis of new onset Parkinson disease (an evidence-based review): report of the Quality Standards Subcommittee of the American Academy of Neurology. *Neurology*. 2006;66:968–975.

The Parkinson Study Group. Effect of deprenyl on the progression of disability in early Parkinson's disease. *N Engl J Med*. 1989;321:1364.

Weiner WJ, Shulman LM, Lang AE. *Parkinson's Disease: A Complete Guide for Patients and Families*. 2nd ed. Baltimore: Johns Hopkins University Press; 2006.

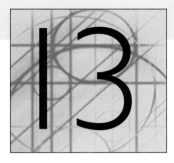

Hyperkinetic Movement Disorders

GONZALO J. REVUELTA, WILLIAM J. WEINER, AND STEWART A. FACTOR

key points

- Dystonia is a movement disorder seen in a variety of genetic, sporadic, and acquired conditions, for which multiple medical therapies and surgical interventions are available.

- Essential tremor (ET) is primarily a postural and kinetic tremor that often responds to medical therapy, but if severe it can be treated effectively with deep brain stimulation (DBS).

- Huntington disease (HD) is a progressive inherited neuropsychiatric disorder for which a definitive genetic diagnosis is available; however, this information is very sensitive and should be handled by multidisciplinary centers experienced with this process.

- Wilson disease (WD) is a hereditary, potentially reversible condition that can be associated with myriad movement disorders, and, if not diagnosed and treated appropriately, is fatal.

- Gilles de la Tourette syndrome (GTS) is a tic disorder associated with a variety of behavioral disorders often necessitating a multidisciplinary treatment approach.

- Tardive dyskinesia (TD) is a choreo-dystonic, persistent movement disorder that occurs as an adverse effect of neuroleptic and antiemetic therapy.

Strange, abnormal involuntary movements are the hallmarks of a number of neurologic diseases; they are collectively termed "hyperkinetic movement disorders" (also referred to as dyskinesias). In such conditions, the movements are easily visible, and observation allows the clinician, in most instances, to suggest the proper diagnosis or class of disorders. The characteristic tremor of Parkinson disease, which is present at rest but markedly diminished during volitional movements, is an example (Chapter 10). In this chapter, six hyperkinetic movement disorders are described. All are dramatic visually because bizarre and abnormal involuntary movements are their major features. The non-neurologist encounters patients with these disorders in an office practice and also identifies them in public (e.g., in parks, trains, and shopping centers).

The disorders discussed in this chapter are dystonia, essential tremor (ET), Huntington disease (HD), Wilson disease (WD), Gilles de la Tourette syndrome (GTS), and tardive dyskinesia (TD).

Definitions

Dystonia: Involuntary sustained muscle contractions producing twisting or squeezing movements and abnormal postures. Dystonia can have stereotyped, repetitive movements that vary in speed from rapid to slow and that may result in fixed postures from the sustained muscle contractions.

Tremor: Involuntary rhythmic oscillating movement that results from the alternating or synchronous contraction of reciprocally innervated antagonist muscles. Tremor may be classified according to its prominence during activity or at rest.

Chorea: Excessive, spontaneous movements that are irregularly timed, nonrepetitive, randomly distributed, and often have a flowing "dancelike" quality that involves multiple body parts.

Tics: Repetitive, brief, rapid, purposeless, stereotyped movements that involve single or multiple muscle groups. The tics can be a patterned sequence of coordinated movements that may be complex or simple, associated with a premonitory urge, and are suppressible.

Myoclonus: Rapid, shock-like, arrhythmic (usually), and often repetitive involuntary movements. Myoclonus can be classified by location (focal, multifocal, or generalized) and by etiology.

Stereotypy: Patterned, repetitive, and purposeless movements that are performed exactly the same way each time.

DYSTONIA

Dystonia is divided into primary (idiopathic) and secondary forms. Several primary dystonic conditions have been identified which are characterized by dystonia as the sole clinical feature. The prevalence of primary dystonia is estimated to be 33 per 100,000. Dystonia of primary origin has a number of unusual but characteristic features. At onset, the movements may occur in relation to specific voluntary actions (such as in writer's cramp) or with varied movements, so-called "action-induced dystonia." It may occur in one body part with movement of another (overflow dystonia). Later, with progression of disease, dystonia becomes present at rest. Dystonic movements typically worsen with anxiety, heightened emotions, and fatigue, whereas they decrease with relaxation and disappear during sleep. There may be diurnal fluctuations in dystonia, which manifest as little or no involuntary movements in the morning (morning honeymoon) followed by severe disabling dystonia in the afternoon and evening. Whereas morning improvement is seen with several types of dystonia, one particular form of childhood-onset dystonia is characterized by this feature (dopa-responsive dystonia [DRD] or Segawa dystonia).

Dystonia may occur in nearly any muscle group. The following terms are used to describe dystonia in varied distributions. When the upper face and eyelids are involved and the eyes are involuntarily closed the clinical symptom is blepharospasm. When the lower face, lips, and jaw are involved and the patient presents with involuntary opening or closing of the jaw, retraction or puckering of the lips, and repetitive contractions of the platysma, the term is "oromandibular dystonia." Pharyngeal dystonia is associated with dysphagia, dysphonia, or dysarthria and is typically action induced. Lingual dystonia may occur at rest, presenting as sustained or repetitive protrusion of the tongue or upward deflection of the tongue against the hard palate, or it may be action induced via speaking or eating. Laryngeal dystonia (involving the vocal cords) causes spasmodic dysphonia in which the speech is tight, constricted, and forced, or it may be whispery, depending on whether the adductor or abductor muscle groups are involved. The smooth flow of speech is lost, and certain sounds are held longer and overemphasized. Spasmodic dysphonia is typically action induced by speech, and it most commonly involves the adductor muscles of the larynx. Abductor dysphonia resulting in a soft whispery voice is less common.

Dystonic contractions of the neck muscles, referred to as spasmodic torticollis or cervical dystonia, result in torticollis, retrocollis, anterocollis, or laterocollis. In spasmodic torticollis, rapid jerking and twisting neck movements may accompany sustained posturing of the neck. Some patients have head tremor and others have a fixed abnormal neck posture without spasmodic movements or tremor. The shoulder on the side of the head tilt typically is elevated. Dystonic movements of the arms (brachial dystonia) commonly present as pronation of the arm, often behind the back. The movements are often action induced as in writing (writer's cramp), manipulating a musical instrument (musician's cramp), and other occupational maneuvers. Truncal or axial dystonia manifests as lordosis, scoliosis, kyphosis, tortipelvis, or opisthotonus. Dystonic movements of the legs (crural dystonia) may occur with action or at rest and present most commonly with equinovarus posturing of the foot while walking, twisting of the foot, or increased elevation of the leg when walking. The knee usually maintains a hyperextended position with crural dystonia. Some patients walk backward, run, or even dance without incident, but when they attempt to walk normally, dystonia recurs. Patients with dystonic disorders often discover ways to suppress or hide the movements using an array of "tricks." These often consist of postural alterations or counterpressure maneuvers that are primarily sensory in nature. Examples include touching an eyebrow in blepharospasm, which leads to eye opening, or the classical *geste antagonistique*, where a finger placed lightly on the chin will neutralize neck-turning in cervical dystonia. There are also motor tasks that may deactivate dystonia, including singing or whistling in blepharospasm or oromandibular dystonia and dancing in cervical or truncal dystonia. Typically, these tricks lose their effectiveness with time.

The pathophysiology of dystonic movements and tricks remain a mystery. However, some clues have emerged. Briefly, it is believed that dystonia is the result of basal ganglia dysfunction. This is primarily based on work involving cases of secondary dystonia and neuroimaging studies in idiopathic cases. There appears to be decreased output from the primary output nucleus of the basal ganglia, the medial globus pallidus. Microelectrode recordings from the globus pallidus in patients undergoing surgery have demonstrated irregular, intermittent group discharges leading to irregular output from that region to the thalamus and cortex. This supports the notion that the basal ganglia are the source of the problem. There also appears to be sensory and motor cortical involvement in the physiology of dystonia. Sensory involvement is suggested by the usefulness of sensory tricks. Physiologic studies also have demonstrated that motor cortex is hyperexcitable and that there is decreased activation of these regions. It is possible that certain patterned or learned tasks (tricks), both sensory and motor, interrupt the production of dystonia through alterations in cortical activity.

Dystonia often is misdiagnosed as hysterical or psychiatric in origin. The basis for this arises from its typical features, including the varied, often bizarre, movements and postures, the fact that they are often action induced, the worsening of dystonia with stress and improvement with relaxation, the diurnal fluctuations, and the effectiveness of various tricks. Knowledge of the unusual characteristics of dystonic disorders will be helpful in avoiding a misdiagnosis.

Classification

Classification of dystonia has been based on (a) age of onset, (b) distribution of movements, and (c) etiology. Clinical and genetic studies have demonstrated that they are all connected. Use of the first two items in the patient's initial assessment can lead to etiology. The age-of-onset classification separates patients into early onset (younger than age 26 years) and late onset (older than age 26 years). Early onset typically begins with limb involvement and carries a worse prognosis than older onset because generalization of the movement disorder is more likely. Early-onset patients more often have hereditary disease, most commonly DYT1. Late-onset patients have focal or segmental dystonia that primarily involves the craniocervical region and does not generalize.

The distribution of dystonia is focal, multifocal, hemidystonia, or generalized. Focal dystonia is dystonia in a single body part. Multifocal dystonia includes dystonic movements in more than one body part yet not fulfilling the criteria for generalized dystonia; segmental dystonia is a form of multifocal dystonia in which contiguous body parts are affected. In hemidystonia, an arm and a leg on the same side are involved. Finally, generalized dystonia refers to the presence of dystonia in at least one leg, the trunk, and an additional body part (cranial, cervical, or brachial) or in both legs and the trunk. This classification

is important in formulating a proper diagnosis. For example, hemidystonia is usually the result of a basal ganglia infarction or space-occupying lesion, whereas generalized dystonia is most likely a primary early-onset disease and has a worse prognosis than focal dystonia or hemidystonia. Early-onset and generalized dystonia appear to be most responsive to deep brain stimulation (DBS) surgery.

Classification by etiology has undergone substantial change in the last decade, primarily because of the linkage (or nonlinkage) of many types of dystonia to a variety of genes (Table 13.1). The primary dystonias (also known as idiopathic torsion dystonias) are

TABLE 13.1	Classification of Dystonia

Primary dystonia
  Early-onset dystonia (Oppenheim dystonia): chromosome 9q (DYT1)
  Non DYT1 autosomal dominant early-onset dystonia with whispering dysphonia (DYT4)
  Autosomal recessive dystonia: DYT2 and DYT16
  Adult-onset familial torticollis
  Adult-onset familial cervicocranial dystonia: chromosome 18p (DYT7)
  Mixed adult- and childhood-onset dystonia: chromosome 8p (DYT6)
  Mixed but predominantly adult-onset segmental dystonia (occasionally childhood onset and generalized): chromosome 1p36 (DYT13)
  Adult-onset sporadic focal dystonia

"Dystonia plus" syndromes
  Dopa-responsive (Segawa) dystonia: chromosomes 14q22 and 11p (DYT5)
  Myoclonus dystonia: chromosome 7q21 (DYT11) or chromosome 18p11 (DYT15)
  Rapid-onset dystonia, parkinsonism: chromosome 19q (DYT12)

Secondary dystonia related to exogenous causes (see Table 13.2)
Hereditary and degenerative diseases associated with dystonia
  Degenerative disorders
  Parkinsonian syndromes including PSP, CBD, MSA, IPD, and juvenile PD
  Huntington disease

TABLE 13.1
Classification of Dystonia (continued)

SCAs such as types 2, 3, 6, 17

Autosomal recessive ataxias:

  AT

  AVED

  AOA

Hallervorden–Spatz disease (NBIA/PKAN)

Lubag (Filipino X-linked dystonia parkinsonism):

  Chromosome Xq13 (DYT3)

Fahr

  DRPLA

  Neuroferritinopathy

Hereditary metabolic disorders

  Wilson disease

  Hexosaminidase deficiency

  Glutaric acidemia

  Gangliosidoses (GM1, GM2)

  Metachromatic leudodystrophy

  Homocesteinuria

  Propionic academia

  Methylmalonic aciduria

  Niemann–Pick type C

  Ceroid lipofuscinosis

  Lesch–Nyhan syndrome

  Neuroacanthocytosis

Hereditary Mitochondrial disorders

  Leber optic neuropathy with dystonia

  Leigh disease

  MERRF

  MELAS

Dystonia related to hereditary dyskinetic disorders

  Dystonic tics

  Paroxysmal kinesiogenic dyskinesia (DYT10)

  Paroxysmal non-kinesiogenic dyskinesia (DYT8)

  Paroxysmal dyskinesia with spasticity (DYT9)

AT, ataxia telangiectasia; AVED, ataxia with vitamin E deficiency; AOA, ataxia with oculomotor apraxia; PSP, progressive supranuclear palsy; CBD, corticobasal degeneration; MSA, multiple system atrophy; IPD, idiopathic Parkinson disease; juvenile PD, juvenile Parkinson disease; SCA, spinocerebellar ataxia; DRPLA, dentatorubral-pallidoluysian atrophy; MERRF, myoclonic epilepsy with ragged red fibers; MELAS, mitochondrial encephalopathy, lactic acidosis, and stroke-like episodes.

defined as syndromes in which the sole manifestation is dystonia, with the exception that tremor may be present. It is unclear if this disorder is purely neurochemical in origin or if some degree of neurodegeneration exists. Primary dystonias are genetically and clinically heterogeneous. Dystonia genes are depicted by the symbol DYT (followed by a number) by the Human Genome Organization/Genome Database. DYT designations have been assigned to a variety of clinically defined dystonic syndromes and unmapped, genetically linked primary dystonias. Dystonia syndromes not classified as primary but with dystonia as a predominating feature are also designated (Table 13.1). Fifteen genetic causes of dystonia have been identified; four are primary dystonias, which are discussed in this chapter.

A second etiological category comprises the dystonia-plus syndromes. These are also considered to be neurochemical in origin, but also have features other than dystonia (e.g., patients with DRD have parkinsonian features). The third category is secondary dystonia, which develops as the result of a wide variety of known etiologies (Table 13.2). The fourth category includes hereditary-degenerative syndromes that have dystonia as part of the clinical spectrum. Examples include Parkinson disease, WD, HD, and X-linked dystonia parkinsonism (Lubag).

Primary Inherited Dystonias Dystonia is the only neurologic abnormality in patients with primary dystonia (although many may have tremor), and any distribution of abnormal involuntary movements may be observed. The primary dystonias have an insidious onset and are progressive. Initially, the movements may be only action induced, but with disease progression they occur at rest and produce fixed and sustained postures. The disorder ultimately plateaus in severity. Five criteria for the diagnosis of primary dystonia are established. These include (a) the development of dystonic movements or postures, (b) a normal perinatal and developmental history, (c) no precipitating illnesses or exposure to drugs known to cause dystonia, (d) no evidence of intellectual, pyramidal, cerebellar, or sensory deficits, and (e) negative results of investigation for secondary causes of dystonia (particularly WD). Two factors are indicators of a

TABLE 13.2
Secondary Forms of Dystonia

Drugs
Dopamine antagonists (i.e., haloperidol, thoridizine, compazine, metoclopramide)
Dopamine agonists (i.e., levodopa, bromocriptine)
Antidepressants (tricyclics, SSRIs, lithium)
Antihistamines
Calcium channel blockers
Stimulants (cocaine)
Buspirone

Vascular disease
Basal ganglia infarction
Basal ganglia hemorrhage
Arteriovenous malformation

Neoplasms
Astrocytoma or glioma of the basal ganglia
Metastatic neoplasm
Cervical spinal cord tumor

Others
Head trauma
Thalamotomy
Anoxia (in adulthood or perinatal)
Meningitis (fungal or tuberculosis)
Syringomyelia
Colloid cyst of the third ventricle
Munchausen syndrome
AIDS (toxoplasmosis abscess of basal ganglia, PML)
SSRIs, PML
Paraneoplastic
Central pontine myelinolysis
Primary antiphospholipid syndrome
Multiple sclerosis
Peripheral injury: complex regional pain syndrome

AIDS, acquired immunodeficiency syndrome; PML, progressive multifocal leukoencephalopathy; SSRIs, selective serotonin reuptake inhibitors.

poor prognosis: onset in childhood and in a crural distribution. Poor prognosis in dystonia refers to increased disability. Most patients with crural dystonia have onset of disease in childhood or early adulthood. The clinical presentation is heterogeneous.

The classical early-onset primary dystonia is DYT1 dystonia. It is the most severe and the most common form of hereditary early-onset dystonia. Oppenheim, who first used the term "dystonia" in 1911, called this particular dis-

order dystonia musculorum deformans and it has since been renamed primary torsion dystonia or Oppenheim dystonia. DYT1 dystonia is inherited in an autosomal dominant pattern, with a 30% to 40% penetrance. The gene is located at chromosome 9q34. The gene abnormality is a unique three–base pair GAG deletion. The resulting protein, torsin A, is characterized by the loss of one of a pair of glutamic acid residues. The function of this protein and its role in altering basal ganglia function to cause dystonia remain unknown. The mutant protein is distorted leading to the formation of cytoplasmic inclusions. There is a high prevalence of early-onset dystonia in Ashkenazi Jewish families, with more than 90% resulting from a single founder mutation in the DYT1 gene. This mutation has been traced back more than 350 years to Lithuania, and the current gene frequency is approximately 1 in 2000. In 50% to 60% of non-Jewish ethnically diverse families with early-onset dystonia, the disease results from the same DYT1 mutation that has arisen independently in varied populations. Apparently, only one variation in the encoded protein can give rise to the DYT1 phenotype.

The clinical spectrum of early-onset DYT1 dystonia is similar in all ethnic populations. Onset of symptoms occurs at an average age of 12 years, but most patients have onset before age 26. The initial presentation is with limb onset, usually leg (crural dystonia). The presence of leg or foot dystonia is the best predictor of a DYT1 mutation. The foot often is twisted and plantar flexed while ambulating, and the patient usually toe-walks. All patients ultimately have leg involvement. The disorder may start in the arm (possibly as writer's cramp), although less frequently. In these cases, the age of onset is a little older than crural onset and the patients are less likely to end up with generalized dystonia. Early-onset dystonia progresses by spreading across or down/up over a period of approximately 5 years; 50% of patients become either bedridden or wheelchair bound. No cognitive problems or other neurologic abnormalities are seen. Spasmodic dysphonia occurs in about 5%; cervical involvement is rare; and cranial involvement is generally not seen. Onset in the neck or vocal cords in early-onset patients, even if they are of Ashkenazi Jewish descent, rarely is caused by the DYT1 gene. These patients rarely generalize. Late-onset (older than age 26) craniocervical dystonia indicates that the patient does not have DYT1 dystonia. The DYT1 patient often stabilizes and may even improve to some degree, but the disorder does not spontaneously remit. Genetic testing is available for DYT1 dystonia and should be considered in early-onset primary dystonias and in late-onset patients with a family history. The specificity of using age 26 as a cutoff age is 63% for Ashkenazi Jews and 43% for non-Jews.

Linkage studies involving several large families with adult- or mixed-onset dystonia of a variety of distributions have excluded the DYT1 locus. However, dystonia families have been linked to other possible genes. DYT6 has been linked to chromosome 8p in two Mennonite families from the midwestern United States with an autosomal dominant form of dystonia with incomplete penetrance. The phenotype of these families includes a broader age of onset (5 to 38 years; mean, 19) and an onset distribution that includes limbs and cervical or cranial areas. There are also differences from typical adult-onset craniocervical dystonia because DYT6 dystonia commonly spreads to the limbs, but the former syndrome does not.

The DYT7 gene is linked to chromosome 18p in a family from northwest Germany. This family has an autosomal dominant form of adult-onset craniocervical dystonia with incomplete penetrance. The average age of onset was 41 years (range 28 to 70 years), and most patients had focal cervical dystonia. Some family members had cranial or laryngeal involvement, and postural hand tremor. Another family was designated DYT13 and linked to chromosome 1p36. This was an Italian family with focal and segmental dystonia usually affecting the craniocervical region. Some had early-onset disease and generalized, indicating a mixed presentation. Other inherited forms of dystonia are listed in Table 13.1.

Adult-Onset Primary Dystonia   Adult-onset primary dystonia is the most common type of dystonia. It presents with brachial and craniocervical dystonia and only rarely as truncal or crural dystonia. Only 18% of these patients develop generalized dystonia, with even a smaller percentage ever becoming wheelchair bound or bedridden. The dystonia usually remains as a focal dystonia, but it may spread to a contiguous body region in some cases, becoming segmental in distribution. The course is usually benign (meaning not life threatening but it can be disabling), and remissions occur in approximately 10% of patients.

Cranial Dystonia   Blepharospasm–oromandibular dystonia (Meige syndrome) was first described by the French neurologist Henry Meige in 1910. Blepharospasm and oromandibular dystonia may occur independently, but the combination is more frequent (in more than 50% of the patients). Pharyngeal, laryngeal, lingual, or cervical dystonia may occur. Blepharospasm in isolation (referred to as benign essential blepharospasm [BEB]) is more common than oromandibular dystonia. Blepharospasm is often preceded by eye irritation, photophobia, and increased blinking. It may start in one eye and spread to the other, or it may start in both. It results in involuntary blinking, repetitive contractions (blepharoclonus), squinting, or sustained closing of the eyes. Approximately 12% of these patients are functionally blind because of their inability to voluntarily open their eyes. Features that aggravate blepharospasm include sunlight (many wear wrap-around dark sunglasses, even indoors), looking upward, feeling stress, fatigue, watching television, walking, driving, talking, and even yawning. Sensory tricks used by patients to open their eyes include forced raising of the eyelids, applying pressure on the superior orbital ridges with a finger, and rubbing the eyelids. In addition, some find that forced jaw opening, neck movements, whistling, and wearing dark glasses are helpful. Some patients use eyeglasses with eyelid crutches to hold the lids open.

Oromandibular dystonia, jaw opening or closing dystonia, is frequently accompanied by lingual protrusion dystonia. It may be aggravated by talking, chewing, or swallowing. Sensory tricks include pressing on the lips or teeth with fingers, pressing on the hard palate with the tongue, or putting a finger in the mouth. About 20% of patients have their ability to eat severely compromised.

Meige syndrome affects women more commonly than men and presents in the sixth decade of life. It often begins with blepharospasm, followed by oromandibular, lingual, and pharyngeal dystonia. Other dystonic movements may occur in some patients, and hand tremor similar to ET may be an associated problem. The severity of dystonia fluctuates from day to day and disappears with sleep. Spontaneous remissions are rare.

Cervical Dystonia (Spasmodic Torticollis) Cervical dystonia is the most common adult-onset focal dystonia, making up about 40% (Fig. 13.1). The age of onset is in the fourth or fifth decade (mean age, 41 years) and women are affected more frequently than men (3 to 1). The disorder is characterized by involuntary neck movements, abnormal postures of the neck and shoulders that are often painful, and hypertrophy of involved neck muscles. Pain is present in about 80% of patients, and hypertrophy is seen in all. Initially, some patients do not perceive their dystonia, and it is brought to their attention by others. This suggests that a problem with perception of head position exists. The movements may be intermittent at first and associated with specific actions. Most patients deteriorate during the initial 5 years and then stabilize. The condition may be characterized ultimately by dystonic postures that are present at rest, worsen with action, and improve in sleep. Spontaneous remissions occur in 10% to 30%, most commonly in the first year. All patients relapse eventually but few have a second remission. Rotation of the neck (torticollis) is the most common posture seen, with lateral flexion (laterocollis), flexion (anterocollis), and extension (retrocollis) occurring in various combinations. Spasmodic (dynamic) movements are not present in all patients despite the commonly used term "spasmodic torticollis." In fact, they occur in only 10% to 15% of patients. Factors that may exacerbate cervical dystonia include emotional stress, fatigue, walking, working with the hands, and attempting to look in the opposite direction of

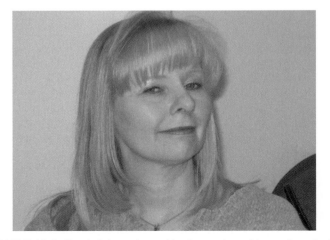

FIGURE 13.1 Cervical dystonia resulting in rotation of the neck to the left.

the dystonic contractions. When the patient tries to overcome the movements and look in the opposite direction, he or she may experience a high-amplitude, jerky tremor referred to as dystonic tremor. Some patients present with bidirectional torticollis because at varying times the head may turn in different directions and muscles of both sides of the neck may be involved.

■ **SPECIAL CLINICAL POINT: Many patients with cervical dystonia (spasmodic torticollis) present with head tremor (40%). The tremor varies in amplitude and, if there is little directional change, the patients frequently are misdiagnosed as having essential tremor (ET). The distinction is important because dystonia does not respond to tremor medications but does respond to botulinum toxin.**

This tremor can be distinguished from essential head tremor by the presence of subtle changes in posture, a jerky nonrhythmic quality, and muscle hypertrophy along with improvement with sensory tricks. Sensory tricks usually involve the use of a light touch or pressure to the chin or cheek with fingers (*geste antagonistique*) (Fig. 13.2) or other objects such as a pen or eye glasses and holding the back of the head with the hand or leaning the head against a wall or a headrest. This lessens the head tilt and

tremor and relaxes the muscles for variable durations of time. Tricks usually lose their effectiveness. Cervical dystonia may be associated with Meige syndrome, writer's cramp, and ET. Complications of prolonged cervical dystonia occur in many patients including those with degenerative osteoarthritis of the cervical spine with the expected sequelae of radiculopathy and myelopathy. These complications could lead to permanent neurologic deficits.

Writer's Cramp   Writer's cramp (Fig. 13.3) is a dystonic spasm induced by a specific task (action-induced or task-specific dystonia). When these cramps occur with a single type of action (such as writing), they are referred to as simple writer's cramp, but when the spasms occur with a variety of activities, they are referred to as dystonic cramps. Writer's cramp occurs in both men and women, and the age of onset ranges from 20 to 70 years. These patients present with a change in handwriting that becomes sloppy and illegible. Some patients squeeze the pen tightly and press down hard on the writing surface, which results in a jerky writing motion and tearing of the paper. In others, the fingers splay and pull away from the pen. Writing is painful in most patients. Initially, the dystonic

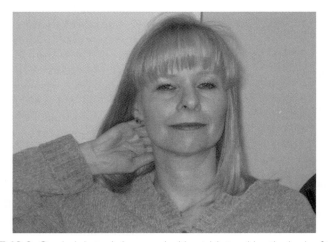

FIGURE 13.2 Cervical dystonia improved with a trick, touching the back of the head.

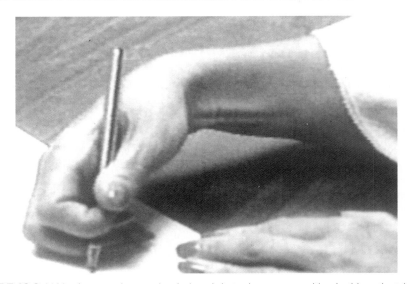

FIGURE 13.3 Writer's cramp is an action-induced dystonic spasm, resulting, in this patient, in wrist flexion, metacarpophalangeal joint extension, extension of the thumb, and flexion of the distal interphalangeal joints, leaving the patient with an inability to continue writing.

contraction occurs with persistence of task, but as the disorder progresses, it occurs with initiation of the task. Initially, other tasks performed with the same hand are normal, but later these too may become involved. The disorder is usually asymmetric, but those patients who learn to write with the opposite hand, the disorder may become bilateral (about 25% of patients). When some patients write with the unaffected hand, the affected hand exhibits involuntary spasms—so-called "mirror dystonia." Writer's cramp may be associated with ET and may be related to the syndrome of primary writing tremor, which is thought by some to be a variant of ET. Other occupational cramps that have been reported include pianist's and violinist's palsy, golfer's palsy, and dart-thrower's palsy. The common factor of these disorders is the occurrence during the performance of a well-learned motor (manual) task and perhaps the overuse of the hand with that particular task. In writer's cramp, there appears to be co-contraction of agonist and antagonist muscles, perhaps related to loss of reciprocal inhibition. Evidence has been mounting to support abnormalities in neuroplasticity as the etiology of task-specific dystonias in genetically susceptible individuals.

Dopa-Responsive Dystonia One "dystonia plus" syndrome that warrants discussion is DRD (DYT5). DRD is characterized by childhood (mean age, 6 years) or adolescent onset, female predominance (four times that of males), foot dystonia in childhood, parkinsonism in adults, and diurnal fluctuation. Patients function well in the morning and deteriorate as the day wears on. They improve with sleep. Purely dystonic limb presentations are most common. Some patients have mixed dystonia and parkinsonism, and the parkinsonism becomes more prominent with age. The clinical spectrum includes developmental delay and spasticity mimicking cerebral palsy. The most characteristic feature is profound and sustained response to levodopa $\leq$ 300 mg/day.

■ **SPECIAL CLINICAL POINT: So profound and sustained is the treatment response in dopa-responsive dystonia (DRD) that all individuals presenting with dystonia should be given a trial of levodopa.**

DRD has been linked to two chromosomes. The most common is chromosome 14q11–24.3—the gene codes for an enzyme in the rate-limiting step in the biosynthesis of tetrahydrobiopterin (GTP cyclohydrolase I), a cofactor in dopamine synthesis, and is dominantly inherited. The other link is to a rare defect seen on chromosome 11p15.5—the gene codes for tyrosine hydroxylase, the rate-limiting step in catecholamine metabolism—and is recessively inherited. The resulting deficiency of biopterin, a cofactor in catecholamine synthesis, leads to decreased levels of dopamine, which explains the long-term responsiveness of patients to levodopa. Dopamine transporter single-photon emission computed tomography (SPECT) scanning is normal in patients with DRD, and this helps differentiate these patients from those with early-onset Parkinson disease. Diagnosis of DRD is based on clinical profile and response to levodopa.

Secondary Dystonia   To make a diagnosis of primary dystonia, known causes of dystonia (i.e., secondary or symptomatic dystonias [Table 13.2] and hereditary degenerative diseases [Table 13.1]) must be excluded. Clues to the diagnosis of a secondary dystonia can be uncovered with a thorough history and physical examination, and radiologic and laboratory testing. Usually, examination findings in addition to dystonia are suggestive of dysfunction of other parts of the central nervous system (CNS), including the cranial nerves, pyramidal system, cerebellar system, and higher cortical function. There is often an abrupt onset to dystonia, and dystonia is present at rest from the start in secondary cases.

■ **SPECIAL CLINICAL POINT: The presence of hemidystonia suggests a focal lesion such as a tumor, infarction, abscess, or arteriovenous malformation in the basal ganglia.**

In patients with a single nonprogressive event such as an infarction or trauma, dystonia will stabilize and not be progressive. The examiner should be cautious because secondary dystonia may mimic idiopathic dystonia. For instance, stroke in the basal ganglia may cause typical-looking cervical dystonia and neuroleptic-induced (tardive) dystonia in adult patients may be symptomatically identical to adult-onset primary dystonia. Clues that tardive dystonia is more likely include retrocollis, a more phasic or dynamic form of torticollis, and the co-occurrence of choreiform movements. These patients also report less effectiveness of tricks and do not often have head tremor. A lack of muscle hypertrophy also suggests drug-induced dystonia.

An important feature of secondary dystonia is that dystonia may have a delayed onset after a cerebral insult. In adults, the most frequent cause of delayed-onset dystonia is cerebral infarction. The duration of the delay can vary from weeks to years and is often associated with an improvement of the original neurologic deficit. In children, the most frequent cause of delayed-onset dystonia is perinatal trauma or hypoxia. The reason for the delay is unclear, but it has been postulated that dystonia in these circumstances is a result of neuronal sprouting stimulated by the original injury. A history of perinatal difficulties must be ruled out if a diagnosis of primary dystonia is made.

■ **SPECIAL CLINICAL POINT: The most important disorder to exclude in a new-onset young dystonia patient is Wilson disease (WD). Screening for WD and an imaging study of the brain should be performed on all young dystonia patients. The rest of the diagnostic evaluation should be tailored to the individual patient.**

It had been suggested that secondary dystonia occurs in genetically susceptible individuals. However, it has been demonstrated that these patients are not genetically susceptible.

Pathology and Neurochemistry

Dystonia is related to basal ganglia dysfunction. Because there have been few neuropathologic examinations of patients with dystonia (most were without abnormality), the pathologic–anatomic basis of this movement disorder has been based

TABLE 13.3 Medical Treatment of Dystonia		
Drug Name	**Initial Daily Dose (mg)**	**Usual Daily Dose Range (mg)**
Levodopa	100	300–600
Trihexyphenidyl	2	12–24
Baclofen	10	60–120
Clonazepam	0.5	3–6
Reserpine	0.1	1–3
Tetrabenazine	25	100–200

almost exclusively on cases of symptomatic dystonia. Abnormalities were seen in the putamen and, to a lesser extent, the caudate nucleus and the thalamus. These findings have been supported by imaging studies. Interestingly, in those rare cases of dystonia with pathologic abnormalities, the microscopic changes were observed in the brainstem. The neurochemical basis of dystonia is also unclear. It has been suggested that the abnormality in this disorder is in the dopamine or acetylcholine systems. Clinical evidence to suggest these hypotheses include the onset of dystonia after treatment with dopamine receptor antagonists and the response of dystonia to anticholinergic medications. In addition, the discovery that DRD is acutely responsive to small doses of levodopa and that it is caused by two genes involved in the biosynthesis of dopamine support a dopaminergic hypothesis. Finally, the expression of torsin A in the substantia nigra pars compacta also implicates the dopamine system. Norepinephrine is a neurotransmitter that, among other actions, inhibits cholinergic neurons. A deficiency of norepinephrine might explain the response of dystonia to anticholinergic medications. Other theories include alterations in γ-aminobutyric acid (GABA) or cerebral somatostatin.

Treatment

Because the etiology and neurochemistry of dystonia is unclear, medical treatment has been less than satisfactory. A number of therapeutic modalities have been tested (for review see Table 13.3). The approach is to treat patients empirically with one agent at a time. Ultimately various combinations may be tried. Unfortunately, less than 50% of dystonic patients respond to medical therapy.

Because of the dramatic effect levodopa has on DRD, it is recommended that every patient with dystonia be tried on levodopa. Patients with DRD usually respond rapidly to low doses (<300 mg/day), but in some cases higher doses are needed. If there is no benefit, the dose is pushed to 600 mg/day over 2 to 3 weeks.

Anticholinergics are the most frequently used agents to treat primary dystonia. In an open-label trial, improvement was seen in 61% of children and 38% of adults. The average daily dose of trihexyphenidyl in children and adults was 41 mg and 24 mg, respectively. Adverse effects include blurred vision, dry mouth, urinary difficulties, constipation, sleep pattern alteration, forgetfulness, weight loss, personality changes, and psychosis. The earlier in the course of disease patients were treated, the better they did.

Tetrabenazine, a dopamine-depleting agent, is effective in patients with Meige syndrome and other types of dystonia. Reserpine, another dopamine-depleting drug, is effective in approximately 30% of patients. The adverse effects of most concern with dopamine-depleting agents include depression (which can be severe, come on suddenly, and have a protracted course), parkinsonism, orthostatic hypotension, and gastrointestinal problems.

Dopamine antagonists should be avoided. Mixed results with baclofen, carbamazepine, benzodiazepines (particularly clonazepam and diazepam), mexiletine, and clozapine have been observed.

In patients failing medical and botulinum toxin (BoNT) therapy, surgical techniques, including both central and peripheral procedures, have been used. Central procedures are used primarily for generalized dystonia. Modern techniques include the use of DBS with electrophysiologic microelectrode cellular recording and mapping to improve localization. Two well-designed, double-blind, controlled trials (22 and 40 patients) demonstrated significant improvement (54% and 39.9% in movement, and 44% and 38% in disability scores) in patients with primary generalized dystonia after DBS using bilateral globus pallidus pars interna as targets. Both studies showed continued improvement up to a year, and a third study of 31 patients showed 79% improvement in movement scores up to 2 years following surgery. Serious complications are rare with DBS, and failures or loss of benefit have rarely been reported. The most important factors for successful treatment with DBS are patient selection, lead placement, and optimal postsurgical programming of the stimulator. Surgical candidates suffer from medically refractory, unequivocal dystonia (diagnosed by a movement disorder specialist), and significant disability.

Peripheral surgical procedures include myectomy of the orbicularis oculi for blepharospasm and selective peripheral denervation for cervical dystonia. Another technique used to treat generalized dystonia is intrathecal baclofen. Baclofen is delivered to the intrathecal space through an inserted catheter with a continuous pump. This has been highly effective in treating spasticity of spinal and cortical origin. In the few patients with dystonia treated, results have been modest. Possible adverse effects include respiratory depression from baclofen overdose, catheter malfunction, and pump infection.

Intramuscular injection of BoNT remains the treatment of choice for focal dystonias, particularly in the craniocervical distribution.

BoNT is one of the most lethal toxins known to man. Of eight subtypes produced by the anaerobic organism *Clostridium botulinum*, three have been linked to human botulism: types A, B, E. BoNT A (Botox) has been used therapeutically since the mid-1980s for treatment of strabismus. In 1990, BoNT A was approved by the U.S. Food and Drug Administration (FDA) for treatment of blepharospasm, strabismus, and hemifacial spasm. In 2000, it was approved for cervical dystonia as was BoNT B. The use of these toxins is more widespread than these indications because they are used to treat all types of focal dystonia, including blepharospasm, oromandibular dystonia, spasmodic dysphonia, and limb dystonias. BoNTs act presynaptically at the cholinergic neuromuscular junction. The toxin attaches to an acceptor protein that is specific for each type of BoNT, is endocytosed into the nerve terminal and blocks the release of acetylcholine. The blockade of the neuromuscular junction results in weakness and atrophy of the muscle and a decrease in muscle spasms, but the effect is transient, lasting 3 to 6 months. If a desirable clinical result is achieved, repeated injections are necessary. BoNT is administered by direct intramuscular injection and all adverse effects are local. In blepharospasm improvement is seen after 3 to 14 days. The response lasts 2 to 4 months and treatment is needed three or four times per year. Adverse effects include ptosis, diplopia, and increased tearing, all of which are transient. Cervical dystonia is the most common disorder treated with BoNT. Multiple studies with both toxins have shown significant improvement in a majority of patients. As with blepharospasm, response occurs in 3 to 14 days and lasts 3 to 6 months. Neck muscles injected are chosen based on the presence of pain and hypertrophy and spasm and in relation to the abnormal posture. Ninety percent of cervical dystonia patients respond. Side effects include transient neck weakness, dysphagia, dry mouth, and a "flu-like" syndrome.

Spasmodic dysphonia of the adductor type, previously poorly responsive to any therapy, responds dramatically to BoNT. The thyroarytenoid muscles are approached through the neck with electromyogram (EMG) guidance. The only adverse effects are a breathy, whispery voice and dysphagia, which improves over days to weeks. Treatment of oromandibular dystonia is also frequently successful. Injections can be made into the pterygoid muscles (medial or lateral) with EMG guidance, and into the masseters, temporalis, and digastric muscles in varied combinations depending on whether the patient has jaw opening, closing, or lateral deviation as the main manifestation. Side effects include dysphagia and weakness of the soft palate that allows fluid regurgitation through the nose. Limb dystonias (writer's cramp) respond with less consistency because the resulting weakness of the hand muscles may be more troublesome than the cramps themselves. BoNT is the treatment of choice for most focal dystonias because of greater efficacy and fewer side effects than standard medical therapies.

Physicians administering BoNT should be familiar with the disorders treated, mechanisms of action, effective doses in each disorder, and the anatomy of the area injected. The disorders treated with BoNT have expanded beyond dystonia and include spasticity, achalasia, anal and urethral sphincter disorders, hyperhydrosis, sialorrhea, and others. BoNT A also has been approved for cosmetic use for facial wrinkles.

There are no alternative medical therapies with proven effect in dystonia. Physical therapy can be a useful adjunct for maintaining mobility and preventing contractures.

When to Refer to a Neurologist

Dystonia is a complicated disorder. Neurologists, especially movement disorder specialists, are most qualified for addressing diagnosis, genetic testing, and therapy. In particular, referral should be made to neurologist well versed in the use of BoNT.

Special Challenges for Hospitalized Patients

Most hospital staff are unfamiliar with dystonia, and because of the bizarre movements, cessation with sleep, and exacerbation with anxiety they are likely to assume or suspect that the movements are psychogenic in origin. This can lead to frustration and anger on the part of the patient. Staff education is required. Patients may be unable to stay still for testing and procedures, and mild sedation may be necessary.

ESSENTIAL TREMOR

Essential tremor is a monosymptomatic (kinetic tremor) syndrome. Tremor is generally classified by its anatomic location, frequency, etiology, or in relation to rest, posture, and action. Resting tremor refers to tremor while the body part is at rest. Resting tremor is seen in Parkinson disease. Postural tremor is seen when the body part maintains posture against gravity, and is frequently seen in ET. Kinetic tremor refers to tremor during goal-directed movements, as typically seen in cerebellar disease. This simple classification can be very useful in developing a differential diagnosis (Table 13.4). ET is the most common tremor disorder and is the subject of discussion in this section.

Clinical Features

ET is a nervous system disorder that occurs in a sporadic or familial form. The familial form is often autosomal dominant with high but not full penetrance. ET is the most common movement disorder, occurring in up to 6% of the population and 13% of people over age 65. It occurs equally in men and women and is characterized by a postural tremor, with or without a kinetic component, which is most evident in the upper extremities. The kinetic component is seen in finger-to-nose testing, although it is often not as dramatic as in cerebellar disorders,

TABLE 13.4
Differential Diagnosis of Tremor

Rest tremors
  Parkinson disease
  Secondary parkinsonism
  Hereditary chin quivering
  Severe essential tremor
  Drug-induced (neuroleptics)

Postural tremors
  Physiologic tremor
  Essential tremor
  Neuropathic tremor (Roussy–Livy syndrome)
  Cerebellar head tremor (titubation)
  Dystonic tremor
  Drug-induced tremor (lithium, valproate,
    neuroleptics, caffeine, theophylline, tricyclic
    antidepressants, amphetamines)

Action tremors
  Classical cerebellar tremor (multiple sclerosis,
    infarction)
  Primary writing tremor

Mixed tremors
  Wilson disease
  Rubral tremor
  Psychogenic tremors

and tremor at rest occurs rarely (in 5% to 10% of patients) in the most severe cases when the patient has a long-standing disease. Tremor frequency ranges from 4 to 12 Hz.

A maneuver to potentiate tremor during physical examination is to have patients hold the fingertips of their two open hands close together under the chin without touching while holding their elbows out like wings. This maneuver can also bring out a more proximal tremor distribution. Another examination technique is the cup test: the patient holds a full cup of water and pours it into another cup or takes a drink. The tremor is often worse as the hand approaches the face. The onset of ET can be at any age from early childhood to age 90, with a mean of 45 years. The patients with a family history appear to have an earlier age of onset (age 40) compared with sporadic cases

(age 51). ET usually affects the fingers and hands first and then moves proximally. Tremor onset may occur bilaterally in the hands or in one hand at a time. When bilateral, it may be symmetric or asymmetric.

Tremor may spread to the head and neck. Approximately 50% to 60% of patients with ET have head involvement, and in some instances head tremor is the sole manifestation. Head tremor may present as a vertical nod (yes-yes) or as a horizontal nod (no-no). Voice tremor occurs in approximately 25% to 30% of patients with ET. The voice is characterized by rhythmic alteration in intensity at the same frequency as the hand tremor. Head and voice tremor tend to be more frequent and severe in women. Tremor of the head or voice should strongly suggest a diagnosis of ET and not Parkinson disease because both are very uncommon in the latter. Less frequently, tremor occurs in the jaw, face (lips, tongue), trunk, and legs (15%). There are also a variety of task-specific tremors (i.e., primary writing tremor), which are variants of ET. ET is a slowly progressive disorder that can remain stable in some patients for decades. It is not unusual for patients to seek medical advice after having the tremor for one or two decades. At first tremor may occur when the limb is placed in a specific posture but later it is aggravated by many different movements or postures. The tremor disappears during sleep and worsens with anxiety, fatigue, temperature changes, local pain, caffeine ingestion, aminophylline ingestion, and possibly hunger.

■ **SPECIAL CLINICAL POINT: Alcohol characteristically improves essential tremor for 30 to 60 minutes, which may be a helpful diagnostic clue.**

A substantial proportion of patients are functionally disabled, with ~20% having impaired job performance and requiring early retirement. This is the reason the term benign has been eliminated from the name. Other patients are embarrassed by the tremor and impose social isolation on themselves.

■ **SPECIAL CLINICAL POINT:** **Essential tremor is a clinically heterogeneous disorder that may go unnoticed by the patient, may simply represent an embarrassment, or actually be disabling, leading to difficulties with writing, drinking, or using kitchen utensils.**

Approximately 5 million people in the United States have this disorder. There are many people with this problem who have not bothered to seek medical advice and therefore are not diagnosed.

Genetics

At least 60% of ET cases have a clear genetic component with an autosomal dominant mode of inheritance. This may be an underestimate because some sporadic cases may represent nonrecognition in family members. Genetic mapping has resulted in the linking of ET to genes on four different chromosomes.

Pathology and Pathophysiology

Because ET is neither life threatening nor life shortening, the opportunity for a postmortem examination of the CNS is not frequent. In those patients who have been examined pathologically, there is no distinctive CNS pathology although Lewy bodies (the hallmark of Parkinson disease) have been reported in brainstem nuclei. The significance of this finding remains to be deciphered. Positron emission tomography (PET) studies have demonstrated an increase in regional cerebral blood flow in the cerebellum and red nucleus, indicating that the neuronal circuitry involving these regions may be the location of the abnormality. One study also demonstrated increased glucose metabolism in the inferior olivary nucleus of the medulla. This structure may be the source of the rhythmic discharge causing the tremors. This notion is supported by the fact that lesions in the cerebellum and thalamus may stop tremor.

Differential Diagnosis

The diagnosis of ET is clinical (Table 13.4). The most common misdiagnosis in ET patients is Parkinson disease. The two disorders can be differentiated by careful history and physical examination. The tremor of Parkinson disease occurs at rest, whereas the ET is postural and kinetic. Patients with parkinsonism have rigidity, bradykinesia, micrographia, and postural and gait difficulties, and ET is associated with none of these. The handwriting in ET is usually big and shaky but not small (see Fig. 12.1).

■ **SPECIAL CLINICAL POINT:** **Sometimes a handwriting sample alone can lead to the correct diagnosis of essential tremor (ET).**

Postural tremor is frequently present in patients with primary dystonia. This tremor can be indistinguishable from ET. A family history of ET is not uncommon in both of these disorders. Some investigators have indicated that this frequent association between postural tremor and dystonia is indicative of a link between ET and primary dystonia, but linkage of ET to the DYT1 gene has been ruled out. Tremor is particularly frequent in patients with cervical dystonia and Meige syndrome.

■ **SPECIAL CLINICAL POINT:** **In cervical dystonia (torticollis), a head tremor is present in approximately 40% of patients and a hand tremor similar to that seen with ET is found in approximately 20% of patients. It is important to differentiate between these disorders because treatments differ.**

Postural and kinetic tremor secondary to cerebellar lesions can be differentiated from ET because of the presence of other signs of cerebellar dysfunction and the difference in severity (cerebellar tremor is generally much more disabling with higher amplitude and lower frequency). There are three types of cerebellar tremor: (a) cerebellar kinetic tremor, (b) cerebellar outflow rubral tremor, and (c) head titubation. The cerebellar kinetic tremor appears with goal-related movements most evident at the beginning and end of the movement. It is much slower than ET, 2 to 5 Hz, and of wider amplitude. The lesion usually includes the dentate nucleus (most common in stroke patients). Outflow tremor is present at rest, when maintaining posture, and with action. Amplitude and frequency are similar to the kinetic tremor, and the lesion includes the outflow pathway from dentate nucleus to the thalamus, with the most common location of the lesion being the midbrain involving the red nucleus. This type of tremor is most commonly seen in young patients as a manifestation of multiple sclerosis and in the elderly as the result of a stroke. Finally, titubation is a head tremor similar to the head tremor of ET. It is generally the result of bilateral cerebellar lesions.

Kinetic tremor, similar to ET, is also seen in the late—adult-onset neurodegenerative disease which affects male carriers of a premutation expansion of the fragile X mental retardation gene (FMR-1). This disorder is called fragile X tremor ataxia syndrome (FXTAS). These patients often present with a kinetic tremor that interferes with handwriting and can be quite disabling. This is followed by the development of progressive ataxia, neuropathy, and psychiatric manifestations.

Evaluation

The diagnosis of ET is based on the history and examination. If the patient presents with the typical history and findings, no laboratory or imaging studies are necessary except for thyroid function studies.

■ **SPECIAL CLINICAL POINT: Hyperthyroidism can worsen an already-existing tremor or cause an enhanced physiologic tremor that may appear similar to ET.**

Any patient with a sudden-onset tremor, unilateral tremor, or other complex features that do not fit with ET or Parkinson disease should be studied further with imaging studies and screening for WD. The diagnosis of WD is extremely important because it is fatal if undiagnosed. All patients under the age of 50 years with atypical ET presentation should have an evaluation for WD.

Treatment

Medical treatment of ET can improve function and relieve embarrassment in a substantial portion of patients. However, effectiveness often is limited (for review of medical therapy of ET see Table 13.5). The two agents considered first-line treatment for ET are propranolol and primidone. Propranolol (standard and long-acting formulations) is a beta-blocker that has been known to be effective for more than 20 years. It is particularly useful in controlling postural and kinetic tremor in the upper extremities and may make a significant difference to the patient in terms of being able to feed themselves or write legibly. This may be true even though propranolol usually does not abolish the tremor but only decreases its amplitude, having little or no effect on frequency. Approximately 40% to 70% of patients show a decrease in amplitude of 50% to 60%. There does not appear to be a correlation between plasma concentration of propranolol or its metabolites and reduction in tremor. There are no apparent features that separate responders and nonresponders. The dose of propranolol may range from 60 to 320 mg/day but usually is less than 120 mg/day. It exerts its effect in 2 to 6 hours after a single dose, and the effects may last as long as 8 hours. Withdrawal from propranolol may result in a rebound increase in amplitude of the tremor, which may last longer than a week. The site of action of propranolol, whether central or peripheral, has not been fully established. There are certain groups of patients with ET in whom the use of propranolol is relatively contraindicated. They include patients with diabetes mellitus, chronic obstructive lung disease, and asthma; propranolol can cause dyspnea and wheezing in these patients. In these instances the substitution of a different beta antagonist, metoprolol, may result in amelioration of the tremor and no bronchospastic symptoms. Metoprolol

TABLE 13.5 | **Medical Therapy for Essential Tremor**

Drug Name	Initial Daily Dose (mg)	Usual Daily Dose Range (mg)
First-line agents		
Propranolol	20	60–320
Primidone	25	50–750
Benzodiazepines		
Alprazolam	0.25	0.75–3
Clonazepam	0.5	1.5–6
Carbonic anhydrase inhibitors		
Acetazolamide	125	250–750
Methazolamide	50	100–200
Anticonvulsants		
Gabapentin	300	900–3600
Topiramate	50	100–400
Phenobarbital	30	60–120

is a beta receptor antagonist that is relatively selective in its action; however, patients who do not respond to propranolol also do not respond to metoprolol, and propranolol is superior. It has been suggested that the selectivity of metoprolol is lost when higher doses are used, and at higher doses bronchospastic symptoms may re-emerge. Acute side effects of beta-blockers include bradycardia and syncope; chronic problems include dizziness, fatigue, impotence, and depression. Propranolol also rarely causes hallucinations.

Primidone, an anticonvulsant, may be as effective as propranolol in the treatment of ET. The major problem has been acute adverse effects that are frequent (30%) and include vertigo, a general ill feeling, unsteadiness, nausea, ataxia, and confusion. These side effects clear spontaneously after 1 to 7 days, so patients can be encouraged to stick with the drug during this time. It has been observed that lower doses (50 to 250 mg/day) are as effective as higher doses and are better tolerated. As with propranolol, response has varied from patient to patient; the reason for this is unknown. However, many patients prefer primidone to propranolol. Plasma levels of primidone and its

metabolites do not correlate with responsiveness. It is likely that a combination of primidone and propranolol will be more effective than each drug used alone.

■ **SPECIAL CLINICAL POINT: A majority of patients respond to either propranolol or primidone. However, patients who do not respond or who are unable to tolerate these agents face more difficult therapeutic choices.**

Several other drugs have been used in the treatment of ET. One feature in the clinical history that an adult with ET will volunteer is the salutary effect of alcohol on the tremor. In fact, alcohol may be the most effective agent; 75% of patients respond quickly and dramatically. The occasional use of alcohol in patients with ET is a reasonable recommendation. Benzodiazepines, particularly alprazolam and clonazepam, also have been demonstrated to be successful in treating ET. Alprazolam is the only one shown to be effective in a small controlled trial and it induced significant reduction in tremor. Some literature suggests clonazepam is particularly useful in kinetic predominant tremor. A major adverse effect of this class of medications is sedation. Alprazolam is less sedating than clonazepam.

Other agents useful in some patients with ET include methazolamide and acetazolamide, gabapentin, phenobarbital, clozapine, and topiramate. Clozapine seems to have a general tremorolytic action, improving tremors in ET, Parkinson disease, and multiple sclerosis. At low doses (<50 mg/day) there was reduction in tremor amplitude and frequency. The major disadvantage of using this drug is the need to monitor white blood counts because 1% of patients develop agranulocytosis. It is also very sedating. Topiramate and gabapentin are both antiepileptic agents reported to be helpful in ET. The dose of gabapentin was up to 3600 mg/day, but typical dosing schedules range from 300 to 600 mg t.i.d. It can cause sedation, dizziness, slurred speech, and gait imbalance. Topiramate is an anticonvulsant that enhances GABA activity. It is a carbonic anhydrase inhibitor that has been reported to be effective in the treatment of moderate to severe ET. Adverse effects include ataxia, fatigue, dizziness, poor concentration, slowing down, weight loss, paresthesias, nausea, and renal stones. The data on carbonic anhydrase inhibitors methazolamide and acetazolamide have been conflicting. In our experience these drugs provide no useful effect. Mirtazapine was suggested as an alternative treatment for ET in open experiences; however, a small randomized, double-blind trial was negative.

Several studies indicated that BoNT A (Botox) injection directly into contracting muscles may be useful in dampening tremor. Pilot studies in patients with head, hand, and voice tremors with moderate to marked functional improvement have shown tremor reduction in approximately 70% of patients. It is not used often for hand or arm tremor because of the trade-off related to weakness. However, it is very useful for the treatment of head and voice tremor.

Thirty percent to 60% of patients do not respond to medication, and the rest have only a partial response. Those who have severe tremor are possible surgical candidates. DBS of the ventral intermediate nucleus nucleus of the thalamus has become the surgery of choice. Chronic stimulating electrodes are implanted through a burr hole in the skull and placed in the thalamus using stereotactic techniques and magnetic resonance imaging (MRI) or computed tomography (CT) imaging. The stimulator is adjustable and reprogrammable depending on patient needs. Significant improvement has been observed in blinded evaluations and maintained for 1 year. In one study efficacy was seen up to 8 years. More than 30% of patients with ET experience complete resolution, and 90% demonstrate moderate to marked improvement. This magnitude of response is not seen with any medication. It improves writing, pouring, drinking, and other activities. Surgical complications include low-frequency occurrence of intracerebral hemorrhage, subdural hematoma, and postoperative seizure. Stimulation-related complications include transient paresthesias, which occur in most patients at the time the stimulator is turned on, headache, gait disequilibrium, limb paresis, dystonia, and dysarthria. These problems may disappear with time. Drawbacks of the procedure include the cost of the stimulators, implantation of a foreign object and the risk of infection, need to replace battery (every 3 to 5 years depending on the parameters), possibility of breakage, and malfunction. There are no alternative therapies that are useful for ET. Occupational therapy suggestions include using either wrist weights to decrease the amplitude of tremor or weighted cups and utensils.

When to Refer to a Neurologist

Most patients are well controlled with propranolol or primidone. However, if tremor is severe and unresponsive to these agents, referral to a neurologist is necessary. This is particularly true if surgery is considered. The referral should be to a specialty center performing DBS. If BoNT injection is considered, then referral should be made to a neurologist with experience with this modality of therapy. Finally, if tremor is complex and diagnosis is unsure, referral to a movement disorders center is suggested.

Special Challenges for Hospitalized Patients

Education of hospital staff should be directed at possible functional impairment. Assistance in feeding and other activities of daily living may be required.

HUNTINGTON DISEASE

Huntington disease is a progressive degenerative disorder of the CNS characterized by involuntary movements (mostly chorea), psychiatric symptoms, and progressive dementia. Prevalence in the United States is approximately 12 per 100,000 population. HD is an autosomal dominant disorder and commonly presents in mid adult life. It is named after George Huntington, who initially described this disease in 1872. The word chorea is derived from the Greek word for dance (*choreia*) and originally was used to describe the dancelike gait and continual limb movements of parainfectious forms of chorea (Sydenham chorea). Choreiform movements disappear during sleep and are exacerbated by nervousness and emotional distress.

Clinical Features

■ **SPECIAL CLINICAL POINT: A patient with HD may manifest disease initially with chorea, psychiatric features, or dementia, although eventually all of these abnormalities are seen.**

HD may begin any time from the first to the eighth decade of life, but it most commonly presents between 35 and 42 years. The onset of chorea is insidious with a few irregular movements of the face and limbs. Patients find themselves to be fidgety and clumsy. The typical history includes slight clumsiness or restlessness that progresses to "piano playing" movements of the fingers and facial grimacing.

Family members notice a peculiar gait associated with irregular involuntary hand movements. The patient may try to mask the involuntary facial movements by chewing gum and the limb movements by sitting on their hands. Carrying out of a continuous movement frequently is impeded by the superimposition of chorea. Reflexes are frequently brisk, but patients rarely have a Babinski sign until the final stages of the disease. Voice often affected is by this condition, and abnormalities of respiratory and articulatory muscles may lead to severe dysarthria and erratic, explosive, speech. As the disorder progresses, the chorea may diminish and rigidity and dystonia emerge. Other movements, including dystonia, parkinsonism, and myoclonus, may predominate instead of chorea.

Approximately 5% of patients have onset in childhood. Of these patients, 60% have parkinsonian features, not chorea. This is known as the Westphal variant. There is an increased incidence of seizures in children with HD (30% to 60%). Children progress more rapidly than adults and die in an average of 9 years. Childhood-onset cases more frequently inherit the disease from their fathers.

Progressive intellectual and psychiatric deterioration can manifest as personality change, depression, or dementia. Some patients show more personality changes than intellectual decline, becoming irritable, agitated, excitable, or apathetic. Inattention, poor concentration and judgment, and eventual memory loss progress until the patient is demented. Other psychiatric features include psychosis and obsessive–compulsive disorder (OCD).

Difficulties include abnormal ocular motor function, gait, and loss of finger and hand dexterity. The ocular motor difficulties include impairment of fixation, increased ocular reaction time with an obvious latency before movement is initiated, loss of smooth pursuit movements, and an inability to look toward an object without accompanying head movements and blinking (impaired saccades). These findings are frequently observed early in the course of the disease. Gait is characterized by a stuttering and dancing character with a wide-based stance, swaying motions, decreased arm swing, spontaneous knee flexion, and variable cadence. The inability to maintain tongue protrusion is a sign of motor impersistence.

■ **SPECIAL CLINICAL POINT: Weight loss can be a serious issue for patients with Huntington disease.**

Patients with HD live 10 to 30 years (average, 17 years) and usually die from pulmonary causes (aspiration pneumonia), sepsis secondary to urinary tract infections, cardiac disease (ischemic heart disease), trauma-related injuries (subdural hematoma) from multiple falls, or nutritional deficiencies. Slower progression of disease is associated with older age of onset and heavier body weight. Since the discovery of the gene, it has become obvious that HD is clinically heterogeneous. For instance, patients with late-onset chorea and no dementia have been shown to have the HD gene. End-stage disease includes loss of ambulatory function, severe dysarthria, dysphagia with aspiration, and dementia.

■ **SPECIAL CLINICAL POINT: The clinical spectrum of Huntington disease is variable, and some patients have more chorea than mental changes, but the reverse is also possible.**

This can lead to difficulties with diagnosis. Because HD is an inherited, progressive, debilitating disorder with no cure, accurate diagnosis is of utmost importance. In the patient with adult-onset chorea, dementia, and a positive family history, the diagnosis can be made easily. However, in patients with chorea and even dementia who have no family history, the diagnosis of HD requires a diagnostic gene test. If a patient has chorea but a definite lack of family history, the chorea may result from some other etiology. However, studies of patients with a sporadic form of chorea resembling HD have shown that a majority of these patients do indeed have the HD gene. A follow-up study of 49 patients suspected to have HD on clinical grounds but without family history revealed that 75% have the disease. Dementia and emotional symptoms are not essential for the diagnosis and are not considered sufficient evidence of HD in a family, but a history of family members hospitalized for these reasons in middle age or because of neurologic problems helps to raise the index of suspicion in patients with choreiform movements. There are a number of disorders that present with chorea (Table 13.6).

Genetics

■ **SPECIAL CLINICAL POINT: Huntington disease is an autosomal dominant disorder with 100% penetrance. Children of an affected parent have a 50% risk of developing the disease.**

The emotional impact of the disease on children of an HD patient is profound. They must watch as a parent deteriorates slowly, inexorably, while facing the prospect of inheriting the same disorder. Enormous advances have been made in the last decade regarding the genetics of HD. In 1993, the HD gene was discovered, and genetic testing became available. The availability of this test has raised a number of ethical questions, most fundamental of which is the following: Why should predictive testing be performed for an illness that has no effective therapy? The impact of revealing to a young healthy person the rather bleak future of HD may be devastating. The results could be marital difficulties leading to disruption of the family and divorce, loss of employment, and psychiatric problems including suicide. However, positive reasons for genetic testing are numerous and include family and financial planning. In at-risk symptomatic patients, genetic testing is the gold standard for diagnosis. Its use will avoid a costly workup for other causes of chorea. In asymptomatic individuals, genetic testing allows for personal and family planning and relieves uncertainty, and in both groups it will prepare patient and physician for treatment possibilities (e.g., clinical trials or new treatment). There are realistic hopes that research in genetics and pathogenesis

TABLE 13.6	Differential Diagnosis of Huntington Disease

Acquired	Inherited
Senile chorea	Benign hereditary chorea
SLE	Familial Alzheimer disease with myoclonus
Antiphospholipid syndrome	Inherited prion disease (including HDL1)
AIDS	Wilson disease
CJD	Neuroacanthocytosis
Tardive dyskinesia in a psychiatric patient	DRPLA (chromosome 11)
Basal ganglia or subthalamic infarction or structural lesion	Spinocerebellar ataxias 1, 3, and 17
Patients with Parkinson disease treated with levodopa	Brain iron accumulation disorders (including PKAN and neuroferritinopathies)
Polycythaemia rubra vera	Friedreich ataxia
Choreoathetotic cerebral palsy	Mitochondrial disease
Chorea gravidarum	MacLeod syndrome
Postinfective (following Sydenham chorea, PANDAS, or herpes simplex encephalitis)	HDL2 (caused by junctophilin mutations)
Other drug-induced choreas (oral contraceptives, anticonvulsants, stimulants, antidepressants, anticholinergics, calcium channel blockers, buspirone)	HDL3 (mutation unknown—extremely rare)
Hyperthyroid chorea	Lysosomal storage disorders
	Tuberous sclerosis
	Amino acid disorders
	Ataxia telangiectasia

SLE, Systemic lupus erythematosus; AIDS, Acquired immunodeficiency syndrome; CJD, Creutzfeldt-Jakob disease; DRPLA, dentatorubral-pallidoluysian atrophy; PANDAS, pediatric autoimmune neuropsychiatric disorders associated with streptococcal infection; PKAN, pantothenate kinase-associated neurodegeneration.

will lead to disease-modifying therapies. There are also legal and social issues related to predictive testing that need to be addressed. Early studies showed that approximately 75% of at-risk patients would be interested in participating in predictive testing, but with the advent of such testing this was found to be a gross overestimation. Experience has demonstrated that less than 5% of at-risk individuals actually request the predictive test.

Huntington disease genetic testing is extremely serious. One can imagine the devastating effect of a positive result on a young asymptomatic person and his or her family, but, surprisingly, a negative result also can cause havoc. Some people live their lives and make decisions based on the probability that they will develop HD. When it is discovered they do not carry the gene, they experience regrets, and this can have a significant impact on family relationships. In addition, there is guilt for being gene negative while other family members suffer with the disease. This may cause the gene-negative persons to either spend inordinate amounts of time helping the affected siblings or distance themselves.

■ SPECIAL CLINICAL POINT: The HD testing process should be performed at a center staffed with the appropriate team of personnel in genetics, neurology, psychiatry, psychology, social work, speech therapy, and nutrition.

The goals of such a program are to ensure that an informed decision is made, to prepare the subject for the result, and to ensure that an adequate support system is in place. The program must have maximal control over whether the patient and his or her family receive this irrevocable information (because of its profound impact); it must provide the opportunity for the patient to withdraw; and it must be able to ensure confidentiality. In most centers, the process of genetic testing for at-risk asymptomatic patients begins with an initial visit to a genetics counselor or psychologist followed by evaluations from neurology and psychiatry. Occasionally, a second genetic visit is required. Once all evaluations are complete, the team meets and addresses whether the patient is already symptomatic, and decides if testing can be performed safely or if it needs to be delayed. The patient then comes in for blood to be drawn and returns for results. Results are never given on phone or by mail. In early symptomatic patients, the process is the same, but in advanced cases, and where a diagnosis is not clear, many of the steps are skipped depending on decisions made by the testing team. In some centers prenatal testing is performed, but this leads to new issues. For instance, a positive test may reveal simultaneously the carrier status in the parent and child (if the parents' status is not known) and counseling regarding the option of terminating the pregnancy. Testing should be avoided under the following circumstances: when not requested by the patient but requested by an employer, insurance company, prison, court, or the military; if the subject is younger than 18 years (debatable); if there is no informed consent; and if the subject has a poor support system. Most clinical geneticists advise against presymptomatic testing of underage patients for adult-onset diseases for which testing provides little or no medical benefit.

The HD gene is on chromosome 4p16.3 and is referred to as IT15 (IT, interesting transcription). The gene product is a protein designated as huntingtin. The abnormality within the gene is a polymorphic trinucleotide repeat sequence $[(CAG)_n]$ that is expanded and unstable and

located on exon 1 of 67. The instability leads to variations (expansion) in length between generations, especially if the father carries the gene. In normal individuals, this sequence repeats up to 29 times. Repeat lengths of 30 to 34 could lead to paternal transmission if expansion occurs, and lengths of 35 to 39 represent an intermediate or a reduced penetrance as well as expansion in offspring. In HD, there are 40 or more copies and every person with this sequence ultimately is affected. Longer segments (55 or greater) are found in juvenile cases, suggesting there is an inverse correlation between repeat length and age of onset of symptoms. This is a statistical correlation, but any given expansion may be associated with a broad range of onset ages and thus is not predictive. The repeat length may expand with each generation if the affected parent is the father and this could lead to the phenomenon of anticipation, when the disease occurs at younger ages with each new generation. There is also a correlation between repeat length and severity of disease and pathology. There are no differences in repeat length in those patients presenting with neurologic or psychiatric symptoms.

Pathology, Neurochemistry, and Pathogenesis

Postmortem examination of brain tissue from patients with HD reveals characteristic pathologic abnormalities. Grossly, the caudate nucleus, putamen, and cerebral cortex are atrophied. In advanced cases brain weight may decrease up to 30%. On microscopic examination, severe neuronal loss and gliosis in the striatum are detected, with the caudate nucleus being more affected than the putamen. Neuronal intranuclear inclusions are seen. Although it has been suggested that early features of disease are related to striatal degeneration, it has been demonstrated that widespread neuronal degeneration occurs early. Occasionally, patients come to postmortem examination with well-documented chorea and no pathologic changes.

Postmortem studies have revealed that levels of many neurotransmitters, biosynthetic enzymes, and receptor-binding sites are abnormal. These studies also indicate that there is selective death of neurons depending on their predominant transmitter type. GABA and glutamic acid decarboxylase (GAD) levels are diminished in the striatum and globus pallidus. A threefold to fivefold relative increase in somatostatin has been discovered in the caudate, putamen, and globus pallidus in patients with HD compared with controls, indicating that the neurons containing it are spared. This indicates that cell death is selective in terms of both regions and cell type. Striatal cholinergic interneurons also appear to be spared. Other neurochemical abnormalities include diminished levels of substance P, cholecystokinin, met-enkephalin, and angiotensin-converting enzyme, plus an increase in neuropeptide Y. All these abnormalities are seen in the basal ganglia. The pathogenesis of the selective neuronal degeneration in the striatum remains unknown.

The study of the pathophysiology of HD has made great progress since the development of transgenic animals. The normal function of huntingtin and the effect of the mutation on that function remain unknown. There are now several transgenic animals including mice, fruit flies, and worms. The key finding in these mice is that they parallel the human disease closely. Clinically they develop a progressive disease with weight loss and a movement disorder, and the pathology is characterized by neuronal loss, gliosis, and neuronal intranuclear inclusions in the striatum. In addition, there is increasing evidence that excitotoxicity, mitochondrial dysfunction, and free radical formation play a role in the pathophysiology of cell death in the animal model. The CAG trinucleotide repeat expansion in the gene results in a polyglutamine (polyQ) stretch within the huntingtin protein near the N-terminus. The protein is necessary for normal growth and development as demonstrated by the fact that knockout animals (not expressing the gene) do not survive. Its role in cell survival may be the result, in part, of enhancement of the transcription of brain-derived neurotrophic factor stimulation. It has been suggested that the mutant gene is less efficient at this task, leading to decreased levels of the nerve growth factor and the development of apoptosis. Huntingtin, in the wild-type form, is ubiquitous, being expressed in the cytoplasm of most cells in the body. In the brain, it primarily is seen in neurons and is associated with several organelles including endoplasmic reticulum, microtubules, vesicles, and mitochondria. The widespread location of the protein begs the question of how selective neuronal degeneration occurs in disease. The mutant protein is found in cytoplasm and the nucleus where it forms aggregates. When the mutant enters the nucleus it is cleaved by caspases, making the protein more susceptible to aggregate formation. The interaction between huntingtin and caspases is an important step in neuronal toxicity. It appears that nuclear aggregates are toxic to cells; in fact, it is suggested that penetration of huntingtin into the nucleus is a necessary step for toxicity. The presence of aggregates disturbs proteolysis within cells. An increased number of polyQ repeats correlates with the number of aggregates. Some additional roles of huntingtin include iron homeostasis, maintenance of perinuclear organelle structure, trafficking of secretory membranes, and gene expression.

Mutant huntingtin potentially affects several pathways to cell death. These include alteration of brain-derived neurotrophic factor activity, excitotoxicity, free radical formation, reduction of energy production, activation of apoptosis, and disruption of gene transcription through varied protein interactions. Entrance of the protein into the nucleus and caspase-induced cleavage and aggregation seem to be important steps in cellular toxicity. All of these mechanisms relate to progression and are being explained as possible disease-altering agents in transgenic animals. Free radical scavengers, glutamate antagonists, creatine, and caspase inhibitors (including minocycline) prolonged life by 20% in mice.

Treatment

Disease-Modifying Agents   The goal of therapy is to find an agent (or agents) that will stop or slow the disease process. Glutamate antagonists have been examined most frequently as disease-modifying therapy. Baclofen, remacemide, riluzole, and lamotrigine all failed. However, remacemide, riluzole, and amantadine have antichoreic effects. Amantadine is readily available, and at 200 to 400 mg/day improvement in chorea can be seen. This drug is better tolerated than neuroleptics in most patients. Free radical scavengers and energy boosters also have been examined in HD. Vitamin E, OPC-14117, and idebenone all failed. However, one study demonstrated possible effects of the supplemental coenzyme Q10. This compound occurs naturally in mitochondria and shuttles electrons between complexes I, II, and III, and it functions as an antioxidant and a respiratory chain activator. Coenzyme Q10 was used in a 30-month, double-blind trial in 360 patients to examine its potential disease-modifying effects. Patients on coenzyme Q10 demonstrated a 13% slowing in total functional capacity decline, which was not significantly different from other groups. Coenzyme Q10 (600 mg/day) was safe and well tolerated. A large scale double-blind, placebo-controlled study of 2400 mg of co-enzyme Q10 is underway (the 2CARE study) and a clinical trial using high-dose creatine has also just begun.

Symptomatic Therapy   The management of HD involves a multidisciplinary approach. HD clinics usually include neurologists, genetic counselors, psychologists, psychiatrists, speech therapists, physiotherapists, nutritionists, and social workers. From the neurologic standpoint the only feature amenable to symptomatic therapy is the movement disorder. Historically, the mainstay of therapy for chorea has been dopamine receptor antagonists. Phenothiazines (e.g., chlorpromazine) and butyrophenones (e.g., haloperidol) share the property of dopaminergic receptor blockade and may be required for relief of chorea.

■ **SPECIAL CLINICAL POINT: In Huntington disease, improvement in chorea may not improve functional ability or quality of life. Frequently a patient with gait disorder and chorea is treated with neuroleptics, but often the gait worsens because of the development of parkinsonism.**

The treatment of chorea should be limited to those in whom it is severe and troublesome. Atypical antipsychotics may have a role because of their potential for fewer extrapyramidal effects. Clozapine (25 to 500 mg/day) yields some improvement in chorea, but is often associated with sedation and little or no improvement in quality of life. Experience with risperidone for symptomatic treatment of chorea is even more limited. It appears to have an effect similar to haloperidol when used at doses between 1 and 6 mg/day. There is no significant literature regarding the use of other atypical agents in HD. Experience from practice has demonstrated that risperidone and olanzapine can be used in a manner similar to standard neuroleptics for the treatment of chorea. Quetiapine has even less effect, but atypical agents should be used prior to standard neuroleptics in the treatment of chorea. Other agents that decrease striatal dopaminergic activity and should reduce chorea include reserpine, alpha-methylparatyrosine, and tetrabenazine. Historically, reserpine was the first agent reported to be of use in the treatment of chorea. Reserpine acts to block intravesicular neurotransmitter reuptake and depletes the brain of dopamine. It also depletes central norepinephrine and serotonin, and is used in the treatment of HD at doses of 0.5 to 3 mg/day because it has a less severe side-effect profile than dopamine antagonists. Tetrabenazine, a dopamine depletor with minor dopamine receptor–blocking effects, is a reversible vesicle uptake inhibitor and is useful in HD. Tetrabenazine adverse events (hypotension and depression) are less severe than those of reserpine. The typical dose is 50 to 200 mg/day. Tetrabenazine is the first drug approved by the FDA for its use in the symptomatic treatment of chorea in patients with HD at doses of up to 100 mg/day.

■ **SPECIAL CLINICAL POINT: Psychiatric symptoms need to be treated aggressively in HD, and pharmacologic therapy may be very helpful.**

Atypical antipsychotics should be the first agents used in treating psychosis. Quetiapine, olanzapine, risperidone, and clozapine all have been shown to be effective in treating HD-related psychosis. These agents also may be of benefit in agitation and irritability. For depression, anxiety, and obsessive–compulsive symptoms serotonin reuptake inhibitors are effective and well tolerated. In the case of depression, particular care should be taken in assessing whether the patient is at risk for suicide. In addition to pharmacotherapy, many of these issues can be addressed with psychologic approaches.

There are several other issues that are addressed routinely at HD clinic visits. These include disability, speech disorders and dysphagia, nutritional status, weight loss, and home safety. These problems require the assessment of physical and speech therapists, nutritionists, and social workers. The goals are improved quality of life and a safe environment at home. There are some nursing homes that specialize in HD care.

■ **SPECIAL CLINICAL POINT: The most difficult decisions surround the need for feeding tubes and nursing home placement.**

When to Refer to a Neurologist or Other Specialist

All patients with HD should be referred to a neurologist or psychiatrist involved in a multidisciplinary clinic to provide comprehensive care. This is particularly true for those with more advanced disease. At-risk patients (affected parent or sibling) who request presymptomatic testing should be referred to a testing center.

Special Challenges for Hospitalized Patients

Hospital staff should be educated regarding variability of chorea and the relationship of severity of chorea to stress. Behavioral abnormalities are frequent in these patients, and staff should be aware of them.

WILSON DISEASE

Wilson disease, or hepatolenticular degeneration, is a rare neurologic disorder of copper metabolism with a prevalence of approximately 5 to 20 per million; its prevalence is higher in countries with increased consanguinity, but it is present worldwide. Copper accumulation becomes toxic and causes signs and symptoms that are neurologic (most notably movement disorders), psychiatric, hepatic, or ocular, but they may occur in variable combinations, making WD a difficult disorder to recognize.

■ **SPECIAL CLINICAL POINT: The importance of recognizing Wilson disease cannot be overstated because it is a treatable and often reversible disorder that otherwise inevitably results in death. The only way to make the diagnosis is to always keep it in mind. Approximately 75% of deaths from WD result from a failure to make the diagnosis.**

Clinical Manifestations

Approximately 40% of patients with WD present with neurologic signs and symptoms. The most common are speech and extrapyramidal disorders beginning at 18 to 20 years of age. WD has a slowly progressive course, often with a single symptom predominating for months or even years before other manifestations appear. However, there may be a sudden dramatic worsening of what appears to be a stable neurologic deficit.

Incoordination involving fine finger movements such as in handwriting and typing is frequently an early manifestation. It may be subtle at first but worsens as the disorder progresses.

Resting tremor is a common early manifestation, and when associated with rigidity, bradykinesia, and/or gait difficulty, WD may mimic Parkinson disease. The tremor may be postural or kinetic. When severe, it takes on a flapping quality at the wrist with high-amplitude oscillations and a "wing beating" appearance at the shoulder, often resulting in significant disability. Some patients present with bradykinesia and rigidity without tremor.

Focal or generalized dystonia is also a common and predominant symptom of WD. Chorea is rare but may result in movements and a gait disorder that resemble HD. Spasticity and ataxia are rare.

Dysarthria is a consistent feature of WD. It sometimes is associated with dysphagia, and frequently patients show frustration because of their difficulty communicating. Often patients develop a characteristic facial expression with retraction of the upper lip, the mouth constantly agape, and upper teeth protruding. This gives the patient the appearance of grinning, or a "vacuous smile."

Approximately 6% of patients have generalized seizures. A majority of the symptoms are exacerbated by emotional stress and ameliorated by calm and sleep. There is also an acute dystonic form of WD. These patients appear ill, and they have a high fever, significant muscle rigidity, rapid emaciation, and confusion, a picture that can be confused with a neuroleptic malignant syndrome. This acute presentation could be a preterminal event, so diagnosis is of utmost importance. Because of the protean nature of WD, it is very important to consider this diagnosis in all patients under the age of 40 years presenting with movement disorders.

Approximately 25% of patients with WD are seen first by psychiatrists for a wide range of emotional difficulties. At least 50% of patients have early psychiatric manifestations. There are no psychiatric manifestations that are specific for WD, and diagnoses may range from adolescent adjustment reactions to depression and schizophrenia. The most common features include abnormal behavior, such as irritability, incongruous behavior, aggression, and personality change. Depression and cognitive impairment are also common, but schizophreniform psychosis is rare. Isolated psychiatric problems may be seen without neurologic deficits, making differentiation from the primary psychiatric disorders quite difficult. However, there frequently are neurologic findings in association with the psychiatric symptoms, and this clinical situation should raise the index of suspicion that WD may be the cause of the patients' problem. In fact, psychiatric symptoms are more closely related to the presence of neurologic features than hepatic features. Some patients with psychiatric manifestations treated with neuroleptics, who later develop movement disorders, are misdiagnosed as having a primary psychiatric disorder and TD.

■ **SPECIAL CLINICAL POINT: Some have advocated that all patients admitted to psychiatric wards under the age of 30 years should be screened for Wilson disease.**

Hepatic disease may be superimposed on neurologic manifestations or may be the presenting problem in 30% to 50% of patients. Hepatic disease usually presents at an earlier age (approximately age 10) than the neurologic symptomatology of WD, and hepatic patients with WD may be psychologically and neurologically normal.

There are four different presentations for hepatic WD. First, there may be a transient acute hepatitis that resolves spontaneously. This is often misdiagnosed as infectious mononucleosis or viral hepatitis because patients present with the typical hepatic symptoms and signs such as jaundice, malaise, and anorexia. The second presentation is fulminant hepatitis, which is seen in adolescents and which presents with sudden onset of jaundice and ascites progressing relentlessly to hepatic failure and death. Third, and most common, is chronic active hepatitis that presents with weakness, anorexia, jaundice, malaise, and abnormal liver function tests. Finally, patients may present with cirrhosis, and nearly all patients have some residual cirrhosis.

■ **SPECIAL CLINICAL POINT: All patients with Wilson disease and neurologic symptoms exhibit a Kayser–Fleischer (KF) ring in the cornea.**

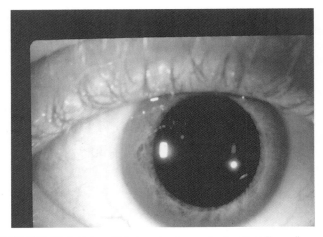

FIGURE 13.4 Kaiser–Fleischer ring in a patient with Wilson disease.

This is a golden or greenish-brown ring that represents copper deposition in Descemet's membrane (Fig. 13.4). The ring is seen easily around the limbus in patients with light-colored or blue eyes but may be quite difficult to see in those with brown eyes. A slit lamp examination should be performed by an experienced ophthalmologist to accurately diagnose a KF ring in all those suspected of WD. Although a KF ring is not pathognomonic for WD, its presence is important in the diagnosis. It fades with adequate chelation therapy.

Another unusual ocular manifestation of WD is the sunflower cataract. This is a disc-shaped opacity with frond-like radiations that often are described as a "cataract like the rays of the Sun."

Other possible manifestations of WD include Coomb negative hemolytic anemia, skeletal changes including pathologic fractures from metabolic bone disease and hypertrophic osteoarthropathy, renal disease including gross hematuria, stones, tubular and glomerular disease, and the Fanconi syndrome, and cardiac symptoms including arrhythmia and cardiomyopathy.

Neuropathology

The lenticular nuclei are involved bilaterally and symmetrically. The lesions vary from softening and discoloration to frank cavitation. Other areas less significantly involved include the subcortical white matter, cerebellum (most commonly the dentate nucleus), and other nuclei that make up the basal ganglia. Excess copper is distributed throughout the CNS. Neuronal loss is observed in the basal ganglia and, to a lesser extent, in the cerebral cortex.

Pathogenesis and Genetics

Excessive accumulation of copper as a result of poor copper excretion leads to organ system dysfunction and clinical stigmata of WD. Ceruloplasmin, a copper-containing polypeptide, is deficient in 95% of patients with WD. Biliary excretion of copper in WD is impaired and copper accumulates in the liver, binding to thiol and carboxyl groups on copper-storage proteins. The copper binding alters both structure and function of storage proteins, disrupting normal cellular activity in a variety of ways. When storage reaches capacity, excess copper begins to move into extrahepatic storage sites, particularly the eye and brain. This explains why KF rings are not seen in 50% of patients with hepatic WD.

Wilson disease is an autosomal recessive disorder with the gene locus located on chromosome

13q14–21. In 1993 the WD gene was cloned, and the gene frequency is 0.6% with a carrier frequency of 1 in 90. The gene codes for a copper-transporting p-type ATPase called ATP7B. ATP7B functions in copper transport coupled with the synthesis of ceruloplasmin in the Golgi apparatus. The abnormal protein from the mutated gene leads to decreased function, which causes failure of the liver to excrete copper into the bile. Since more than 300 gene mutations have been identified, genetic testing is not available.

Diagnosis

■ **SPECIAL CLINICAL POINT: It can never be said enough that a high index of suspicion is very important in making the diagnosis of WD. This is especially true when evaluating patients 40 years or younger who present with extrapyramidal disorders, psychiatric disorders (especially when associated with neurologic signs and symptoms), and hepatic disease.**

In addition, a family history of WD (particularly a sibling) or hepatic disease at a young age should alert the physician to a possible diagnosis of WD. Once suspected, the diagnosis of WD can be confirmed using four tests: (a) a slit lamp examination for KF rings (the specificity of KF rings for patients with neuropsychiatric WD is nearly 100%), (b) a serum ceruloplasmin level (usually low in 80% of patients with WD), (c) 24-hour urinary copper excretion (elevated in WD to more than 100 µg), and (d) a liver biopsy with quantitation of copper concentration—the most definitive of all tests (copper levels higher than 250 mg/g of dry tissue are considered diagnostic).

Clinical evaluation and the first three tests are usually sufficient to make the diagnosis of WD in symptomatic patients, and liver biopsy is not required. A normal serum ceruloplasmin level (often used to screen for WD) by itself should not convince the treating physician that WD is ruled out because 5% to 20% of patients with WD have normal levels. This is due, in part, to overestimation of ceruloplasmin concentrations with immunologic (as opposed to enzymatic) assays, as well as due to false elevation of ceruloplasmin in acute inflammation, pregnancy, estrogen supplementation, and use of oral contraceptives. Low ceruloplasmin levels are not diagnostic of WD, especially if the clinical presentation is not consistent. Other conditions where there is marked protein loss, copper deficiency, or rarely Menkes disease and aceruloplasminemia will also exhibit low ceruloplasmin levels.

If ceruloplasmin level is low, examination for KF ring and 24-hour urine copper excretion must be performed. If ceruloplasmin is normal and KF ring is present, a liver biopsy should be performed to make the diagnosis. Hepatic WD is the most difficult presentation to diagnose because ceruloplasmin may be falsely elevated or normal in WD hepatitis and a KF ring may be absent.

■ **SPECIAL CLINICAL POINT: If confusion remains after serum ceruloplasmin levels, slit lamp examination, and 24-hour urinary copper concentration, liver biopsy is required.**

Wilson disease is inherited as an autosomal recessive disorder, so each sibling of a patient with WD has a 25% chance of having the disease.

■ **SPECIAL CLINICAL POINT: All siblings of patients with Wilson disease should be screened. If they have WD, treatment will prevent onset of clinical stigmata.**

At-risk siblings should have slit lamp examination and 24-hour urinary copper and ceruloplasmin determination, along with physical and neurologic examinations at regular intervals. If a KF ring is present, ceruloplasmin level is low, and urinary excretion of copper is elevated, the diagnosis of WD is clear and liver biopsy is not required. However, if the serum ceruloplasmin level is low but KF ring is absent, the patient may be a heterozygote for WD and liver biopsy will be necessary to make a definitive diagnosis. Ten percent to 20% of heterozygotes have low serum ceruloplasmin levels, but these patients do not require treatment.

Following the discovery of multiple polymorphic DNA markers close to the gene on chromosome 13, multilocus linkage analysis makes possible accurate and informative testing of potential carriers in families with WD in whom the mutation has been found. Such testing is now commercially available from certain clinical laboratories. With these techniques, one could discriminate between carriers and presymptomatic patients. Advantages of this technique include its noninvasive nature and early (possibly prenatal) diagnosis. Direct mutation analysis by whole-genome sequencing is also feasible and can be integral to the diagnosis in patients where clinical and biochemical investigations have been unrevealing.

Neuroimaging techniques are not diagnostic in WD, but typical lesions can be observed. On CT scanning, cortical and brainstem atrophy are seen in nearly all patients. Hypodensity of the head of the caudate and putamen is seen early, and cavitation of the putamen is seen late. Sometimes, hypodensities are seen in other areas including cerebellum, brainstem, thalamus, and cerebral cortex. These lesions do not enhance with contrast. On MRI scanning, hypointense lesions are observed in the lenticular nucleus, thalamus, caudate nucleus, cerebellum, brainstem, and subcortical white matter on T1-weighted images whereas hyperintense lesions are observed on T2-weighted images (Fig. 13.5). The accumulation of copper leads to areas of hypointensity adjacent to the hyperintense regions (Fig. 13.5B). These changes are seen in all patients with neurologic symptoms and represent edema, gliosis, or cystic lesions.

Treatment

Once the diagnosis of WD is confirmed, treatment should be instituted without delay. There is now a choice of agents including chelating agents such as D-penicillamine, trientine, or zinc acetate, all of which are now FDA approved (Table 13.7). There is also an experimental agent that shows great promise, tetrathiomolybdate

(TTM). D-penicillamine, a potent chelating agent with thiol groups to bind copper and remove it from organ systems via urinary excretion, had been the treatment of choice for decades. Penicillamine has a rapid action in mobilizing and clearing copper through the urine. Four divided doses of 1 to 2 g should be given 30 minutes before or 2 hours after meals to ensure maximal absorption. Pyridoxine, 25 mg/day, should be added because of an antipyridoxine effect of penicillamine. Improvement begins 2 weeks to 1 year after the institution of therapy. Of patients with WD, 75% to 80% respond successfully to penicillamine. In the first 2 months of therapy, complete blood count, urinalysis, and liver enzyme levels should be examined frequently. Some patients initially worsen with penicillamine therapy.

Adverse effects of penicillamine are many and occur early and late. Early adverse effects include hypersensitivity reactions, fever, rash, adenopathy, leukopenia, thrombocytopenia, collagen vascular disorders, and bone marrow suppression. Late adverse effects occurring after a year of therapy include nephrotic syndrome, agranulocytosis, thrombocytopenia, Goodpasture syndrome, pemphigus, myasthenia gravis, elastosis perforans serpiginosa, and dermopathy. Serious intolerance to penicillamine occurs in only 3% to 5% of patients, and these patients require alternative therapy.

Trientine, like penicillamine, is a copper-chelating agent and is the alternative chelation therapy of choice. The dose is 1 to 1.5 g/day 30 minutes before or 2 hours after meals. Trientine is effective for the treatment of WD, apparently has fewer side effects than penicillamine, and only rarely causes acute worsening. Adverse effects include collagen vascular disorders and iron-deficiency anemia.

Two newer therapies have changed the approach to these patients. Zinc acetate, approved by the FDA in 1997, induces excretion of copper via the gastrointestinal tract by increasing the concentration of metallothionein in the bowel mucosa by 25-fold. As the tissue content

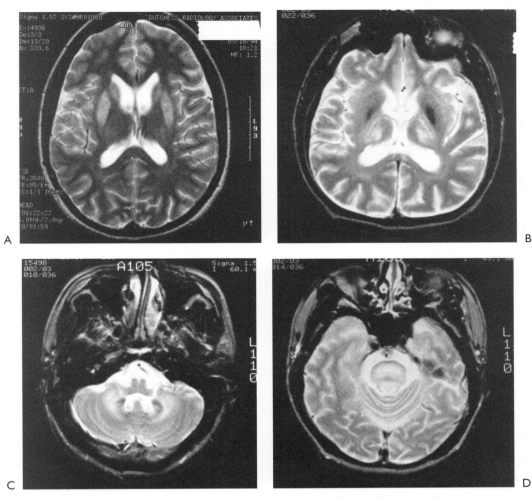

FIGURE 13.5 A: T2-weighted magnetic resonance imaging (MRI) scan of a patient with early symptomatic Wilson disease, demonstrating hyperintensity in the caudate nucleus and putamen. **B:** T2-weighted MRI scan of a more advanced patient with hypointensity in the striatum. The same scan as seen in **(B)**, showing hyperintensity in the dentate nucleus of the cerebellum **(C)** and the pons **(D)**.

of this protein increases, the proportion of copper in the cells increases. Then, as the mucosal cells are sloughed and lost in the stool, copper is excreted. Metallothionein levels also increase in the liver; this increases liver copper levels, but the copper is stored in a nontoxic form. Initially, zinc has a slower effect on copper excretion than the chelating agents. The dose is started at 50 to 100 mg three times a day 1 hour after or before food or beverage in adults and 50 mg twice a day in children, and the ultimate daily dose ranges from 300 to 1200 mg/day. Patients are monitored by following urinary copper levels. Monitoring should be performed within the first 2 weeks, and if no change is seen the dose is increased. The final dose is individualized. Zinc is less toxic than penicillamine and does not cause paradoxical worsening of

TABLE 13.7 Medical Treatment of Wilson Disease		
Drug Name	Initial Daily Dose	Usual Daily Dose
Penicillamine	125 mg q.i.d.	250 mg q.i.d.
Trientine	250 mg q.i.d.	250 mg q.i.d.
Zinc acetate	50 mg t.i.d.	50 mg t.i.d.
Tetrathiomolybdate[a]	20 mg 6 times	20 mg 6 times

[a]Currently experimental.

symptoms as penicillamine can. The side effects include gastrointestinal irritation, elevation of serum amylase, and decreased high-density lipoprotein. Rarely, copper deficiency can occur, leading to leukopenia and anemia. It has been used successfully as both initial treatment and maintenance.

The newest treatment is tetrathiomolybdate (TTM). When given with meals it prevents absorption of copper, and when given between meals it is absorbed into the blood and forms complexes with copper and albumin, rendering the copper nontoxic. It has a rapid action in relation to copper metabolism and does not cause worsening of symptoms. It has been studied for initial therapy but not for maintenance. The daily maintenance dose is 20 mg six times a day, three doses with and three without meals. One side effect is a reversible anemia. The drug is experimental and has limited availability.

Initial treatment of WD has become controversial. Currently, most recommend that a chelating agent should be included in initial treatment. Some argue that the old reliable treatment of penicillamine chelation therapy, based on decades of experience (since the 1950s), should not be abandoned. Others argue that zinc is the appropriate choice because it is equally effective, is much better tolerated, and does not cause paradoxical worsening. For hepatic presentations, it is suggested that zinc and a chelating agent be used concurrently. Some suggest trientine because it is less toxic than penicillamine. For neuropsychiatric presentations, zinc and a chelating agent should be initiated unless TTM is available. For maintenance, zinc is the treatment of choice. No formal controlled trials were conducted to examine this issue. Zinc has become the treatment of choice in presymptomatic and pregnant patients. Copper-rich foods particularly shellfish and liver should be avoided.

Frequently, patients whose neurologic symptoms have resolved are tempted to stop their chronic medication. It may become difficult for asymptomatic patients to connect their good health to their chronic medication. Discontinuing chelation therapy invariably results in disaster for these patients, many of whom die of fulminant hepatitis within 3 years. It is the physician's job to reinforce the need for medication and to inform these patients of the disastrous results that lie ahead should the medication be stopped. Response to medication should be monitored using 24-hour urinary copper levels. Chelating agents will cause an increase in urinary copper output before a decrease.

For patients with liver failure the standard measures taken should include lactulose, neomycin, and protein restriction. Liver transplant is sometimes the only treatment alternative in patients with fulminant hepatitis and cirrhosis with liver failure. The 1-year survival rate is about 80% and the 5-year survival rate is 40% to 70%. These numbers are quite respectable, especially in this situation in which all patients will otherwise die.

There is no role for alternative therapies in WD. Physical, occupational, and speech therapy may play a role. Speech therapy and assistive devices can be helpful for the dysarthria that characterizes WD. Physical therapy may be useful for treating dystonia and gait disorders, perhaps with the addition of assistive devices such as walkers. Occupational therapy can help patients who have dystonia and tremor to continue to function.

When to Refer to a Neurologist or Other Specialist

Wilson disease is a complex disorder with regard to diagnosis and assessment of siblings. Any patient with neuropsychiatric symptoms should be referred to a neurologist. Treatment is also a complicated matter best handled by a neurologist with experience. When the diagnosis is suspected and an evaluation for a KF ring is sought, it should be performed by an experienced ophthalmologist. Finally, all patients should have an evaluation by a gastroenterologist.

GILLES DE LA TOURETTE SYNDROME

Gilles de la Tourette syndrome is a movement disorder dominated by tics and various behavioral abnormalities. It is seen in approximately 1% to 3% of school children and is three times more common in males than females.

Tics are sudden, brief, intermittent, stereotyped involuntary movements or sounds. They are classified according to whether they are motor or vocal (phonic), simple or complex. Simple motor tics are abrupt, brief, purposeless, isolated (single muscle or muscle group) movements that are jerky or clonic emerging out of a background of normal activity. Examples of simple motor tics are eye blinks, head or limb jerks, and shoulder shrugs. Complex motor tics are more coordinated, sequential, and complicated movements or gestures that almost may appear purposeful but are inappropriately intense and timed. Examples of complex motor tics include eye deviation, facial grimacing, hand shaking, waving arm movements, muscle flexing and posing with isometric or tonic movements, touching, jumping, hitting, kicking, squatting, truncal bending or gyrating, copropraxia (making obscene gestures), and echopraxia (mimicking the movements of others).

Sometimes, a cluster of simple tics will appear to be complex. In extreme cases tics may be so forceful as to cause self-injurious behavior such as cervical injury with neck tics or lip biting. Simple vocal tics are a variety of inarticulate noises and sounds. Examples include sniffing, snorting, barking, throat clearing, and grunting. Complex vocal tics are linguistically meaningful utterances. They can include the utilization of words (no-no), phrases (oh boy), or even sentences. Classical forms of complex vocal tics include palilalia (involuntary repetition of words or sentences), echolalia (involuntary repetition of words or sentences just spoken by another person), and coprolalia (involuntary utterances of curse words). This latter phenomenon is perhaps the best known feature in GTS, but it occurs in less than 10% of patients. Coprolalia is distinguished from emotion-driven swearing by its cadence, volume, and context. Vocal tics tend to occur at phrase junctions in speech and can cause blockage or hesitation of speech patterns.

Although motor tics are commonly clonic or rapid in nature, when they are slow, twisting, and result in brief sustained postures (resembling dystonia), they are referred to as dystonic tics. A common type involves slow shoulder shrugging with rotational scapular movements. Others include blepharospasm, ocular deviations, and torticollis. Sensory tics (premonitory sensations) are patterns of somatic sensations that have been variously described as a pressure, a tickle, a temperature change, paresthesias, or an uncomfortable feeling, localized to specific body regions, and resulting in dysphoric feelings. These uncomfortable sensations may provoke a motor or a vocal tic such as limb stretching, blepharospasm, and throat clearing. This indicates that the tic itself actually may be a voluntary movement under conscious control (sometimes referred to as "unvoluntary"). The uncomfortable sensation is usually relieved by this movement, but relief is only temporary, leading to repeated movements.

Tics have a number of characteristic features that help to differentiate them from other movement disorders. They are suppressible to some extent. Often, when patients with GTS come into the physician's office, their history of tics is a better indication than just observation because patients can suppress their tics (and often do) in the office. In addition, tics tend to wax and wane, so they can vary in intensity over time and occur in bouts. This can have a significant bearing on clinical trials. They also tend to change location over time. More frequently, tics begin in the eyes with eye blinking and then move so that there are neck movements or shoulder shrugs or other types of movements. Patients often will describe an inner tension or urge that is transiently relieved by the tic itself. When patients suppress the tics, the inner tension grows and there often will be a flurry of tics once the suppression is released. Patients often will give a history of having few tics during work but a flurry of them once they return home at the end of the day. Tics, in general, increase with stress, anger, and excitement and decrease with relaxation, concentration, distraction, and sleep. The urges or sensations may be disabling by themselves.

Tics usually begin between the ages of 3 and 8 years, although GTS is defined by onset prior to age 21. They start as facial movements, especially blinking, and then move to other regions including neck and shoulders. Vocal tics typically occur after the motor tics. Tics reach peak severity in the early to mid second decade and then diminish by the beginning of the third decade. By 18 years, up to 50% of patients may be tic-free. In the rest the movement disorder persists into adulthood but with diminished severity. There are occasional cases with adult-onset tics. The severity of tics in childhood has no bearing on severity in adulthood because even the most severe cases can improve or even disappear. Moderate to severe tics in late adolescence, however, can be an indication that patients will have more severe tics in adulthood. Despite difficulties in school at younger ages, most people with tics are employed or complete their education as young adults and become very well adjusted. The need for treatment diminishes in adulthood.

Clinical Spectrum of Tic Disorders

■ SPECIAL CLINICAL POINT: Tic disorders represent a continuum from a mild transient form to a potentially devastating neurobehavioral disorder.

Transient tic disorder is probably the most common and mildest form of the disorder. It is defined as the duration of the tic disorder of less than 12 months. As such, the diagnosis is often retrospective. In these patients, tics are usually the simple motor type. Chronic multiple tic disorder is a more severe form than transient tic disorder. Patients have multiple motor or vocal tics but not both. Multiple motor tics are much more common. The duration of this syndrome is longer than 1 year. GTS represents the full expression of the tic disorder. Estimates of the prevalence of GTS are probably significantly lower than actual prevalence because, in milder cases, a large percentage of patients are unaware that they have a tic disorder and in many the tics are not bothersome so they do not seek medical assistance.

Associated Behavioral Disturbances

■ SPECIAL CLINICAL POINT: Obsessive–compulsive disorder is present in 20% to 60% of patients with Gilles de la Tourette syndrome.

This behavioral disorder appears to be linked genetically to GTS and may represent an alternate expression of this disorder. Symptoms can result in significant stress and disability. Examples of compulsive symptoms include ordered arranging habits, rituals of decontamination, including repeated hand washing, checking rituals (locks on doors or cars and stove switches), and ritualistic counting. Obsessive thoughts often intrude on conscious thoughts and interrupt daily routines. Compulsions relieve the obsessions. Examples of obsessions include fears and images of injuries to loved ones, fear of contamination with germs, dirt, or disease, feelings of responsibility for misfortune of others, feelings of doubt that one has performed tasks that are already completed, and need for exactness and symmetry. Compulsive behavior and tics, particularly complex ones, can overlap and they may be difficult to differentiate. OCD symptoms, like tics, wax and wane and increase with stress.

Another common behavioral disturbance associated with GTS is attention deficit hyperactivity disorder (ADHD). In these patients, the disorder can result in a short attention span, restlessness, poor concentration, diminished impulse control, and hyperactivity.

■ **SPECIAL CLINICAL POINT: Attention deficit hyperactivity disorder (ADHD) may be present in 40% to 70% of children with Gilles de la Tourette syndrome, and it is not uncommon for ADHD to precede the onset of tics.**

Attention deficit hyperactivity disorder seems to be more common in patients with severe tic disorder. Increased irritability, rage attacks, vulnerability to drug abuse, depression, and antisocial behavior are common in patients with ADHD. Stimulant medications used for primary ADHD were believed to provoke or exacerbate tics. A study by the Tourette Study Group using methylphenidate (MPH) dispelled that myth and demonstrated that MPH can be used in this population with no risk of inducing tics.

Other behavioral abnormalities include learning disabilities, oppositional defiant disorder, anxiety (separation anxiety), depression, mania, conduct disorders, self-injurious behavior, phobias (simple, social, agoraphobia), dyslexia, and stuttering.

■ **SPECIAL CLINICAL POINT: Behavioral disorders occur 5 to 20 times more commonly in patients with Gilles de la Tourette syndrome than in the general population.**

It is difficult to know whether these disorders are secondary to the primary aspects of the disease (tics, OCD, ADHD) or they are neurobiologically linked. Sleep disorders including somnambulism, night terrors, nightmares, disturbances in sleep initiation, and maintenance are present in about 50% of the patients.

Diagnosis and Differential Diagnosis

The diagnosis of GTS is based on clinical symptoms; there are no diagnostic laboratory tests. Because the features can be so varied, there is often a delay in diagnosis. Many patients diagnose themselves based on what they see on television or read on the Internet. Often when patients recognize their own symptoms they seek a medical opinion. The Tourette Syndrome Classification Study Group formulated diagnostic criteria for GTS, which include the following: (a) both multiple motor and one or more phonic tics must be present sometime during the illness, not necessarily concurrently; (b) tics must occur many times per day, nearly every day, for a period of more than a year; (c) the anatomic location, number, frequency, type, complexity, or severity of tics must change over time; (d) the onset is earlier than the age of 21 years; (e) the symptoms must not be explainable by other medical conditions; and (f) the tics should be witnessed by a reliable examiner at some point.

Tics may be secondary to other etiologies. Tics have been seen in patients after stroke, tumor, head trauma, peripheral trauma (neck or face), encephalitis (and postencephalitic syndrome of encephalitis lethargica), and carbon monoxide poisoning. Lesions in these disorders include frontal and temporal lobe and basal ganglia. The most common cause of secondary tics is chronic use of neuroleptic medications (tardive tics). These patients usually have onset in adulthood and a clear history of neuroleptic exposure prior to the onset of the disorder. Other drugs that cause tics include anticonvulsants (phenytoin, carbamazepine), stimulants (including cocaine), and antihistamines. Finally, tics can be a manifestation of chronic neurodegenerative disorders; examples include HD and neuroacanthocytosis. They also can be a manifestation of developmental diseases or chromosomal disorders; examples include Klinefelter syndrome, Down syndrome, and fragile X disease.

Genetics and Pathophysiology

Evidence from the study of multiple large families and twins has suggested that GTS is an autosomal dominant disorder. It has variable expressivity, including transient tic disorder, chronic multiple tic disorder, GTS, and OCD, and is sex influenced because males are affected more than females. Several methods have been used to isolate genes linked to GTS. The nature of GTS genes that lead to the development of the disorder remains elusive. Other disease aspects suggest a genetic pattern different from a major dominant gene and that it is more likely to be a complex polygenetic pattern. It has also been suggested that genomic imprinting, in which gene expression is altered by whether the gene is inherited from the father or mother, may play a role in GTS. GTS appears to be genetically heterogeneous, relating to the interaction of several genes and influenced, to some extent, by nongenetic factors.

Despite clear genetic influences, there appear to be nongenetic developmental factors that influence the form and severity of the disorder. Such factors include maternal life stresses during pregnancy, smoking during pregnancy, gender of the child, severe nausea and/or vomiting in the first trimester, and birth weight.

One possible environmental cause of GTS that is currently a matter of debate involves its relationship with streptococcal infection. It is proposed that an antibody response results in the development of cross-reactive antibodies against neuronal substrates, so-called "antineuronal antibodies." Some have argued that the development of tics or OCD falls into the spectrum of childhood-onset disorders called PANDAS (pediatric autoimmune neuropsychiatric disorders associated with streptococcal infection). Although some patients with GTS have been found to have antistreptococcal antibodies and antineuronal antibodies in the sera, the connection between the two remains to be proven. There is no association between antibody titer and severity of tics, no clear temporal association between infection and exacerbation of symptoms, and no occurrence of inflammatory symptoms such as polyarthritis or mitral valve disease. Although it is possible that tics may result from a postinfectious process in a subgroup of patients much the way chorea does (Sydenham chorea), it seems unlikely that this is the cause of GTS.

The neuroanatomic location of the abnormality resulting in GTS is unknown. It is suspected from cases of secondary tic disorders and imaging with PET, SPECT, and MRI that the basal ganglia (particularly striatum), midbrain, frontal and medial temporal lobes, and limbic structures may be involved. The biochemical basis of GTS is also not clearly understood. However, there is evidence to suggest that increase in activity of the dopamine systems is involved. This evidence includes (a) response to dopamine antagonist medications, (b) response to dopamine-depleting medications (reserpine, tetrabenazine), (c) occurrence of tardive tics, (d) presence of alterations in dopamine metabolites in the cerebrospinal fluid of patients with GTS, and (e) possible increase in density of presynaptic dopamine transporters and postsynaptic D_2 receptors. Two hypotheses related to this increase in dopamine stimulation have been suggested. The more prominent one is that there is dopamine receptor supersensitivity in the basal ganglia, similar to that described in TD. There is also the possibility that there is an increase in dopamine input into the striatum. However, the recent discovery that dopamine agonist medications actually may alleviate tics has placed the hyperdopaminergic hypothesis in question. Pathologic studies, which are few, have demonstrated various neurochemical alterations in the brain. Dynorphin levels (from the opiate system) have been found to be reduced in the lateral globus pallidus; serotonin levels are low in the brainstem; and glutamate was found to be diminished in the globus pallidus.

Treatment

Effective pharmacologic treatment is available for GTS and its many behavioral manifestations. Multidisciplinary treatment involving a neurologist, psychiatrist, and social worker is the best approach, with patient education as a key component. It may be that many patients with this disorder do not need treatment because their symptoms are mild. If symptoms are not disruptive or disabling, patients should be treated supportively. Some patients may do well with behavioral therapy, such as relaxation training and self-monitoring. However, benefits of such therapies are usually temporary. Nevertheless, they may be useful when used in conjunction with pharmacotherapy. Pharmacologic treatment should be used only in those patients who are severely troubled by their symptomatology.

■ **SPECIAL CLINICAL POINT: A team approach to evaluating patients with Gilles de la Tourette syndrome can dictate which group of symptoms require treatment (i.e., tics or behavioral disorder). Treatment should be individualized and directed toward those specific symptoms that are most troublesome (Table 13.8).**

With regard to tic control, dopamine receptor antagonists (neuroleptics) historically have been the most frequently used and effective drugs. Haloperidol (0.25 to 2.5 mg/day) at bedtime can be effective in up to 80% of patients. Adverse effects can be limiting and include sedation, dysphoria, weight gain, TD, acute movement disorders (akathisia, acute dystonia, parkinsonism), depression, poor school performance, and school phobias.

Other neuroleptic medications with fewer side effects include pimozide (1.5 to 10 mg/day). This drug can cause prolongation of the QT interval, which could lead to cardiac dysrhythmias. An electrocardiogram is required at baseline and should be repeated periodically. Atypical neuroleptics including clozapine have been used in a limited number of patients with GTS with mixed results. Risperidone demonstrated efficacy in several case reports, short-term open trials, and placebo-controlled trials in treating motor tics and perhaps OCD. Approximately 30% to 60% of patients had tic improvement. A 12-week, double-blind, randomized comparison with pimozide was reported in 50 patients with GTS. The final mean doses were 3.8 mg/day for risperidone and 2.9 mg/day for pimozide. Both treatments resulted in a significant improvement in tic measures with no difference between groups. Results were similar for children and adults.

TABLE 13.8	Medical Therapy for Tics	
Drug Name	**Initial Daily Dose (mg)**	**Usual Daily Dose Range (mg)**
Neuroleptics		
Haloperidol	0.25	0.25–20
Pimozide	1	1.5–10
Atypical antipsychotics		
Risperidone	0.5	0.5–4
Olanzapine	2.5	2.5–10
Ziprasidone	20	20–80
Aripiprazole	5	5–30
Others		
Clonidine	0.1	0.1.3
Guanfacine	1	1–4
Clonazepam	0.25	0.5–3
Topiramate	25	25–100
Donepezil	5	10

Extrapyramidal symptomatology (EPS) was reported in 15% of patients treated with risperidone and 33% of patients in the pimozide group. Somnolence, fatigue, weight gain, and depression were seen with both therapies. These results indicate that risperidone improves tics as well as OCD to an equal or better level than pimozide and causes fewer EPSs.

■ **SPECIAL CLINICAL POINT: Neuroleptics should be used in children only when tics are severe, and should be avoided if possible in adults, particularly women, who are at greatest risk for tardive dyskinesia and other extrapyramidal effects.**

Olanzapine, ziprasidone, quetiapine, and aripiprazole all have been reported to suppress tics but to a lesser extent. Further studies are needed with all three of these drugs. These agents can be associated with weight gain, diabetes, hypertension, and dyslipidemia as well as sedation.

Neuroleptics are the most potent treatment for tics; however, the adverse event profile suggests they should be used with caution. Clonidine is a useful alternative for GTS. This drug is an alpha2-adrenergic agonist that inhibits presynaptic norepinephrine release. It can be useful for tics, and also for behavioral aspects of the disorder, particularly ADHD. Daily doses range from 0.15 to 0.5 mg. It is available as oral medication or transdermal patches. Guanfacine is a similar class agent but has less sedation. Adverse events include sedation, dry mouth and eyes, headaches, and postural hypotension. Alpha2-adrenergic agonists are good first-line drugs because of their better side-effect profile.

Other agents used with some success, which have not been studied in controlled trials, include clonazepam, reserpine, tetrabenazine, selegiline, baclofen, donepezil, topiramate, nicotine patches, calcium channel blockers, and opiate.

Facial and neck tics, especially dystonic tics, can be treated with carefully placed intramuscular BoNT injections. In some patients the injections decrease the tic number and severity, eliminate the associated urge to perform the tic, and decrease the pain associated with tics.

When treating OCD, cognitive behavioral techniques can be useful; however, pharmacologic intervention is often necessary. Selective serotonin reuptake inhibitors are the treatment of choice for this behavioral disorder. Fluoxetine (20 to 60 mg/day), a bicyclic antidepressant, can be useful. Clomipramine, sertraline, paroxetine, venlafaxine, citalopram, escitalopram, and fluvoxamine are other selective serotonin reuptake inhibitors that have been used in primary OCD with favorable results and may be useful in GTS. These drugs also may be effective in treating associated anxiety, depression, and social phobias.

Attention deficit hyperactivity disorder can be disabling in GTS. Primary ADHD is often treated with stimulant medications, such as MPH, dextroamphetamine, and pemoline. A multicenter, double-blind trial randomized 37 children to MPH, 34 to clonidine, 33 to clonidine and MPH, and 32 to placebo. ADHD significantly improved in all three active groups, with the most significant change in the combination group. Clonidine was most useful for impulsivity and hyperactivity; MPH was most useful for inattention. A similar degree of tic worsening was seen with MPH and placebo, and tic severity actually lessened in all active groups. In patients with GTS with ADHD and tics, the treatment of choice is MPH (long acting or short acting, the former is preferred) plus clonidine. Selegiline, a monoamine oxidase B inhibitor that is metabolized to methamphetamine, tricyclic antidepressants, and norepinephrine reuptake inhibitors, is useful in treating ADHD and tics.

The role of DBS for GTS is unknown. Data have been accumulated for 10 years regarding this therapeutic option for adults with severe and medically refractory disease. Several studies using different targets have reported benefit in both tics and behavioral symptoms with DBS. Targets have included centromedian parafascicular, ventralis oralis complex of the thalamus, globus pallidus interna, and nucleus accumbens, but which is a preferable target remains to be seen. Sustained benefit has been reported for up to 17 months. GTS patients represent a particular challenge with this procedure because of behavior issues and the nature of the tics. There are no data to support the use of alternative medications or physical therapy for GTS.

When to Refer to a Neurologist

Tic disorders are often complex, especially with the associated behavioral disorders, and may represent diagnostic and therapeutic dilemmas. Simple tics are quite common, often do not require treatment, and need not be referred to a neurologist. If the movements are more severe and associated with behavioral problems, patients should be referred to a neurologist or psychiatrist for diagnostic clarification and treatment.

Special Challenges for Hospitalized Patients

The hospital is a stressful place for patients. Stress can make tics worse, so physicians should anticipate an escalation. This is particularly pertinent to those who have had surgery. Wound infection and tearing of sutures are not unusual. Proper arrangements should be made to avoid these problems.

TARDIVE DYSKINESIA

Tardive Dyskinesia is an iatrogenic movement disorder related to treatment with dopamine receptor antagonists (neuroleptics and antiemetics). The term "tardive" was coined to describe two features of the illness: (a) that it occurs after chronic therapy with these drugs (arbitrarily 3 months for patients younger than age 60 and 1 month for those older than 60) and (b) that the disorder is persistent. Relative persistence of the dyskinesia is a characteristic feature.

A number of clinical variants of TD exist. The most common is characterized by stereotypic or choreiform movements of the orofacial musculature, which constitutes at least half of all tardive syndromes. Others are classified by the movement disorder that dominates the clinical picture—tardive dystonia, tardive akathisia, tardive tics, and tardive myoclonus. Although all these variants occur and can be present at the same time, there are differences beyond clinical phenomenology (including natural history and pharmacology) and separation of these syndromes is important from a practical standpoint.

Clinical Features

■ **SPECIAL CLINICAL POINT: Tardive dyskinesia occurs in approximately 20% (0.5%-65%) of patients treated with first-generation antipsychotic medications.**

The incidence of new cases of TD associated with first-generation antipsychotics increases 5% per year. Approximately 10% to 20% of patients can be severely disabled. Incidence with the newer atypical (second-generation) antipsychotics is reported to be lower than with first-generation medications. Despite a lower incidence, the prevalence of TD remains the same or higher with atypical antipsychotics. There are several factors that may explain this, such as the perceived safety of atypical antipsychotics that leads to increased use in higher risk patients and off-label use. All atypical antipsychotics with the exception of clozapine have been implicated in causing TD.

TD is characterized by patterned, stereotypic orobuccolingual (OBL) chewing-type movements or dyskinesias. The tongue often has a writhing-type movement that can result in pushing out the cheeks (bonbon sign), but there also may be stereotypic repetitive protrusions (flycatcher's tongue). The movements range in severity from extremely mild (the movements simply look like an exaggeration of normal movements such as lip wetting), in which the patients may be unaware of the movements, to severe enough to cause dysarthria and dysphagia to the point of requiring a feeding tube. On examination, the tongue movements tend to decrease with protrusion. In addition, patients can have jaw dystonia or stereotypies (opening, closing, deviations), facial grimacing, blepharospasm, cheek retraction and puffing, pouting, puckering, and lip smacking.

Choreiform movements also may be present in limbs (piano playing movements of the fingers) and in the axial regions (dancelike movements). Involvement of intercostal and diaphragm musculature results in respiratory dyskinesia. These patients have grunting, sighing, air gasping, and belching sounds, and they may become short of breath because of irregular breathing patterns. Respiratory dyskinesias usually occur in conjunction with OBL and affect about 15% of patients with TD. Choreic movements can also include pelvic thrusting and twisting movements (copulatory dyskinesia). TD movements may be exacerbated by activating tasks such as testing dexterity maneuvers (finger or toe tapping, rapid alternating movements) and having patients walk and perform cognitive tasks. Anxiety and fatigue also increase the movements.

TD reaches maximal intensity fairly quickly, and in 50% of patients, the movement disorder is persistent. The intensity of TD varies depending on a number of factors such as the age of the patient, the drug administered, and the duration of exposure. In patients in whom the inciting agent is discontinued, TD may disappear gradually, but this may take years (as long as 5 years).

■ **SPECIAL CLINICAL POINT: In some patients with choreiform movements, the continued administration of neuroleptics will result in progression.**

In these patients, isolated OBL dyskinesias may spread to involve the axial, limb, or diaphragmatic musculature. Another example of progression might be an increase in the severity and amplitude of the choreiform movements. For these reasons, the use of a neuroleptic to treat TD is inappropriate and unwarranted. The fact that many patients who develop this syndrome have an irreversible problem is an indication of the serious nature of this disorder.

TD can occur in any patient chronically exposed to dopamine-blocking agents, including those who are neurologically and psychiatrically normal. Nevertheless, there are factors that seem to increase a patient's risk for the development of this disorder.

■ **SPECIAL CLINICAL POINT: Age is the most consistent risk factor for tardive dyskinesia.**

After age 40, there is a dramatic rise in relative risk. There appears to be a direct relationship between age and severity, and an inverse correlation between age and remission rate. Other possible patient-related risk factors include female gender, diagnosis of affective disorders, history of drug-induced parkinsonism, concomitant use of anticholinergics, and presence of diabetes mellitus. There are also a number of treatment-related risk factors, including the use of depot formulations of neuroleptics and duration of exposure to these drugs. Genetic risk factors also have been the subject of study; TD is associated with mutations in the cytochrome P450 2D6 (CYP2D6) gene, a major drug-metabolizing enzyme.

Pathophysiology

Investigations have focused on alterations in dopaminergic function as a possible mechanism for TD. It has been proposed that the chronic administration of neuroleptics results in a chronic blockade of striatal dopamine receptor sites and that this chronic blockade ultimately induces alterations in the sensitivity and number of dopamine receptors. This hypothesis is supported by the exacerbation of TD with dopaminergic medications, suppression of TD with dopamine antagonists, and enhancement of the movements with anticholinergics. In addition, a study of atypical antipsychotics has demonstrated that those with the lowest risk for extrapyramidal side effects are atypical antipsychotics that do not chronically bind to dopamine receptors. Clozapine and quetiapine bind loosely to these receptors and are easily dissociated by the presence of endogenous dopamine. This phenomenon is referred to as "loose binding" or "fast dissociation" and equates to lower binding affinity. In the simplest conceptual terms, TD has been proposed to be the result of chemical denervation supersensitivity.

Although choreiform movements may begin when the neuroleptic is chronically administered without a change in dose, the most common clinical setting in which the movement disorder emerges is after the dose is lowered or discontinued. This latter setting is in keeping with the postulate of lowering the pharmacologic blockade of the dopamine receptor and allowing normal dopaminergic mechanisms to resume their interaction with the already hypersensitized receptor. Although there is much evidence in animal models to support this notion, there have been inconsistencies. For this reason, examination of other neurotransmitter abnormalities and mechanisms related to TD have been recommended, such as a decrease in GABA activity in the basal ganglia. Some studies have indicated that an overactivity of norepinephrine is present and that decreased activity of serotonin (both of which modulate dopamine transmission) and increased glutamatergic transmission also may occur. Finally, there has been some suggestion that a decrease in acetylcholine activity in the striatum might play a role.

Another possible pathophysiologic mechanism for TD is direct neurotoxicity of neuroleptic medications. It has been theorized that the blockade of dopamine receptors results in an increase in dopamine turnover. This, in turn, results in the formation of increased free oxyradicals that ultimately damage striatal neurons. Neuroleptics also may be toxic to mitochondrial complex I.

Prevention

As in all iatrogenic disorders, prevention is better than treatment. This is especially true for TD in which the symptoms and signs may be irreversible. There are a series of simple steps that may help to limit the development of TD in the general population.

First, the number of patients at risk should be limited. This implies that standard neuroleptics should be used to treat only appropriate illnesses such as schizophrenia, other forms of psychosis, and GTS syndrome. These agents should not be used for minor episodes of anxiety, restlessness, insomnia, minor psychiatric disturbances, or other off-label problems. With antiemetics they should only be used for intractable nausea and for short durations of time. Metoclopramide is approved for gastroparesis and should not be used for nausea or acid reflux. The development of TD does not depend on any preexistent brain damage or psychiatric history, and patients who are normal psychiatrically can develop TD if exposed to neuroleptic agents.

Other methods of decreasing the incidence of TD would be to limit the dose and duration of treatment with neuroleptics.

Finally, if an antipsychotic agent is needed, the choice should be one with less risk of extrapyramidal side effects—atypical agents. These include olanzapine, quetiapine, aripiprazole, and clozapine. Although data suggest a lower incidence of extrapyramidal side effects with these drugs, it should be remembered that it is not zero.

All of these recommendations are commonsense approaches and seem realistic, although there is little information in the literature to confirm these concepts. It is always wise to limit the dose of a pharmacologic agent to the symptoms being treated or controlled. Neuroleptic administration is no exception, and the dose of neuroleptic administered should be tailored to each patient. This is also true for the atypical agents.

When neuroleptics are withdrawn from patients with relapsing psychosis, the relapse rate is significant. However, an initial episode of psychotic behavior does not necessitate chronic lifelong administration of neuroleptics.

■ **SPECIAL CLINICAL POINT: Avoid the concomitant administration of anticholinergic and neuroleptic medication, particularly on a chronic basis.**

The problem of chronic administration of neuroleptics and anticholinergics concomitantly is that there is some retrospective clinical evidence that patients who take both have a slightly greater risk for the development of TD than those taking neuroleptics alone. The only reason for the concomitant use of anticholinergics and neuroleptics is to treat or prevent drug-induced parkinsonism. The drugs should be used symptomatically, not preventatively and prudently. If drug-induced parkinsonism has resolved, there is no point in administering a pharmacologic agent that is no longer indicated.

Another step to limit the development of TD is early recognition of the syndrome and discontinuation of neuroleptics, if psychiatrically possible. The continued administration of neuroleptics in the face of developing TD may result in progression and permanence of the syndrome.

■ **SPECIAL CLINICAL POINT: The best chance of halting progression and reversing TD resides in early detection of abnormal movements.**

Patients should be routinely monitored for emergence of abnormal movements. A final approach to prevention relates to the use of antipsychotic agents that are associated with a lower risk of TD—atypical antipsychotics. Clozapine does not appear to cause D_2 dopamine receptor supersensitivity and causes significantly fewer chewing-type movements than standard neuroleptics in animal models. Clinical trials demonstrated that this drug is much less likely to cause TD. There has not been a case of de novo TD in a patient treated with clozapine. Clozapine is not used as first-line therapy despite its unique and potent antipsychotic properties. It has been approved for use in patients who have unresponsive psychosis and in cases where typical neuroleptics are contraindicated. Serious adverse effects are associated with this medication. The most important is agranulocytosis. For this reason, a weekly white blood count is required for patients taking this drug for the first 6 months, and then blood counts are required every other week.

Other atypical antipsychotics used to treat psychosis include risperidone, olanzapine, quetiapine, ziprasidone, and aripiprazole. All have a higher risk for TD than clozapine.

Treatment

The management of the patient with TD is difficult. Medical therapies are frequently inadequate. In particular, the longer TD is present, the less likely it is to respond. The first approach to these patients should be careful review of whether the neuroleptics (or antiemetics) that have been or are being administered are psychiatrically (or otherwise) indicated. In many instances, there is no indication for the use of these drugs. If this is true, these dopamine receptor-blocking agents should be tapered.

In many patients, the movement disorder initially becomes worse when the drugs are discontinued. This should not be surprising because if TD is related to increased dopamine receptor site sensitivity secondary to chronic dopamine antagonist blockade, and if the patient is already having involuntary movements (indicating dopamine receptor site sensitivity alteration is present) while on the neuroleptics, and the drug is discontinued with abolition of the blockade, the abnormally hypersensitive dopamine receptor would be exposed to normal dopaminergic physiology. This is expected to result in increased involuntary movements. This time period is often difficult to manage.

■ **SPECIAL CLINICAL POINT: Worsening of symptoms with discontinuation of neuroleptic medication should not be confused with worsening of the disease process itself. This**

rebound of tardive dyskinesia on withdrawal of neuroleptic medication may persist for only 2 to 6 weeks.

At the end of this period, assessment of the extent of the baseline disorder is possible. TD has been reported to be irreversible in 30% to 50% of cases, depending on the age of the patient and other factors. Pharmacologic intervention in this choreiform movement disorder is based on pathophysiologic mechanisms that indicate that agents that decrease dopaminergic activity within the brain will decrease chorea. Consequently, agents such as reserpine or tetrabenazine, which deplete the brain of dopamine, will ameliorate this movement disorder. Doses of reserpine (1 to 5 mg/day) and tetrabenazine (25 to 200 mg/day) are reached with a gradually increasing dose schedule.

Side effects of these agents include orthostatic hypotension, parkinsonism, depression, and gastrointestinal problems. Tetrabenazine differs from reserpine because it is shorter acting and causes fewer side effects, particularly orthostatic hypotension and depression.

Other drugs that interfere with dopaminergic activity include neuroleptics. Despite the fact that if the neuroleptic dose is raised the chorea of TD can be ameliorated, this is an incorrect approach because it will place the treating physician in a position of using the etiologic agent to treat the disorder. The movements are simply masked. The only time that neuroleptics would be appropriate to treat TD is if it is life threatening, and this is very rare.

Atypical antipsychotics may also have a therapeutic benefit. Clinical trials evaluating the effectiveness of clozapine in psychosis not only suggested that the drug is less likely to cause TD, but also indicated that there may be a therapeutic potential in treating TD. Numerous single case reports and larger studies have addressed the therapeutic usefulness of clozapine in TD.

Some patients appear to have improvement of TD with clozapine, indicating a therapeutic effect. Variability of response may relate to the heterogeneity of TD. However, considerable caution must be taken when interpreting results of the literature because of methodologic limitations. Studies were open-label treatment protocols with inadequate controls. Properly controlled double-blind studies will be necessary before definitive conclusions can be made. Still, the use of clozapine is strongly recommended as treatment of choice in psychotic patients with TD, with discontinuation of all standard neuroleptics. The recommended dose ranges from 100 to 900 mg/day, and the side effects most commonly seen include sialorrhea, orthostatic hypotension, weight gain, and seizures.

Dopamine agonists, such as levodopa or bromocriptine, have been tried based on the hypothesis that they would "downregulate" dopaminergic hypersensitivity. Studies have shown variable results with these agents, and they should not be used. Other pharmacologic approaches to the treatment of TD are based on manipulation of other neurotransmitter systems that may be abnormal in TD. Increasing cholinergic activity may decrease chorea. The use of a variety of GABA-agonist medications including valproate, diazepam, clonazepam, and baclofen has been disappointing, but some patients respond. Noradrenergic antagonists such as propranolol and clonidine have also been occasionally successful. These drugs are safe and reasonable choices in the treatment of TD. Glutamatergic agents such as amantadine may be helpful in controlling movements. Facial and neck tardive dystonia may be amenable to intramuscular BoNT injections.

Vitamin E, an antioxidant, has a very mixed record in improving TD symptoms. In addition, retrospective epidemiological study suggested that Vitamin E (over 400 IU/day) may result in increased mortality. This has led to limited use. The roles of physical, occupational, and speech therapy are varied depending on patient needs, but they can be helpful.

When to Refer to a Neurologist

TD is often complex clinically and may present diagnostic and therapeutic dilemmas. Patients with TD should be referred to a movement disorder specialist for diagnostic clarification and treatment. In mild cases medication can be withdrawn and the patient observed, but in those in whom the symptoms are troublesome, referral is recommended.

Special Challenges for Hospitalized Patients

Because the movements can be bizarre in appearance and influenced by stress and anxiety, staff education is required so that they understand that this is a neurologic disorder.

Always Remember

- In patients with young-onset dystonia, rule out Wilson disease and consider a trial of levodopa.
- When evaluating patients with possible essential tremor, it is crucial to differentiate alternate etiologies, since this may change your treatment approach.
- Treatment of chorea in patients with Huntington disease does not always result in functional improvement and should be reserved for selected patients.
- A high index of suspicion for Wilson disease should be present when evaluating patients under the age of 40 with a neuropsychiatric presentation.
- Treatment in Gilles de la Tourette syndrome should be individualized to target only the most disabling symptoms, which may or may not be the tics themselves.
- Limit the dose, duration, and overall use of neuroleptics in order to avoid potentially irreversible side effects.

QUESTIONS AND DISCUSSION

1. Match the neurologic term with the appropriate description:

   A. Tremor   1. Excessive, spontaneous movements irregularly timed, nonrepetitive, randomly distributed, and "dancelike"

   B. Chorea   2. An abnormal sustained posture

   C. Dystonia 3. Involuntary, rhythmic, oscillating movement resulting from alternating or synchronous contraction of reciprocally innervated antagonist muscles

   D. Tic   4. Patterned sequence of coordinated movements that may be simple or complex

   The correct matches are A and 3, B and 1, C and 2, D and 4.

2. A patient presents with sustained involuntary eye closure and forced involuntary mouth opening. Which diagnosis is correct?
   A. Meige syndrome
   B. Parkinson disease
   C. Gilles de la Tourette syndrome
   D. Essential tremor

   The correct answer is A. The description is that of Meige syndrome. Parkinson disease, ET, and GTS do not present with dystonic facial movements.

3. A 19-year-old patient complains of the recent onset of shaking, which occurs when he lifts a cup to drink or tries to retrieve food with a fork. When his index fingers are approximated, the tremor worsens. His mother has a similar problem. This description suggests
   A. Essential tremor
   B. Huntington disease

C. Wilson disease

D. Parkinson disease

The correct answer is A. The description is of a postural and kinetic tremor. This is the most common presentation of ET. ET can be familial or sporadic and frequently occurs in adolescence or early adult life. The fact that her mother has a similar tremor suggests the diagnosis.

4. Which drug is most effective in reducing essential tremor?
   A. Levadopa
   B. Ropinirole
   C. Amphetamine
   D. Propranolol
   E. Rasagiline

The correct answer is D. Amphetamines may induce a postural kinetic tremor. Levodopa, ropinirole, and rasagiline all affect the dopaminergic system and are used to treat PD. Propranolol, a beta-blocker, is very useful in treating ET.

5. A patient presents with a generalized choreiform disorder that began at the age of 45 years. He denies any neurologic or psychiatric problems before the onset of his current problem and never received neuroleptic medications. He denies a family history of any similar movement disorder, but his mother was institutionalized at the age of 55 for psychiatric reasons. What is this patient's probable diagnosis?
   A. Huntington disease
   B. Parkinson disease
   C. Essential tremor
   D. Primary dystonia

The correct answer is A. Huntington disease is an autosomal dominant disorder with onset typically in the middle age. Although psychiatric symptoms are insufficient for making a diagnosis of Huntington disease, a family history of a parent with psychiatric disease in a patient with a choreiform disorder may be very suggestive. The diagnosis can be confirmed with genetic testing.

6. Which of the following is not inherited in an autosomal dominant fashion?
   A. Primary childhood-onset (Oppenheim) dystonia
   B. Huntington disease
   C. Essential tremor
   D. Wilson disease

The correct answer is D. Wilson disease is inherited as an autosomal recessive disorder.

7. Botulinum toxin is used in therapy for which of the following?
   A. Spasmodic torticollis
   B. Muscle weakness
   C. Paresthesias
   D. Myoclonus

The correct answer is A. Botulinum toxin therapy is accepted as safe and effective for the treatment of spasmodic torticollis.

SUGGESTED READING

Bressman SB. Genetics of dystonia: an overview. *Parkinsonism Relat Disord.* 2007;13:S347–S355.

Factor SA, Lang AE, Weiner WJ. *Drug-Induced Movement Disorders.* 2nd ed. New York, NY: Blackwell Futura; 2005.

Gasser T, Bressman S, Durr A, et al. Molecular diagnosis of inherited movement disorders: Movement Disorders Society Task Force on Molecular Diagnosis. *Mov Disord.* 2003;18:3–18.

Louis ED. Essential tremor. *N Engl J Med.* 2001;345:887–891.

Lyons KE, Pahwa R. Deep brain stimulation and tremor. *Neurotherapeutics.* 2008;5:331–338.

Ondo WD, Jankovic J, Connor GS, et al. Topiramate in essential tremor, a double-blind, placebo-controlled trial. *Neurology.* 2006;66:672–677.

Ostrem JL, Starr PA. Treatment of dystonia with deep brain stimulation. *NeuroRx.* 2008;5:320–330.

Pffeifer RF. Wilson's disease. *Semin Neurol.* 2007;27:123–132.

Quartarone A, Rizzo V, Morgante F. Clinical features of dystonia: a pathophysiological revisitation. *Current Opinion in Neurology.* 2008;21:484–490.

Rezai AR, Machado AG, Deogaonkar M, et al. Surgery for movement disorders. *Neurosurgery.* 2008;62(suppl 2):809–838.

Roberts EA, Schilsky ML. Diagnosis and treatment of Wilson disease: an update. *Hepatology*. 2008;47(6):2089–2111.

Shprecher D, Kurlan R. The management of tics. *Mov Disord*. 2009;24:15–24.

SuttonBrown M, Suchowersky O. Clinical and research advances in Huntington's disease. *Can J Neurol Sci*. 2003;30(suppl 1):S45–S52.

Tarsy D, Baldesserini RJ. Epidemiology of tardive dyskinesia: is risk declining with modern antipsychotics? *Mov Disord*. 2006;21:589–598.

The Huntington Study Group. Tetrabenazine as antichorea therapy in Huntington disease. *Neurology*. 2006;66:366–372.

Young AB. Huntingtin in health and disease. *J Clin Invest*. 2003;111:299–302.

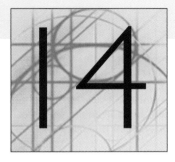

14

Alzheimer Disease and Other Dementias

NEELUM T. AGGARWAL AND RAJ C. SHAH

key points

- Dementia is a common age-related condition with a prevalence of about 5% in persons over age 65 years and up to 50% in persons over the age of 85 years.

- Alzheimer disease is the most frequent type of dementia in the United States and Europe, comprising approximately 60 to 80 percent of persons who present with dementing disorders. Other forms of dementia, such as Lewy Body disease, frontotemporal dementia, and vascular dementia, also are increasingly being recognized.

- Facing increasing numbers of older patients with cognitive symptoms, primary care physicians need to have a practical approach for recognizing and managing Alzheimer's disease and other dementias.

- The goal of this chapter is to present a framework diagnosing individuals with cognitive concerns and developing a tailored care plan.

OVERVIEW

Dementia (or chronic loss of cognitive function) associated with old age was recognized in antiquity. For most of history, dementia of older persons was attributed to the effects of aging or to the effects of cerebral artherosclerosis (hardening of the arteries). In the early 20th century, Dr Alois Alzheimer presented the clinical history of a 54-year-old woman with a progressive dementia that he ascribed to the accumulation of senile plaques and tangles found on postmortem examination. Based on his case study, the term "Alzheimer disease" (AD) referred to a relatively uncommon progressive dementia in middle-aged persons. However, over the past 30 years, it has become apparent that most of the older people with dementia have the same condition described by Alzheimer almost 100 years ago.

287

Only a small proportion of people with dementia are managed in specialized dementia centers. Because physicians often do not look for or recognize the signs of dementia, many people with dementia remain undiagnosed. Timely diagnosis allows for the person with dementia to be a part of important care decision-making processes. It also permits early pharmacologic and nonpharmacologic intervention. Finally, it can prevent medical emergencies resulting from behavioral disturbances and other superimposed medical problems. Therefore, increased awareness of dementia offers neurologists and nonneurologists an opportunity to improve the lives of patients with dementia and their caregivers.

■ **SPECIAL CLINICAL POINT: Up to two thirds of older people with dementia are not detected.**

NORMAL AGING AND MILD COGNITIVE IMPAIRMENT

Physicians often are faced with the dilemma of trying to determine the importance of complaints such as "senior moments" or "forgetfulness" voiced by their patients. In individuals who ultimately develop dementia and AD, one can presume that there is a gradual progression of an underlying process, which begins with "normal aging," that can culminate into pathologically proven AD. Between the state of normal cognition and mild dementia is a zone often referred to as "mild cognitive impairment" (MCI). In the past, this zone has been referred to as "benign senescent forgetfulness," "age-associated memory impairment," or "cognitive impairment no dementia." In recent years, MCI has been increasingly used to describe individuals who typically have mild memory impairment noted on neuropsychological testing, with general cognitive functioning that is otherwise normal for age and normal activities of daily living. The clinical evaluation for subjects with suspected MCI is virtually identical to that for clinical AD, but may involve more detailed neuropsychological testing.

■ **SPECIAL CLINICAL POINT: In persons with MCI, the mini-mental status examination (MMSE) scores often will appear normal (scores of 26 to 28). Yet, on neuropsychological examination, persons will show impairment on tests of verbal and nonverbal delayed recall, a finding that is often seen in early AD.**

As characterization of MCI continues, research now has focused on identifying potential risk factors for the development of dementia and AD in those with MCI. Recent data suggest that persons who have been diagnosed with MCI are likely to be at an increased risk of developing AD and of cognitive decline. Further, they frequently have the pathology of AD, suggesting that MCI represents preclinical AD in many cases. The apolipoprotein e4 allele has been associated with the development of AD among persons with MCI in multiple studies, and some small samples have shown that elevated levels of tau in the cerebrospinal fluid may have the potential to predict the development of AD in MCI patients.

■ **SPECIAL CLINICAL POINT: The rates of progression of MCI to AD are highly variable depending on the study; however, it is in the 10% to 15% per year range.**

DEMENTIA

Dementia refers to acquired intellectual deterioration in an adult. Evaluating a person for dementia involves determining whether there has been a loss of cognition relative to a previous level of performance. The clinical evaluation for assessing memory complaints has four objectives: (a) to determine if the person has dementia; (b) if dementia is present, to determine whether its presentation and course are consistent with AD; (c) to assess evidence for any alternate diagnoses, especially if the presentation and course are atypical for AD; and (d) to evaluate evidence of other, coexisting, diseases that may contribute to the dementia, especially conditions that might respond to treatment. The section titled "Differential Diagnosis of Primary Neurodegenerative Dementias" will provide details on important features in the patient's history, key physical examination findings, and ancillary tests to conduct on an individual with memory concerns. An algorithm highlighting three decision point questions for clinically triaging a person with memory concerns is shown in Figure 14.1.

Typically, evidence is obtained through the clinical history from a knowledgeable informant (a family member or close friend) and should be documented by mental status testing. When the clinical history is not available, test results from a single evaluation can be contrasted with the estimated premorbid level of ability based on the patient's education and occupation. In some cases, formal neuropsychologic performance testing on two or more occasions over a period of 12 or more months may be necessary to document cognitive decline. For clinical purposes, loss of cognition should be sufficiently severe to interfere with an individual's usual occupational or social activities and the cognitive deficit cannot be present in the setting of an altered sensorium such as in delirium or an acute confusional state.

Differential Diagnosis for Conditions Presenting with Cognitive Impairment

The differential diagnosis of dementia should emphasize common potentially treatable disorders that may cause or exacerbate cognitive impairment, which occur in the elderly. Reversible conditions including delirium, depression, structural conditions, and toxic or metabolic disorders, often are cited as potential causes of cognitive impairment. A thorough evaluation of each condition is justified for persons suspected of having dementia. If one of the conditions described below is identified as a potential cause of the cognitive impairment, appropriate treatment should be started. However, it is important to re-evaluate an individual

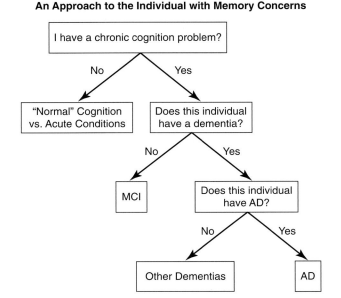

An Approach to the Individual with Memory Concerns

FIGURE 14.1 An algorithm for clinically triaging a person with memory concerns. MCI, mild cognitive impairment. AD, Alzheimer disease.

after treatment is completed to determine if cognitive difficulties have resolved. If resolution is not achieved fully, an underlying primary neurodegenerative cause for cognitive decline may also be present.

Delirium   Delirium differs from dementia by the onset and duration of cognitive impairment and by the level of consciousness. The onset of cognitive impairment in delirium typically is hours to days, and it lasts days to weeks. In addition, individuals often are either hyperalert or hypo-alert. However, in older persons, altered consciousness may be less evident. A delirium may be the initial manifestation of an underlying, unrecognized dementia. Thus, data suggest that delirium in the elderly may take many months to resolve or may not resolve at all. The occurrence of delirium in the hospitalized elderly has been associated with excess mortality.

Depression   Loss of interest in hobbies and community activities, apathy, weight loss, and sleep disorders may be interpreted by the family as depression, although they actually may be the result of the dementia itself. Among the elderly, depression and dementia coexist and do not always present as two distinct entities. Although it is useful to ask the caregiver about symptoms suggesting dysphoric mood such as crying, complaining, and depression in the elderly may present with agitation or increased irritability. Depression may contribute to impairment of activities of daily living and rarely to the cognitive deficits. If impairment in activities of daily living exceeds what is expected for the severity of cognitive dysfunction, the possibility of a coexisting depression should be considered.

Structural Conditions   Brain tumors rarely present with a degenerative dementia. When they do, there usually are other major focal findings and signs of increased intracranial pressure. Although rare, brain tumors in the "silent" areas of the brain may present only as a personality change and/or intellectual decline. Subtle focal findings usually can be demonstrated on the neurologic examination, but they occasionally are lacking. Similar comments may be applied to subdural hematomas, especially in the geriatric age group. Thus, some type of neuroimaging procedure remains warranted for all patients being evaluated for dementia.

No other syndrome causing dementia has generated such intense interest (and frustration) among neurologists as normal pressure hydrocephalus (NPH). The classic syndrome consists of gait disturbance, dementia, and incontinence. However, this triad is also seen commonly in AD and other degenerative dementias.

■ **SPECIAL CLINICAL POINT: NPH typically presents first as a gait disorder, and over time cognitive impairment and urinary incontinence can occur.**

The onset can progress over months or years. The dementia is mild, often "subcortical" with slowing of thought and relative preservation of "cortical" features such as naming and language skills. Often there is no profound short-term (or episodic) memory deficit that distinguishes this dementia from AD. Brain scans typically demonstrate hydrocephalus with enlargement of ventricles out of proportion to sulci enlargement. Numerous studies have attempted to determine predictors of improvement following ventricular shunting, without much success. Perhaps the most useful piece of clinical information is the history of a reason for hydrocephalus (such as meningitis or subarachnoid hemorrhage from either a ruptured aneurysm or, more commonly, a previous traumatic head injury). Some patients with gait problems or dementia improve with cerebrospinal fluid shunting procedures; however, the insertion of a shunt is not a benign procedure, especially in geriatric patients. Although the diagnosis of NPH rarely, if ever, can be made with complete confidence, an etiology for the hydrocephalus should be sought prior to recommending shunting.

Toxic or Metabolic Disorders   Drug toxicity is a common reversible cause of delirium in the elderly. Older persons may be more susceptible than younger persons to drug side effects on cognition. This is the result of many factors, including altered drug kinetics and use of multiple medications in older persons with several illnesses or complaints (polypharmacy). Clinicians also should be alert to the possibility of drug side effects further impairing cognition in persons with preexisting cognitive impairment. A typical presentation is the rapid worsening of dementia following the administration of a new drug (or following the reinstitution of a previous medication that the patient has not taken for some time), with or without altered level of consciousness.

■ **SPECIAL CLINICAL POINT: Psychotropic (including neuroleptic), sedative–hypnotic, anticholinergic, and antihistaminic medications are common agents associated with cognitive impairment.**

Hypothyroidism has been recognized for many years as being associated with altered mental state, although it is currently quite rare in the United States. Similar cases are seen with disorders of calcium metabolism, especially hypercalcemia, and also with an electrolyte imbalance. Chronic liver and renal diseases frequently are associated with an altered mental state; however, it is unusual for these diseases to be present without prominent manifestations of the primary illnesses. Finally, Korsakoff syndrome, a result of thiamine deficiency, also can present with an amnestic syndrome mimicking a dementia. It classically develops in the wake of an acute Wernicke encephalopathy with confusion, ophthalmoplegia, and ataxia. However, many patients with Korsakoff syndrome do not present with a Wernicke encephalopathy. Although alcoholism is the most frequent setting for this syndrome in developed countries, it also may be associated with other conditions leading to nutritional deficiency, including starvation, malnutrition, protracted vomiting, and gastric resection. It also can be precipitated by administration of carbohydrates to patients with marginal thiamine stores.

Cognitive impairment is among the most common neurologic manifestations of acquired immunodeficiency syndrome (AIDS) and may precede the development of other signs of infection with the human immunodeficiency virus (HIV). Persons with AIDS dementia complex present with forgetfulness and poor attention, generally over several months with the memory impairment significantly less striking than that seen in AD. Chronic meningitis, especially cryptococcal meningitis, also can present as dementia, although there are almost always other associated signs and symptoms. The same can be said for neurosyphilis. Brain abscesses, like brain tumors, can present solely with dementia, although focal findings are usually present.

Differential Diagnosis of Primary Neurodegenerative Dementias

Once the conditions presenting with cognitive impairment have been ruled out, the clinician then must determine the underlying nature of the dementia. It is at this time, referrals sometimes are made to a neurologist, as diagnosing of the exact neurodegenerative cause of a dementia may be problematic.

Generally speaking, if an elderly person presents with a gradual progression of a memory disorder, which is now advanced to involve other nonmemory cognitive domains and these changes have affected daily functioning, AD is the most likely diagnosis. Vascular dementia (VaD) can involve abrupt changes in cognition if large vessels are affected, or can be present insidiously if subcortical ischemia is responsible for the change in function. In subjects with parkinsonism, hallucinations, and wide fluctuations in behavior, dementia with Lewy bodies (DLB) might be more likely than AD. Alternatively, if the initial presentation is one of the changes in personality or behavior instead of memory, a frontotemporal dementia (FTD) should be considered. Finally, if the time course of the dementia is relatively rapid over months and the clinical features include psychiatric symptoms and motor function abnormalities, a prion disorder such as Creutzfeld–Jakob disease (CJD) should be considered.

Alzheimer Disease   In 2000, it was estimated that there were approximately 4.5 million individuals with AD in the United States and this number has been projected to increase to 14 million by 2050. Prevalence estimates suggest that AD affects about 10% of persons over the age of 65, making it one of the most common chronic diseases of the elderly. The occurrence of AD is strongly related to age, with the incidence doubling every 5 years after the age of 65.

■ **SPECIAL CLINICAL POINT: From the ages 65 to 85, the prevalence of AD doubles approximately every 5 years.**

Other than age, there are few well-documented risk factors for AD. There is some evidence that women may be more likely to develop the disease than men. However, this observation appears to be attributed, in large part, to the fact that women live longer than men. Years of formal education have been associated with a reduced risk of disease in many, although not all studies. The mechanism linking education to risk of disease is unclear, but recent evidence suggests that participation in cognitively stimulating activities also reduces the risk of disease.

The first-degree relative appears to have a slightly greater risk of inheriting disease. In rare families, however, AD is inherited as an autosomal dominant disease in which half of the family members are affected. In these families, the disease has been linked to mutations on one of three different chromosomes: 21, 14, and 1 and often age of onset is very young (<65 years). The majority of cases of AD are "late onset" and in some of these cases, chromosome 19 has been implicated. Chromosome 19 is thought to code for the apolipoprotein E alleles. The presence of one apolipoprotein E e4 allele approximately doubles an individual's

risk of developing AD, and the risk is even higher among those homozygous for the allele. By contrast, the apolipoprotein E e2 allele appears to lower risk of the disease. The mechanism whereby this allele causes the disease is unknown, but recent data suggest that it increases the deposition of AD pathology.

■ **SPECIAL CLINICAL POINT: Familial autosomal dominant cases comprise 5% to 10% of all the cases with AD.**

Clinical Symptoms

■ **SPECIAL CLINICAL POINT: The most common initial sign of AD is difficulty with episodic memory (the ability to learn new information). Old memories are often accurate and intact until the mid to later stages of the disease.**

The clinical history should focus on the temporal relationship between the loss of different cognitive abilities and the development of behavioral disturbances and impairment of motor abilities. At the onset, this disease may be almost imperceptible, but it typically will progress to become a more serious problem in a few years' time. The family will report that the patient frequently repeats himself or herself. He or she leaves important tasks undone, such as bills unpaid and appointments not kept. After the memory disorder becomes apparent, the family will notice other disorders of cognition. Confusion in following directions also can be a common earlier symptom. If the person is driving a car, he or she may get lost or "turned around" (an event that frequently precipitates the first evaluation by a physician), have an increase in minor "fender benders," or use poor judgment while driving. Frightening lapses of memory, such as leaving on a gas stove, also may occur.

As the disease progresses, the person may have difficulty in remembering simple words or names and may be unable to participate in normal conversation. Often family members comment that the individual has become a "listener" instead of actively participating in conversations. Reading and writing also will be impaired, as will simple activities of daily living, such as bathing and dressing.

Agitation, hallucination, delusions, and even violent outbursts may be seen at any time during the course of the illness. Previous personality traits may be exaggerated or may be obscured completely by new behavior patterns. Changes in sleep–wake patterns also may disrupt normal living patterns. These types of symptoms are particularly difficult for the family and place a great burden on the caregiver. Parkinsonian signs such as unsteady gait and slowed movements are common.

■ **SPECIAL CLINICAL POINT: A general physical decline is not seen until the latest stages of the illness. If decline occurs rapidly, which is associated with a change in gait, parkinsonian signs, or weakness, other dementing illnesses need to be considered (Fig. 14.1).**

Incontinence may be seen at any time and initially may reflect the patient's inability to find the bathroom. As the illness progresses, there seems to be a true loss of bladder control and, ultimately, a loss of bowel function. Inability to walk is also a common occurrence seen at the late stages of the illness. Seizures and an inability or unwillingness to eat also may occur in the later stages of AD.

The typical history in AD is a gradually progressive dementia over several years. The average patient with AD survives about a decade from the time of diagnosis, although the variation may be from a few years to 20 years. There may be plateau periods during which deterioration is not obvious; however, a lengthy plateau would be unusual. There is no clear evidence that the age of onset determines the natural history. However, younger patients generally tend to have more speech disorders as the illness progresses. Older patients are more prone to age-related medical problems associated with morbidity and mortality.

Neurologic Examination Formal, standardized assessment of cognition is required to make a diagnosis of dementia and AD. Wide ranges of measures are available for this purpose. Several brief measures (e.g., the MMSE and the blessed orientation, memory concentration test) are suitable for use at the bedside or in the physician's office. Although they may help distinguish persons with dementia from persons without dementia, they are less effective in distinguishing AD from other dementias. In these cases, full neuropsychological testing is recommended.

In the office or hospital, routine mental status testing should include checking the person's orientation by asking for his or her full name, the day of the week, the day of the month, the month and the year, where he or she is, and also his or her age and date of birth. Show the individual four or five objects and then ask him or her to name them twice (e.g., a coin, a safety pin, keys, and a comb). Tell the person that you will ask him or her to recall the objects in a few minutes. Then check the individual's knowledge of common events by asking for the names of well-known public figures (e.g., the president, governor, or mayor). Ask the person to repeat some numbers (the typical patient can remember six numbers forward and three or four backward) and then have him or her do some simple calculations (e.g., multiplication, addition, and serial sevens). Have the individual to repeat a simple phrase, to follow a two-step direction (e.g., point to the ceiling, then point to the floor), and to do something with his right hand and then his left hand (e.g., make a fist with your left hand, followed by salute with your right hand). Ask the individual to write his or her name, to write a brief phrase to dictation (e.g., today is Monday), and then to draw something (usually a clock). Also, ask the person to read a simple phrase. Finally, have the patient recall the four or five objects that you showed him or her previously. This mental status test can be administered in a few minutes and should be part of the routine clinical evaluation of all older persons. Recommended education-adjusted cutoffs have been developed for the MMSE and the results can serve as guidelines to direct further evaluation, and also provide valuable screening information.

■ **SPECIAL CLINICAL POINT: To make a diagnosis of dementia, a deficit should exist in more than one area of cognition. Patients with early AD may have profound memory problems with only mild deficits in other aspects of cognition. As the disease progresses, however, language and other aspects of cognitive dysfunction typically become more obvious.**

The most important function of the neurologic examination in evaluating persons with dementia is in diagnosing conditions other than AD. The general physical examination and neurologic examination (excluding the mental status testing) is usually normal in AD. Minor parkinsonian features, myoclonic jerks, frontal lobe signs (grasp reflex, snout and glabellar signs), and similar abnormalities occasionally may be seen on examination, especially later in the course of the illness. However, these features noted in persons with mild memory problems should alert the physician of a diagnosis other than, or perhaps in addition to, AD. If a person has parkinsonian signs, changes in gait and tone suggestive of rigidity in addition to memory complaints, the possibility of DLB exists. If a person has limb weakness, a visual field cut, or asymmetric reflexes, one could consider VaD or a mixed dementia (AD/VaD). Myoclonic jerks in addition to unsteady gait could signify a rapidly progressive dementia such as CJD.

Ancillary Tests

■ **SPECIAL CLINICAL POINT: Currently there is no reliable diagnostic test for AD.**

The purpose of laboratory testing is to identify other conditions that might cause or exacerbate dementia and include a brain scan and blood tests (Table 14.1). The use of lumbar puncture in the routine evaluation of elderly patients for dementia or AD is not recommended. However, if the clinical picture is associated with an acute change in mental status, nuchal rigidity, or fever, a lumbar puncture

TABLE 14.1	Laboratory Aids in the Differential Diagnosis of Dementia	
Routine Tests	**Optional Tests**
Chemistry panel	Sedimentation rate
Complete blood count	Electrocardiogram
Thyroid function studies	Urinalysis
Vitamin B_{12} level	Chest x-ray
Syphilis serology	Drug levels
CT/MRI of the head	Twenty-four hour urine for heavy metal
	Electroencephalogram
	Cerebrospinal fluid (LP)
	PET/SPECT
	HIV testing

should be done to rule out a possible infectious etiology for the cognitive impairment.

Morphologic neuroimaging with magnetic resonance imaging (MRI) or computed tomography (CT) is used to look for evidence of another disease that can cause or contribute to cognitive impairment, such as a cerebral infarct or tumor. MRI is superior to CT because it is less subject to artifact, it provides greater contrast between gray and white matter, and coronal images can provide excellent views of the mesial temporal lobe structures vital to mnemonic function. Over the years there has been a strong research interest in using morphologic imaging (quantitative structural neuroimaging) as a direct diagnostic tool for AD. In particular, atrophy of the medial temporal lobe structures, for example the hippocampus, has been found in patients with AD.

Another area of neuroimaging research has centered around the detection of amyloid deposition in the brain through the use of radioligand for positron emission tomography (PET) imaging studies of amyloid in the brain of living subjects. Similarly single photon emission computed tomography (SPECT) and PET scanning have shown promise in its ability to differentiate among dementias. There is literature attesting to the utility of FDG-PET (fluorodeoxyglucose-positron emission tomography) in differentiating AD from other dementias, specifically that of FTD and the Centers for Medicare and Medicaid Services have approved for reimbursement the use of FDG-PET for this purpose. *In the clinical setting, these tests are used to confirm an underlying suspicion of an atypical dementia, to aid in the treatment and management of the patient and to assist the family with long-term care issues. However, it is probably better for a primary care physician to arrange a patient consultation with a dementia specialist prior to ordering an FDG-PET scan.*

As noted earlier there appears to be a genetic component to the development of AD. Genetic testing can be considered in young onset suspected familial AD. Often these types of cases are referred to a neurologist and may be further referred to a specific AD research center for more detailed investigation, in addition to appropriate genetic counseling. In the more typical variety of late onset AD (onset occurring after the age of 65 years), genetic testing for specific mutations is not useful.

■ **SPECIAL CLINICAL POINT:** **The current recommendations by the Academy of Neurology suggest that APOE testing should not be done routinely in asymptomatic individuals.**

Pathology Data suggest that the progressive loss of memory and other cognitive abilities from AD is a complex function of the accumulation of pathology (amyloid plaques and neurofibrillary tangles) and neurochemical deficits (deterioration of cholinergic system), leading to a loss of neurons and synapses within selectively vulnerable neural systems. Grossly, there is atrophy and dilatation of the ventricles and marked atrophy of the hippocampal formation. Microscopically, there are large numbers of neuritic plaques and neurofibrillary tangles. Although both of these lesions can be seen in the brains of older persons without dementia, they are found in greater numbers in the hippocampal formation and neocortex in persons with AD. Tangles also accumulate in the basal forebrain, the major source of cholinergic neurons that project to the hippocampal formation and neocortex. Plaques are composed of a central extracellular proteinaceous amyloid core, surrounded by dystrophic axon terminals. Amyloid comes from a larger precursor protein coded on chromosome 21. Processing of this protein by various secretases (alpha, beta, and gamma secretases) can result in either the putative toxic fragment that is deposited in the brain or another smaller, benign fragment.

The major constituents of neurofibrillary tangles are paired helical filaments. Evidence suggests that these tangles are composed of the microtubule associated protein tau, which is in an abnormal hyperphosphorylated state.

Vascular Dementia As alluded to earlier not all cases of dementia are that of AD. VaD is often considered by some to be the second most common cause of dementia in older persons accounting from 10% to 20% of the dementia cases. VaD includes all dementia syndromes resulting from ischemic, anoxic, or hypoxic brain damage. Thus, it is not simply an AD-type dementia caused by stroke but a constellation of cognitive syndromes that may or may not mimic AD. The most consistent risk factor for VaD has been advanced age, with some studies suggesting that the prevalence of VaD is higher in Asians and African-Americans. Similar to AD, it appears that higher education is a protective factor. Risk factors for VaD include hypertension, smoking hypercholesterolemia, and diabetes.

The traditional teaching and description of VaD is that of a stepwise progression with abrupt stroke-like episodes causing abrupt decline and then stabilization until the next stroke-like episode. In clinical practice, this is not always readily seen, causing difficulty at times in making the diagnosis. In addition, because VaD is often combined with AD (mixed dementia) signs and symptoms may overlap and clinical diagnosis may prove to be difficult.

Although there is no typical neuropsychologic profile of persons with VaD (because the behavioral manifestations are dependent on the vascular territory involved), the cognitive pattern in VaD tends to differ as compared to patients with AD. Rather than the prominent short-term memory loss (episodic memory loss) that is seen in persons with AD, those with VaD tend to have difficulties with tasks that focus on frontal executive dysfunction (such as motor planning). Because the MMSE does not focus on executive dysfunction, it may not be the best screening test for the diagnosis.

One of the most important clinical signs noted in VaD is a history or neurologic examination consistent with a focal neurologic event such as a stroke. Ideally, the event should have occurred proximate to the onset of cognitive impairment and is confirmed by neuroimaging.

■ **SPECIAL CLINICAL POINT: The temporal relation between a clinical stroke and the onset of cognitive impairment and dementia is the best predictor of VaD.**

Because subcortical vascular disease often involves pathology in multiple subcortical areas, symptoms are often varied and include slowness (parkinsonian signs), changes in speech (aphasia or dysarthria), mood (depression) in addition to urinary incontinence, or gait disturbance. White matter lesions commonly are found on MRI or CT in elderly persons, but their etiology and significance remain controversial. Many persons with dementia with white matter changes on MRI or CT have AD at autopsy. Therefore, although the presence of VaD should be supported by evidence of vascular disease on CT or MRI, the presence of these lesions does not necessarily indicate that the dementia is of vascular origin.

Cholinesterase inhibitors have been shown to be beneficial in patients with VaD. Some studies have shown that persons with VaD treated with either galantamine or donepezil compared to persons treated with placebo have shown a treatment effect to be similar to that seen in patients with AD.

Dementia with Lewy Bodies   In some situations, the dementia and parkinsonian signs appear to develop simultaneously. These cases often are referred to as having DLB, diffuse Lewy body disease, or the Lewy body variant of AD. These are all rather unfortunate terms because they implicate a specific pathology rather than a dementia syndrome.

DLB is considered by some to be the third most common neurodegenerative dementia and tends to be under diagnosed. In some studies, DLB accounts for 15% to 20% of the hospital autopsy cases and 35% of the dementia cases in population studies. As with AD, the incidence of DLB appears to increase with age. There may be a slight increase in males; however, other differences, such as racial and ethnic trends, are not known. The mean survival time appears to be similar to AD and like AD some persons may show rapid progression with 1 to 2 years survival.

People with well-established Parkinson disease who subsequently develop dementia often are simply referred to as having Parkinson disease with dementia. Although in many cases this is the result of concomitant AD, persons with Parkinson disease also can develop a dementia that appears to be the result of the invasion of the limbic system and neocortex with Lewy bodies.

There have been two workshops on criteria for DLB. In addition to dementia and parkinsonian signs, these patients have fluctuating cognition, depression, REM (rapid eye movement) sleep disturbances, hallucinations, sensitivity to neuroleptics, and changes on PET scanning (cerebral hypometabolism in the primary and association visual cortices). The hallucinations can be black or white, often involve animals and people, and can be very frightening at times.

Finally, many persons with AD also develop parkinsonian signs. These signs often are the result of concomitant Lewy bodies in the substantia nigra as seen in Parkinson disease but also can result from AD changes in the substantia nigra or subcortical ischemic cerebrovascular disease. One feature of DLB is that these patients may be subject to onset of parkinsonian signs and symptoms with modest doses of neuroleptic medications, and use of neuroleptics should be limited.

▪ SPECIAL CLINICAL POINT: Three defining features useful in making the diagnosis of DLB are the presence of marked fluctuations in cognition and behavior, the occurrence of vivid hallucinations, and the development of parkinsonism within one year after the onset of dementia.

There is substantial evidence that the cholinergic dysfunction is a prominent abnormality in DLB. Therefore, it is not surprising that evidence suggests that cholinesterase inhibitors, the mainstay treatment in patients with AD, may be even more efficacious in patients with DLB. Reports of improvement in apathy, somnolence, and hallucinations are all noteworthy. In addition, cholinesterase inhibitors have been shown to improve cognition and behavior without worsening of extrapyramidal symptoms. Although levodopa does not work particularly well in patients with DLB and has the potential to worsen hallucinations, and other behavioral symptoms, a cautious trial can be considered in those with prominent motor impairment.

FRONTOTEMPORAL DEMENTIA

FTDs are a rare group of conditions that include Pick disease, primary progressive aphasia, and motor neuron disease (MND) with dementia. Patients typically are younger than those with AD, with a typical age of onset in the late 50s. They present with neurobehavioral or "psychiatric features" that are thought to be of frontal and/or temporal lobe dysfunction such as socially inappropriate behavior or a progressive language deficit, as opposed to the memory impairment that characterizes AD. Often patients are seen by psychiatrist first because of behavioral changes and are then referred to a neurologist for further evaluation.

On neurologic examination, early signs may include frontal release signs such as a snout, grasp, or palmomental reflex. Other abnormalities include the presence of early MND or parkinsonian signs. The families with autosomal dominant FTDs with parkinsonism have been linked to chromosome 17 and are thought to be due to an aberrant coding of the tau protein. The motor findings in persons with FTD-MND are similar to that seen in pure MND, and may precede, coincide with, or follow the development of cognitive behaviors.

▪ SPECIAL CLINICAL POINT: Spontaneous parkinsonism and clinical MND may be encountered in some patients with FTD.

The pattern of abnormality on neuropsychological testing is different from that seen in AD, VaD, and DLB. It can reveal relatively isolated dysfunction of frontal abilities (impaired set shifting or shifting from one set or rules to another) or dysfunction of language abilities (e.g., naming). Structural brain imaging, especially MRI, can support the diagnosis and demonstrate focal and sometimes very marked atrophy of the frontal and or anterior temporal lobes, which is often asymmetrical. FDG-PET recently has been approved by the Centers of Medicare and Medicaid Services to distinguish FTD from AD.

The pharmacologic treatment of FTD is currently aimed at behavioral management, with "off-label" use of acetylcholinesterase inhibitors, antidepressants, and neuroleptics. Several studies have evaluated the use of acetylcholinesterase inhibitors for behavior in FTD and suggest that some patients may benefit from these agents, including donepezil and rivastigmine. Other small studies have utilized serotonin uptake inhibitors, such as paroxetine or trazodone, and monoamine oxidase inhibitors, such as as moclobemide, and have had mixed results with regards to behavior management.

Prion Diseases

Prion diseases are a heterogeneous group of fatal neurodegenerative conditions of sporadic, infectious, or genetic origin. The transmissible agent appears to be composed solely of the prion protein, encoded by a gene on chromosome 20, without any nucleic acid, making it unlike any other known viral or bacterial agent. The most common prion disease is CJD.

■ SPECIAL CLINICAL POINT: CJD is a rapidly progressive dementia that leads to death within a year.

Sporadic CJD presents as a rapidly progressive dementia with myoclonus, cerebellar dysfunction, parkinsonian signs, and pyramidal tract signs. Iatrogenic CJD can follow corneal or dural transplants or use of implanted stereotactic electrodes or human growth hormone. Several forms of autosomal dominant familial prion diseases can result from mutations in the prion protein gene on chromosome 20. Familial CJD tends to present younger and has a long preclinical period. In its prodromal stage, behavioral symptoms such as mania, paranoia, or psychosis can occur.

MANAGEMENT OF ALZHEIMER DISEASE

Once AD is diagnosed, the clinician assists individuals in developing a network of personal care, medical, social service, and legal providers that will become their support foundation. The network attempts to maintain cognitive abilities, preserve functional abilities, control behavioral difficulties, and reduce caregivers' burden through education, social and legal services, and treatment interventions (Fig. 14.2).

Pharmacotherapy

Five agents are approved by the U.S. Food and Drug Administration (FDA) for the symptomatic treatment of AD. Four drugs work to enhance cholinergic transmission in the brain by reducing the degradation of acetylcholine through inhibition of the enzyme acetylcholinesterase (AchE). The first drug approved in this class of agents, tacrine, is no longer clinically used because it induces liver toxicity and requires

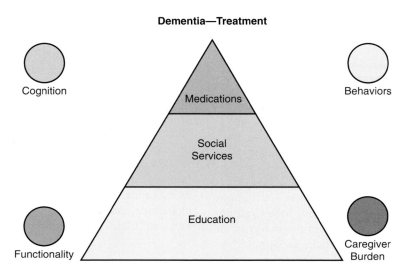

FIGURE 14.2 A diagram depicting the need to develop a treatment plan for individuals with dementia that includes education, social and legal services, and medications to maintain cognitive abilities, preserve functional abilities, control behavioral difficulties, and reduce caregiver burden.

dosing four times a day. Therefore, it is not discussed further. One drug works by being a partial glutamate antagonist.

Acetylcholinesterase Inhibitors Rivastigmine inhibits both AchE and butyrylcholinesterase (BuChE), whereas donepezil and galantamine inhibit AchE but have only minimal inhibition of BuChE. All of the AchEs except rivastigmine are eliminated via the liver. Rivastigmine is eliminated in the urine and may need to be adjusted in individuals with chronic kidney disease.

Donepezil administration is once a day starting at 5 mg and increasing to 10 mg after 4 to 6 weeks. Rivastigmine is administered twice daily, starting at 1.5 mg twice a day, and increased to 3 mg a day every 2 weeks, as tolerated, until a dose of 6 mg twice daily is reached. Because of significant nausea and vomiting, dose escalation frequently is done more slowly. A patch version of rivastigmine is currently available in doses of 4.6 and 9.5 mg/day for those individuals with difficulty taking oral medications or medications more than once a day. Galantamine is started at 4 mg twice a day and increased to 8 mg twice a day after 4 weeks. Galantamine can be further increased to 12 mg twice a day. An extended release formula of galantamine in 8, 16, and 24 mg doses to be taken once daily is also available. Oral solutions of rivastigmine and galantamine and a rapidly dissolvable tablet of donepezil are available for individuals with swallowing difficulties.

All of these drugs have similar efficacy for the symptomatic treatment of mild-to-moderate AD. Donepezil has received additional approval for the treatment of moderate-to-severe AD. None of these drugs are thought to slow down the progression of the underlying disease. Thus, patients should be monitored for improvement with both formal mental status testing and discussions with the patient's family and/or caregiver. In addition, none of these medications have proven efficacy among persons with MCI.

■ **SPECIAL CLINICAL POINT: Most experts agree that all of the cholinesterase inhibitors have had "modest" effects on cognitive, functional, and behavioral function in patients with AD and none are thought to slow down the progression of the underlying disease.**

There are several medical contraindications to cholinesterase inhibitors. Patients with serious liver disease or active alcohol abuse are not candidates for treatment with these agents. These inhibitors increase gastric secretions and should not be used in patients with active peptic ulcer disease. They also can increase bronchial secretions and should be avoided in patients with severe chronic obstructive pulmonary disease or asthma. They are vagotonic and can cause bradycardia, and they should not be used in patients with preexisting bradycardia or sick sinus syndrome. Donepezil metabolism is inhibited by quinidine and ketoconazole. Medications such as carbamazepine, phenytoin, phenobarbital, rifampin, and dexamethasone may increase donepezil's elimination from the body.

Partial Glutamate Antagonist Memantine is an uncompetitive, N-methyl-D-aspartate (NMDA) receptor channel antagonist that blocks the excitatory effects of glutamate. Memantine is excreted via the kidney and has a half-life of 60 to 80 hours. Memantine is titrated over the course of 4 weeks from 5 mg once daily to 10 mg twice a day. It is also available in an oral solution formulation. Memantine has received FDA approval for the treatment of moderate-to-severe AD alone or in combination with an AchE agent (clinical trials for the indication were done in addition to donepezil only). Memantine has the main side effects of constipation and sleepiness. No drug–drug interactions are known. However, memantine is chemically similar to amantadine and has the potential to interact with dextromethorphan, which is commonly found in over-the-counter cough suppression agents.

Other Agents Multiple other agents have been tested to see if they can slow down the progression of AD. Estrogen did not slow down the decline of memory loss in women with AD. In the Women's Health Initiative

Memory Study, use of a combination of estrogen and progesterone did not reduce the incidence of AD. Anti-inflammatory agents such as prednisone, and celecoxib, a Cox-2 selective anti-inflammatory agent, did not slow down the decline of AD. Use of naproxen to prevent the onset of AD in Cache County, UT, was stopped due to safety concerns of use of Cox-2 inhibitors; however, it did not show a prevention of the incidence of AD. The phase 3 studies of flubriprofen and tramiprosate did not slow down cognitive loss with AD. Statin agents, specifically simvastatin, have been studied with results pending.

Alternative Treatments   One study suggested that a high-dose vitamin E supplement (2000 IU/day) delayed overall time to one of the following outcomes: death, institutionalization, loss of the ability to perform basic activities of daily living, or severe dementia. The mechanism of this effect, and its specificity, remains to be elucidated because vitamin E did not appear to have an effect on cognitive function. Some, but not most, studies suggest that *Ginkgo biloba* may be of benefit in AD. A placebo controlled trial funded by the National Center for Complementary and Alternative Medicine and the National Institute on Aging of 3000 older individuals without memory complaints, showed that G. biloba was not effective in reducing the incidence of AD in these individuals. High doses of vitamins B_{12}, B_6, and folic acid to reduce homocysteine levels were not found to slow down the progression of cognitive loss in individuals with mild-to-moderate AD.

Other alternative medications such as huperzine, a Chinese herbal medicine with properties similar to AchE inhibitors, curcumin, a chemical compound in tumeric, and docosahexaenoic acid, an omega-3 fatty acid, are currently being evaluated in clinical trials at various stages.

Pharmacologic Treatment of Behavior Symptoms Associated with AD   The course of AD often is punctuated by neuropsychiatric disturbances. Although psychotic symptoms may present at

any time during the course of the dementing illness, they are more common in the middle and late stages. Common psychotic symptoms include delusions (e.g., theft of belongings, abandonment by family, and spousal infidelity), misinterpretation of delusions (e.g., characters on television are real, others are living in the house [phantom boarders]), or hallucinations.

Physical aggression that may result can have the most severe consequences for the family, eventually leading to institutionalization of the patient. Numerous studies have addressed the pharmacologic management of behavioral disturbances among patients with AD. High-potency antipsychotic agents, such as haloperidol and fluphenazine, have predominantly extrapyramidal adverse effects and have fallen out of favor in the treatment of psychosis in patients with AD. The atypical antipsychotics (risperidone, olanzapine, quetiapine, and clozapine) have replaced conventional neuroleptics as initial pharmacotherapy for psychosis associated with AD. However, these agents have been associated with increased death in clinical trials of individuals with dementia and have a "black box" warning regarding their use in older individuals with dementia. Also, the first phase of the CATIE-AD study sponsored by the National Institutes of Mental Health did not show any significant benefit of the atypical antipsychotics in reducing the intensity of behavioral symptoms over a 6-week time period. Therefore, these agents are used "off-label" for the treatment of behavioral symptoms associated with AD. These agents should be used only if environmental interventions have failed, at the lowest doses possible, with documented counseling of the risks, benefits, and alternatives to treatment with the individual and their family, and with careful monitoring for metabolic syndrome (including weight gain, diabetes, elevated cholesterol, and high blood pressure).

■ SPECIAL CLINICAL POINT: The main behavioral disturbances seen in AD are agitation, psychosis, depression, anxiety, and insomnia, all of which are treatable.

Depression and alterations of sleep–wake cycles respond to pharmacologic intervention and should be treated. Few controlled studies exist from which to guide the dose and duration of pharmacotherapy. In persons with dementia and depression, agents such as sertraline, citalopram, paroxetine, and mirtazapine have been used. A low dose, sedating narcoleptic may be preferable for the nondepressed AD patient with a significant sleep disorder. Some studies suggest that melatonin, or phototherapy, may be beneficial for sleep disorders associated with AD. However, data on the efficacy of these agents in AD are limited.

Other Interventions

There are many areas in which intervention can improve the quality of life for both the patient and the caregiver. Successful intervention requires that the physicians work effectively with providers of many other medical and nonmedical services. In general, five issues should be discussed with the family: (a) community resources, (b) advocacy, (c) pharmacotherapy, (d) behavior management, and (e) prognosis.

Community Resources   Most patients with AD in the mild-to-moderate stage can be cared for at home, assuming a caregiver is available and willing to assume this responsibility. This decision can be made only by the family. It is not appropriate for the physician (or others not involved in daily care) to insist on home care when the family finds this objectionable. Adult day-care centers provide a structured, comprehensive program in a protective setting. They offer respite for short periods but can provide care up to 7 days a week for 12 hours a day. Most centers serve mixed populations, but some are dementia specific. Many patients do well in the day-care setting, and the use of day centers for patients with dementia results in lower levels of stress and improved psychologic well-being for caregivers. The caregiver's mental and physical health must be maintained. This ultimately benefits the patient because a

healthy caregiver can manage a patient with AD longer and better than one who is overwrought and exhausted. The caregiver must have rest, and other family members should be urged to take turns in caring for the patient. Family support groups, often sponsored by the Alzheimer's Association (www.alz.org), are also helpful. The National Adult Day Services Association (www.nadsa.org) or the Eldercare Locator (www.eldercare.gov) has information on local or nationwide day-care centers.

Special care units (SCUs) have emerged over the last few years in an attempt to maximize the independence of patients by creating a 24-hour supervised environment that is safe for disoriented residents and provide structure. Nursing home placement with dementia care units can exist in rest homes or skilled nursing facilities and often are chosen by most families at the later stages of the illness. The family should be advised to seek out a nursing home where activities and exercise are stressed and where tranquilizers and restraints are minimized.

AD places a tremendous social, economic, physical, and psychologic burden on the family. The psychologic stress on the family is frequently not dealt with adequately. Stress is placed on the family in general, and particularly on the caregiver. The physician should be available and supportive throughout the course of the illness and urge the family to contact the local chapter of the Alzheimer's Association (contact information available from the national headquarters at www.alz.org). The association provides information regarding local support services for both the patient and the caregiver from other people facing similar problems. The National Institute on Aging also maintains the Alzheimer's Disease Education and Referral Center (ADEAR) (www.nia.nih.gov/Alzheimers/), which has information for both family members and physicians.

Persons with AD eventually may lose all decision-making capabilities. At the time of initial diagnosis, it is important that the physician alert the individual and family of the need to make decisions regarding advance directives, living wills and trusts, power of attorney, and guardianship. Advance directives should include an open discussion of the person's wishes regarding nursing home placement and aggressive intervention at the end of life, including feeding tubes, intubations, and resuscitation. The determination of power of attorney or guardianship is fundamental to making economic or ethical decisions regarding the care of the individual. Many persons with MCI are legally competent to execute a valid power of attorney, placing in the hands of another person decisions regarding his or her health and estate. A separate power of attorney for health care and property must be completed. In addition, the power of attorney should be "durable," which means that it remains effective if the individual becomes incompetent. Guardianship must be imposed on a person who has become incompetent and is no longer able to sign for power of attorney. In the event of family discord, the physician should avoid siding with one family member over another and should refer the family to a competent and sympathetic attorney.

Prognosis   One question that is asked frequently by the family is whether the physician can predict the course of the illness. No proven methods are yet available to make accurate predictions, but a few guidelines are available. First, clearly, AD is associated with increased risk of death among patients in institutions. However, data from community based studies has shown that persons with AD (with mild to moderate impairment) have survival rates comparable to that of persons without the disease. Finally, persons with any of these three signs—severe cognitive impairment, cachexia, or parkinsonian signs—have a much greater risk of dying.

Special Considerations for Hospitalized Patients

There are three special considerations regarding hospitalized patients. First, because many persons with AD are not diagnosed, hospital staff must be sensitive to the possibility of

unrecognized dementia among subjects admitted to the hospital for an unrelated reason. Because the hospital setting can be very disorienting, this situation can easily unmask a mild, unrecognized dementia. Thus, in the evaluation of conditions that can cause a delirium, the physician should seek detailed information regarding the patient's premorbid function. Second, patients with dementia frequently become agitated in the hospital setting, often to the point of needing physical and/or chemical sedation that can frighten patients,

---

Always Remember

- Increased awareness of dementia offers neurologists and non-neurologists an opportunity to improve the lives of patients and their caregivers.
- The clinical evaluation for assessing memory complaints has four objectives: (a) to determine if the person has dementia; (b) if dementia is present, to determine whether its presentation and course are consistent with AD; (c) to assess evidence for any alternate diagnoses, especially if the presentation and course are atypical for AD; and (d) to evaluate evidence of other, coexisting, diseases that may contribute to the dementia, especially conditions that might respond to treatment.
- After diagnosis, the clinician assists individuals with cognitive concerns to develop a network of personal care, medical, social service, and legal providers that will become their support foundation. The network attempts to maintain cognitive abilities, preserve functional abilities, control behavioral difficulties, and reduce caregiver burden through education, social and legal services, and treatment interventions.
- In general, five issues should be discussed with the family upon diagnosis of a dementia: (a) community resources, (b) advocacy, (c) pharmacotherapy, (d) behavior management, and (e) prognosis.

staff, and family. Thus, whenever possible, one should avoid hospitalizing patients with a known dementia. When hospitalization is necessary, a geriatric psychiatry unit may be preferred over a medical floor because the nurses, staff, and setting may be better prepared to care for these problems. Family should be encouraged to stay with the patient, and the use of infusing tubes and machines, including intravenous lines and urinary catheters, should be brief.

QUESTIONS AND DISCUSSION

1. A 75-year-old man is brought to the physician by his wife for evaluation of memory problems. She states that over the last few years he has become more forgetful and is having difficulty in doing some household tasks. Initially his wife felt this was just the result of getting older, but she became more concerned when her husband got lost driving to a store that they both go to regularly. In addition, at a recent party he had noticeable problems recalling friends' names and did not participate in conversations as much as he had in the past. Family members mentioned that the patient appears "sad" at times, but no changes in the patient's hobbies, sleep, or appetite have occurred. Medical history includes hypertension for 5 years (controlled with enalapril) and a history of angina. Physical and neurologic examinations are unremarkable except for an MMSE score of 25/30. Psychometric testing reveals mild short-term memory impairment. Attention and orientation are mildly impaired, and language, and visual perception are in the normal range. Mood is not suggestive of depression. A workup for reversible causes of dementia (including thyroid-stimulating hormone and vitamin B_{12} levels) is normal. An MRI of the brain reveals mild cortical atrophy with no evidence of stroke. Which of the following is the most likely diagnosis?
   A. Mild cognitive impairment
   B. Depression
   C. Alzheimer disease
   D. Frontotemporal dementia

The answer is (C). Recent literature suggests that individuals evolving to dementia generally will go through a transitional phase of MCI. In its purest form, memory impairment is the most prominent feature of MCI on cognitive testing, with relatively sparing of other cognitive functions. This patient's neuropsychologic profile suggests that more than one cognitive domain is affected (in addition to memory problems), and thus an MCI diagnosis is incorrect. Because of the lack of depressive symptomatology, depression is also not thought to be a major contributor to the patient's memory problem. *The notable lack of marked behavior or personality changes, and intact language abilities, make the diagnosis of FTD less likely.* The patient's history and clinical and neuropsychologic examinatins are consistent with the early stages of AD.

2. The patient described in question 1 above is diagnosed with mild Alzheimer dementia. A drug with which of the following actions is most appropriate for this patient?
   A. Acetylcholinesterase inhibitor
   B. Anticholinergic
   C. Dopamine blocker
   D. Serotonergic agonist

The correct answer is (A). The levels of acetylcholine, noradrenaline, serotonin, gamma aminobuyric acid (GABA), glutamate, somatostatin, and substance P have all been documented to be reduced in the brains of AD patients. However, reductions in acetylcholine and choline acetyltransferase are the most profound and are thought to be the most important with regards to cognitive function. Acetylcholine reductions may be due to the neuronal loss in the basal forebrain, which is the major region from which cholinergic projections originate. For the symptomatic treatment of AD, there are currently three commonly used drugs that enhance cholinergic transmission in the brain by reducing the degradation of acetylcholine through inhibition of the enzyme AchE. Rivastigmine inhibits both the AchE and BuChE, whereas donepezil and galantamine inhibit AchE but have only minimal inhibition of BuChE. Anticholinergic compounds would reduce the action of acetylcholine on receptors in the brain and would be more harmful than helpful. Symptomatic improvement in mood but not cognitive improvement has been noted with serotonergic agonists. Presently, there is no role for the use of dopamine blockers in the symptomatic treatment for AD.

3. The patient described in question 1 starts donepezil, but on his first return visit to the clinic 1 year later, his MMSE score drops to 18. His wife reports that he has been experiencing behavior changes—mainly mild agitation, hallucinations, and delusions. On examination, he has very mild parkinsonian signs with no evidence of tremor. Which of the following intervention(s) is (are) suitable for the management of psychosis in this patient?
   A. Selective-serotonin reuptake agents
   B. Atypical antipsychotics
   C. Typical antipsychotics
   D. Caregiver education and environmental interventions
   E. Hospitalization

The answer is (D). Caregiver education and environmental interventions are key nonpharmacologic interventions to reduce the effects of behavioral syndromes associated with dementia. Selective-serotonin reuptake inhibitors are useful in depression and are being systematically evaluated in the control of behavioral symptoms in an ongoing National Institute of Mental Health study. Atypical antipsychotics have shown mixed results in clinical trials for the long-term management of psychosis in dementia but

have significant mortality and morbidity risks in older persons with dementia. Typical antipsychotics have significant extrapyridamidal side effects commonly are not utilized for long-term treatment of psychosis in dementia. The risk of drug-induced parkinsonism and tardive dyskinesia is high, and this patient already is having very mild parkinsonian signs. As the symptoms are mild at this point and there is no indication that the patient or caregiver is at significant risk for harm, hospitalization is not warranted.

SUGGESTED READING

Aisen PS, Schafer KA, Grundman M, et al. Alzheimer's disease cooperative study. Effects of rofecoxib or naproxen vs. placebo on Alzheimer disease progression: a randomized controlled trial. *JAMA*. 2003;289: 2819–2826.

Aisen PS, Schneider LS, Sano M, et al. Alzheimer disease cooperative study. High-dose B vitamin supplementation and cognitive decline in Alzheimer disease: a randomized controlled trial. *JAMA*. 2008;300: 1774–1783.

Aggarwal NT, Wilson RS, Beck TL, et al. Mild cognitive impairment in different functional domains and incident Alzheimer's disease. *J Neurol Neurosurg Psychiatr*. 2005;76:1479–1484.

Bennett DA, Wilson RS, Schneider JA, et al. Natural history of mild cognitive impairment in older persons. *Neurology*. 2002;59:198–205.

Bennett DA, Wilson RS, Schneider JA, et al. Apolipoprotein E e4 allele, Alzheimer's disease pathology, and the clinical expression of Alzheimer's disease. *Neurology*. 2003;60:246–252.

Boyle PA, Wilson RS, Aggarwal NT, et al. Mild cognitive impairment: risk of Alzheimer disease and rate of cognitive decline. *Neurology*. 2006;67:441–445.

Callahan CM, Boustani MA, Unverzagt FW, et al. Effectiveness of collaborative care for older adults with Alzheimer disease in primary care: a randomized controlled trial. *JAMA*. 2006;295:2148–2157.

Cummings JL. Alzheimer's disease. *N Engl J Med*. 2004; 351(1):56–67.

Cummings JL, Cherry D, Kohatsu ND. Guidelines for managing Alzheimer's disease: part II. Treatment. *Am Fam Physician*. 2002;65(12);2525–2534.

Cummings JL, Frank JC, Cherry D. Guidelines for managing Alzheimer's disease: part I. Assessment. *Am Fam Physician*. 2002:65(12);2263–2272.

DeKosky ST, Williamson JD, Fitzpatrick AL, et al. Ginkgo evaluation of memory (GEM) study investigators. *Ginkgo biloba* for prevention of dementia: a randomized controlled trial. *JAMA.* 2008;300: 2253–2262.

Doody RS, Stevens JC, Beck C, et al. Practice parameter: management of dementia (an evidence-based review). Report of the Quality Standards Subcommittee of the American Academy of Neurology. *Neurology.* 2001; 56:1154–1166.

Ellison JM. A 60-year-old woman with mild memory impairment: review of mild cognitive impairment. *JAMA.* 2008;300(13):1566–1574.

Hachinski V. Shifts in thinking about dementia. *JAMA.* 2008;300:2172–2173.

Hebert LE, Scherr PA, Bienias JL, et al. Alzheimer disease in the US population: prevalence estimates using the 2000 census. *Arch Neurol.* 2003;60(8): 1119–1122.

Hebert LE, Scherr PA, McCann JJ, et al. Is the risk of developing Alzheimer's disease greater for women than for men? *Am J Epidemiol.* 2001;153:132–136.

Holsinger T, Deveau J, Boustani M, et al. Does this patient have dementia? *JAMA.* 2007;297:2391–2404.

Inouye SK. The dilemma of delirium: clinical and research controversies regarding diagnosis and evaluation of delirium in hospitalized elderly medical patients. *Am J Med.* 1994;97:278–288.

Knopman DS, DeKosky ST, Cummings JL, et al. Practice parameter: diagnosis of dementia (an evidence-based review). Report of the Quality Standards Subcommittee of the American Academy of Neurology. *Neurology.* 2001;56:1143–1153.

Kuhn, D. *Alzheimer's Early Stages: First Steps for Families, Friends and Caregivers.* Alameda, CA: Hunter House; 2003.

Mace NL, Rabbins PV. *The 36 Hour Day, 4th Edition: A Family Guide to Caring for People with Alzheimer Disease, Other Dementias, and Memory Loss in Later Life.* Baltimore, MD: John Hopkins University Press; 2006.

McCann JJ, Hebert LE, Li Y, et al. The effect of adult day care services on time to nursing home placement in older adults with Alzheimer's disease. *Gerontologist.* 2005;45:754–763.

McKeith IG, Galasko D, Kosaka K, et al. Consensus guidelines for the clinical and pathologic diagnosis of dementia with Lewy bodies (DLB): report of the Consortium on DLB International Workshop. *J Alzheimers Dis.* 2006;9(suppl 3):417–423.

McKhann GM, Albert MS, Grossman M, et al. Clinical and pathological diagnosis of frontotemporal dementia: report of the Work Group on Frontotemporal Dementia and Pick's Disease. *Arch Neurol.* 2001;58:1803–1809.

Mendez MF, Shapira JS, McMurtray A, et al. Accuracy of the clinical evaluation for frontotemporal dementia. *Arch Neurol.* 2007;64(6):830–835.

Mittelman MS, Ferris SH, Shulman E, et al. A family intervention to delay nursing home placement of patients with Alzheimer disease: a randomized controlled trial. *JAMA.* 1996;276:1725.

Mulnard RA, Cotman CW, Kawas C, et al. Estrogen replacement therapy for treatment of mild to moderate Alzheimer disease: a randomized controlled trial. Alzheimer's Disease Cooperative Study. *JAMA.* 2000; 283:1007–1015.

Petersen RC, Stevens JC, Ganguli M, et al. Practice parameter: early detection of dementia: mild cognitive impairment (an evidence-based review). Report of the Quality Standards Subcommittee of the American Academy of Neurology. *Neurology.* 2001;56:1133–1142.

Petersen RC, Thomas RG, Grundman M, et al. Alzheimer's Disease Cooperative Study Group. Vitamin E and donepezil for the treatment of mild cognitive impairment. *N Engl J Med.* 2005;352:2379–2388.

Qaseem A, Snow V, Cross JT Jr, et al. American College of Physicians/American Academy of Family Physicians Panel on Dementia. Current pharmacologic treatment of dementia: a clinical practice guideline from the American College of Physicians and the American Academy of Family Physicians. *Ann Intern Med.* 2008; 148:370–378.

Roman GC, Tatemichi TK, Erkinjuntti T, et al. Vascular dementia: diagnostic criteria for research studies. Report of the NINDS-AIREN International Work Group. *Neurology.* 1993;43:250.

Sano M, Ernesto C, Thomas RG, et al. A controlled trial of selegiline, alpha-tocopherol, or both as treatment for Alzheimer's disease. *N Engl J Med.* 1997;336:1216.

Schneider JA, Arvanitakis Z, Bang W, et al. Mixed brain pathologies account for most dementia cases in community dwelling older persons. *Neurology.* 2007;69: 2197–2204.

Schneider LS, Dagerman KS, Insel P. Risk of death with atypical antipsychotic drug treatment for dementia: meta-analysis of randomized placebo-controlled trials. *JAMA.* 2005;294:1934–1943.

Schneider LS, Tariot PN, Dagerman KS, et al. CATIE-AD Study Group. Effectiveness of atypical antipsychotic drugs in patients with Alzheimer's disease. *N Engl J Med.* 2006;355:1525–1538.

Schulz R, Belle SH, Czaja SJ, et al. Long-term care placement of dementia patients and caregiver health and well-being. *JAMA.* 2004;292:961–967.

Shumaker SA, Legault C, Kuller L, et al. Conjugated equine estrogens and incidence of probable dementia and mild cognitive impairment in postmenopausal women: Women's Health Initiative Memory Study. *JAMA.* 2004;291:2947–2958.

Tangalos EG, Smith GE, Ivnik RJ, et al. The mini-mental state examination in general medical practice: clinical utility and acceptance. *Mayo Clin Proc.* 1996;71:829.

Tanzi RE, Bertram L. New frontiers in Alzheimer's disease genetics. *Neuron.* 2001;32:181–184.

Tariot PN, Farlow MR, Grossberg GT, et al. Memantine treatment in patients with moderate to severe Alzheimer disease already receiving donepezil: a randomized controlled trial. *JAMA.* 2004;291:317–324.

Teri L, Gibbons LE, McCurry SM, et al. Exercise plus behavioral management in patients with Alzheimer disease: a randomized controlled trial. *JAMA.* 2003;290:2015–2022.

US Preventive Services Task Force. Screening for dementia: recommendation and rationale. *Ann Intern Med.* 2003;138(11):925–926.

Wilson RS, Mendes de Leon CF, Barnes LL, et al. Participation in cognitively stimulating activities and risk of incident Alzheimer's disease. *JAMA.* 2002;287:742–748.

Yaffe K. Treatment of neuropsychiatric symptoms in patients with dementia. *N Engl J Med.* 2007; 357:1441–1443.

Zaccai J, McCracken C, Brayne C. A systematic review of prevalence and incidence studies of dementia with Lewy bodies. *Age Ageing.* 2005;34(6):561–566.

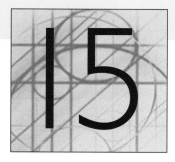

15

Behavioral Neurology

ROBERT S. WILSON AND
CHRISTOPHER G. GOETZ

key points

- Disease involving the Papez circuit often results in aberrant emotional behavior, memory dysfunction, or both.

- Temporal lobe epilepsy is characterized by sudden loss of contact with the environment and brief behavioral changes.

- Temporal lobe epilepsy may be ushered in by a stereotypic sensory experience (i.e., aura) and involve stereotypic motor behaviors (i.e., automatisms).

- All individuals with a sudden change in language function should be referred to a neurologist.

- Fluent aphasia is usually the result of dominant temporal or temporoparietal damage, and because of the temporal lobe involvement, behavioral changes are often seen.

- All patients with suspected Wernicke encephalopathy should immediately receive thiamine.

- Transient global amnesia involves the abrupt onset of a dense anterograde amnesia that typically completely resolves within 24 hours.

- Anterograde amnesia and bizarre behavioral and emotional changes are common sequelae of herpes simplex encephalitis.

B izarre or altered behavioral patterns traditionally are felt to relate to psychiatric disorders or generalized delirium from drugs, toxins, or metabolic imbalances. However, some specific neurologic conditions present with remarkably consistent behavioral abnormalities. These conditions have equally consistent anatomic substrates, and, when identified by an astute diagnostician, they suggest specific causes and treatments. In this chapter, five conditions are discussed, each with a prominent behavioral and seemingly psychiatric presentation but with a pathologic basis related to a specific neurologic dysfunction. These conditions are temporal lobe epilepsy (TLE), fluent aphasia, Wernicke encephalopathy, transient global amnesia, and herpes encephalitis.

These strange disorders are not rare, and their complexity often relates not to management problems but to accurate identification. The topic is thus particularly pertinent to the non-neurologist, who is most likely to be the first person to interview and evaluate these patients.

ANATOMIC BASIS—PAPEZ CIRCUIT

It is well recognized that the ability to recall and engender memories is intimately linked to the emotional makeup of such memories. Furthermore, several clinical conditions demonstrate combined and prominent memory–emotional alterations, suggesting that the anatomic basis of these two functions may be linked. In 1937, the neuroanatomist Papez published a treatise describing an anatomic circuit that linked those nuclei and paths that appear important to many aspects of emotional–behavioral integration. This circuit, the Papez circuit, is probably the most important circuit for clinicians dealing with behavioral abnormalities; familiarity with it allows them to think systematically about the anatomic foundations of behavioral neurology.

The circuit is diagrammed schematically in Figure 15.1A, with anatomic nuclei and paths identified in the sagittal brain section of Figure 15.1B. As indicated, the pathway is circular, providing continual reintegration of information. The two focal cortical areas most prominently involved are the cingulate cortex and the hippocampus of the temporal lobe. Diffuse cortical impulses travel into the hippocampus, an area felt to be particularly important to memory and emotional expression. This information travels forward in the fornix path to the mammillary bodies of the hypothalamus and continues to the anterior lobe of the thalamus, and further to the midline cingulate cortex, which finally projects diffusely to cortical regions.

Familiarity with this circuit is useful because disease anywhere along the pathway can be expected to result in aberrant emotional behaviors, although not necessarily the same patterns. This knowledge allows the clinician to focus immediately on a finite number of nuclei and connecting paths to explain abnormal behavioral symptoms that may have a focal

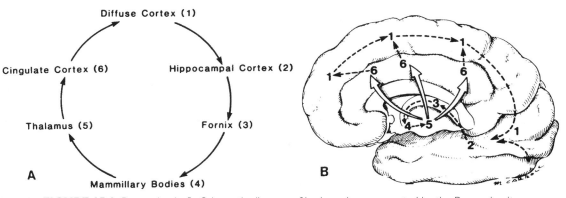

FIGURE 15.1 Papez circuit. **A:** Schematic diagram of brain regions connected by the Papez circuit. **B:** Anatomic diagram of brain regions numbered in **(A)**, with arrows indicating the direction of general informational flow.

anatomic basis. The term diffuse cortical input is important because toxic and metabolic encephalopathy often present with agitated behavior or a change in personality. The other areas, however, are focal, and identification of disease at these levels can lead to rapid intervention. Reference will be made to this circuit throughout this chapter.

TEMPORAL LOBE EPILEPSY

Also referred to as psychomotor epilepsy and partial complex seizure, psychomotor or psychosensory variety, TLE may manifest itself with intermittent spells of bizarre behavior, including babbling nonsense and frank visual and auditory hallucinations, all related to organic disease of the central nervous system. Differentiation of this disorder from psychotic disorders such as schizophrenia can be difficult, yet it is essential because their treatments are drastically different. Certain specific characteristics are helpful in establishing abnormal behavioral patterns as probable epilepsy, and they are the focus of this discussion.

TLE represents an abnormal electrical discharge that begins in one temporal lobe and usually crosses rapidly to involve both sides of the brain. To recognize TLE in a patient, the clinician should attempt to elicit specific information in four areas. If information in even one of these areas is characteristic of TLE, the diagnosis is suggested.

1. The distinctive temporal pattern of the spells.
2. The presence of an aura, a distinctive feeling, or sensation that regularly precedes or begins the spells.
3. The presence of peculiar motor behaviors called automatisms.
4. The specific type of loss of consciousness.

The distinctive temporal pattern of TLE refers to repeated, but intermittent, and paroxysmal changes in behavior, not necessarily linked to any emotional provocation. The behavioral changes are brief, lasting seconds to

TABLE 15.1 Temporal Lobe Foci and Related Auras	
Anatomic Focus	**Clinical Symptoms of Aura**
Uncus	Smell, taste
Cingulate cortex	Change in emotional perception—déjà vu (strange familiarity with the environment), jamais vu (strange sense of never being in current environment), euphoria, sense of sudden doom
Insula	Epigastric rising sensation
Amygdala	Pupillary dilatation, photophobia, automatisms
Temporal cortex including auditory cortex and association areas	Hallucinations

minutes. Often, before any visible behavioral change can be appreciated by an observer, the patient experiences a stereotypic and fixed sensation, known as an epileptic aura. The aura represents the beginning of the seizure and can help in localizing the focus, or source, of the seizure activity. The aura may be olfactory, in which the patient suddenly smells a strange, often pungent odor, or it may be a gustatory sensation or a strange abdominal "butterflies" feeling, also called epigastric rising. Emotional changes of sudden unfamiliarity with one's environment (jamais vu) or sudden intense familiarity with the surroundings (déjà vu) are seen, and there may be intense and vivid auditory or visual hallucinations. The aura and the area of the temporal lobe cortex that are felt to relate to the seizure focus are listed in Table 15.1. The presence of this stereotypic aura and sudden unprovoked change in behavior help to quickly identify a patient with TLE. The aura is sensed by the patient and is not identified by the clinician except by interview. The patient may not necessarily link the strange aura to his spells, so that information must be solicited specifically.

■ **SPECIAL CLINICAL POINT: The very first perceived abnormality related to a seizure has key importance to localizing the source of the epilepsy, so careful interviewing of a typical spell, step-by-step is essential.**

The presence of automatisms is also useful in the diagnosis of TLE. These activities appear as the seizure spreads in the amygdala region of the temporal lobe. The movements may range from rather primitive movements (lip smacking, eye blinking, or chewing motions) or may be highly complex (dressing and undressing, piling objects on top of one another). These are stereotypic and rather fixed from one spell to another, so a detailed record of two or more episodes helps to establish the pattern of behavior.

The peculiar characteristic of the loss of consciousness seen in TLE is also helpful. After the aura, which the examiner cannot see unless it involves automatisms, there is a sudden loss of contact with the environment in TLE. Unlike patients who have other generalized seizures, these patients only rarely fall to the floor, shake all over, urinate, or bite their tongue. Instead, when they lose consciousness, they maintain body tone and may walk around but "in a daze, out of contact" with the environment. When the spell is over, the patient is usually amnestic for the seizure, except that he may recall its beginning and be able to recount, if specifically asked, the details of the aura. Immediately after the spell, the patient is usually confused and sleepy. If restrained during this period, he may strike out randomly at people who try to assist. However, these patients are generally not violent in a goal-directed manner, either during or after their seizures. As strange as their behaviors may be, focused violence, such as tracking a person with a gun or retrieving a kitchen knife out of a drawer and stabbing a victim, is far outside the repertoire of TLE. Table 15.2 serves as a summary and outlines additional guidelines for differentiating TLE episodes from psychotic bizarre behaviors of schizophrenia. These patterns are clinically useful, although no absolute rules hold true. The following example demonstrates that TLE patients can be misdiagnosed.

Case: A 16-year-old boy on the psychiatric unit with a diagnosis of schizophrenia and hallucinatory behavior is evaluated by the neurologist because of a single generalized seizure. On being interviewed, this patient says, "It's just like before, but this time much worse." Several times each week, this patient sees "the man," a blurry but discernible bearded man who beckons him forward verbally. As this happens, everything in the patient's environment becomes suddenly more distinct, clearer, and more colorful, with a clear sense of familiarity and warmth. Then a strange feeling of dread and a "fog" come over the patient, who

TABLE 15.2 Clinical Distinctions Between TLE Behavior and Schizophrenia

	TLE	Schizophrenia
Environmental precipitants	Rare	Frequent
Duration of attack	0.5–5 minutes	May be days
Aura	Usual	Lacking
Injury to others	Rare and undirected	Unpredictable—may be directed or undirected
Disturbance of consciousness	Present	Lacking or mildly clouded
Symptoms and signs after attack	Sleepy, confused	Lacking

then appears to lose touch for approximately 5 minutes. He has no recollection of this period of losing touch, but his family says that he walks around in the house mumbling strange noises that are sometimes prayers, and at the same time he bows his head back and forth in a seemingly ritualistic manner. After this, he lies down and sleeps for approximately 2 hours. The same stereotypic pattern occurred immediately before the generalized seizure.

This patient again shows the stereotypic aura, which is hallucinatory this time, along with the sense of emotional familiarity with the environment. Stereotypic repetition of episodes and the automatisms with amnesia and sleepiness afterward strongly suggest TLE. In regard to this latter episode in which there was a generalized motor seizure with bilateral shaking, this pattern can be seen with TLE when the seizure activity spreads throughout both sides of the brain. An EEG study with nasopharyngeal recordings demonstrated abnormal epileptiform activity. On medication, the patient has shown remarkable improvement. This case demonstrates the important interface between psychiatric symptoms and clear focal neurologic disease.

■ **SPECIAL CLINICAL POINT: The distinctive behavioral manifestation of these seizures is a stereotypic loss of contact with the environment, often a "dazed" look while otherwise apparently awake.**

ANATOMY AND CLINICAL FINDINGS

The anatomic lesions of TLE naturally relate to the temporal lobe and, depending on the area damaged, will give rise to different auras (Table 15.1). As can be seen, some of these nuclei are primary portions of the Papez circuit and the others have direct input into the circuit.

In examining a patient with TLE, if there is a tumor, stroke, or space occupying lesion, a finding may include a homonymous hemianopia, or a homonymous quadrantanopsia, especially in the superior fields (Fig. 15.2). Because the visual fibers pass through the temporal lobe en route to the occipital cortex, the superior quadrantanopsia should be specifically sought.

Much has been written about psychopathology in patients with TLE. Although the seizures and bizarre behavior are intermittent, interictal or between-seizure abnormalities are often attributed to TLE. Problems such as sedation, inattention, and depressed mood may be seen as dose-related side effects of antiepileptic medications. If toxicity can be ruled out, the most common psychiatric problem in epilepsy is depression. Although not specific to TLE, research suggests rates of depression as high as 75% in some clinical samples. Paradoxically, depression may appear after seizure control is accomplished, suggesting that seizures, like electroconvulsive therapy, may serve to elevate mood, possibly through opioid mechanisms.

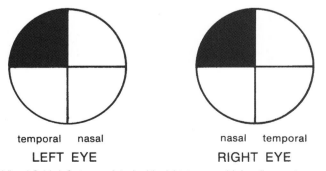

FIGURE 15.2. Visual field defect associated with right temporal lobe disease, termed left superior quadrantanopsia.

Aggressive behavior is often attributed to TLE. There is, however, no good evidence of a disproportionate level of aggressive or violent behavior in TLE or epilepsy. Aggressive behavior may be seen following a seizure, but it is typically nondirected and random, occurring when the patient is aroused or restrained. The hypothesis that TLE is characterized by a distinct personality profile has not been supported by recent research. However, psychiatric signs and symptoms in general are seen more commonly in TLE than in other forms of epilepsy, particularly in patients with severe, uncontrolled TLE.

ETIOLOGY

TLE is often seen in patients with a history of birth trauma. Brain tumors, both primary and metastatic, also may involve the temporal lobe and present early with characteristic TLE. Subacute onset of TLE with fever should suggest encephalitis, specifically resulting from herpes simplex, which has a predilection for the temporal lobes. EEG findings are discussed in Chapter 8. Treatment drugs useful in the control of TLE are listed in Table 15.3, along with usual doses, plasma levels, and common side effects. There are no specific rehabilitation or alternate medical therapies that are applicable to the treatment of TLE.

When to Refer Patients to a Neurologist

TLE is a complicated neurologic condition, and all patients should be referred to a neurologist at least once to obtain expert opinion on the nature of the condition and its management. The neurologist can provide guidelines to the non-neurologist for drug management

TABLE 15.3 Drugs Used in the Control of TLE: Dosages, Therapeutic Plasma Levels, and Common or Important Side Effects

Drug	Adult Dosage (mg/day)	Plasma Level (mg/mL)	Toxicity
Carbamazepine[a]	600–1200	4–10	Diplopia, nausea, vomiting, sedation, ataxia
Phenytoin	300	10–20	Ataxia, nausea, vomiting, sedation folate deficiency
Valproic acid[a]	750–1500	50–150	Tremor, nausea, weight gain
Lamotrigine	300–500	2–15	Dizziness, diplopia, ataxia, insomnia
Phenobarbital	90–180	15–40	Sedation, hyperactivity in children, depression
Gabapentin	900–3600	4–8	Somnolence, nausea, weight gain, vomiting, sedation, depression, impotence
Primidone[a]	750–1000	7–15 primidone 20–40 phenobarbital	See Phenobarbital toxicity
Topiramate	300–600	2–20	Confusion, dysphasia, weight loss
Oxcarbazepine	600–1800	5–50	Diplopia, nausea, dizziness
Zonisamide	200–600	10–40	Confusion, irritability
Levetiracetam	1000–3000	20–60	Irritability, confusion
Pregabalin	300–600	Not applicable	Weight gain, confusion

[a]Drug preferentially recommended for TLE as opposed to other forms of seizures.

and behaviors that fall within and outside the realm of TLE. Because the government guidelines for driving are different in each state, the neurologist also can provide the non-neurologist with the specific rules regarding driving limitations for patients who have seizures.

Special Challenges for Hospitalized Patients

Hospital personnel are unlikely to be familiar with the behaviors that typify TLE; therefore, the admitting physician must outline the sequence of behaviors of the seizure episodes. Seizure precautions and seizure treatment as outlined in Chapter 8 should be followed throughout the hospitalized period. When patients have surgery and cannot take medications by mouth, alternate routes of medication delivery must be used, as outlined in Chapter 8.

FLUENT APHASIA

Aphasia is a specific language deficit that occurs without weakness of the articulatory muscles, and it is caused by cortical brain disease. The two basic types of aphasia are subfluent and fluent. The former group is not difficult to diagnose and would not be confused with psychiatric disease because in most cases an obvious right hemiparesis accompanies the change in speech pattern. The fluent aphasias, however, are not associated with motor problems, so that these patients present with behavioral alterations in the form of strange speech. The adage taught to young neurologists—when evaluating an acute behavioral change, one must always rule out fluent aphasia—is applicable to all clinicians.

Aphasic problems occur with focal dominant hemisphere disorders. For most people, the left hemisphere is dominant for speech, although in a small percentage of left-handed people, the right hemisphere may be dominant. Subfluent aphasias relate to frontal lobe disease, and fluent aphasias relate usually to dominant temporal or temporoparietal damage. Because the temporal lobe is involved in the Papez circuit, behavioral alterations in fluent aphasias are expected and characteristic.

In contrast to the frustration and depressed affect common in subfluent aphasia, patients with fluent aphasia are often seemingly unaware of their deficit and are unconcerned. Patients may not realize that their speech is incomprehensible to others. In extreme cases, these patients may blame their inability to communicate to others on the point of frank paranoia. Impulsivity is also observed. The combination of such behaviors can result in serious management problems.

The evaluation of aphasia is usually rapid and requires no unusual implements. Table 15.4 outlines the manner of examination, which has three focal points. First, by listening to the patient's spontaneous speech, the clinician decides whether the speech is subfluent, slow, and sparse or fluent, rapid, and free flowing. This evaluation makes no judgment on content of speech; instead it judges rhythm and ease of word production. Second, the examiner asks the patient to follow a verbal command—"Show me a spoon," "Raise your left hand," and so forth—which tests ability to comprehend. This integration of auditory information helps to distinguish various aphasias and localizes the disease. The command must be verbal, and the investigator must discipline himself not to use nonverbal communication during this task. Third, the patient is asked to repeat a sentence—first a reasonable phrase, such as "Today is Tuesday; tomorrow I will phone Bill," and then a nonsense phrase, such as "No ifs, ands, or buts." These three simple maneuvers can be performed by patients who are confused or intoxicated and by patients with short attention spans. However, they are not performed by patients with aphasia. Furthermore, the pattern of disability in the three tasks isolates the specific areas of dominant cortical dysfunction.

■ **SPECIAL CLINICAL POINT: Patients with dominant hemisphere temporal lobe disease and fluent aphasia babble incoherently, but are**

TABLE 15.4 | **Major Types of Aphasia and Guides to their Rapid Identification**

Names	Fluency	Follow Commands	Repeat	Focal Damage	Associative Problems
Broca	Subfluent	Yes	No	Dominant frontal lobe	Right hemiparesis
Wernicke	Fluent	No	No	Dominant temporal lobe	Visual field abnormalities, no weakness
Conductive	Fluent	Yes	Yes for short phrases; cannot repeat "no ifs, ands, or buts"	Dominant connecting fibers between Broca and Wernicke area	Visual field abnormalities or mild weakness, decreased sensation on right side of body and face

often emotionally undisturbed by their language difficulty.

A patient with fluent aphasia, known classically as Wernicke aphasia (not to be confused with Wernicke encephalopathy, discussed later in the text under Wernicke-Korsakoff Syndrome), is often first diagnosed as confused, agitated, and sometimes even schizophrenic. The following case history helps to typify this syndrome, and it emphasizes the common confusion between this condition and the word salad of schizophrenia.

Case: A 65-year-old hypertensive right-handed woman was well until 3 hours before an evaluation in the emergency room. Her family lived with her and reported that after lunch the patient took a 40-minute nap; on awaking, she "began speaking nonsense—crazy talk." Her past medical and psychiatric histories were negative, and no similar events had ever occurred.

The patient is alert and talkative, but her speech has no discernible sense. Phrases such as "oh, me," "why not," "should we," "what now," and "amen Moses" are spoken rapidly and spontaneously. She can follow no verbal commands nor will she repeat simple phrases. The family feels she may be poisoned or has gone crazy.

The highlights of this case are the patient's age, the acute onset, the characteristic speech pattern, and the easily retrieved results of an accurate aphasia testing screen. It is important to note that in a patient who is 65 years old without prior psychiatric history, the new onset of schizophrenia, regardless of how bizarre the behavior or speech may be, would be exceptional.

ETIOLOGY

Wernicke fluent aphasia is usually seen with dominant temporal lobe disease in the form of cerebrovascular accidents or sometimes tumors. The rapid onset in an elderly individual suggests the former, whereas a more indolent course can be seen with tumors. When this speech pattern is encountered, the clinician immediately should focus attention on the dominant temporal lobe. Associated findings often include the superior quadrantanopsia (Fig. 15.2), and temporal lobe seizures may be an associated phenomenon.

The other fluent aphasia, conduction aphasia, does not appear to be a psychiatric illness; thus, it will not be discussed in detail. These patients speak fluently and usually make sense, except that they mix up words or make new words (paraphasic errors). Although they can repeat simple sentences, they have trouble with nonsense phrases such as "no ifs, ands, or buts." This disease localizes to the arcuate fasciculus of the parietal lobe connecting the temporal and frontal speech areas. Strokes and tumors are again the likely causes, although sometimes Wernicke aphasia, as it resolves, tends to become a conduction aphasia. Anomic aphasia, in which the patient is fluent and behaviorally appropriate but has trouble finding the proper word, is seen as other forms of aphasia resolve.

Treatment

The treatment of aphasia focuses on two elements: rehabilitation of the speech deficit and treatment of the underlying cause. Because patients with fluent aphasia often do not recognize their speech problems, they are difficult rehabilitation patients. Speech therapy is used, but until the patient becomes motivated to communicate more effectively, the speech exercises are often fruitless. No medications or alternate medical treatments are specifically useful. Diagnostic tests, such as MRI scans, will identify the anatomic lesion in the dominant (left) temporal lobe, and the contours of the lesion will help in suggesting a vascular etiology (stroke) from tumor, where there is often extensive edema or multiple discrete lesions. An EEG will help define if there are seizures. The treatments will be directed to the most likely cause; stroke treatment is outlined in Chapter 6, tumor therapy is discussed in Chapter 20, and seizure management is covered in Chapter 8.

When to Refer the Patient to a Neurologist

In contrast to subjects with subfluent aphasia, in which the patient cannot produce speech, patients with Wernicke aphasia speak excessively and typically are unconcerned about their speech and behavioral abnormalities. The family and medical staff, however, readily recognize the incoherent language, although they may not be able to interpret the problem as an aphasia. In an emergency room or office setting, the physician must always be alert to the possibility of a focal neurologic lesion when there is a sudden change in language function. Once the diagnosis and underlying cause are defined, the management often can be directed by the non-neurologist with intermittent consultation back to the neurologist.

■ **SPECIAL CLINICAL NOTE: All patients with a sudden change in language content should be referred to a neurologist for a consultation.**

Special Challenges for Hospitalized Patients

In the hospital, patients with aphasia are a particular challenge. Usually, they are hospitalized at the onset of the aphasia, and the staff will not understand the language abnormality or its origin. Staff must be educated to be compassionate and solicitous of the patient's needs despite the seemingly nonsensical language. In a patient with a chronic Wernicke aphasia who must be hospitalized, the family often will be more familiar with the speech deficit than a professional staff, and their aid must be sought to maximize communication efficiency between staff and patient. Because patients with fluent aphasia have specific difficulty understanding language, when the physician or staff need to explain a procedure, treatment, or test, the family member with authority for the patient's care must be included for proper consent.

WERNICKE–KORSAKOFF SYNDROME (WERNICKE ENCEPHALOPATHY)

Wernicke–Korsakoff syndrome, also known as Wernicke encephalopathy or, in its extreme form, Korsakoff psychosis, represents a neurologic emergency. The important triad of Wernicke encephalopathy includes behavioral alterations, extraocular movement abnormalities, and ataxia. These symptoms occur to a greater or lesser extent with selective memory impairment, and when this memory impairment is marked, the syndrome is called Korsakoff psychosis. The two diseases are the same but are referred to with different terms depending on the degree of memory deficit. The pathogenesis of this syndrome relates to vitamin deficiency in the form of vitamin B_1 (thiamine). The primary patients at high risk for this syndrome are alcoholics who obtain calories through the alcohol but do not receive essential vitamins. Patients with prolonged emesis or with gastric bowel resection or bariatric surgery also can suffer with thiamine deficiency. Occasionally, voluntary starvation in the form of political protest, psychotic disturbances, or unsupervised treatment of obesity also can induce this syndrome. Finally, and important to surgical patients, hyperalimentation can be associated with Wernicke encephalopathy when water-soluble B vitamins are not included in the formula.

■ **SPECIAL CLINICAL POINT: When a patient presents with behavioral changes and has a gait abnormality and abnormalities of eye movements, Wernicke encephalopathy must be considered and rapid treatment with thiamine supplementation is essential to treat this medical emergency.**

The behavioral picture of Wernicke encephalopathy–Korsakoff psychosis has three different presentations. The patient with acute Wernicke encephalopathy shows global confusion, and his or her demeanor is usually quiet and apathetic. He or she is alert and responsive but inattentive, and the patient appears fatigued. Occasionally, a patient may be more agitated, especially if he or she is undergoing delirium tremens associated with alcohol withdrawal. The usual presentation, however, is one of an affable but dull affect.

In the partially treated patient or in the early stages of chronic disease, the affect becomes more bright, and the patient becomes more loquacious. The memory deficits become more apparent as the patient is less globally confused. The patient is nonhesitant in his speech, and it is at this point that the famed confabulatory aspects of Korsakoff psychosis may be

seen. Confabulation is not an essential component of Korsakoff psychosis; the characteristic trait of this condition is the preferential loss of recent memory.

The patient with chronic Wernicke–Korsakoff syndrome is typically alert and oriented but displays characteristic deficiencies in recent and remote memory. The recent memory deficit is usually profound and consists of an inability to make an enduring record of daily experiences. The remote memory deficit is temporally graded such that more remote events are relatively more accessible to recall. Thus, a patient asked to name presidents since World War II may recall Truman and Eisenhower but not their successors. Confabulation is not typically seen in chronic patients. Behaviorally, such patients are usually apathetic and indifferent, with occasional outbursts of irritability.

■ **SPECIAL CLINICAL POINT: Memory loss is the key behavioral abnormality seen in Wernicke encephalopathy.**

In diagnosing this syndrome, the neurologic signs of extraocular muscle palsy or nystagmus and ataxia are important features to recognize. In many ways, the patient with acute Wernicke encephalopathy looks like a drunkard with trouble walking, nystagmus, and altered affect. Because of the similarity, it is a common adage that a drunk patient seen in the emergency room should be given an injection of thiamine (a) to treat possible Wernicke encephalopathy and (b) to prevent a future episode of the condition. The chronic patient is difficult to manage because, although the extraocular movements improve quickly with thiamine therapy and the ataxia improves to a moderate extent, the memory problems are least abated by thiamine therapy.

ANATOMIC BASIS

The unifying basis for this disorder involves the Papez circuit where there is capillary proliferation at the level of the mammillary bodies. In some cases in which the mammillary bodies are spared, the anterior lobe of the thalamus is involved. Additional pathologic findings may involve cerebellar and diffuse cortical degeneration. Although the clinical picture of Korsakoff psychosis should immediately suggest vitamin deficiency and disease that at least includes the mammillary bodies, it can be seen in diseases that involve other aspects of the Papez circuit. The same syndrome has been reported in patients who recover from a viral encephalitis with prominent hippocampus involvement. Such clinical overlap again emphasizes the importance of the Papez circuit in localizing diseases that involve both memory and affective disorders.

Treatment

All patients with suspected Wernicke encephalopathy must immediately receive thiamine. At least 100 mg intravenous thiamine should be given, followed by 100 mg IM daily for 3 to 5 days, with a chronic dose of oral thiamine (50 mg daily) and a multivitamin.

Once thiamine has been given and good nutrition is reestablished, physical and occupational therapy can be recommended to help in gait training and coordination. Full neuropsychologic testing will help in establishing specific mental deficits and provide data that will be useful for discharge planning. No alternative medical therapies are recommended.

When to Refer to a Neurologist

The non-neurologist should never hesitate to treat a patient with components of Wernicke encephalopathy with thiamine. Clear documentation on the chart of the mental status, the presence of nystagmus or ophthalmoplegia, and a description of the gait should be noted. Therefore, the neurologist can be consulted to corroborate the diagnosis and suggest other treatment or diagnostic evaluations.

Special Challenges for Hospitalized Patients

Because so many patients with Wernicke encephalopathy are heavy alcohol users, the risk of alcohol withdrawal in the hospital and its consequences including delirium tremens is high. The hospital staff must be aware of these problems and appropriately protect the patient against injury and medical complications of alcohol withdrawal, especially in the first 72 hours of hospitalization, as outlined in Chapter 12. These include a careful attention to the diagnosis of infection or associated injuries, such as meningitis or subdural hematomas. Further, maintenance of fluid and electrolyte balance is essential, as well as a watchful attention to the possibility of hypoglycemia. Control of agitation is essential to avoid patient and staff injury. Specific recommendations are outlined in Chapter 12.

TRANSIENT GLOBAL AMNESIA

The syndrome of transient global amnesia occurs in middle-aged or elderly patients. A characteristic triggering event, such as physical or emotional stress or sexual intercourse, often precedes the amnestic episode.

When the spell has begun, the patient is unable to learn new information until it is over. His memory for events that day and the preceding day are almost always poor. Memory for prior events will be better, although memory loss during the event sometimes will be detectable even for events that took place years before the amnestic spell. The syndrome of transient global amnesia typically clears completely within 24 hours, except for a permanent amnesia for the episode itself. Significantly, the patient's affect is often bland during the episode, although family members are distressed.

Patients with transient global amnesia are often brought to medical attention when the family notes that they repeatedly ask the same questions and seem unable to remember the answer and sometimes deny that an answer has been given. At the same time, these patients may perform complex tasks during an episode without difficulty, as long as these tasks were learned prior to the event.

These patients are not globally confused. In testing orientation, however, they may report the wrong answer because they cannot integrate changes in place and time. When asked to do arithmetic calculations or use logical processing, they respond appropriately.

■ **SPECIAL CLINICAL POINT: A sudden change in behavior that involves continual questioning with the inability to retain new information in a patient who is otherwise alert should immediately suggest transient global amnesia.**

Memory testing during an attack of transient global amnesia demonstrates a marked inability to establish new memories despite preserved attention, language, and higher cognitive functioning. If the physician leaves the room of a patient with this disorder, he will have to reintroduce himself when he returns. Recent memory function is deficient in such patients regardless of which sensory system is used in the memory tasks, so that visual, tactile, and auditory memories are disturbed. The retrograde amnesia is such that the activities of the previous days may be only dimly recollected during the episode. The retrograde amnesia is occasionally more extensive, affecting memories formed years before the episode. Confabulation is notably lacking in these patients. On recovery, there is no recollection of the episode itself, and there is typically a permanent retrograde amnesia for events occurring in the moments prior to the episode.

This syndrome with its peculiar constellation of memory and behavioral features can be highly confusing unless it is recognized.

In patients whose amnesic episodes are brief (e.g., less than 1 hour) and/or recurrent, TLE should be considered, and treatment with anticonvulsant medications can be successful. In patients with focal neurologic signs or symptoms during or subsequent to the amnesic episode, tumors and cerebrovascular disease should be considered, and the prognosis may be more guarded. If the amnesia includes additional disorientation and/or inattention, drug ingestion, especially of anticholinergic or sedative drugs, may be the cause.

Transient global amnesia is most often confused with psychogenic amnestic states. Hysterical amnesia may occur abruptly but is frequently associated with a specific precipitating event, with retention of memory for other events within the time interval. One does not see the profound yet selective deficit in recent memory, nor the temporally graded retrograde amnesia.

In the more severe hysterical amnesia, such as in fugue states, there is the characteristic dissociative behavior with an additional loss of personal identity, a feature not seen in transient global amnesia. In contrast to the transient global amnesia patient, the hysterical patient will often acknowledge that the memory is poor but will have an inappropriate affect, "la belle indifférence."

Anatomic Basis

Because the episodes of transient global amnesia tend not to recur, no extensive pathologic studies have been performed on patients. The anatomic basis of this syndrome, however, is felt to relate to temporal lobe dysfunction in the area involved in the Papez circuit. MRI studies have shown that, despite the transient nature of the syndrome, some patients with transient global amnesia show small unilateral or bilateral changes on diffusion-weighted MRI in the hippocampal regions within the first 24 to 48 hours following the event. The etiology of transient global amnesia remains uncertain, but current hypotheses include transient venous or arterial ischemia to the hippocampi, and migraine. As noted above, patients with epilepsy as the cause of transient amnesia (transient epileptic amnesia) tend to have briefer and more recurrent attacks than patients with classic transient global amnesia.

Treatment

For most patients, the dramatic events of transient global amnesia never recur, and therefore, treatment is not required. Diagnostic tests to examine for cerebrovascular disease, epilepsy, and migraine are important, and MRI and EEG are both useful tests. A second attack occurs in less than 25% of subjects, and fewer than 5% have more than three episodes. The frequency of seizures or subsequent strokes is not different from that of a comparable age-matched group without a prior episode. Unless a specific etiologic diagnosis is made, no treatment is needed.

When to Consult a Neurologist

The isolated event is rarely seen by the neurologist, and often only the emergency room physician actually witnesses the amnestic episode. In such cases, the neurologist is best utilized as a consultant to interpret the description of events and guide the non-neurologist in the limited diagnostic tests needed and the usual lack of needed intervention. A follow-up appointment after the event with a neurologist is useful to document the absence of static neurologic signs; at this appointment, the neurologist can review with the family the relative statistics on recurrence and the signs or symptoms of stroke, migraine, and epilepsy that should alert the family to a second consultation.

Special Challenges for Hospitalized Patients

Most of these patients are seen in emergency room settings; therefore, acute care personnel must be aware of the distinctive features of this syndrome. The combination of sudden memory loss without superimposed confusion and without language abnormalities should alert nurses and physicians to this entity. Very specific and rapid documentation on the memory loss, affect, and preservation of other mental capacities is essential because the syndrome clears quickly. Because of its very good prognosis, transient global amnesia must be considered and specifically diagnosed while the signs are still present, not afterward when the neurologic examination is normal.

HERPES SIMPLEX ENCEPHALITIS

Herpes encephalitis affects primarily the temporal lobes and leads to necrosis and hemorrhagic destruction of brain tissue. The mortality rate in herpes simplex encephalitis has been reduced, but the prevalence of neurologic deficits among survivors remains high. These deficits are almost exclusively in the behavioral realm. Temporal lobe seizures already described are a common presenting feature of this disease. Acute or subacute behavioral changes, including cognitive and memory impairment, mood alterations, and psychiatric symptoms, may be the first signs of encephalitis. The most common behavioral sequel of herpes encephalitis is an amnesia that can be isolated, with sparing of other cognitive functions. The amnesia consists of an inability to form enduring memories. In more severe cases, the deficit in recent memory is accompanied by alterations in language, perception, and intelligence such that global dementia is seen. This linguistic disorder typically resembles a fluent aphasia with poor comprehension and paraphasic or nonsensical speech. Profound perceptual problems may also be seen: patients may be unable to recognize family members or friends (prosopagnosia) or common objects (visual agnosia).

The most striking potential sequelae of herpes simplex encephalitis are a series of often bizarre behavioral and emotional changes that, in the extreme, resemble those reported by Kluver and Bucy in primates after bilateral removal of the temporal lobes. In humans, the syndrome is sometimes referred to as a limbic dementia and consists of (in addition to the visual agnosia) emotional placidity, distractibility, and alterations in sexual behavior. Thus, patients are often apathetic with flat affect and may show childlike compliance. In humans, the hypermetamorphosis consists of manual and oral exploration of the environment with placement of objects in the mouth. Episodes of bulimia may be seen along with ingestion of inappropriate material. The sexual changes consist primarily of inappropriate comments and overtures. The Kluver–Bucy syndrome is not diagnostically specific; the symptom complex may also be seen with head trauma, Alzheimer disease, and Pick disease. The behavioral alterations in herpes simplex encephalitis are typically less extreme than the full Kluver–Bucy syndrome, and they consist of episodically inappropriate behavior, personality changes, delusions, and hyposexuality. Such behavioral sequelae frequently are viewed as psychogenic by the family and may be resistant to traditional forms of psychiatric treatment.

■ SPECIAL CLINICAL POINT: Memory loss is typical of Herpes encephalitis, and many other behaviors and personality changes can occur in the acute infection.

Anatomic Basis

For unknown reasons, herpes encephalitis has a predilection for the temporal lobes of the brain; therefore the cortical regions of the Papez circuit are involved. The encephalitis is not isolated to the temporal lobe, but the major involvement occurs in this area often in an asymmetric pattern, with one lobe showing more hemorrhagic involvement than the other.

Treatment

Acyclovir is the drug of choice for the treatment of herpes simplex encephalitis, and the standard care is 30 mg/kg/day for a minimum of 14 days. Higher doses and longer courses (3 weeks followed by an oral antiviral agent) are being investigated. Brain biopsy generally is reserved for subjects whose diagnosis remains unclear despite the diagnostic studies that include MRI scans and polymerase chain reaction (PCR) assays of cerebrospinal fluid. Anticonvulsant medications may be needed for seizure treatment or prevention. After recovery, physical, occupational, and speech therapy may be important to maximize rehabilitation. No alternative medical therapies are indicated for this acute infection.

When to Refer the Patient to a Neurologist

The main experts in this condition are infectious disease specialists and neurologists. Rapid consultation is essential to order the appropriate cerebrospinal tests and initiate therapy without delay. With this guidance, the non-neurologist often will manage the case with appropriate reconsultation of these specialists as needed.

Special Challenges for Hospitalized Patients

Most patients with herpes encephalitis are hospitalized during the acute illness, and special attention must be given to the identification of seizures and preherniation syndromes. Nursing staff must be vigilant to the level of consciousness of the patient, vital signs, the strength of arms and legs, and the size of the pupils. Because temporal lobe swelling can occur, the development of a large pupil, contralateral weakness of the arm and leg, and change in level of consciousness are significant neurologic changes and call for emergency intervention. Staff must be educated to observe the patient for involuntary jerking movements, sometimes very subtle, that can indicate seizures.

The unifying points of this chapter have been that abnormal behavior can be a manifestation of focal neurologic disease and the lesions responsible for such behaviors mainly are predictably located somewhere in or near the Papez circuit. Using the Papez circuit as the foundation provides two major diagnostic advantages. First, behavior can be analyzed with a systematic, rigorous discipline provided by neuroanatomy. Second, because this is an anatomic circuit, there is the plasticity to integrate diseases that may be of different etiologies or that may affect different nuclei in the brain and yet that present with similar clinical presentations.

Future Perspectives

There has been new interest in the treatment of memory deficits with presumed cholinergic precursors such as lecithin or choline chloride, but these agents have not been tested extensively. Future diagnostic tools with greater anatomic precision will help delineate the exact area of involvement in the Papez circuit for the entities discussed. The use of such tools as function magnetic resonance imagery (fMRI) will allow patients to be tested during memory or other tasks to define the functional deficits related to this anatomy. A greater understanding of the neurochemical transmitters that link each nucleus in the circuit will help to design therapies that are more specific to lesions within this neurologic circuit.

Always Remember

- Damage to the Papez circuit often leads to emotional and memory dysfunction.
- An abrupt change in language function should trigger a neurological consultation.
- Suspected Wernicke's encephalopathy should be immediately treated with thiamine.
- Memory disorders in conditions involving the Papez circuit are primarily characterized by an inability to form an enduring record of recent experience (i.e., anterograde amnesia).

QUESTIONS AND DISCUSSION

1. Patients at high risk for developing Wernicke encephalopathy include:
   A. Patients with posthepatitis cirrhosis
   B. Hospitalized patients receiving intravenous hyperalimentation
   C. Patients with Parkinson disease
   D. Health food advocates who consume large quantities of B vitamins

The correct answer is B. Wernicke encephalopathy relates to thiamine deficiency. Patients who do not receive vitamins in hyperalimentation eventually will become depleted, as will patients whose dietary caloric intake involves only alcohol. Cirrhosis per se is not associated with water-soluble vitamin problems, and patients ingesting megavitamins may develop many other problems but certainly not Wernicke encephalopathy. Parkinsonian patients are usually slender, but are not thiamine deficient.

2. A patient says he has a seizure disorder. He is under arrest for having destroyed his friend's apartment and beaten up his girlfriend. He says, "I didn't mean to. I don't remember a thing." This behavior could represent TLE, or it could be antisocial behavior by a patient trying to plead ignorance. Along with an EEG, which of the following supports a likely seizure disorder?
   A. After an argument, the patient raced after his girlfriend, caught her in the parking lot, and beat her up.
   B. He was observed to exhibit picking movements of his hands and lip smacking before any belligerent behavior began.
   C. The fighting and destructive behavior occurred when the topic of visiting his college roommate for the weekend was broached.
   D. The patient says this happened three times before: "I know when I'm going into a spell because I hear my mother whispering in my ears something about my credit card debt."

The correct answer is B. Automatisms like those described in B are common in TLE; the aura of primitive auditory sensation like a buzzing sound can be part of a seizure, but a complex and condemning whispering from the patient's mother is more complex than typical seizure auras. The destructive combative behavior seen in epilepsy is not common and when it occurs, it is nondirected. Patients will not chase after someone in the midst of a seizure, although if they are restrained or confined, they may possibly be combative. Running after his girlfriend in the midst of an argument and searching for her in a dark parking lot is a highly directed violent activity far outside the realm of epilepsy. Epileptic spells can be triggered by hyperventilation and other stimuli, but a specific topic like a visit to the former roommate is far too specific to suggest epilepsy.

3. Transient global amnesia is felt to relate to dysfunction in which of the following brain regions?
   A. Frontal lobes
   B. Parietal lobes
   C. Hippocampal regions
   D. Occipital lobes

The correct answer is C. Transient global amnesia occurs due to transient dysfunction of the hippocampal regions of the temporal lobes, brain regions involved in recent memory.

4. Other conditions, besides transient global amnesia, that are part of the differential diagnosis of amnestic syndromes include:
   A. Anticholinergic drug effect
   B. Psychomotor epilepsy
   C. Head trauma
   D. Migraine headaches
   E. All of the above

The correct answer is E. It is important to consider all of the listed options in dealing with the differential diagnosis of amnestic syndromes.

5. During or after herpes encephalitis, which of the following occur?
   A. Temporal lobe seizures
   B. Aphasia
   C. Amnesia
   D. Childlike affect and hypersexual behavior
   E. All of the above

The correct answer is E. During the encephalitis, and as a residual, seizures may occur and they may be difficult to control. Because there may not be generalized shaking, tongue biting, or incontinence associated with the spells, they may not be appreciated as epileptic aphasia. Especially fluent forms can occur because the dominant temporal lobe may be diseased, and when both temporal lobes are affected, amnesia and the Kluver–Bucy syndrome may occur.

SUGGESTED READING

Benson DF. *Aphasia, Alexia, and Agraphia*. New York: Churchill Livingstone; 1979.

Benson DF, Ardila A. *Aphasia: A Clinical Perspective*. New York: Oxford University Press; 1996.

Bogen JE. Wernicke's region—where is it? *Ann NY Acad Sci*. 1976;280:834.

Edwards S. *Fluent Aphasia*. Cambridge: Cambridge University Press; 2005.

Engel J, Caldecott-Hazard S, Bandler R. Neurobiology of behavior: anatomic and physiological implications related to epilepsy. *Epilepsia*. 1986;27(suppl 2):53.

Flor-Henry P. Lateralized temporal-limbic dysfunction and psychopathology. *Ann NY Acad Sci*. 1976;280:777.

Gabrieli JDE. Memory systems analyses in aging and age-related diseases. *Proc Nat Head Sci*. 1996;93:13534–13540.

Geschwind N. Aphasia. *N Engl J Med*. 1971;284:654.

Greenwood R, Bhalla A, Gordon A, et al. Behaviour disturbance during recovery from herpes simplex encephalitis. *J Neurol Neurosurg Psychiatry*. 1983;46:809.

Hanibert G. Emotional disturbance and temporal lobe injury. *Compr Psychiatry*. 1978;19:441.

Hodges JR, Warlow CP. The aetiology of transient global amnesia: a case–control study of 114 cases with prospective follow-up. *Brain*. 1990;113:639.

Kinsella LJ, Riley DE. Nutritional deficiencies and syndromes associated with alcoholism. In: Goetz CG, ed. *Textbook of Clinical Neurology*. 2nd ed. Philadelphia: WB Saunders; 2003:873–888.

Luria AR, Hutton JT. Modern assessment of the basic forms of aphasia. *Brain Lang*. 1977;4:190.

Miller JW, Peterson RC, Metter EJ. Transient global America: clinical characteristics and prognosis. *Neurology*. 1987;37:733.

Papez JW. A proposed mechanism of emotion. *Arch Neurol Psychiatry*. 1937;38:725.

Pierce CJ. The anatomy of language: contributions from function neuroimaging. *J Anat*. 2000;197:335–359.

Pincus JH, Tucker GJ. *Behavioral Neurology*. New York: Oxford University Press; 1974.

Pritchard PB, Lombroso CT, McIntyre M. Psychological complications of temporal lobe epilepsy. *Neurology*. 1980;30:227.

Quinette P, Guillery-Girard B, Dayan J, et al. What does transient global amnesia really mean? Review of the literature and thorough study of 142 cases. *Brain*. 2006;129:1640–1658.

Roos K. Viral infections. In: Goetz CG, ed. *Textbook of Clinical Neurology.* 3rd ed. Philadelphia: Saunders-Elsevier; 2007:919–942.

Sander K, Sander D. New insights into transient global amnesia: recent imaging and clinical findings. *Lancet Neurol.* 2005;4:437–444.

Sechi G, Serra A. Wernicke's encephalopathy: new clinical settings and recent advances in diagnosis and management. *Lancet Neurol.* 2007;6:442–445.

Verfaellie M, O'Conner M. A neuropsychological analysis of memory and amnesia. *Seminars Neurol.* 2001;20:455–462.

Victor M, Adams RD, Collins GH. Wernicke–Korsakoff's syndrome—a clinical and pathological study of 245 patients. *Contemp Neurol Sci.* 1971;1:1.

Wyllie E, ed. *The Treatment of Epilepsy: Principles and Practices.* 3rd ed. Philadelphia: Lippincott Williams & Wilkins; 2001.

16

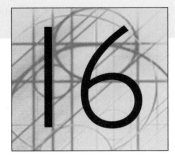

Traumatic Brain Injury

MICHAEL J. MAKLEY

---

key points

- Traumatic brain injury (TBI) is the leading cause of death and disability in young adults.

- The two primary mechanisms of injury in acceleration/deceleration brain trauma are focal cortical contusion and widespread neuronal damage called diffuse axonal injury (DAI).

- The duration of amnesia and confusion termed posttraumatic amnesia (PTA) is the best predictor of outcome following TBI.

- Disrupted sleep cycles play a major role in the cognitive and behavioral deficits that are the hallmarks of emergence from a moderate-to-severe TBI.

- Although patients with TBI are at an increased risk for seizures, use of prophylactic anticonvulsants should not continue beyond one week after injury in most cases.

EPIDEMIOLOGY AND OVERVIEW

The wide spectrum of possible presentations in traumatic brain injury (TBI) offers several challenges to the clinician. Often the clinician is asked not only to manage the patient medically but also to prognosticate regarding outcome and return to former activities such as school, work, or driving. Managing each of these patients is complicated additionally by various factors that will affect outcome and recovery, such as the extent and severity of injury, age, genetic factors, premorbid learning disability, or substance abuse history. This chapter will discuss this wide spectrum of patient presen-

tations with TBI. Topics covered will range from the patient in coma to guidelines for dealing with sports-related concussion. This overview will provide the reader with a sense of the breadth of the disease process; an understanding of some basic terminology and pathophysiology; and finally, some fundamental concepts of managing these patients at various levels of disease severity.

The aftermath of brain injury has a huge impact not only on individuals and families but also on society. It has been estimated that 1.5 to 2 million people suffer a TBI each year, with nearly a million of these being treated in an emergency room. In relative terms this is greater than the yearly incidence of stroke, spinal cord injury, and multiple sclerosis combined. The incidence of severe TBI is 14 per 100,000 people, with nearly 60% of these people dying from their injury. The incidence for moderate and mild TBI is 15 and 131 per 100,000, respectively.

There is a bimodal distribution in regard to age and TBI. The first peak, in the second and third decade of life, is predominantly related to motor-vehicle accidents (MVA); the second peak, in the sixth decade of life, is predominantly related to falls. In the younger age groups it is a male disease (2:1), whereas in the older age groups it becomes more evenly distributed between genders. TBI is the leading cause of death and disability in young adults, affecting this population in their peak income-producing and reproductive part of their lives. The economic impact in the United States has been estimated for both direct and indirect costs of lost wages and productivity at $39 billion per year. Despite this incidence and cost to society there are very few well-controlled clinical trials to guide the clinician in the management of these patients after acute resuscitation. Often treatment is based on small trials, case reports, and anecdote. The need for the development of effective treatment is made all the more compelling with the return of soldiers from Afghanistan and Iraq. It is estimated that 10% to 20% of soldiers involved in these two wars have sustained a head injury. The enormity of the cost of long-term care and management of these veterans is only beginning to be realized.

■ **SPECIAL CLINICAL POINT: Traumatic brain injury in the younger population is primarily young males having car and motorcycle accidents while in the older population brain injury is generally related to falls and is more evenly distributed between males and females.**

PATHOPHYSIOLOGY AND OPERATIONAL TERMS

To understand TBI at any injury severity level it is important to understand some fundamental pathophysiology. The two main mechanisms of injury considered to be at work in acceleration/deceleration injury are related to impact injury or focal cortical contusion and diffuse axonal injury (DAI). In Figure 16.1, an impact injury, the point of impact is primarily the bilateral frontal and temporal poles, which correspond to the brain overlying the inside of the skull's orbitofrontal ridge and each wing of the sphenoid bone, which cradles the temporal lobes. These areas of damage ultimately will lead to long-term behavioral sequelae of TBI as manifested by executive dysfunction, specifically deficits in behavior modulation, attention, and memory encoding and retrieval. Other focal injuries to motor, language, and visual cortex will lead to more obvious neurologic syndromes such as spastic hemiparesis, aphasia, and hemianopsia.

The pathologic hallmark of DAI on a cellular level is the presence of axonal retraction balls (Fig. 16.2). Originally it was thought that

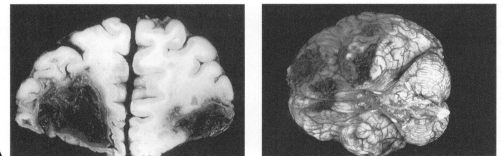

A   **B**

FIGURE 16.1 Hemorrhagic contusion at frontal and temporal lobes after traumatic brain injury.

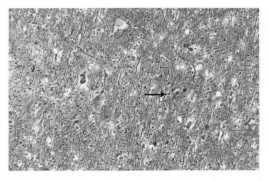

FIGURE 16.2 Axonal retraction ball formation seen in diffuse axonal injury (DAI).

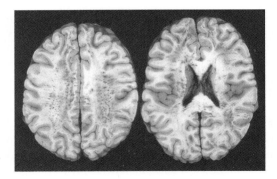

FIGURE 16.3 Diffuse white matter petechial hemorrhage seen in diffuse axonal injury (DAI) on gross section.

these occurred with shearing forces to the axon at the moment of impact and that these "balls" were just the effect of the axon rolling up like a window shade that was wound too tightly. Postmortem studies, however, have shown that these retraction balls are not evident for 12 to 24 hours postinjury. It is now thought that impact causes a perturbation in axoplasmic transfer that, over several hours, leads to axonal swelling and finally disconnection and Wallerian degeneration. This disconnection leads to widespread deafferentation, which is thought to be one of the most significant factors in terms of long-term morbidity and recovery. Although DAI is a pathologic, postmortem diagnosis, patients who survive TBI are described as having had axonal injury when there is a prolonged loss of consciousness with a normal computed tomography (CT) scan or neuroimaging findings that show diffuse petechial intraparenchymal hemorrhage (Fig. 16.3).

■ **SPECIAL CLINICAL POINT: The primary mechanism of brain injury in acceleration/ deceleration trauma is focal cortical contusion and diffuse axonal injury (DAI).**

Other factors that contribute to injury severity include extra-axial and intraparenchymal hemorrhage, anoxia, and impact depolarization with widespread release of excitatory neurotransmitters and generation of free radicals.

For every level of injury this secondary cascade of events also will have an impact on outcome and recovery. Anoxic injury in addition to TBI is associated with the worst outcome, and the prognosis for a good recovery is poor. Finally, in considering outcome, it is important to keep in mind that the extent of each person's recovery from TBI may be determined by an individual's genetic makeup. Some research suggests that patients carrying a mutant allele of apolipoprotein E have increased beta amyloid deposition in the brain and a significantly longer recovery following TBI.

Before discussion of patient management, it is helpful to define certain terms commonly used by specialists who treat brain-injured patients. Because of the current lack of any specific functional or structural imaging test that can reliably define the extent of injury, the field has relied primarily on descriptor scales to describe brain injury severity. Two of the most commonly used scales in TBI are the Glasgow Coma Scale (GCS) and the Rancho Los Amigos Scale (RLAS) (Figs. 16.4 and 16.5) . The GCS is widely used in trauma centers to describe the level of awareness in the patient with TBI. This scoring system occurs over three domains of motor, verbal response, and eye opening. The lower scores (3–8) are associated with coma or the minimally responsive patient, and the higher scores (13–15) describe a person who may be a little confused

PATIENT'S RESPONSE

SCORE

EYE OPENING

- Eyes open spontaneously............................... 4

- Eyes open when spoken to 3

- Eyes open to painful stimulation 2

- Eyes do not open 1

MOTOR

- Follows commands 6

- Localizes to pain 5

- Withdrawal to pain 4

- Flexor posturing to pain 3

- Extensor posturing to pain.............................2

- No motor response to pain..............................1

VERBAL

- Oriented to place and date.............................5

- Converses but is disoriented...........................4

- Utters inappropriate words............................3

- Incomprehensible nonverbal sounds 2

- Not vocalizing...1

TOTAL_____

FIGURE 16.4 The Glasgow Coma Scale Scoring Sheet.

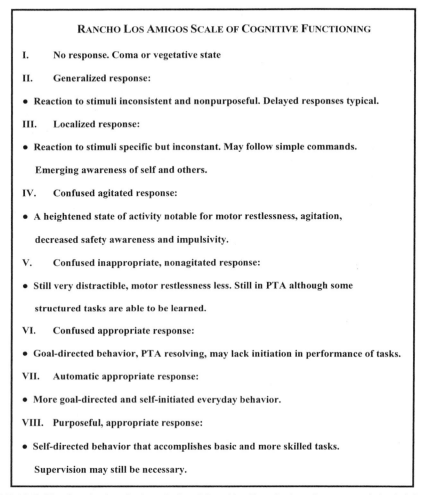

RANCHO LOS AMIGOS SCALE OF COGNITIVE FUNCTIONING

I.   No response. Coma or vegetative state

II.   Generalized response:

• Reaction to stimuli inconsistent and nonpurposeful. Delayed responses typical.

III.   Localized response:

• Reaction to stimuli specific but inconstant. May follow simple commands.

    Emerging awareness of self and others.

IV.   Confused agitated response:

• A heightened state of activity notable for motor restlessness, agitation,

    decreased safety awareness and impulsivity.

V.   Confused inappropriate, nonagitated response:

• Still very distractible, motor restlessness less. Still in PTA although some

    structured tasks are able to be learned.

VI.   Confused appropriate response:

• Goal-directed behavior, PTA resolving, may lack initiation in performance of tasks.

VII.   Automatic appropriate response:

• More goal-directed and self-initiated everyday behavior.

VIII.   Purposeful, appropriate response:

• Self-directed behavior that accomplishes basic and more skilled tasks.

    Supervision may still be necessary.

FIGURE 16.5 The Rancho Los Amigos Scale of Cognitive Functioning after traumatic brain injury.

but is oriented and following commands. The GCS also has been used to grade severity of TBI (Fig. 16.6). Although commonly used to grade severity, a number of recent studies have shown that initial GCS is a poor predictor of long-term functional outcome.

The RLAS is used primarily in the postacute or rehabilitation setting, in which the bottom of the scale, I and II, is associated with a vegetative state and the top of the scale at VIII is associated with only mild cognitive deficits. This scale is a narrative description of emergence stage by stage from DAI where the duration of each stage on the scale is directly proportional to the severity of injury. In the least severe injury, such as concussion, passage through the first stages may be fairly rapid. In the more severe cases the passage up these stages can be months to years, and for some patients their progress can stall at any point on the RLAS.

Traumatic brain injury is unique among acquired brain disease because of the predominance of behavioral and memory deficits over motor and sensory deficits. Because of this, it is important to understand the concept of post-traumatic amnesia (PTA), a unique memory

GRADE OF TBI	GLASGOW COMA SCORE
MILD	13–15
MODERATE	9–12
SEVERE	< 9

FIGURE 16.6 Severity of brain injury graded by Glasgow Coma Scale (GCS).

disorder of TBI. PTA is a compound amnestic syndrome in which a person has lost both previously acquired memory (retrograde amnesia) as well as the ability to lay down new memory (anterograde amnesia). PTA is more than a memory disorder. It is a constellation of behavioral symptoms, which in addition to amnesia includes poor safety awareness and insight into deficits, decreased attention, as well as impulse dyscontrol. In many ways this state could be considered a delirium. Patients with ongoing PTA are very difficult to discharge into the community because of the need for 24-hour supervision. Because of this, many patients will be discharged to nursing homes or specialized behavioral units until this resolves.

Obviously the inability to lay down memory has implications for any rehabilitation-training program, but the duration of PTA also has been used to describe severity of TBI as well as predict outcome in terms of disability. One neuropsychologic screening test to determine the duration of PTA is called the Galveston Orientation and Amnesia Test (GOAT), in which a score of 75 or greater is associated with resolution of PTA. Another commonly used tool to measure PTA in the rehabilitation setting is called the Orientation Log or O-LOG. The O-LOG is less cumbersome than the GOAT and can be administered by a clinician other than a neuropsychologist. This particular test scores the patient from 0 to 30 and the threshold for clearance of PTA is a score of 25. Serial testing using either the GOAT or the O-LOG provides the length of time spent in this amnestic state. Length of PTA can be estimated retrospectively by a neuropsychologist.

While the initial GCS score is a poor prognostic marker, the duration of PTA has been linked to severity of injury, long-term functional outcomes, and resource utilization. PTA longer than 24 hours is associated with severe TBI. Data from Katz and Alexander showed that for those with PTA of less than 2 weeks, 76% reached a level of good recovery, whereas 22% were moderately disabled and 2% were severely disabled at 1 year. For survivors with 8 to 12 weeks of PTA, only 12% had a good recovery at 1 year, whereas 75% suffered moderate disability and 13% were severely disabled. No one with PTA longer than 12 weeks had what was described as a good recovery.

Information about long-range needs for patients following head injury is often identified by loved ones and families of brain-injured individuals as essential information they expect from the clinician. However, the traditionally quoted percentage breakdown between good recovery and disability, as discussed above, can often be confusing for families. Kothari and colleagues recently completed a review of the literature on TBI outcomes in order to develop evidence based "threshold values" for prognostication following head injury based on duration of both PTA and coma. These values can be helpful to the clinician in discussions with families regarding long-term outcomes. According to this review, severe disability, or being functionally dependant for most care, is unlikely with a period of PTA less than the threshold value of 2 weeks. Conversely duration of PTA greater than 3 months is unlikely to be associated with a return to previous level of functioning and independence. With regards to the comatose patient, Kothari's review supports the observation that the longer the duration of coma the worse the outcome. In terms of coma threshold values Kothari suggests that for coma less than 2 weeks severe disability is unlikely while a good recovery is improbable for patients in coma longer than 3 months.

■ **SPECIAL CLINICAL POINT: Families of people with head injury identify prognostic information on long-term outcomes as the most important information they need from the clinician after the acute period. Threshold values based on duration of PTA and coma can help present this information in an understandable way.**

ACUTE HOSPITALIZATION

Most patients who experience a brief loss of consciousness and present to the emergency department with a GCS of 13 to 15 will have routine evaluations that should include a complete neurologic examination, CT scan looking for evidence of extra-axial blood, and radiographic clearance of any neck injuries. Those with a normal neurologic and radiographic examination often will be sent home after a period of observation. The acute hospitalization of moderate-to-severe TBI typically will be managed in a trauma center and will be provided by a neurosurgeon or an experienced team of trauma specialists and intensivists.

In the acute hospitalized setting the primary focus of care often will be the management of increased intracranial pressure and intracranial hemorrhage. Patients with expanding epidural hematomas will be taken to the operating room immediately. Subdural and intraparenchymal blood will be assessed for evacuation according to the grade and severity as well as the underlying neurologic examination. The blood generally may be removed when it is associated with mass effect and shift of midline structures or a deteriorating neurologic examination.

With severe impact injury the secondary cascade of widespread depolarization can lead to an overwhelming increase in intracranial pressure from intraparenchymal edema. Even without an expanding mass lesion this type of diffuse swelling can rapidly lead to herniation and death. Typically neurosurgeons monitor this with an intracranial pressure monitor that is passed through the skull. Patients may be given hypertonic saline or mannitol and may be hyperventilated to bring their P_{CO_2} down to 25 mmHg. Pentobarbital coma is often the next step when these measures fail to bring down the pressure. Even with all of these interventions, patients with severe trauma can continue to have unrelenting elevated pressures. The most drastic measure to reverse this process is craniectomy and duraplasty. This surgery removes the cranium and places a duraplastic patch on the dura that allows the brain to expand unimpeded by the calvarium. The skull flap is frozen in the pathology lab and replaced after the swelling has subsided. Although many patients survive the acute edema, carefully controlled studies have not been done for this dramatic intervention and long-term outcome data are unknown.

Another issue that arises in the acute care setting is seizure prophylaxis. People with closed-head injury (CHI) are at a greater risk of developing seizures. Various studies have found between 2% and 12% of patients with CHI will develop posttraumatic seizures. For those with dural-penetrating injuries, the rate may be more than 50%. In the early 1990s Temkin and colleagues investigated seizure prophylaxis using a double-blind, placebo-controlled paradigm in patients presenting with TBI. Their results showed there was no benefit to phenytoin after the first 7 days in terms of preventing the development of posttraumatic seizures. However, patients with penetrating head injury, because of the higher risk of developing posttraumatic seizures, should be maintained on seizure prophylaxis for 6 months to 1 year, depending on the severity of injury.

SPECIAL CLINICAL POINT: While patients with closed head injury should be taken off

prophylactic seizure medication after 7 days, those patients with dural penetration injury (i.e., a bullet) should be maintained on seizure medications for 6 months to 1 year.

POSTACUTE HOSPITALIZATION

As methods for acute resuscitation improve with the development of acute trauma centers there has been a dramatic increase in brain-injured patients at the lowest level of responsiveness. Data from the National Traumatic Coma Data Bank demonstrated that nearly 10% of the patients discharged from an acute trauma center are in a minimally responsive state, yet there is no consensus on their appropriate management. Often these patients are discharged to nursing homes poorly equipped and trained to manage the complex needs of these patients. Although functional goals are limited in the minimally responsive patient, there is a role for an interdisciplinary approach to the management of these low-level patients (i.e., RLAS I to II), particularly just after acute hospitalization. In one study, 60% of patients admitted to a specialized low-level head-injury program emerged and progressed to an acute rehabilitation program with age being the most significant predictor of successful emergence.

In these low-level patients the most important medical management issues revolve around complications that come from an immobile, minimally responsive patient. Such a patient needs provision of aggressive pulmonary toilet, treatment of infections, prevention of decubitus ulcers, maintenance of adequate nutrition, management of spasticity, and access to comprehensive family education. The role of the interdisciplinary therapy team within a specialized low-level brain injury program is not only for passive range of motion and sensory stimulation. Trained therapists also assess the person's level of responsiveness to his or her environment using a systematic scoring tool such as the JFK Coma Recovery Score or other scoring system. The physician, in addition to treating medical issues and spasticity, often will introduce various neurostimulants, such as methylphenidate, amantadine, bromocriptine, or levodopa/carbidopa (Table 16.1). These agents are thought to enhance arousal and attention primarily through augmentation of the dopaminergic system. Another agent used to treat attention-deficit disorder called atomoxetine is getting wide use in the low-level brain-injured patient. This agent is thought to primarily work at the noradrenergic receptor by selectively inhibiting reuptake of norepinephrine. Exactly how these neurostimulants work in the low-level TBI patient is not clear, although they may correct a severe disturbance of sleep–wake cycle. Although there is widespread use of these agents in this patient

TABLE 16.1 Commonly Used Neurostimulant Agents for Low-Level Responsive Patients Following TBI		
Medicine	**Effects**	**Dosing**
Amantadine	Both presynaptic and postsynaptic dopaminergic effect	100 mg b.i.d. Max. dose 300 mg/day
Bromocriptine	Dopamine agonist	1.25–2.5 mg b.i.d.
Carbidopa/levodopa	Primary targets are mesial and prefrontal dopaminergic pathways	Starting dose of 25/100 t.i.d. and titrate up to 1–1.5 g of levodopa
Methylphenidate	Indirect catecholamine agonist	Starting dose at 2.5–5 mg b.i.d. Can titrate up to 20 mg/day Dose at morning and noon

TBI, traumatic brain injury.

population, there are no large-scale, placebo-controlled trials that guide their use.

After emerging from coma, patients with severe TBI may progress to RLAS III to VII behavior. At this stage they will exhibit emerging awareness and evolving communication; however, they will have severe cognitive deficits as well as deficits in attention, self-monitoring, and safety awareness. The early part of this period also is marked by motor restlessness, sleep–wake cycle disturbance (SWCD), and continued anterograde amnesia. This phase of an emerging head-injured patient's recovery is best managed in an acute rehabilitation setting with a dedicated staff of interdisciplinary specialists experienced in brain injury providing physical therapy, occupational therapy, and speech and language therapy. In addition, a neuropsychologist or behavioral psychologist who can address the behavioral aspects of these patients is an essential part of the multidisciplinary team.

As their working memory returns and patients move on to the RLAS VII and VIII levels, they frequently are discharged from an acute rehabilitation setting to their families with continued outpatient therapy in the community. Almost all patients, when discharged from a rehabilitation setting after a moderate-to-severe injury, will require 24-hour supervision, which is often a very large burden on the family and caregivers.

Once in the community, patients should be connected with resources for vocational or educational re-entry. There are regional advocacy groups for patients and families with TBI that offer resources and support groups to assist in this transition. Frequently school systems have programs in place to reintegrate adolescents with TBI into the classroom. Some states have funded programs for vocational evaluation and placement following head injury. In terms of motor-vehicle operation, each state has individual requirements and protocols for return to driving after a head injury, and the physician should investigate these particulars before clearing the person. In CHI the biggest risk for driving is the risk of seizures. In those states without a formal medical review board determining when a person can return to driving, it may be prudent to refer the patient to a neurologist for an opinion.

SPECIAL CHALLENGES OF THE HOSPITALIZED PATIENT

Sleep–Wake Cycle Disturbance (SWCD)

SWCD is often observed during the subacute period of recovery from moderate-to-severe TBI. Populations of neurons implicated in sleep–wake cycle generation have been found to be widespread across the neural axis. These neurons range from the raphe nucleus of the brainstem, and the thalamic reticular nucleus, to the basal forebrain nuclei. Given acceleration/deceleration forces common to TBI it should not be surprising that these centers could be individually or collectively injured. In addition, neurotransmitter and second messenger system derangements are likely involved in this clinical phenomenon. A study in patients with moderate and severe TBI reported low cerebrospinal fluid (CSF) levels of hypocretin 1, an excitatory hypothalamic neuropeptide involved in regulation of sleep–wake cycles and known to be reduced or absent in patients with narcolepsy.

Following resuscitation from moderate-to-severe head injury most patients will be sent to a rehabilitation center for intensive therapy. In this setting, daytime drowsiness can affect a patient's participation in therapy, while nighttime wakefulness makes a patient more prone to adverse events when less staff is on duty. There is little description in the medical literature of SWCD during this early period of recovery. Most studies of sleep disturbance in brain injury have focused on 6 months to 1 year postinjury. SWCD reported during this chronic phase after injury includes excessive daytime somnolence, sleep phase cycle disturbance, narcolepsy, and sleep apnea. Problems with sleep are also common in the early phase of recovery from TBI. In fact,

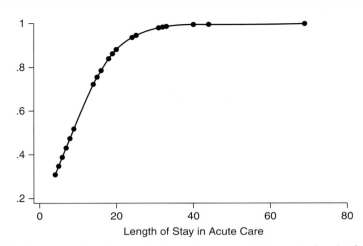

FIGURE 16.7 The probability of sleep disturbance increases with increasing length of stay in the acute care hospital. This graph suggests that after 25 to 30 days in the acute care hospital disrupted sleep is almost certain to be present.

disrupted sleep may play a central role in the memory and behavioral deficits common to this period of recovery. It has recently been shown that 68% of patients admitted to a rehabilitation unit with the diagnosis of moderate-to-severe CHI had disrupted nighttime sleep. Despite similar admission Glasgow Coma Score (GCS), patients identified with SWCD had longer stays in the acute trauma center and the rehabilitation hospital and had lower functional scores on admission to rehabilitation suggesting that SWCD may be a marker for a more severe injury. As Figure 16.7 shows, the longer the patient is in the acute trauma center the more likely they are to have disrupted nighttime sleep and the clinician should be aware of this when treating patients in this postacute setting.

The problem of disrupted sleep in CHI patients on an inpatient rehabilitation unit is not trivial. Confused patients who are awake at night are often physically restrained by nursing staff to prevent falls and unsafe behavior like ambulating on a broken limb. Restraints in a confused, emerging head-injured patient frequently lead to more agitation, which in turn often requires pharmacologic interventions such as benzodiazepines or even antipsychotics. Such

medications have been shown in both animal models and human subjects to be detrimental to the recovering central nervous system after injury. Patients with excessive daytime somnolence have poor attention, which may make rehabilitation efforts fall short and in some cases lead to transfer of the patient to a lower level of care such as a nursing home.

Poor sleep, regardless of the underlying pathology, can have a significant impact on cognitive functioning and behavior. Several studies have shown that sleep fragmentation in healthy adults can lead to an increase in daytime sleepiness, decrease in psychomotor performance, depressed mood and sleep apnea. Similarly, a study of soldiers during simulated combat training found that sleep deprivation led to severe degradation in cognitive and executive function, including memory, reaction time, attention, and reasoning. Gathering evidence in the field of sleep research suggests that sleep plays a significant role in memory consolidation. Interestingly, poor memory consolidation, impaired attention and executive function seen with disrupted sleep circumscribe the same constellation of symptoms that are the hallmarks of PTA in emerging brain-injured patients.

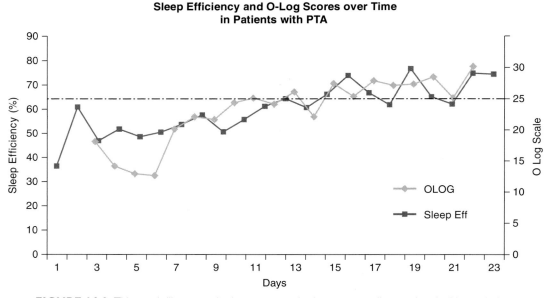

Sleep Efficiency and O-Log Scores over Time in Patients with PTA

FIGURE 16.8 This graph illustrates the improvement in sleep temporally correlated with resolution of posttraumatic amnesia (PTA is considered resolved at an O-LOG score of 25).

It is of primary importance for the clinician to be aware of the high prevalence of disordered sleep following brain injury and be alert for its presence. Appropriate treatment of SWCD in these patients will hinge on the clinician correctly identifying the specific type of sleep derangement. SWCD in the subacute period of recovery can manifest as either hypersomnolence, hypervigilance, or a shift/inversion of normal sleep phase. A recent study has shown that as sleep improves in these patients their memory improves and the syndrome of PTA resolves (Fig. 16.8). Identification of the specific type of sleep disruption can be accomplished by simple nursing observational logs. A more objective measure of a patient's complete circadian cycles, however, can be obtained using actigraphy. An actigraph is a small wristwatch-sized accelerometer which has been used in sleep research for more than 20 years. This device differentiates between sleep and waking based on the amount of movement in the limb and has been correlated with polysomnography (Fig. 16.9).

Hypersomnolence is typically treated with neurostimulants or modafinil a medication commonly used in narcolepsy. Clinicians use typical sedative hypnotics for their patients with insomnia such as zolpidem or eszopiclone. Trazodone is frequently used in these patients and may have some beneficial effect on reducing daytime agitation. In TBI patients it is

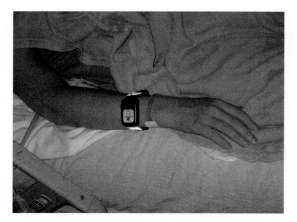

FIGURE 16.9 This is an actigraph on a patient's wrist.

best to avoid anticholinergic medications such as diphenhydramine as this may add to their confusion. The clinician should be alert to the possibility that some patients will have a severe form of insomnia or hypervigilance where they literally do not sleep for consecutive days. Many of these patients will subsequently develop acute psychotic symptoms such as paranoid delusions, hallucinations, and severe, directed agitation. In these patients the use of sedating atypical neuroleptics such as quetiapine is often helpful. Treatment of circadian shift of sleep cycles is often accomplished by using a combination of sedative and stimulant medications. Some sleep specialists would advocate the use of light therapy to try to reset sleep cycles in these patients. While trials in nursing home patients with dementia have shown some benefit of this approach, there are no trials of this intervention in the emerging head-injured patient. Although there appears to be an association between disrupted sleep and PTA in the early stage of recovery following moderate-to-severe brain injury, it is unclear if aggressively treating SWCD leads to a shorter duration of this period of confusion or better long-term outcomes.

■ **SPECIAL CLINICAL POINT: Sleep–wake cycle disturbance is prevalent in traumatic brain injury and may contribute to the patient's confusion, agitation, and poor memory.**

Dysautonomia

In patients with moderate-to-severe head injury it is not uncommon to observe tachycardia; tachypnea; hypertension; profuse neurosweats; and persistently and markedly elevated temperature, particularly in patients at low levels of responsiveness (GCS of less than 8 or an RLAS of I or II). These symptoms are often attributed to being centrally mediated, although it must be remembered that, for the most part, this is a diagnosis of exclusion. Prior to this clinical conclusion the patient should be evaluated thoroughly for infection, dehydration, pain, pulmonary em-

bolus, thyroid disease, and other clinical entities. Centrally mediated symptoms are thought to be related to hypothalamic damage and most often are treated symptomatically and observed. Typically these symptoms remit after emergence from coma. Beta-blockers often are used for this condition and serendipitously may help with agitation as the patient emerges to the next level on the RLAS. In patients with neurosweats the physician should watch for dehydration, particularly in the patient receiving nutrition and hydration through a feeding tube because the dietitian calculating the diet for the patient frequently overlooks this.

Hyponatremia

Low serum sodium is a fairly common occurrence in people with TBI related to their brain injury or medications. Most often electrolyte analysis of serum and urine will show that it is related to the syndrome of inappropriate antidiuretic hormone (SIADH) secretion from the anterior hypothalamus.

Drugs often are implicated in SIADH, particularly carbamazepine, so a complete review of the patient's pharmacology should be performed. Management involves removal of potential pharmacologic etiologies such as carbamazepine, selective serotonin reuptake inhibitors (SSRIs), and nonsteroidal anti-inflammatory drugs (NSAIDs). For SIADH, the patient is typically fluid restricted to 1500 cc of fluid per day. In refractory cases, demeclocycline, a tetracycline that blocks the effect of vasopressin on the renal collecting duct, is used.

Late-Onset Hydrocephalus

Another late complication in TBI is hydrocephalus. Subarachnoid blood blocking the egress of CSF in the arachnoid villi is thought to be the etiology. This diagnosis should be considered in a patient who does not progress in terms of recovery or who was progressing and then stops or regresses. At least one follow-up CT scan should be performed on patients in a vegetative state following their acute hospitalization or in any patient who regresses in their rehabilitation program without a clear etiology. It remains controversial as to who will benefit from a shunt procedure because it is often not clear whether the widened ventricles are ex vacuo changes from diffuse neuronal loss and atrophy or indeed a result of a high-pressure system in need of shunting. Therapeutic spinal taps are rarely conclusive to determine whether a person needs a shunt, but they often are performed. Some neurosurgeons will place a temporary lumbar drain to evaluate for clinical improvement. Others have advocated placing a shunt as a trial for 4 to 6 months.

▪ **SPECIAL CLINICAL POINT: Regression or failure to progress in recovery following a brain injury in the subacute period should prompt a head CT to evaluate for late-onset hydrocephalus.**

Agitation

One of the major management problems for the clinician dealing with patients emerging at an RLAS III to V level is agitation. Typically the agitation is generalized and related to their amnestic state and their impulse dyscontrol. This type of agitation is very similar to delirium, and causes for delirium should be explored in each of these patients before attempting to treat agitation thought to be related to emerging head-injury behavior. Specific entities the clinician should watch out for include infection, drug or alcohol withdrawal, metabolic abnormality, and adverse drug reaction. The clinician should also look for sleep–wake cycle abnormalities, particularly severe insomnia or hypervigilance, as this may be playing a role in the patient's agitation. In the low level and confused patient pain is a commonly overlooked although prevalent problem in individuals who are often involved in a multitrauma injury with concomitant orthopedic and musculoskeletal injuries.

If possible, agitation should be treated nonpharmacologically by removing all identifiable triggers for the patient's agitation. For example, limit the number of friends and family who visit and keep environmental stimuli to a minimum (i.e., turn down the lights, turn off the Jerry Springer show on the television). Part of agitation can be iatrogenic, caused by attempts to keep the patient safe because of their poor insight, memory, and poor safety awareness. Restraints and locking belts invariably escalate problems in the patient who is confused and delirious, and their use should be minimized, although at times they are unavoidable.

A number of theories have been put forth about the agitation in TBI. One behavioral theory holds that because of severe frontal lobe injury, the patient becomes stimulus bound. In other words, because of frontal injury the patient has no block or filter on their reaction to their environment or internal needs. This is compounded by several factors, including their confusional/amnestic state, the strange environment of a rehabilitation hospital, and restraint use.

Another theory of agitation in head injury holds that it is related to attentional deficits. Analogous to the child with attention-deficit hyperactivity disorder, the patient with TBI is overwhelmed with sensory stimuli, and that causes random, generalized striking out or hostile behavior. Advocates of this school of thought prescribe stimulant medication to try to hone attention and reduce agitation. Although seemingly paradoxical, for some patients with prominent attentional deficits, giving stimulants works.

Although commonly used for agitation in this patient population, it is thought that one should avoid neuroleptic medications in patients with TBI because of experimental evidence suggesting that these agents have a detrimental effect on brain recovery. The exception to this rule is the patient with paranoid delusions or the violently agitated patient whose actions endanger staff or themselves. For the patient who is acutely agitated, the use of haloperidol intramuscularly or intravenously is indicated. For patients with paranoid delusions but who are not an imminent safety or health risk, one of the atypical neuroleptics is preferred.

When nonpharmacologic measures fail to control symptoms, stepwise progression through beta-blockers, antiepileptic drugs, and SSRIs is indicated (Fig. 16.10). The primary aim should be patient and staff safety, and in time most people will pass through this phase. For the small minority whose behaviors do not improve, they often are referred to a specialty program with specific expertise and experience in dealing with the refractory behavioral sequela of TBI. In some places this might be a psychiatric hospital or a chronic neurorehabilitation center.

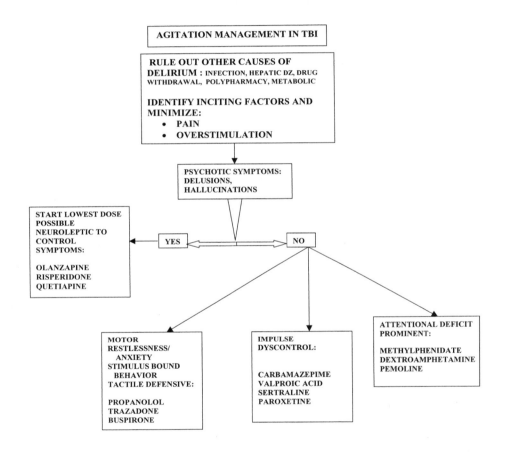

FIGURE 16.10 Agitation management in traumatic brain injury.

■ **SPECIAL CLINICAL POINT: Pharmacology should be used to treat agitation only after other measures have been tried.**

Lack of Initiation

At the other end of the spectrum of agitation is the patient with TBI without any motivation or self drive, which is described as abulia, derived from the Greek word meaning "without will." This describes a patient who is awake but wholly disconnected from his or her environment. In the most extreme cases the person is completely without motivation or initiation and, in fact, will starve to death if not fed. As in the patient who is comatose or in a vegetative state, these individuals primarily are treated with dopaminergic agents or serotonergic reuptake inhibitors.

Spasticity

Spasticity is a frequent and difficult problem for patients, particularly those with severe head injury. With the onset of increasing tone the therapist in the acute or rehabilitation center will begin using conservative measures to try and counteract spasticity. These measures include passive range of motion, weight bearing, and serial casting, in which the affected limb is casted into a more neutral, or functional position in the upper or lower extremity. When conservative measures fail to control spasticity, more aggressive pharmacologic interventions will need to be used.

In patients with TBI in general one should avoid baclofen because of its gamma-aminobutyric acid (GABA)-agonist activity as well as the significant sedation that it frequently causes. GABA is the primary inhibitory neurotransmitter in the central nervous system, and many studies have suggested that GABA agonists may slow the recovering brain. Also, baclofen may be so sedating as to obscure a person's emergence from a low level of responsiveness. For these reasons the first-line agent is considered to be dantrolene sodium. This medication works peripherally on the muscle by inhibiting the release of calcium from the sarcoplasmic reticulum, thereby inhibiting excitation contraction coupling between the myosin and the myosin light chain kinase. To treat focal spasticity or to try and improve positioning of the upper and lower extremities, focal blocks are useful with either botulinum toxin or phenol. These are often very helpful while the therapists try measures such as serial casting. Although systemic spasmolytics such as baclofen and tizanidine are avoided in brain injury, there are times when spasticity becomes so overwhelming that these agents must be utilized. An intrathecal baclofen pump should be considered in cases of unrelenting spasticity when systemic spasmolytics cause intolerable sedation. This is a small programmable pump device that is implanted into the abdomen wall. A silastic catheter comes off the pump reservoir and is tunneled around the abdomen and inserted into the lumbar cistern. The pump can deliver continuous microgram amounts of baclofen directly to the spinal column capillary beds, thus providing spasticity relief at a much smaller total dose while leaving cortical neurons relatively unaffected. A center specializing in the management of intrathecal pumps will be needed in this case.

Mild TBI

Mild TBI, or those patients with a presenting GCS of 13 to 15, compose the largest percentage of all occurrences of brain injury. It is a significant public health problem and probably the most common brain injury presentation to face the primary care physician or non-neurologist. The American Congress of Rehabilitation Medicine delineates specific components of the diagnosis of mild TBI (Fig. 16.11).

The postconcussive syndrome that follows a mild head injury has a myriad of associated symptomatology with the most common being headache, vertigo, depression, fatigue, irritability, sleep disturbance, slowed reaction time, slowed information processing, and loss of

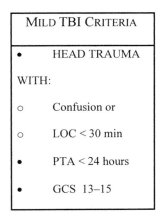

MILD TBI CRITERIA
• HEAD TRAUMA WITH:
o Confusion or
o LOC < 30 min
• PTA < 24 hours
• GCS 13–15

FIGURE 16.11 The American Congress of Rehabilitation Medicine's specific components of the diagnosis of mild traumatic brain injury.

concentration and memory. Subdural or epidural blood, seizures, tremor, or dystonia are rare occurrences that also have been reported following mild TBI.

Typically these patients present with many subjective symptoms but with a normal neurologic examination and unremarkable imaging studies. That litigation is not infrequently involved often colors the clinician's opinion in these cases. It is important to keep an objective sense of this symptomatology despite lack of hard objective findings on examination or conventional neuroimaging studies.

Headaches Posttraumatic cephalgia is one of the most common complaints after a mild TBI. These often are described with components of both a tension-type and a vascular- or migraine-type headache. For instance, a patient may complain of a daily headache that is pressure in character and associated with photophobia and nausea and vomiting. These "mixed-type" headaches respond to low-dose amitriptyline at bedtime in a dosage range of 25 to 50 mg. It is important to inform patients that amitriptyline is not a pain reliever and should be taken consistently at bedtime for at least 1 week before titrating up. For pain relief NSAIDs are often beneficial. Typical migraine headache will respond to conventional migraine interventions but perhaps would be handled better by a neurologist or headache specialist. Posttraumatic cephalgia that does not respond to tricyclics and NSAIDs should be referred to a specialist.

■ **SPECIAL CLINICAL POINT: Headaches are common after head injury and respond well to low-dose tricyclic antidepressants and NSAIDs.**

Vertigo Vertigo, or the sensation of movement with any turn of the head, is quite common after head injury of any severity even in minor concussive injury. It often comes to light in the outpatient clinic after the person with moderate-to-severe injury is discharged from the rehabilitation center. In mild TBI it often can be a presenting complaint. Symptoms are thought to be related to concussive forces knocking otolith crystals off of hair cells in the inner ear. Typically patients will report that when they are lying in bed or when they turn their head suddenly either they will have a sensation of spinning or have the sensation that the room is spinning around them. Nearly all patients will recover after 6 months, and often symptoms are mild and the only treatment necessary is gentle reassurance. For patients whose symptoms interfere with function, any of the vestibular suppressants such as anticholinergics or benzodiazepines can be used; however, all of them have the side effect of drowsiness, which may worsen other symptoms associated with mild TBI such as fatigue and mental slowness (see Chapter 21).

Sports-Related Concussive Injury The non-neurologist often is asked to clear an athlete following concussive injury for return to sports. That decision should be based on the severity of the concussive injury and the duration of concussive symptomatology. The clinician also should keep in mind that the effects of concussive injury are thought to be additive. Guidelines published by the American Academy of Neurology can help with these decisions. Concussive injury is described by grades. Those with transient confusion, no loss of consciousness, and concussive symptoms that last less than 15 minutes are rated as grade 1. People with transient confusion and no loss of consciousness but concussive symptoms or mental status abnormalities that last greater than 15 minutes are considered grade 2. Grade 3 concussive injury is anyone with loss of consciousness of any duration. Any athlete with grade 3 concussion should be transported to an emergency room for a full evaluation to include a CT scan of the head and neck. It should be kept in mind that under most circumstances the neck should be immobilized until this evaluation. Grade 2 concussions should eliminate the athlete from the contest or sporting activity, whereas an athlete with a grade 1 injury should be watched carefully and only permitted to return to play if all symptoms clear in less than 15 minutes. CT imaging of grade 2 concussive injuries should be done for those with persistent postconcussive symptoms.

■ **SPECIAL CLINICAL POINT: A loss of consciousness of any duration would require immediate removal from play and transport to an emergency department for a full evaluation which should include a CT scan of head and neck.**

WHEN TO REFER TO A NEUROLOGIST OR OTHER SPECIALIST

Refractory Headaches

Posttraumatic cephalgia is common in CHI and is usually self-limited or treatable with a combination of low-dose tricyclic antidepressants and NSAIDs. Those patients with headaches that do not respond to doses of tricyclics at 100 mg/day probably should be sent to a neurologist or a headache specialist who might use other therapeutic options such as occipital nerve block, transcutaneous electrical nerve stimulator (TENS) units, or antiepileptic medications. Also, patients who develop migraine-type symptoms following their head injury, such as pulsatile headache with photophobia, scintillating scotoma, and nausea and vomiting, also should be referred to a specialist for treatment.

Posttraumatic Epilepsy

All patients with moderate-to-severe head injury should be informed of their increased risk for epilepsy as a result of their injury, and family members or significant others should be counseled on basic seizure first aid. First-time seizure patients should be instructed to go for evaluation in an emergency room, including a CT scan. Follow up with an evaluation by a neurologist that should include an electroencephalogram. Carbamazepine is the current drug of choice for focal seizures with secondary generalization that result from CHI. Carbamazepine is also a mood stabilizer, and for patients with impulse dyscontrol or agitation this may have a secondary benefit. Levetiracetam is becoming more widely used mainly for its ease of administration. Levels do not need to be followed and there is little in the way of drug interactions or side effects of liver toxicity. The clinician should be aware that one of the major adverse reactions is hostility and aggressive behavior, which may already be a problem for a patient with brain injury. One antiepileptic drug that should be avoided in this patient population, particularly in the acute recovery phase, is phenobarbital, which has the side effects of both cognitive and motoric slowing that only compounds already existing problems for the brain-injured patient.

Neuropsychologic Testing

Formal neuropsychologic testing is always indicated in patients returning to school or any type of high-level management or professional occupation. Information from such testing may be helpful to reintegrate the student into their academic track or help modify a work environment that allows successful return to employment or professional life. This testing is of no use in a period of ongoing PTA and is best-utilized 4 to 6 months after injury. Sometimes it is helpful to have the tests repeated at 1 year to see if there are improvements in any domains of intellect.

Severe Behavioral Disorder/Depression

In all levels of TBI there are patients who emerge with severe and refractory behavioral disorders that do not resolve. Patients with severe impulse dyscontrol, aggression, agitation, or depression should be referred to a neurologist with experience in TBI or a neuropsychiatrist who can manage these difficult patients with appropriate pharmacology. Unfortunately, some of the most impaired of these patients will not be able to function outside of a structured institutional setting.

Depression is a common occurrence among survivors at all injury levels. Depression complicated by psychotic features or unresponsive to first-line agents such as the SSRIs should be referred to a psychiatrist for further evaluation and treatment.

SUMMARY

TBI is a common problem with life-changing consequences for those affected and their families. The cost to society is equally large. Although there has been some suggestion of a decline in head injury incidence in the United States, there is still a great deal to learn on how to effectively treat survivors of TBI to return them to their highest level of functioning within their community. These patients have a number of problems at every level of severity that the physician is asked to manage—from headaches to agitation and impulse dyscontrol. Very often victims of CHI are relatively young and can have a normal life span while living with symptoms and the after effects of their brain injury. On the horizon are new treatments in both the acute center and the outpatient arena that may change the ultimate outcome and quality of life for survivors of TBI.

QUESTIONS AND DISCUSSION

1. A 26-year-old man is discharged to a rehabilitation facility after sustaining a severe closed-head injury after wrecking his motorcycle. His blood alcohol level was elevated, and he had an open book fracture of his pelvis, a right femur fracture, and a T4 compression fracture. He is transferred, after 5 weeks at the trauma center at what the speech therapist is calling "Rancho 4 level." He exhibits a great deal of motor restlessness in bed and frequently is found by the nursing staff to be attempting to climb out of the bed. He is nonverbal. The nurses are requesting medication for agitation. The most likely cause of this agitation is:
   A. An acute meningeal infection
   B. Part of his brain injury
   C. Alcohol withdrawal
   D. Pain
   E. Acute paranoid delusions

The correct answer is D. Part of the emergence from severe head injury does involve generalized agitation and motor restlessness, but it is important for the physician not to overlook treating musculoskeletal pain in patients, particularly those who have multi-trauma injury and who might not be able to communicate their needs. It is well past the point for him to be going through acute alcohol withdrawal at 5 weeks.

2. A 20-year-old man is involved in a severe motor-vehicle accident and is admitted to a rehabilitation center in a vegetative state. The therapists who are working with him report steady gains in the coma recovery scoring tool that they are using until week 5, which is 9 weeks after his injury. They tell you he actually is regressing in some parts of the scoring system. The most likely cause is:
   A. Vasospasm and infarct
   B. Drug-related encephalopathy
   C. Hydrocephalus
   D. Depression
   E. Expanding epidural hemorrhage

The correct answer is C. Hydrocephalus is a late-onset complication from severe head injury and is thought to be related to subarachnoid blood blocking the egress of CSF from the arachnoid villi. Communicating hydrocephalus should be suspected in anyone with a decline in function but should be a particular concern in those at the lowest level of responsivity. Often these patients will respond to ventriculoperitoneal shunting. Expanding epidural hematoma would be a much more dramatic change in neurologic functioning and would, under most circumstances, need rapid neurosurgical intervention.

3. A 32-year-old mother of a newborn comes in with complaints of dizziness. She was involved in a motor-vehicle accident 1 week before, and she reports that she was knocked unconscious for a brief period. She was taken to a local emergency room for evaluation, where a head CT was done that was negative. She was sent home after a brief period of observation. She has little recollection of any events before being in the hospital. She reports that when she is lying down on the sofa and turns her head a certain direction she feels as if the room is spinning. Her neurologic examination is normal. She most likely has:
A. Postpartum depression
B. Subdural hematoma that was missed on the first CT scan
C. Dislodged otolith crystals
D. Complicated migraine
E. Postconcussive syndrome

The correct answer is C. Although it can be part of a postconcussive syndrome, this patient is describing a type of positional vertigo that is common after concussive injury.

The most appropriate treatment for this patient is:
A. Gabapentin
B. Diazepam
C. Meclizine
D. Reassurance and possibly an otolith repositioning maneuver

The correct answer is D.

4. You are at your daughter's lacrosse game, which is the last game of the season against their archrivals. One of the senior forwards, and leading scorers, takes a stick to the head (National Collegiate Athletic Association women's lacrosse rules do not mandate helmets) and for a brief moment is knocked unconscious. On the sidelines she briefly is confused, but this clears quickly (<5 minutes) and she wants to get back into the game. She denies headache, dizziness, nausea, or vomiting. She is alert and oriented. The coach looks at you standing on the sidelines and, knowing you are a physician, asks your opinion. Your recommendation is that:
A. She should be observed for 15 to 30 minutes before being allowed to return to the field.
B. She should not be allowed back in the game and should be taken to the emergency room immediately for evaluation.
C. She can return to play, but if she suffers another blow to the head she should be taken out of the game.
D. She should be removed from the contest and not allowed to return that day.

The correct answer is B. Any loss of consciousness is considered a grade 3 or severe concussion, and an evaluation in an emergency room is warranted. One also should keep in mind that if the athlete went down there could be a spine injury, and cervical immobilization would be prudent until this can be evaluated in an emergency room. After a brief grade 3 concussion the athlete should be withheld from play for a minimum of 2 weeks.

5. A 50-year-old dairy farmer is up early milking his cows 1 day and falls off his tractor, approximately 15 feet, suffering a closed-head injury and a fractured right humerus. A CT scan in the emergency room shows a right temporal contusion. His posttraumatic amnesia resolves within 1 week, and he is discharged from the acute hospital to home and outpatient therapies. His wife brings him in to your family

practice for an office visit the week after his discharge and wants to know how long he needs to be taking the phenytoin. She says it makes him "foggy." She relates that to her knowledge he never had a seizure and there is no one in the family who has seizures. Your response:

A. Because of his advanced age and the location of his contusion he is at a high risk for seizures and should be maintained for 1 year.

B. He needs to see a neurologist to determine this.

C. He can stop taking phenytoin.

D. He needs to be switched to carbamazepine, which works better than phenytoin.

The correct answer is C. There is evidence that there is no benefit to the use of anti-seizure medications beyond the first week in TBI. The patient should be reminded that he is still at risk for having a seizure because of their head injury, and the patient and family should be informed of this and counseled in what to do should their family member have a seizure.

SUGGESTED READING

Brown AW, Elovic EP, Kothari S, et al. Congenital and acquired brain injury. 1. Epidemiology, pathophysiology, prognostication, innovative treatments, and prevention. *Arch Phys Med Rehabil.* 2008;89(3 suppl 1): S3–S8.

Chang BS, Lowenstein DH. Practice parameter: antiepileptic drug prophylaxis in severe traumatic brain injury. *Neurology.* 2003;60(1):10–16.

Katz DI, Alexander MP. Traumatic brain injury: predicting course of recovery and outcome for patients admitted to rehabilitation. *Arch Neurol.* 1994;51:661–670.

Makley MJ, English JB, Drubach DA, et al. Prevalence of sleep disturbance in closed head injury patients in a rehabilitation unit. *Neurorehabil Neural Repair.* 2008; 22(4):341–347.

Makley MJ, Johnson-Greene L, Kreuz A, et al. Return of memory and sleep efficiency following moderate to severe closed head injury. *Neurorehabil Neural Repair.* 2009;23(4);320–326.

Mysiw WJ, Sandel ME. The agitated brain injured patient. Part 2: pathophysiology and treatment. *Arch Phys Med Rehabil.* 1997;78(2):213–220.

Nathan DZ, Douglas IK, Ross DZ, eds. *Brain Injury Medicine: Principles and Practice.* New York: Demos; 2007.

Practice parameter: the management of concussion in sports (summary statement). *Neurology.* 1997;48(3):581–585.

Report of the Consensus Development Conference on the Rehabilitation of Persons with Traumatic Brain Injury. Bethesda, MD: National Institutes of Health; 1998.

Temkin NR, Dikmen SS, Wilensky AJ, et al. A randomized, double-blind study of phenytoin for the prevention of posttraumatic seizures. *N Engl J Med.* 1990;323(8):497–502.

Zafonte RD, Mann NR. Cerebral salt wasting syndrome in brain injury patients: a potential cause of hyponatremia. *Arch Phys Med Rehabil.* 1994;78(5):540–542.

Zaloshnja E, Miller T, Langlois JA, et al. Prevalence of long-term disability from traumatic brain injury in the civilian population of the United States, 2005. *J Head Trauma Rehabil.* 2008;23(6):394–400.

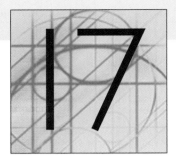

17

Neuromuscular Diseases

DIANNA QUAN AND STEVEN P. RINGEL

> ## key points
> - Neuromuscular disorders include diseases affecting muscle, neuromuscular junction, peripheral nerve, and their nerve cell bodies.
> - Pace of onset and patterns of weakness help guide a focused evaluation.
> - It is important to identify neuromuscular disorders that have specific disease-modifying therapy.
> - For disorders that have no disease-modifying treatment, accurate diagnosis is important to ensure appropriate supportive care.

Disorders that result from abnormalities of spinal cord motor neurons, peripheral nerve, neuromuscular junction, or muscle constitute "neuromuscular disease." Weakness is a common symptom, but unlike central nervous system (CNS) disorders, neuromuscular diseases may be accompanied by muscle atrophy and diminished muscle tone. Patients also may develop muscle pain, stiffness, cramps, twitching, limb deformities, or myoglobinuria.

This chapter begins with an overview of the variable clinical presentations of neuromuscular disease and a description of the tests commonly used to aid in the diagnosis of neuromuscular conditions. Subsequent sections include more detailed descriptions of specific neuromuscular disorders, excluding disorders of peripheral nerve, which will be covered in a separate chapter. For each condition, pertinent diagnostic investigations including genetic testing (Table 17.1), outpatient treatment principles (Table 17.2), special problems in managing hospitalized patients, and suggestions on when to refer to a neurologist will be discussed.

CLINICAL PRESENTATIONS

Weakness

■ **SPECIAL CLINICAL POINT: A useful clinical generalization for neuromuscular disorders is as follows: all motor neuron, neuromuscular junction, and muscle diseases have no sensory changes accompanying weakness.**

Coexisting sensory loss, dysesthesias, or paresthesias strongly suggest a peripheral nerve disorder (see Chapter 18, Peripheral Neuropathy).

TABLE 17.1 | Gene Abnormalities in Neuromuscular Disease

Disorder	Chromosome	Recessive (R) or Dominant (D)	Gene Product	Special Features
Motor Neuron Disease				
Spinal muscular atrophy				
SMA 1, 2	5	(R)	SMN and rarely NAIP protein in SMA 1, 2, 3	SMN protein mutation in 95% of Type 1, 2, 3
SMA 3	5	(R) and (D)		
SMA 4 (adult)	Unknown	(R) and (D)	SMN defect in some	Clinical overlap with progressive muscular atrophy
Spinal and bulbar muscular atrophy (Kennedy's disease)	X	(R)	Androgen receptor	Androgen receptor gene enlarged (multiple CAG repeats)
Amyotrophic lateral sclerosis				
Sporadic (90%–95%)	No known defect		None known	See text
Familial (5%–10%)				
SOD-1 mutation	21	(D)	More than 90 known mutations	SOD-1 mutation in only 20% of familial cases
Other mutations	2, 9, 15, 18	(D) or (R)	Unknown	Mutations very rare
Peripheral Nerve (See Chapter 18)				
Neuromuscular Junction				
Acquired MG	No gene defect	—	—	
Congenital MG	17	(R)	Subunit of acetylcholine receptor protein	No antibodies to the receptor protein, and immunosuppression is ineffective
Muscular Dystrophies				
Duchenne/Becker dystrophy	X	(R)	Dystrophin	Gene deletion (60%–70%); point mutation in rest
Facioscapulohumeral dystrophy	4	(D)	Unknown	Specific deletions in 95% on chromosome 4, but gene itself is still unknown
Limb–girdle dystrophy (recessive)	2, 4, 5, 13, 15, 17	(R)	2A Calpain 2B Dysferlin	LGMD2A mildly weak LGMD2B proximal and distant weakness (Myoshi)
LGMD 2A, 2B, 2C, 2D, 2E, 2F, 2G, 2H, 2I, 2J			2C, D, E, F sarcoglycan defect 2G Telethonin defect 2H E-3 Ubiquitin defect 2I Fukutin-related protein 2J Titan-related protein	LGMD 2C-J tend to have severe symptoms, some resembling Duchenne dystrophy (see text)

(continued)

TABLE 17.1   Gene Abnormalities in Neuromuscular Disease (continued)

Disorder	Chromosome	Recessive (R) or Dominant (D)	Gene Product	Special Features
Limb–girdle dystrophy (dominant)				
LGMD1A	5	(D)	Myotilin	Dysarthria seen
LGMD1B	1	(D)	Laminin	Cardiac involvement
LGMD1C	3	(D)	Caveolin	"Rippling" muscle
Emery-Dreifuss muscular dystrophy	X	(R)	Emerin	Elbow contractures and cardiac changes
Congenital muscular dystrophy	1, 6	(R)	Absent merosin in some	Normal mentation
	9	(R)	Fukutin defect	Severe mental and developmental retardation
Oculopharyngeal dystrophy	14	(D)	Protein regulates polyadenylation and mRNA size	Ptosis, swallowing defects
Myotonias				
Myotonia congenita	7	(D) and (R)	Muscle chloride channel	Autosomal recessive form most common; dominant forms rare (Thomsen's disease)
Myotonic dystrophy (DM1)	19	(D)	Myotonin	Gene has triplet (CCTG) repeats. Disease worse with increasing number of repeats
Myotonic dystrophy (DM2 or PROMM)	3	(D)	An mRNA binding protein	Gene has multiple CCTG repeats
Inflammatory Myopathies				
Inclusion body myositis	9	(R)	Unknown	Rare autosomal dominant form (most IBM is sporadic)
Glycogen Storage Diseases				
Phosphorylase deficiency (McArdle's)	11	(R) and (D)	Muscle phosphorylase	Exercise intolerance, cramps
Acid maltase deficiency	17	(R)	Acid maltase	Fatal in infants; moderately severe in adults
PFK deficiency	1	(R)	Phosphofructokinase	Exercise intolerance
PGAM-M deficiency	7	(R)	Phosphoglycerate mutase	Exercise intolerance
PGK deficiency	X	(R)	Phosphoglycerate kinase	Myopathy rare
LDH deficiency	11	(R)	Lactic dehydrogenase	Myopathy rare

Disease	Chromosome	Inheritance	Gene product	Clinical features
Debranching enzyme deficiency	21	(R)	Debranching enzyme	Survival to adulthood common
Branching enzyme deficiency	3	(R)	Branching enzyme	Early death common
Phosphorylase b kinase deficiency	X, 16, 7, 6	(R)	Phosphorylase b kinase	Fatal in infancy, moderately severe in adults
Lipid Storage Disorders				
CPT II deficiency	1	(R)	Carnitine palmitoyl transferase II	Diagnosis by muscle biopsy and CPT enzyme assay
Carnitine deficiency	Unknown	(R)	Unknown	Diagnosis by muscle biopsy and muscle carnitine assay
Mitochondrial Myopathies				
Kearns-Sayres syndrome (KSS)	Mitochondrial DNA	Maternal inheritance	Various mitochondrial proteins	Extraocular muscle paresis, cardiac conduction block
MELAS	"	"	tRNA	Lactic acidosis, stroke
MERRF	"	"	tRNA	Myoclonus epilepsy, ataxia / Diagnosis by distinctive muscle biopsy changes
Congenital Myopathies				
Myotubular myopathy Neonatal, late infantile, adult-onset forms	X in some / Unknown	(R) and (D) / (R) and (D)	Myotubularin in neonatal form / Unknown in adult form	Neonatal often fatal
Central core disease	19	(D)	Ryanodine receptor	Same gene as for malignant hyperthermia
Nemaline myopathy	1, 2, 19	(R) and (D)	Mutations reported in nebulin, alpha actin, alpha and beta tropomyosin, troponin	Respiratory problems common
Channelopathies				
Hypokalemic periodic paralysis	1	(D)	Muscle calcium channel	Diaphragm never involved
Hyperkalemic periodic paralysis/paramyotonia congenital/potassium aggravated myotonia	17	(D)	Muscle sodium channel	Different mutations of sodium channel gene define unique clinical features of each

SMA, spinal muscular atrophy; SMN, survival motor neuron; NAIP, neuronal apoptotic inhibitory protein; CAG, cytosine-adenine-guanine; SOD, superoxide dismutase; MG, myasthenia gravis; LGMD, limb–girdle muscular dystrophy; mRNA, messenger ribonucleic acid; CTG, cytosine-thymine-guanine; DM, myotonic dystrophy; PROMM, proximal myotonic myopathy; PFK, phosphofructo kinase; PGAM-M, phosphoglycerate mutase; PGK, phosphoglycerate kinase; LDH, lactic dehydrogenase; CPT, carnitine palmitoyl transferase; MELAS, mitochondrial myopathy, encephalopathy, lactacidosis, stroke; tRNA, transfer RNA; MERF, myoclonus epilepsy with ragged-red fibers.

TABLE 17.2   Pharmacologic Treatments

Disorder	Drug Start Dose; Expected Effect	Stable Dose Range	Interactions/Side Effects
Motor Neuron Disease			
Amyotrophic Lateral Sclerosis Sporadic or familial	RILUZOLE 50 mg bid Extends life 2–3 months	50 mg bid	Abnormal hepatic enzymes in 5%—stop drug
	ANTIOXIDANTS (theoretic value—no trials)		
	Vitamin E 800 IU/day	800 IU/day	None
	Vitamin C 1000 mg/day	1000–3000 mg/day	None
	Coenzyme Q10–50 mg/day	50–300 mg/day	None
	PSEUDOBULBAR AFFECT		
	Nortriptyline 10 mg bid	Up to 50 mg tid as tolerated	Excessive sleepiness
	Dextromethorphan 25 mg and quinidine 25 mg	Recent trial using this dose (unpublished)	Nausea, dizziness, sleepiness, loose stools
	CRAMPS		
	Baclofen 10–20 mg bid	20–40 mg qid	Muscle weakness at higher doses
	Quinine 325 mg/day	325 mg bid to tid	Ringing in ears
	EXCESS SALIVA		
	Nortriptyline 10 mg bid		Sleepiness
Neuromuscular Junction			
Myasthenia gravis	Prednisone 50 mg/day	50–80 mg/day depending on patient weight. Try tapering dose after strength back to normal. Use with azathioprine.	Weight gain, mood changes, cataract, osteopenia, diabetes, hypertension
	Azathioprine 50 mg/day	Increase each week by 50 mg increments until taking 50 mg qid. Add on to stable prednisone dose and after 2–3 months, try tapering the prednisone.	May cause leukopenia and liver function abnormalities, so monitor with weekly studies until maximal dose reached. Then, can do blood safety studies every 3 months. Also may cause skin rash.
	mycophenolate mofetil 0.5 g/day	Increase over 2–3 weeks to 1 g bid	Not authorized by FDA for MG. Used primarily as antirejection drug for organ transplant but occasionally of use in MG when other drugs fail. Major side effect is GI distress.

	Pyridostigmine 60 mg q4hr	60–120 mg q4hr, 180 mg timespan appropriately spaced	Symptomatic only and used primarily for mild ocular symptoms when risk of immunosuppression is unacceptable. Overdosage and cholinergic crisis can occur, however.
	Plasma exchange IVIG 400 mg/kg	3–5 daily exchanges and repeat as needed 400 mg/kg × 5 days, reassess; repeat as needed	Used for acute worsening if best pharmacologic treatment fails. Used in patients totally refractory to all other therapy.
Muscular Dystrophies Duchenne and Becker	Prednisone 0.65 mg/kg	Maintain at this dose for months to years depending on side effects	Treatment is controversial, and there are steroid side effects, as described for MG. In addition, there is growth retardation in children.
Myotonias Myotonia congenita	Mexilitine 150 mg bid	Increase by 50 mg increments every week to a maximum of 200 mg tid	GI distress, lightheadedness, tremor are side effects. Drug interactions with phenytoin, phenobarbital, rifampin, cimetidine, and theophylline.
Lipid Storage Disorders Carnitine deficiency	L-carnitine 2–4 g/day in adults 100 mg/kg/day (children)	Maintain at starting doses	
Channelopathies Hypokalemic periodic paralysis	Acetazolamide 250 mg bid	Increase to 250 mg tid as needed	Interactions with various drugs. Taste change, anorexia, nausea, drowsiness, kidney stones.
Hyperkalemic periodic paralysis	Hydrochlorthiazide 25 mg/day in AM	Increase to 50 mg/day in AM, and add 12.5 mg in PM, if necessary	Interactions with various drugs. Weakness, hypotension, electrolyte disturbance.

FDA, Food and Drug Administration; MG, myasthenia gravis; GI, gastrointestinal; IVIG, intravenous immune globulin.

The rapidity of onset, location, and progression of weakness are important diagnostic features. Rapidly developing weakness (hours to several days) is characteristic of diseases of the neuromuscular junction, Guillain–Barré syndrome, toxic myopathies, and acute electrolyte disturbances. Acute remissions and relapses may be seen with myasthenia gravis (MG), periodic paralysis, and other channelopathies. Insidious and slowly progressive weakness occurs in many diseases affecting muscle or spinal cord motor neurons. Three major patterns of weakness can be encountered: proximal, distal, or cranial. Each pattern is associated with typical symptoms related by the patient and with some signs easily observed even before individual muscles are tested.

Proximal weakness is characteristic of many muscle disorders, the spinal muscular atrophies, and MG. These patients report difficulty in climbing stairs or arising from low chairs. When arising from a chair, they will lean forward and "push off" with their hands on the armrests. In arising from the floor or a squatting position, they may require one or more supports with the hands on the floor, knees, and thighs (Gowers maneuver; Fig. 17.1). The gait of a person with proximal weakness has a waddling appearance because of hip girdle weakness. Knee extensor weakness may cause the leg to "give out." Patients may lock their knees to compensate, gradually leading to hyperextension (back-kneeing), which in turn produces an exaggeration of the lumbar lordosis. Shoulder girdle weakness produces difficulty in elevating the arms and may be accompanied by scapular winging (Fig. 17.2). With the arms hanging at the sides, the scapulae may slide laterally to produce a curving inward of the shoulders with the backs of the hands facing forward and an associated oblique "axillary crease" (Fig. 17.3). The high-riding scapulae produce a conspicuous "trapezius hump"; the clavicles may slope downward and stand out prominently from the atrophic neck musculature (Fig. 17.3).

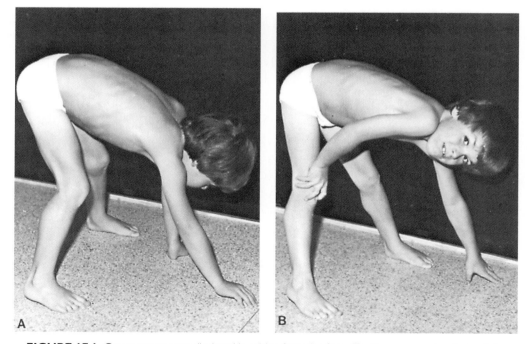

FIGURE 17.1 Gowers maneuver displayed in arising from the floor (Duchenne muscular dystrophy).

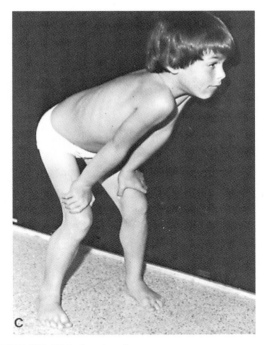

FIGURE 17.1 *(continued)*

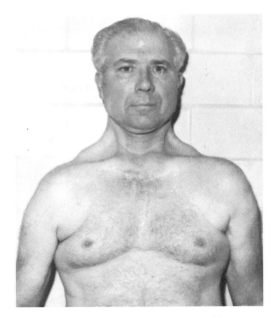

FIGURE 17.3 Shoulder girdle weakness with "trapezius hump," "step-sign" with prominent downsloping clavicles, and an oblique anterior axillary crease (LGD).

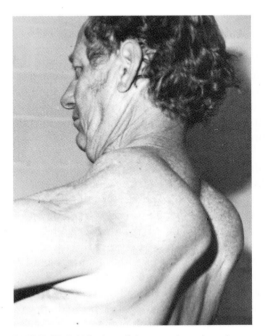

FIGURE 17.2 Winging of the scapulae when the arms are elevated (fascioscapulohumeral dystrophy [FSH]).

Distal weakness in the presence of atrophy is commonly seen in amyotrophic lateral sclerosis (ALS) (Fig. 17.4), inclusion body myositis (IBM), and myotonic dystrophy. Patients with ALS or IBM may present with unilateral symptoms but eventually develop weakness bilaterally. These patients find it difficult to manipulate small objects such as buttons or writing or eating utensils. They may complain of "dragging" their legs because of "foot drop" or of frequent tripping, particularly on uneven ground. With each step, the knees are raised high while the feet flap limply; shoe soles may show asymmetrical wear.

Cranial weakness may manifest as extraocular, facial, or oropharyngeal muscle weakness and is an important differential feature in diagnosis of various dystrophies (Figs. 17.5 and 17.6). Ptosis and ophthalmoparesis occur in several myopathic disorders and are very common in MG. Swallowing and speech changes can also be early signs of either ALS or MG.

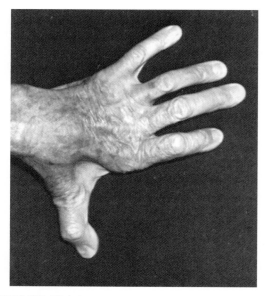

FIGURE 17.4 Marked atrophy of the first dorsal interosseous muscle in motor neuron disease.

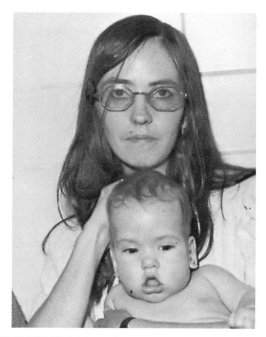

FIGURE 17.6 Myotonic dystrophy in mother (note "hatchet face") and infant (note "shark mouth"). Diagnosis first made in the child suggested the same diagnosis in the mother.

Atrophy and Hypertrophy

The disuse of a limb will produce modest muscle atrophy, as is seen in nonneuromuscular conditions such as after casting of a bone fracture. The muscle retains much of its strength in disuse atrophy, and the apparently atrophied limbs of an elderly person may be surprisingly strong. In contrast, the striking muscular atrophy in patients with neuromuscular disease is associated with obvious weakness.

Atrophy of the muscles around the shoulder girdle commonly reveals underlying bony prominences. Flattening of the thenar eminence and guttering of the interossei can produce a wasted, clawlike deformity of the hand (Fig. 17.4). Several disorders produce characteristic appearances. Examples include "Popeye arms" (very atrophied biceps/triceps with a normal-appearing forearm) in facioscapulohumeral dystrophy, the "hatchet face" (temporalis wasting) appearance in myotonic dystrophy (Figs. 17.5 and 17.6), and

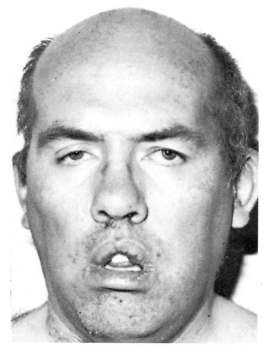

FIGURE 17.5 Typical facial appearance in myotonic dystrophy with frontal balding, temporalis and masseter atrophy, ptosis, and protuberant lower lip.

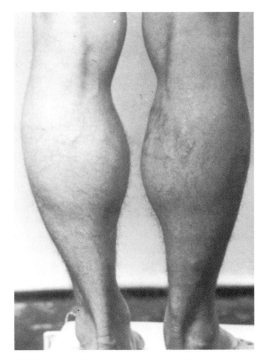

FIGURE 17.7 Pseudohypertrophy of the calves (Duchenne dystrophy).

the enlarged calves of Duchenne dystrophy (DUD; Fig. 17.7). Diffuse hypertrophy of all limb muscles is commonly seen in myotonia congenita, rarely in hypothyroidism, or very rarely in amyloidosis.

Pain, Stiffness, and Cramps

Pain is a nonspecific symptom that may be seen in many neuromuscular conditions. Inflammatory myopathies and other collagen vascular diseases may produce muscle pain and tenderness, but the absence of these symptoms does not exclude the diagnosis. Some patients may have difficulty distinguishing between pain and weakness because pain limits their ability to perform motor tasks. This may result in perceived weakness. Such individuals often prove to have normal strength or a "give-away" pattern of weakness, which suggests lack of full voluntary effort.

■ **SPECIAL CLINICAL POINT: Most patients with limb aching and pain without objective weakness or abnormally elevated muscle enzymes do not have a neuromuscular disease, and other possibilities should be considered, such as joint or soft tissue pathology.**

In older patients, pain, aching, and stiffness in the shoulder and hip girdle muscles should suggest polymyalgia rheumatica, and this disorder is associated with a very high sedimentation rate. It is important to recognize because of its very specific treatment and rapid response to steroid medications. The diagnosis of fibromyalgia often is evoked, particularly in otherwise healthy individuals who have diffuse aches and pains without objective signs of weakness; however, the pathologic foundation of this entity remains controversial.

Stiffness may be a nonspecific symptom, or it may be a symptom of myotonia, a phenomenon consisting of a delayed relaxation of the muscle following voluntary contraction or percussion. This produces difficulty in releasing the grip or initiating movements after a period of rest and may point to a myotonic dystrophy or myotonia congenita.

Muscle cramp, a prolonged involuntary contraction, is a universal and generally benign symptom that occurs with increased frequency during unaccustomed exercise, "body building," pregnancy, or electrolyte disturbance. It also may occur in hypothyroidism, partial denervation due to ALS or other less sinister types of nerve injuries, tetany (with hypocalcemia, hypomagnesemia, or alkalosis), and certain metabolic myopathies.

Muscle Twitching

Fasciculations are contractions of muscle fibers in a single motor unit. Fasciculations appearing in a strong muscle are usually benign and are exacerbated by many factors, including fatigue and caffeine intake. When they occur in a weak muscle, they may be associated with ALS, but they also may occur in the setting of root compression or peripheral nerve injury.

Infantile Hypotonia

The most frequent abnormality causing infantile hypotonia or a "floppy baby" is CNS disease, such as seen after perinatal asphyxia. The hypotonic infant may exhibit normal muscle strength, with the ability to lift its head or limbs against gravity. In the absence of other abnormalities, the prognosis for normal development may be excellent. In infants with obvious weakness, the underlying disorder may be spinal muscle atrophy or one of the congenital myopathies. Weakness of sucking and respiration are serious concomitant findings, which are usually fatal if undiagnosed and untreated.

Deformities

Neuromuscular disorders often are associated with skeletal deformities and should be suspected in a patient with unexplained hip dislocation, scoliosis (Fig. 17.8), contracture, or malformation of the feet (e.g., clubfoot, equinovarus, or pes cavus deformity). Arthrogryposis or multiple congenital limb deformities may occur with various diseases affecting any part of the motor unit.

The syndrome of myoglobinuria consists of weakness and painful swelling of affected muscles in association with headaches, nausea, and vomiting. The urine turns reddish brown within 24 hours and is positive for benzidine and Hemastix. An elevation of serous creatine phosphokinase (CK) peaks at 5 to 7 days after the initial muscle injury. Most episodes are related to acute muscle necrosis due to unusual circumstances, such as vigorous exercise (particularly in deconditioned individuals) or exposure to myotoxic agents such as alcohol, cocaine, amphetamines, heroin, neuroleptics, and halothane in susceptible individuals. A patient with recurrent myoglobinuria should be evaluated for an underlying metabolic neuromuscular disease.

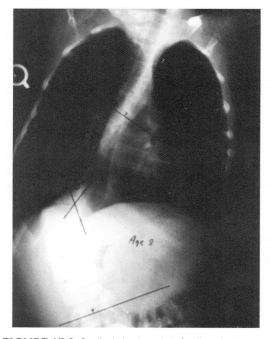

FIGURE 17.8 Scoliosis in chronic infantile spinal muscular atrophy. The angle of curvature is measured and followed closely (55 degrees in this patient).

EXAMINATION FINDINGS

Observing the pattern and distribution of weakness and reflex findings is an important first step in formulating a differential diagnosis for patients with neuromuscular disorders. Table 17.3 and Figure 17.9 provide some general guidance.

DIAGNOSTIC LABORATORY INVESTIGATIONS

Enzyme Elevation

Muscle necrosis results in elevated levels of serum CK. Other enzymes including aldolase may also be elevated. The highest levels occur in the syndrome of myoglobinuria, Duchenne muscular dystrophy, and polymyositis with slightly to moderately elevated values in most of the other dystrophies and motor neuron disorders. The most common causes of a modest CK elevation include recent vigorous

TABLE 17.3 | **Characteristic Examination Findings and Helpful Tests in Neuromuscular Disorders**

	Motor Neuron Disorders	Neuromuscular Junction Disorders	Myopathic Disorders
Pattern of weakness	• May be focal in onset especially in acquired motor neuron disorders • May begin in arms, legs, or bulbar region	• Symmetrical weakness • Bulbar symptoms, e.g., diplopia and ptosis common in MG • Limb weakness eventually occurs in majority and proximal weakness is prominent • Mostly limb and little bulbar weakness in LEMS	• Usually symmetrical proximal weakness • Occasionally other characteristic patterns
Reflexes	• Hyperactive reflexes common in ALS • Normal in lower motor neuron syndromes	• Normal in MG • Sometimes mildly depressed in LEMS	Normal except with severe weakness
Sensory changes	No sensory loss	• No sensory loss in MG • Occasional mild sensory loss in LEMS	No sensory loss
Helpful diagnostic tests	• Nerve conduction studies and electromyography • Spine imaging to exclude stenosis or radiculopathy	• Acetylcholine receptor or muscle-specific tyrosine kinase antibodies in MG • Calcium channel antibodies in LEMS • Nerve conduction studies with repetitive stimulation or single-fiber electromyography	• Creatine phosphokinase level • Nerve conduction studies and electromyography

exercise in an otherwise normal individual and hypothyroidism.

Electrodiagnostic Studies

Electrophysiologic investigations including nerve conduction studies (NCS), needle electromyography (EMG) examination, repetitive nerve stimulation, and single-fiber EMG provide both qualitative and quantitative information about neuromuscular disease states.

NCS broadly differentiate between primary demyelinating and axonal neuropathies and provide quantitative data for following the course of disease. In conditions affecting only muscle, NCS are abnormal only if significant loss of muscle tissue causes low-amplitude compound motor action potential recordings.

Needle EMG is an essential complement to NCS and helps to differentiate neuropathic from myopathic disorders (Fig. 17.10). Neuropathic disorders resulting from loss of anterior horn cells or peripheral nerve leave fewer motor units available to generate muscle force. This manifests on EMG as a decrease in the electrical interference pattern. In the acute period of neuron or axon loss, spontaneous electrical activity from denervated muscle

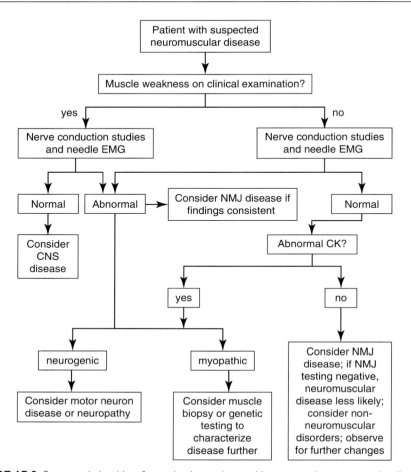

FIGURE 17.9 Suggested algorithm for evaluating patients with suspected neuromuscular disease.

fibers may be recorded in the form of fibrillation potentials and positive sharp waves. Following chronic denervation, surviving motor axons develop collateral sprouts that reinnervate muscle fibers. Spontaneous electrical activity disappears, and the electrical potentials produced by these large motor units have high amplitudes, long durations, and an increased number of phases.

In myopathic disorders, the random loss of individual muscle fibers results in decreased motor unit potential amplitudes (Fig. 17.10, item 2). To generate the same amount of force as a healthy muscle, more of the smaller myo-

pathic motor units are needed. During voluntary contraction, this is seen as "early recruitment" of motor unit potentials and the early development of a maximum interference pattern.

In disorders of the neuromuscular junction, more specialized testing such as repetitive stimulation studies or single-fiber EMG can be performed. Repetitive stimulation of a peripheral nerve in these conditions may produce a characteristic decrease or increase in the amplitude of the compound motor action potential, depending on the type of defect. Single-fiber EMG may reveal increased "jitter," a measure

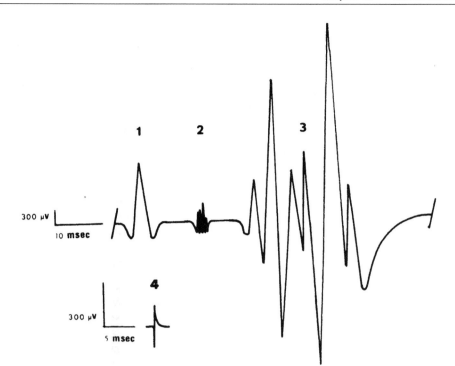

FIGURE 17.10 Single motor unit action potentials recorded by electromyography in a voluntarily contracting skeletal muscle. 1: Normal motor unit action potential. 2: The myopathic potential is brief, has small amplitude, and is polyphasic. 3: The neuropathic potential is prolonged, has high amplitude, and is polyphasic. 4: A fibrillation potential is spontaneously produced by a denervated muscle fiber at rest.

of the synchrony of depolarization occurring in muscle fibers from the same motor unit.

Muscle and Nerve Biopsy

Muscle biopsy is performed easily under local anesthesia as an outpatient procedure, allowing for rapid histologic and histochemical preparation to aid in diagnosis. Characteristic changes are well described for many conditions affecting the motor neuron and muscle.

Genetic Testing of Neuromuscular Diseases

Molecular biology techniques have produced a torrent of information describing gene abnormalities underlying many neuromuscular disorders. Table 17.1 summarizes the more common

gene mutations that produce motor neuron diseases, dystrophies, muscle storage disorders, congenital myopathies, and channelopathies. Further genetic details are provided in subsequent descriptions of specific diseases.

SPECIFIC NEUROMUSCULAR DISORDERS

The following section will describe clinical features of specific diseases, commonly used diagnostic tests, genetics, prognosis, and, when appropriate, specific drug treatment. For the motor neuron disorders and genetically determined muscle diseases that have limited or nonexistent disease-modifying treatments, we will cover general rehabilitation principles for outpatients and hospitalized patients in a later section.

Motor Neuron Diseases

The diagnostic confirmation of motor neuron disease relies heavily on accurate electrodiagnostic studies, which should demonstrate denervation with needle EMG testing of affected myotomes; changes may be acute or chronic depending on when the test is performed in the course of disease. Depending on the time course and severity of disease, motor NCS may be abnormal but are frequently surprisingly normal, especially in more chronic or slowly progressive conditions. Sensory NCS are normal unless another superimposed peripheral nerve disorder is present. When muscle biopsy is carried out in patients with motor neuron disorders, abnormalities will include distinctive muscle fiber group atrophy and type grouping, a reflection of motor unit loss and reorganization. Invasive testing has become less necessary with the increasing ease and availability of genetic testing for some conditions. In all the motor neuron disorders, serum CK may be modestly elevated but rarely rises above 1,000 IU/L.

Spinal Muscular Atrophies   The spinal muscular atrophies (SMA) constitute a group of hereditary disorders characterized by a severe reduction in spinal cord and cranial motor neurons. Patients have normal sensation but chronic progressive weakness. Virtually all cases are autosomal recessive. Four major clinical phenotypes are recognized on the basis of age of onset and severity of disease (Table 17.1). Types 1, 2, and 3 are autosomal recessive, resulting from variable mutations of the survival motor neuron (SMN) gene on chromosome 5. Defects in both SMN alleles are present in about 95% of patients with the SMA phenotype. Rarely, there may be mutations of a closely adjacent neuronal apoptotic inhibitory protein (NAIP) gene. Patients with type 4 SMA are rare, and of the few studied, SMN mutations are found inconsistently. Currently, no specific drug treatments are available for SMA, but several agents are in various phases of clinical trial testing.

X-Linked Spinal and Bulbar Muscular Atrophy (Kennedy Disease)   X-linked spinal and bulbar muscular atrophy (Kennedy disease) is an unusual disorder that can be confused with ALS. Patients in their thirties and forties present with swallowing dysfunction, slurred speech, perioral and tongue fasciculations, facial weakness, mild limb weakness, hand tremor, gynecomastia, and impotence. The disorder is very slowly progressive and, unlike ALS, life expectancy is only minimally shortened.

The disorder results from a gene abnormality on the X chromosome. Thus, only males are affected. There is never male-to-male transmission; and females, although unaffected clinically, are carriers. The disease is caused by multiple cytosin–adenin–guanine (CAG) trinucleotide repeats in the androgen receptor gene. As numbers of CAG repeats increase, the age of disease onset is earlier, but there is no correlation with disease severity. The treatment is supportive since no specific drug therapies are currently available.

Amyotrophic Lateral Sclerosis   ALS is characterized by progressive muscle wasting and weakness resulting from degeneration of brain stem and spinal cord lower motor neurons. There is coexisting spasticity and hyperreflexia caused by degeneration of upper motor neurons in the brain. Although the vast majority of cases are sporadic, between 5% and 10% are familial. Initial clinical symptoms may be limited to asymmetric limb weakness in the presence of fasciculations. Foot drop or marked hand deformity resulting from interossei wasting (Fig. 17.4) can be seen. Speech may become slurred or spastic. In addition to hyperreflexia, there are other pathologic reflexes (Hoffman response and crossed adductor responses) and in some cases extensor plantar responses. Sensation is normal. Frank dementia is uncommon in ALS, but sophisticated psychological test batteries reveal that cognitive deficits, especially executive dysfunction, may be seen in as many as 30% of patients.

The spread and involvement of different muscles in ALS occurs in a characteristic pattern, first moving to involve both sides in one region of the body, and then to contiguous areas caudally and rostrally. Facial weakness may be seen, but eye movement is never affected. Weight loss is common as swallowing becomes increasingly impaired. Diaphragm weakness often leads to a critical time in the disease, as vital capacity drops progressively. The average survival after diagnosis is 3 to 4 years, but 10% survival at 10 years has been reported.

The vast majority of ALS cases are sporadic and have no demonstrable genetic defect. Of the 10% of patients with ALS who have a positive family history, approximately 10% to 20% have a dominant superoxide dismutase (SOD1) gene mutation on chromosome 21; more than 110 mutations have been reported. The ALS phenotype in these individuals results from a toxic "gain of function" which may trigger reactions that cause premature neuronal death (apoptosis). Additional families with non–SOD-1 gene mutations on chromosomes 2, 9, 15, 16, 18, 20, and X have been described, though the phenotypes described in many of these kindreds have features that may not represent classic ALS.

The treatment of ALS is primarily symptomatic (Table 17.2). Of the many drugs and trophic factors tried, only the oral agent riluzole is of value, prolonging survival by an average of 2 to 3 months. Numerous clinical trials testing other agents are in progress. A troublesome symptom in up to 30% of patients with ALS is inappropriate laughing or crying, termed "pseudobulbar affect." Amitriptyline or the combination of quinidine and dextromethorphan may be helpful in this situation. For cramps, baclofen, quinine, or benzodiazepines are sometimes successful. For excessive salivation, nortriptyline or glycopyrrolate can help.

Infections Affecting Motor Neurons Acute poliovirus infection in nonimmunized individuals leads to a nonspecific febrile illness, followed by paralytic symptoms in a minority. Although widespread immunization in the latter half of the 20th century has reduced the frequency of new cases in industrialized countries, many individuals who contracted the disease in earlier times have permanent weakness in regions of the body where the infection destroyed spinal cord motor neurons. With normal age-related attrition of the motor neuron pool, progressive weakness may develop after many years of compensated static deficit, the so-called "postpolio syndrome." There is no evidence for viral reactivation, and the condition is best treated with symptomatic rehabilitative measures.

In the last decade, there have been an increasing number of human West Nile virus infections. Most of those infected develop a nonspecific febrile illness and recover uneventfully. Less than 1% develop a neuroinvasive form of the disease characterized by meningoencephalitis and sometimes anterior horn cell inflammation and destruction. As in poliovirus infection, more severe loss of anterior horn cells may lead to permanent weakness of the affected myotomes. No vaccine or specific treatment is currently available.

Disorders of the Neuromuscular Junction

Myasthenia Gravis MG is an autoimmune disorder associated with a postjunctional defect of the acetylcholine receptor (AChR). It may occur at any age but is most frequent in young women and older men. Fluctuating weakness and fatigue in cranial, limb, or trunk musculature are characteristic. Ocular symptoms, including alternating ptosis, diplopia, and blurred vision, are present initially in more than 50% of patients and eventually in 90%. Facial muscles are often weak, producing a snarling appearance when laughing. Speech becomes increasingly slurred, nasal, or hoarse as the patient continues to talk, and progressive dysphagia with choking and aspiration of food may occur. Neck muscle weakness may be so prominent that the patient resorts to using a hand to prop up the head. Generalized MG frequently involves the respiratory muscles, producing shortness of breath. The clinical course occasionally is fulminant but gradual progression of symptoms with frequent remissions and relapses is more common. Myasthenic "crisis" or sudden worsening of symptoms to life-threatening severity may occur with emotional or physiologic stress, such as superimposed infection, electrolyte disturbance (especially hypokalemia), pregnancy, or other systemic illness.

A diagnosis of MG is confirmed by the presence of AChR antibodies found in the serum of 85% to 90% of patients with generalized MG. Approximately 35% of patients who have no AChR antibodies may have antibodies to muscle-specific receptor tyrosine kinase (MuSK). Many patients with MuSK antibody–related MG are clinically indistinguishable from those with AChR antibodies. However, others may have especially severe oculobulbar weakness, some with striking facial and tongue atrophy. Other patients may have prominent neck, shoulder, and respiratory muscle weakness without ocular weakness.

In instances of negative antibodies, electrodiagnostic testing by repetitive stimulation of a motor nerve may produce a characteristic decremental response in the evoked compound motor action potentials. Single-fiber EMG to look for increased "jitter," a reflection of unstable neuromuscular transmission, may help if other tests are negative but is only available at centers with specialized neuromuscular expertise. A diagnostic intravenous injection of edrophonium (Tensilon) should briefly correct ptosis, ophthalmoparesis, or limb weakness but may be easily misinterpreted.

The treatment of MG has changed considerably in the last several decades, with increasing recognition of the primary autoimmune disturbance. High-quality clinical trial data is not available for most of the treatments used in MG; however, older agents have a long track record of use and empiric evidence of efficacy. The anticholinesterase agent pyridostigmine (Mestinon) is used for symptomatic relief but has no long-term disease-modifying effect. In most cases, prednisone is the initial immunosuppressant

of choice. Initiation of doses greater than 20 to 30 mg/day may result in a transient exacerbation of weakness during the first 2 weeks, with a potential for respiratory failure; slow titration of prednisone to target doses is therefore recommended. High-dose long-term prednisone therapy is not desirable because of the side effects of weight gain, cataracts, diabetes, hypertension, and osteopenia. Steroid-sparing immunosuppressants such as azathioprine, mycophenolate mofetil, cyclosporine, and cyclophosphamide take longer to work than prednisone, but have been used successfully in many patients with MG.

Thymic tumors in patients with MG should be surgically removed. Even in patients without thymoma, the thymus is recognized to play a role in disease pathogenesis. For many decades, thymectomy has been commonly performed as a means of reducing disease severity and dependence on immunosuppressive medications, even among patients without thymic tumors. Retrospective data suggest that there is a beneficial effect on disease in patients who have AChR antibodies and generalized weakness, but no prospective studies have corroborated these observations. The role of thymectomy in older patients with more surgical risk factors, patients with purely ocular MG, and those with seronegative or MuSK antibody MG is even less clear and requires further study.

In the setting of myasthenic crisis with acutely worsening weakness, problems with secretions, or respiratory distress, artificial ventilatory support may be necessary until emergency treatment takes effect. Plasmapheresis or intravenous immune globulin is accepted treatment for MG crisis. Neither modality is clearly superior to the other; both improve symptoms, but the effects generally last only a few weeks, and oral immunosuppression must be continued to achieve sustained remission.

Patients with isolated ocular symptoms (ocular MG) may develop generalized MG, but the risk is low after 2 years. These patients may not require surgery or intensive immunosuppression.

MG in childhood differs little from the adult form but is treated conservatively because aggressive treatment may retard growth.

Lambert–Eaton Myasthenic Syndrome Lambert–Eaton myasthenic syndrome (LEMS) is a rare paraneoplastic or autoimmune disease resulting from antibodies directed against presynaptic voltage-gated P/Q-type calcium channels (VGCC) at the neuromuscular junction. About half of patients have small cell lung carcinoma. Non–small cell lung cancer, thymoma, breast, colon, prostate, and a variety of other cancers have also rarely been associated with LEMS. In contrast to MG, muscles innervated by the cranial nerves usually are spared. Patients may complain of weakness, fatigue, distal paresthesias, or dry mouth. Slow (2 to 3 Hz), repetitive electrical stimulation of motor nerves demonstrates a decrement in compound motor action potential amplitudes at rest, but after brief muscle exercise or rapid (30 to 50 Hz) repetitive stimulation large incremental responses are seen. The diagnosis mandates a search for malignancy, but some patients may have a strictly autoimmune basis for disease and no identifiable cancer. Symptoms may improve with removal of the cancer if one is found. Pyridostigmine, guanidine, and 3,4-diaminopyridine (DAP) may ameliorate symptoms. Guanidine and DAP require frequent monitoring of hepatic, renal, hematologic, and cardiac function, and DAP is only available through special arrangement with the manufacturer, Jacobus Pharmaceutical Company. Immunomodulatory treatments such as plasmapheresis, prednisone, or azathioprine are other options in refractory cases.

Myopathies

Muscular Dystrophies

Duchenne and Becker Muscular Dystrophy These are X-linked recessive disorders. Boys who are affected have a clumsy waddling gait. Examination reveals a protuberant abdomen resulting from accentuation of lumbar lordosis, pseudohypertrophy of the calves (Fig. 17.7), and tight heel cords with a tendency toward toe walking. When arising from the floor, these children demonstrate a Gowers maneuver (Fig. 17.1). Eye movements, swallowing, and sensation are unaffected.

Patients with Duchenne muscular dystrophy have earlier onset and more severe disease; cognitive developmental delay is common. By age 9 to 12 years, increasing proximal weakness makes independent walking progressively unsteady and unsafe. Once in a wheelchair, patients develop progressive kyphoscoliosis, joint contractures, and equinovarus deformities of the feet. In subsequent years, these children become virtually immobile and require comprehensive, around-the-clock care. The combination of weak respiratory muscles and kyphoscoliosis drastically reduces pulmonary reserve, and patients generally succumb by the late teens or early twenties. Becker muscular dystrophy has a later onset, and the course is more benign with survival well into adulthood. Some patients may remain ambulatory, and mental impairment is less common.

Diagnosis is aided by myopathic changes on electrodiagnostic testing and a sometimes incidental observation of serum CK elevation (20 to 100 times normal), even before the disease is clinically evident. Genetic testing to detect a deletion or mutation of the dystrophin gene is routine currently. Although less commonly performed for diagnosis in recent decades, muscle biopsy will show characteristic dystrophic features.

Weakness is caused by a variety of deletions and point mutations affecting the muscle membrane protein dystrophin. Mutations in the X-linked dystrophin gene may lead to a total absence of dystrophin (Duchenne) or the production of a smaller molecular weight dystrophin in diminished quantity (Becker). For children suspected of having the disease, a blood specimen will demonstrate a deletion or duplication in 60% to 70% of cases. The abnormality detected may be specific for either the Duchenne or Becker form of the disease. For the remaining 20% to 30% where no deletion or duplication is found, a small specimen of skeletal muscle can be obtained and used to determine the quantity and quality of dystrophin by immunohistochemistry. Female carriers can be identified by testing peripheral blood for DNA deletions or duplications in the dystrophin gene. Prenatal diagnosis of the fetus may be achieved by using cells obtained at amniocentesis or chorionic villus biopsy.

Facioscapulohumeral (FSH) Dystrophy This is an autosomal dominant disorder characterized by slowly progressive weakness with predominant involvement of the shoulder girdle muscles and variable degrees of facial and foot dorsiflexion weakness. Symptoms may begin insidiously in the first two decades of life and progress slowly or may not be noted until later decades. Common symptoms include difficulty whistling, blowing up a balloon, or drinking through a straw. The lips often are pouting (bouché de tapir), and the smile is transverse. During sleep, the eyes may remain slightly open. The clavicles are prominent and downsloping, and the shoulders droop to produce an oblique axillary crease. The scapulae wing out when the patient attempts to elevate the arms (Fig. 17.2), and the trapezius muscles can be pushed up prominently. Atrophy of the triceps and biceps contrasts with preserved forearm muscles, producing a "Popeye arm" appearance. Foot dorsiflexion weakness results in foot drop in some patients, but hip muscles generally are spared and patients retain the ability to walk. The characteristic clinical findings in a patient with a positive family history make diagnosis fairly straightforward. EMG and muscle biopsy usually show mild but nonspecific myopathic changes.

A mutation in a gene localized on chromosome 4 is thought to lead to the clinical weakness seen in FSH dystrophy, but the gene has not been identified to date. Deletions near the telomeric end of chromosome 4 occur in 85% to 95% of FSH cases and provide laboratory confirmation of the disease.

Limb Girdle Muscular Dystrophy (LGMD) This is a clinically heterogeneous group of disorders with symptom onset ranging from early childhood to middle age. Numerous inheritance patterns have been identified. Research into muscle protein abnormalities underlying the limb girdle dystrophies has resulted in a very complex picture for what was once thought to be a single disease. There are currently at least 14 identified gene loci in families with recessively inherited disease (LGMD 2A-2N) and five gene loci in families exhibiting autosomal dominant inheritance (LGMD 1A-1E). In recent decades, there has been a steady advance in the understanding of the genetics of this heterogeneous class of muscular dystrophies.

In the most common autosomal recessive forms, LGMD 2A and 2B, weakness usually begins in the proximal legs and later is seen in the arms, along with scapular winging. Facial, tongue, and pharyngeal weakness is usually absent. An anterior axillary fold and neck flexor weakness is common. Respiratory muscle involvement may occur in some patients. Clinical variation of the disorder may be seen within families, where the proximal pattern is expressed in some individuals and distal leg weakness is the first and most prominent finding in others. Some families consist entirely of patients with predominantly distal weakness, so-called "Miyoshi myopathy." Depending on the gene mutation involved, the patient may be severely weakened at an early age and resemble DUD or simply display mild limb weakness. Electrodiagnostic studies can confirm an underlying disorder of muscle, but diagnosis rests on molecular diagnostic techniques on blood and immunohistochemistry on muscle biopsy samples. Treatment is supportive and similar to that of other inherited muscle disorders; details are outlined at the end of this chapter.

Oculopharyngeal Muscular Dystrophy Patients with oculopharyngeal dystrophy are normal until their forties or fifties. Symptoms usually begin with progressive ptosis developing over several years accompanied by increasingly restricted eye movements without diplopia. Swallowing difficulties usually develop, and aspiration can be a serious problem in a minority of patients. Mild proximal limb weakness occurs frequently. Often, these patients recall similarly afflicted family members and the pattern of an autosomal dominant disease emerges. Electrodiagnostic studies show nonspecific chronic myopathic changes. The diagnosis is confirmed by the presence of a polyalanine triplet (GCG) repeat expansion or unique exon duplication in the PABP2 gene on chromosome 14. Muscle biopsy shows distinctive red-rimmed vacuoles. Treatment is directed at the surgical correction of ptosis and the prevention of aspiration. A gastrostomy feeding tube occasionally is needed.

Myotonic Disorders and Channelopathies Myotonia refers to a clinical phenomenon of delayed muscle relaxation after voluntary contraction or muscle percussion. The clinical suspicion for a myotonic disorder can be confirmed electrodiagnostically. Needle EMG examination of affected muscles demonstrates spontaneous myotonic discharges with a characteristic waxing and waning amplitude and frequency. Some examiners have compared the auditory recording of these discharges to a dive-bomber or revving motorcycle. In some myotonic disorders, there is also significant muscle weakness, while in others myotonia is predominant.

Myotonic Dystrophy Two forms of myotonic dystrophy have been identified. The most common, myotonic dystrophy 1 (DM1), usually presents in children or young adults with finger grip and foot dorsiflexion weakness. This distal weakness is unlike most other dystrophies that begin proximally. Advanced cases have a characteristic facial appearance with ptosis; temporalis and masseter wasting; protuberant lower lip; and thinning of the sternocleidomastoid muscle, with a typical "hatchet face" appearance (Figs. 17.5 and 17.6). Percussion and grip myotonia are distinctive findings. Speech is often dysarthric and nasal, and the patient may complain of dysphagia. As in other autosomal dominant disorders, mild and severe cases may appear in the same family; however, a commonly observed feature is that patients often are unaware that there are other affected family members, even in obvious cases. About 10% of patients present with severe hypotonia, weakness, and mental retardation in infancy.

In nearly all patients, other organ systems are involved. Cataract formation, impairment of gastrointestinal motility, and endocrine abnormalities are common. Patients frequently are noted to have low intelligence, poor goal orientation, uneven work histories, and bizarre personalities. Progressive cardiac conduction block may lead to sudden death. Serial electrocardiograms (EKGs) are recommended, and a pacemaker–defibrillator should be considered for patients with significant abnormalities. A reduced ventilatory drive may produce symptoms of alveolar hypoventilation including disturbed sleep. General anesthesia should be given cautiously because patients are unduly sensitive to barbiturates and other medications that depress ventilatory drive.

Patients who have myotonic dystrophy 2 (DM2 or proximal myotonic dystrophy) show distinctive proximal weakness as well as percussion myotonia, cataracts, and, rarely, cardiac conduction defects. Pain may be a prominent symptom.

Genetic testing confirms the disease. DM1 is an autosomal dominant disorder linked to excessive CTG trinucleotide repeats in a noncoding part of a gene on chromosome 19. The clinical severity of the disease increases as the number of repeats becomes larger, but the exact defect produced in the protein kinase gene product is uncertain. In the DM2, the gene mutation is found on chromosome 3 and involves a CCTG repeat expansion of a section of the gene coding for a ribonucleic acid–binding protein; the DM1 gene region of chromosome 19 is normal in DM2 patients.

Treatment is symptomatic. Weakness of foot dorsiflexion may be improved with ankle foot orthotics. Individuals with proximal weakness that interferes with walking may need motorized scooters or wheelchairs. All patients should receive regular follow-up and treatment for the nonneurologic manifestations of their disease.

Myotonia Congenita   Impaired muscle relaxation, especially in the legs, is the cause of prominent "stiffness" in patients with myotonia congenita. Patients complain of difficulty in rapidly opening a clenched fist and slowness in initiating activity after a prolonged rest. They also may describe reduction in stiffness after exercising a muscle ("warm-up" phenomenon). Muscle hypertrophy is frequent and occasionally produces a Herculean appearance.

Muscle biopsy is not helpful, and CK levels are usually normal. More than 50 mutations of the chromosome 7 gene coding for the skeletal muscle chloride channel (CLCN1) have been described. Most cases are autosomal recessive (Becker disease), but autosomal dominant cases are well described (Thomsen disease). Diagnostic DNA tests are available for some mutations. In patients who have no identifiable DNA mutation, specific diagnosis relies primarily on clinical and EMG data. Medications such as mexiletine, phenytoin, and tocainide may be helpful in reducing myotonia, but no rigorous clinical trial data exist to support their use.

Channelopathies Affecting Skeletal Muscle   In recent years, a number of skeletal muscle membrane gene mutations causing sodium, calcium, and chloride channel abnormalities have been shown to cause distinctive clinical syndromes, many with episodic muscle weakness. Some of these may be associated with clinical or electrophysiologic myotonia. These disorders are summarized in Table 17.1.

Inflammatory Myopathies   An autoimmune disturbance underlies polymyositis (PM) and dermatomyositis (DM). Other syndromes of muscle inflammation may be caused by coxsackie virus, pyogenic bacteria, trichinosis, sarcoid, or tuberculous granuloma. True inflammatory myopathies should be distinguished from polymyalgia rheumatica (PMR), an inflammatory process that may involve fascia rather than muscle and

may present with similar symptoms of muscle pain and stiffness. PMR is not a primary disorder of muscle, and CK is normal.

Polymyositis and Dermatomyositis   DM and PM have similar clinical symptoms and signs, with the exception of the characteristic rash seen only in DM. The latter disorder may indicate the presence of a neoplasm in adults. In patients with an associated collagen vascular disease (i.e., systemic lupus erythematosus, rheumatoid arthritis, Sjögren syndrome), inflammatory myopathy may be a minor or major manifestation of the disease.

DM is seen in both children and adults, whereas PM is almost exclusively an adult disease occurring in patients in middle and later life. Both diseases may begin insidiously with systemic features such as fever, arthralgias, and myalgias; Raynaud phenomenon may be seen in DM. Weakness may begin relatively suddenly and may become profound, but more commonly there is a subacute progression of proximal weakness that is not readily distinguishable from other limb girdle syndromes. The presence of muscle tenderness is variable. The rash of DM may take several forms, appearing before, after, or in association with the onset of weakness. The upper eyelids often have a lavender or heliotrope discoloration in children, and periorbital edema and flushing of the cheeks occur in advanced cases. The chest and neck may become reddened and develop telangiectasia. Gottren papules are thickened erythematous patches that occur over the knuckles and other joint extensor surfaces. Skin nodules may break down and exude calcium.

The disease often has a variable course. Occasional patients have an acute episode with complete recovery, even without treatment. Other patients demonstrate a relapsing, remitting course with incomplete recovery between episodes or a chronic progressive course that responds poorly to treatment. The serum CK is elevated in most cases, particularly those with acute onset. Electrodiagnostic testing typically shows myopathic changes and may help to identify the best area for muscle biopsy. In both DM and PM, biopsy shows necrosis of muscle fibers and scattered inflammatory infiltrates. In DM, perifascicular atrophy and overt vasculitis are common.

Corticosteroids are the usual initial treatment once a diagnosis is confirmed. Treatment is usually required for several months. Other immunosuppressants can be added, and once strength improves, a gradual steroid taper may be attempted. By reducing the steroids to the lowest possible levels, side effects are minimized. All adult patients who have DM should be screened periodically for an occult malignancy. A home exercise program or physical therapy program may be helpful.

Inclusion Body Myositis (IBM)   IBM is a disorder most commonly seen in men older than age 50, but familial and even juvenile cases have been documented. Symptoms include asymmetric handgrip weakness along with proximal leg weakness. The CK level is only modestly elevated. Electrodiagnostic studies in such patients, some of whom may be suspected of having motor neuron disease, show a mixed neurogenic and myopathic pattern. On muscle biopsy, there are distinctive findings of increased connective tissue, variation in fiber size, isolated patches of inflammatory cells, and small red-rimmed vacuoles containing amyloid deposits, other degenerative proteins, and aggregates of proteinaceous material of unknown significance within individual muscle fibers. No specific drug therapy is available for these patients, though helpful rehabilitative measures are discussed below.

The vast majority of IBM cases are sporadic. In recent years, there have been reports of families with multiple affected siblings whose biopsies show typical IBM findings. Inheritance is mostly autosomal recessive with a gene mutation on chromosome 9, but rare families have shown an autosomal dominant pattern.

Metabolic Myopathies

Glycogen Storage Diseases   These rare autosomal recessive disorders exhibit the common finding of excess glycogen in skeletal muscle and sometimes other organ systems. Symptoms do not arise from the presence of glycogen but, rather, from a defect of energy metabolism involving the conversion of glycogen to glucose.

McArdle disease is the most common of those listed in Table 17.1 and presents in childhood or early adulthood with symptoms of exercise intolerance because of cramping and myoglobinuria. Limb weakness is common in McArdle disease and acid maltase deficiency but is rare in the other glycogen storage diseases. Fixed proximal weakness rather than exercise-induced cramping is a particular feature of acid maltase deficiency, in which early diaphragm involvement in adults may bring the patient to medical attention because of breathing difficulty. The other glycogen storage disorders are either fatal in infancy or present at any age, with exercise intolerance and varying degrees of muscle weakness (Table 17.1).

Diagnosis of these disorders can be made by muscle biopsy, which will show distinctive glycogen storage and abundant lysosomal material. The serum CK is elevated in symptomatic individuals. Gene loci for these disorders are known and inheritance is usually autosomal recessive or X-linked (Table 17.1). McArdle disease can occur as an autosomal dominant disease as well, but this is uncommon. Diagnostic assays for specific enzyme deficits are available commercially.

Disorders of Lipid Metabolism   Carnitine palmitoyl transferase deficiency (CPT II) may present at any age. Patients may show symptoms at birth with a rapidly fatal course. When onset is in childhood, there are severe but reversible metabolic crises. These early onset cases are quite rare. Onset in adolescence mimics the presentation in glycogen storage diseases; patients may develop stiffness and pain (although no cramping) with exercise and then myoglobinuria. Recurrent myoglobinuria may be precipitated in these patients by general anesthesia, infection, or a high-fat meal. The diagnosis of CPT II is not always obvious because muscle biopsy may be surprisingly normal (except after an episode of myoglobinuria). The specific CPT II enzyme defect can be detected in muscle specimens. The gene locus for this autosomal recessive disorder is on chromosome 1. Treatment is directed at preventing attacks by avoiding extreme exercise and consuming a high-carbohydrate, low-fat diet divided into frequent small meals.

A carnitine deficiency disorder results from reduced or absent carnitine, a carrier protein vital to the transport of fatty acids into mitochondria. The disease may present with only limb muscle weakness or as a more serious systemic illness. The myopathic form usually begins in childhood or young adulthood with painless, proximal weakness; exercise intolerance; and rarely cardiomyopathy and diaphragm weakness. The more severe systemic form has earlier onset; encephalopathy is common, and sometimes severe cardiomyopathy and rapid death occur. Primary carnitine deficiency is autosomal recessive and related to defective activity in the OCTN2 carnitine transporter encoded by the SLC22A5 gene on chromosome 5. On biopsy, the major change is a massive accumulation of fat within skeletal muscle, and biochemical assay can detect low or absent carnitine levels. Treatment of either form of the disease entails reducing dietary fat and taking supplements of oral L-carnitine.

Mitochondrial Myopathies   All of the mitochondrial myopathies share the common feature of excessive numbers of abnormal mitochondria in skeletal muscle and often in other tissues, arising from mutations in mitochondrial and nuclear DNA. An ever-increasing number of phenotypes caused by the resulting faulty energy production in the mitochondrial respiratory chain have been identified.

Besides symptoms and findings of muscle disease such as weakness, muscle pain, exercise intolerance, and rhabdomyolysis, other problems such as myoclonus, developmental delay or progressive dementia, ataxia, pigmentary retinal degeneration, cardiac conduction block, stroke-like episodes, diabetes, and hearing loss may provide clues suggesting an underlying mitochondrial disorder.

Muscle biopsy may demonstrate excessive subsarcolemmal collections of mitochondria (ragged-red fibers) or abnormal staining patterns with succinate dehydrogenase (SDH) or cytochrome c oxidase (COX) reactions. The inheritance pattern may be maternal via mitochondrial DNA, autosomal dominant, autosomal recessive, or X-linked. On the basis of common phenotypic patterns, known mutations can be assessed using blood or other tissue samples.

Malignant Hyperthermia   Patients with malignant hyperthermia are free of symptoms unless they are exposed to certain anesthetic agents, particularly halothane and succinylcholine. The syndrome results from abnormally increased release of calcium from sarcoplasmic reticulum and manifests with increased minute ventilation, muscular rigidity, tachycardia, marked lactic acidosis, myoglobinuria, elevation in temperature, and refractory cardiac arrhythmias. Untreated cases may be fatal. Anesthesia and the surgical procedure must be terminated immediately, while dantrolene sodium is administered with cooling measures.

The disease is autosomal dominant in many patients, and there may be subtle evidence of an underlying myopathy. The caffein–halothane contracture test is the gold standard to confirm susceptibility. Genetic testing is available to identify mutations in the ryanodine receptor gene on chromosome 19; approximately 25% of susceptible individuals have an identifiable mutation in this gene, but the absence of a mutation does not exclude susceptibility to the problem.

Toxic Myopathies   A wide variety of medications and toxic compounds can produce either acute muscle necrosis or a slowly progressive chronic myopathy. Alcohol can produce both of these syndromes in the same patient and is the most common myotoxin. The acute myopathy usually follows a binge of drinking and may be accompanied by myoglobinuria. Other drugs and toxins associated with acute myopathy include ipecac, amiodarone, clofibrate, heroin, aminocaproic acid, chlorthalidone, vincristine (where a sensorimotor neuropathy usually is superimposed), zidovudine, and any substance that produces hypokalemia including diuretics, purgatives, licorice, carbenoxolone, or amphotericin B. A chronic proximal myopathy is associated with prolonged corticosteroid therapy, particularly with dexamethasone and fluorinated steroids. The aforementioned drugs associated with acute myopathy also may produce a chronic myopathy.

The increasingly widespread use of statin cholesterol–lowering agents warrants particular discussion. Although significant myopathy is observed in only about 5 per 100,000 statin-treated patients per year, myalgias with or without CK elevations may occur in up to 7% of treated individuals, and asymptomatic CK elevations are common. The exact cause of statin-related myopathy remains uncertain, but may relate to reduced sarcolemmal cholesterol, mitochondrial dysfunction, or depletion of isoprenoids that control myofiber apoptosis. Some individuals may have increased genetically mediated susceptibility to statin myopathy related to polymorphisms in cytochrome P450 enzymes or disease-causing mutations for various metabolic myopathies.

■ **SPECIAL CLINICAL POINT: The treatment for all toxic myopathies is to eliminate the offending toxin.**

In cases where rhabdomyolysis occurs, supportive therapy with hydration should be provided. Most patients improve with these measures, though the time to recovery varies.

Endocrine Myopathies   Thyroid and parathyroid dysfunction are the main considerations among endocrine causes of myopathy. Hypothyroidism is associated with cramps, mild weakness, and "hung-up" reflexes. Hyperthyroidism may produce mild weakness, and

Graves disease may result in weakness and ophthalmoplegia. Hypoparathyroidism may lead to carpopedal spasm or tetany. Hyperparathyroidism may combine weakness with brisk reflexes, which are reminiscent of ALS.

Congenital Myopathies   Congenital myopathies constitute a heterogeneous group of muscle disorders defined by unique structural changes easily identified in histopathologic preparations on muscle biopsy material. The three most common congenital myopathies are summarized in Table 17.1.

OUTPATIENT TREATMENT PRINCIPLES

■ **SPECIAL CLINICAL POINT: The initial reaction of a patient and family to the diagnosis of a neuromuscular disease is often one of despondency and hopelessness. In time, with support and understanding, they may understand that a well-balanced rehabilitative approach will maximize function, prolong ambulation, limit complications, and create a more optimistic environment.**

The treatment of patients with chronic neuromuscular weakness is a team effort requiring the expertise of primary care physicians; neuromuscular specialists; physical, occupational, and respiratory therapists; orthotists; podiatrists; orthopaedists; nutritionists; social workers; and psychiatrists.

Special Considerations in Children

For patients with Duchenne or Becker muscular dystrophy or SMA, most clinicians will opt to work with an experienced team of child rehabilitation specialists. The central goal is to improve quality of life for these patients. For children able to handle controls responsibly, a power-drive wheelchair gives tremendous and welcomed autonomy. Education is a must for all children with these neuromuscular disorders. The child with SMA is generally of above-average intelligence and will find school enjoyable as long as there is sufficient intellectual challenge. Patients with Becker dystrophy fall into the same category and often possess surprising levels of intelligence and insight into their illness. In contrast, patients with Duchenne muscular dystrophy commonly have cognitive delay, difficulty in school, and usually require special education courses.

The prevention of contractures, particularly of the Achilles tendon and iliotibial band, is important early in all of these diseases. A surgical release of contractures along with the use of long leg braces can prolong independent, although somewhat precarious, walking for several years in Duchenne or Becker muscular dystrophy but is rarely an option in children with SMA.

Adequate and good quality rest is important. Patients with severe limb weakness sleep more comfortably on an air or water mattress designed to distribute weight evenly, preventing unrelenting pressure and decubiti.

When the patient becomes confined to a wheelchair, the development of kyphoscoliosis (Fig. 17.8) can be slowed with proper upright positioning and external chest bracing. A great deal of mobility and comfort is possible for individuals confined to a wheelchair, provided the wheelchair is properly designed and fitted. Detachable arm rests and swing-away elevating leg rests facilitate transferring and prevent lower-extremity contractures and edema that may develop if the legs are constantly dependent. Once in the wheelchair, however, the central aim is to prevent the development of restrictive lung disease as pulmonary reserve drops with age. The use of assistive cough devices, chest percussion, measurements of forced vital capacity, and blood gas measurements are all useful and best coordinated by a pediatric pulmonologist. In some children, scoliosis reaches a critical level where spinal fusion must be done to sustain life. This is not always an easy decision to make in children for whom the risk is high but whose life expectancy might be dramatically increased by such a procedure.

The intake of food may present special challenges in these children. Patients with SMA 2 may show poor weight gain, particularly during the first 2 years; even in later years, despite a relatively sedentary existence, weight can plateau despite continuous growth. In contrast, patients with Duchenne or Becker muscular dystrophy may exhibit substantial weight gain and obesity, especially in the preteen age years. Once the weight is there, it is virtually impossible to lose. Advice from dietitians is critical to prevent extremes of weight gain or loss. Often, however, despite everyone's best efforts, the child continues to eat and is indirectly encouraged to do so by the fact that it is one of few pleasures left in an increasingly circumscribed world.

For children with other primary muscle diseases marked by stable but weak limbs or gradual deterioration of strength, or in whom strength is stabilized by drugs (e.g., DM), the principles of strength building and range-of-motion maintenance are the same as for the patients with SMA and Duchenne and Becker muscular dystrophy. Referral to specialists in children's rehabilitation is key to maximizing a child's quality of life. All the principles described here may apply to anyone with chronic neuromuscular disorders.

Special Outpatient Problems in Adults

The patient with ALS probably best exemplifies the need for multiple symptomatic treatments that improve quality of life during progressive loss of strength. Early in the disease every patient needs detailed instruction on a home program of exercise for maintaining strength and range of motion. The "frozen shoulder" is a particularly painful complication that can be minimized by simple range-of-motion exercises. Use of adaptive equipment and bracing, when indicated, is also helpful. Patients initially may need a cane for balance but can be expected to move on to a walker and a standard push- or battery-powered wheelchair. In patients with hip weakness, raising the height of seats with a toilet seat elevator or electric lift chair makes standing without assistance easier. Patients rely heavily on well-anchored hand supports for getting up from the toilet, getting out of a tub, or going up stairs. Weakness of the hands impairs the fine dexterity required for eating, writing, and dressing. Various pieces of adaptive equipment are designed to splint the hand and allow easier grasping. Large-handled utensils, a buttonholer, or a pencil attached to the hand with a Velcro strap may be useful. The patient who has shoulder weakness can use a long-handled reaching device to get objects from cabinets or high shelves. Patients who have severe dysarthria can develop alternate means of communication with relatively inexpensive electronic devices available with the help of a speech therapist.

Because pharyngeal weakness is common in ALS, progressive swallowing dysfunction must be identified early. Clues to swallowing dysfunction come from continuing weight loss in the face of claims that "everything is eaten," prolonged eating time (30 to 60 minutes per meal), and recurrent pneumonias. If aspiration is suspected, a barium swallow can be confirmatory. A first step in addressing swallowing problems is to get the patient "safe swallowing" counseling from a speech therapist and advice on caloric intake from a dietitian. At this point, a frank discussion of the pros and cons of gastric tube placement should be undertaken. Gastric tubes are being recommended earlier and earlier in the course of the disease, although precise guidelines for optimal timing of the procedure are still not available. As a rough rule, weight loss of more than 3 pounds per month and more than one pneumonia episode in the face of demonstrable aspiration when drinking a glass of water in the office are reasonable grounds for bringing the subject to the attention of patient and family.

Early use of noninvasive ventilation (Bi-PAP) is thought to be beneficial but will have to be evaluated in a controlled trial. The failure of breathing in patients with ALS as a result of diaphragm weakness presents specific challenges best handled by a pulmonologist working closely with the neuromuscular neurologist. Nocturnal Bi-PAP using an external face mask is readily available to and tolerated by most patients. By removing carbon dioxide buildup, nighttime sleep is facilitated, daytime sleepiness is avoided, and overall quality of life is improved. With increasing bulbar weakness and difficulty with secretions, a cough assist device should be tried; however, a tracheostomy usually is needed if aspiration is to be prevented and adequate ventilation is to be ensured. The thought of prolonging life on a respirator is unacceptable for many patients, but for others considerable satisfaction still can be gained if the environment is supportive. The physician, patient, and family should discuss these options well in advance. Family counseling and end-of-life decisions are critical to the care of a patient with ALS.

Specific Issues in Other Neuromuscular Disorders

■ **SPECIAL CLINICAL POINT: Palpitations or unexplained syncope resulting from heart block can occur with various neuromuscular disorders, particularly myotonic dystrophy, and some limb girdle dystrophies and mitochondrial disorders. These patients may require periodic EKGs or Holter monitoring, and a pacemaker may be indicated.**

With acute generalized weakness, pulmonary and swallowing function should be monitored carefully. In some conditions like MG, respiratory failure or aspiration can develop rapidly and should be treated in an intensive care unit.

Apart from minimizing the physical handicap, the physician must be aware of the patient's social, emotional, and sexual needs. A severely handicapped patient who relies on others for eating, hygiene, and elimination understandably will become depressed over this extreme dependency. Active counseling of the patient and family should be directed toward solutions to the various problems in "personal space" and independence that arise.

SPECIAL CHALLENGES IN THE HOSPITALIZED PATIENT

Because neuromuscular disorders can impair such vital functions as speaking, swallowing, breathing, and cardiac output, the hospitalized patient must be carefully monitored for these life-threatening complications. For patients with end-stage weakness, treatment decisions must consider patient and family wishes.

Swallowing Dysfunction

Acute onset of swallowing dysfunction can occur in MG and other uncommon neuromuscular syndromes such as botulism or organophosphate poisoning. Recurrent aspiration from chronic progressive dysphagia is a continual concern in patients with ALS, MG, oculopharyngeal dystrophy, myotonic dystrophy, adult forms of SMA, and (rarely) inflammatory myopathies. The integrity of the swallowing mechanism can be tested by asking patients to swallow water from a small glass at the bedside. Patients who choke on thin liquid may have a serious swallowing problem, indicating that oral food intake can lead to aspiration and pneumonia. A tailored barium swallow should be done to confirm such swallowing problems. If aspiration risk is high, a simple "chin tuck" maneuver may be all that is needed. With more frequent and persistent aspiration, an endoscopically placed gastrostomy tube may be needed to guard against pneumonia and to maintain proper nutrition.

Respiratory Complications

Respiratory depression is to be expected and anticipated in most hospitalized patients with neuromuscular disease. Weakness of the diaphragm and accessory intercostal muscles of respiration compromises ventilation. Symptoms of respiratory distress can be mild and nonspecific and include restlessness, irritability, and confusion. Arterial blood gases and pulmonary function tests should be monitored closely for dropping vital capacity and poor inspiratory and expiratory pressures. When the vital capacity falls below 50% of predicted and the disorder appears to be progressing, Bi-PAP or more invasive ventilatory support should be considered. Bulbar dysfunction results in a poor cough and increased risk of aspiration so that early intubation may be warranted to protect the patient's airway. Infrequently, patients with neuromuscular disease have a superimposed central hypoventilation syndrome that further compromises breathing. A patient with limited movement of the extremities is susceptible to deep vein thrombosis and pulmonary embolism, which can further limit adequate oxygenation. Performing range-of-motion exercises, wearing compression stockings, and taking subcutaneous heparin may help mitigate these risks.

Cardiac Complications

In a few neuromuscular disorders such as Duchenne or Becker dystrophy and some limb girdle dystrophies, myocardial involvement leads to impaired contractility and congestive heart failure. Cardiac conduction disturbances are frequent in myotonic dystrophy and some limb girdle dystrophies and mitochondrial myopathies. A demand pacemaker and defibrillator can be life sustaining.

Infectious Complications

Although pneumonia is more likely in patients with bulbar dysfunction and/or respiratory muscle weakness, patients with MG and inflammatory myopathies are at even greater risk because of pharmacologic immunosuppression. Common sites of infection include the urinary and respiratory tracts, but septicemia, peritonitis, meningitis, and other types of infections also may occur. Prophylactic influenza and pneumococcal immunizations are essential.

Rhabdomyolysis and Myoglobinuria

Acute muscle destruction (rhabdomyolysis) may occur from a variety of insults, including extreme physical overexertion, trauma, and toxins, and far less commonly from inherited neuromuscular disorders. Muscle breakdown releases myoglobin, which can cause acute renal failure from tubular necrosis. The resultant electrolyte imbalances can produce life-threatening cardiac arrhythmias. Careful attention should be given to maintaining adequate blood volume, urine flow, and electrolyte balance. Renal dialysis may be needed.

End-of-Life Care

The role of the physician in the care of dying patients has been the subject of renewed interest and intense debate in recent years. Although physicians understand the importance of relieving suffering, some remain uncomfortable with a competent, terminally ill patient's right to refuse life-sustaining treatment, including ventilation, hydration, and nutrition. Similarly, a patient's request for morphine or similar agents to relieve pain or dyspnea can be disconcerting in the face of ventilatory failure. In such circumstances, physicians can benefit from consultation with experts in palliative care and end-of-life decision making.

WHEN TO REFER TO A NEUROLOGIST

Primary care physicians often ask themselves when they should refer the patient with neuromuscular symptoms to a neuromuscular specialist. There is a tendency in this day of restrictive managed care plans to simply ask the specialist for informal advice by phone or during a chance meeting over coffee in the hospital cafeteria. This can be a prescription for disaster. Usually, not all of the critical information is passed to the would-be consultant who is asked to render an opinion without either direct questioning or a complete neurologic examination.

A formal consultation with an experienced neuromuscular consultant serves two important purposes. First, among patients with non-neuromuscular problems, it may stop the otherwise endless chain of self-referrals, which add unnecessarily to medical care costs, and needless patient anxiety. This is a particularly important function in these times when easy access to the medical world via the Internet may compound patient anxieties and lead to "doctor shopping." Second, in patients with an organic neurologic disease, an appropriate consultation can prevent diagnostic delays that might be either overtly dangerous or seriously compromise appropriate therapy.

■ **SPECIAL CLINICAL POINT: Knowing when to refer a patient to a neuromuscular specialist is not a terribly scientific decision. Sometimes it is a reflexive action that occurs when a physician realizes that the problem is beyond his or her capabilities.**

Occasionally, it results from the physician's frustration with a patient who returns repeatedly with symptoms that do not respond to treatment or as a result of complaints from unhappy relatives or caregivers.

Finally, when confronted with a patient who seems to fit the diagnostic criteria for a neuromuscular disorder, ordering one or two laboratory tests is appropriate (e.g., a CK for suspected dystrophies and inflammatory myopathies, anti-AChR antibody for suspected MG). Electrodiagnostic testing is often very helpful to distinguish neuromuscular from nonneuromuscular disease processes and to distinguish neurogenic from myopathic conditions.

■ **SPECIAL CLINICAL POINT: Electrodiagnostic testing is best performed by neuromuscular specialists or physicians with specialty qualifications in electrophysiology.**

More expensive or esoteric tests may be deferred until the patient is seen by the specialist. In this age of cost awareness, allowing the neurologic consultant to direct the focused ordering of these specialty tests can result in considerable savings, both medical and economic.

The referral of a patient is a cooperative venture designed to reach a diagnostic conclusion and offer effective treatment. Referring physicians and neuromuscular consultants must work in partnership for the good of the patient. These guidelines are meant to be the first step in developing such a partnership.

Always Remember

Objective signals that a patient might benefit from a neuromuscular consultation include the following "red flags."

In children:

- The floppy infant or hypotonic infant—think SMA, congenital myopathy
- Child with delayed motor milestones—think muscular dystrophy, SMA, congenital myopathies, metabolic myopathies
- Child with frequent falls, clumsy gait, abnormal use of hands to assist self, trouble getting up from a fall—think muscular dystrophy, DM, congenital myopathies
- Child with toe walking—think muscular dystrophy

In adults:

- Muscle pain—think inflammatory myopathy, PMR
- Trouble with arising from a chair, climbing stairs, lifting objects over head ("trouble with chairs, stairs, and into the air")—think proximal limb weakness as in MG and inflammatory myopathy
- Tripping while running/walking—think foot drop resulting from peripheral neuropathy, ALS, myotonic dystrophy
- Grip weakness—think ALS, myotonic dystrophy, IBM
- Slurred speech—think early ALS, MG, Kennedy disease
- Swallowing difficulties, especially with thin liquids—think ALS, MG, Kennedy disease, IBM, oculopharyngeal dystrophy
- Dark urine—think myoglobinuria resulting from excessive exercise, glycogen storage disease, CPT deficiency
- Muscle atrophy and/or visible twitches—think ALS

QUESTIONS AND DISCUSSION

1. A 61-year-old man presents with insidious and painless progression of left foot weakness. His medical history is unremarkable. His examination shows atrophy of the anterior compartment of the left foreleg, left foot dorsiflexion weakness, hyperactive leg reflexes, and extensor plantar responses. Cognition, cranial nerves, and sensation are normal. Which of the following is the most likely diagnosis?
   A. Myasthenia gravis
   B. Peripheral neuropathy
   C. Amyotrophic lateral sclerosis
   D. Inclusion body myositis

The correct answer is C. Painless weakness in the setting of preserved sensation and hyperactive reflexes are ominous symptoms and signs of possible ALS. Alternate considerations include a focal nerve or nerve root lesion, distal myopathy, or a peripheral neuropathy predominantly affecting motor nerves, but these would not be expected to cause hyperactive reflexes, and focal nerve or root lesions are usually accompanied by sensory symptoms. A less likely possibility is a localized central nervous system lesion, but this would not cause significant muscle atrophy.

A nerve conduction study with needle electromyography would be extremely helpful to distinguish between a neurogenic disorder as would be expected with ALS or a myopathic condition. Other useful studies include serum CK and a sedimentation rate to screen for systemic inflammatory disease or significant muscle disease. The life-changing implications of a suspected ALS diagnosis require that the patient be referred to a neuromuscular specialist for further evaluation and treatment.

2. A 19-year-old pregnant woman reports that two maternal uncles died of muscular dystrophy at the ages of 15 and 16. Of the choices below, which neuromuscular

condition was the most likely condition affecting the uncles?

A. Becker muscular dystrophy
B. Limb girdle muscular dystrophy
C. Fascioscapulohumeral muscular dystrophy
D. Duchenne muscular dystrophy

The correct answer is D. Some cases of muscular dystrophy actually may have been misdiagnosed SMA. SMA is usually an autosomal recessive disorder, and the risk of the woman or her children developing this disease would be low. Among the muscular dystrophies, death occurring in the teenage years is characteristic of Duchenne dystrophy. This illness in two male siblings would not be the result of a spontaneous mutation and indicates that their mother, the patient's grandmother, was a carrier. Genetic linkage analysis requires blood samples from the affected uncles but is not an option in this case.

Blood samples on the patient as well as fetal cells obtained by amniocentesis can be screened for the abnormal dystrophin gene. If no deletion is found, linkage analysis can be carried out to determine the probabilities of family members having the identical X chromosome, but without linkage information from the two deceased uncles of the pregnant patient, no accurate probability can be given concerning her being a carrier or having passed the abnormal gene on to her fetus. The situation might be clarified if the patient's CK were significantly elevated, arguing for her being a carrier, but normal values would not be helpful. In such a complex situation, the assistance of an experienced genetic counselor is advised.

3. A 51-year-old woman is admitted to the hospital with symptomatic bradycardia. She reports frequent "dizzy spells" for about 1 year, but she has never fainted. She also has had lifelong stiffness in her hands and a nasal voice, and she trips frequently. Which of the following is the most likely diagnosis?

A. Duchenne muscular dystrophy
B. Myotonic muscular dystrophy

C. Becker muscular dystrophy
D. Fascioscapulohumeral muscular dystrophy

The correct answer is B. Myotonic dystrophy is suggested by the history of grip myotonia and systemic complaints. Recurrent abdominal pain, gallstones, chronic diarrhea, dyspepsia, and dysphagia are common symptoms. Cardiac conduction disturbances may present with dizziness or may be discovered on a routine EKG. A careful examination for clinical myotonia, as well as for the characteristic facial features, would support the diagnosis in this case. Myotonic dystrophy is a common disorder, although it frequently is overlooked.

4. In the clinical scenario outlined in question 3, an EKG demonstrates complete heart block. What is the most appropriate immediate course of action?

A. Discharge: She has a genetic condition and nothing can be done.
B. Observe for 24 hours and schedule for outpatient follow-up in 3 months.
C. Obtain a cardiac electrophysiology consultation.
D. Contact the patient's family and have everyone genetically tested.

The correct answer is C. A pacemaker may need to be implanted. Bilateral foot drop is relieved with ankle bracing. All relatives of this patient should be evaluated clinically for signs and symptoms of this autosomal dominant disorder. Symptomatic relatives can be counseled and followed as needed for the disorder. Asymptomatic individuals can be given information regarding the disease. Should they wish to know their carrier status with certainty, a DNA analysis of blood can provide definite information regarding the presence or absence of trinucleotide repeat sequences. This information would be of use particularly to asymptomatic mutation carriers who are planning families. However, the first priority is to address the medical needs of the symptomatic patient.

SUGGESTED READING

Aggarwal S, Cudkowicz M. ALS drug development: reflections from the past and a way forward. *Neurotherapeutics*. 2008;5:516–527.

Chahin N, Klein C, Mandrekar J, et al. Natural history of spinal–bulbar muscular atrophy. *Neurology*. 2008; 70:1967–1971.

Engel AG, Franzini-Armstrong C. *Myology*. 3rd ed. Vols 1 and 2. New York: McGraw-Hill; 2004.

Groh WJ, Groh MR, Saha C, et al. Electrocardiographic abnormalities and sudden death in myotonic dystrophy type 1. *N Engl J Med*. 2008;358:2688–2697.

Guglieri M, Straub V, Bushby K, et al. Limb-girdle muscular dystrophies. *Curr Opin Neurol*. 2008;21:576–584.

Kanagawa M, Toda T. The genetic and molecular basis of muscular dystrophy: roles of cell-matrix linkage in the pathogenesis. *J Hum Genet*. 2006;51:915–926.

Karpati G, Hilton-Jones D, Griggs RC. *Disorders of Voluntary Muscle*. 7th ed. New York: Cambridge University Press; 2001.

Klopstock T. Drug-induced myopathies. *Curr Opin Neurol*. 2008;21:590–595.

Litman RS, Rosenberg H. Malignant hyperthermia: update on susceptibility testing. *JAMA*. 2005; 293:2918–2924.

Longo N, Amat di San Filippo C, Pasquali M. Disorders of carnitine transport and the carnitine cycle. *Am J Med Genet C Semin Med Genet*. 2006;142C:77–85.

Lynch DR, Farmer JM. Neurogenetics. Introduction. *Neurol Clin*. 2002;20(3):xi–xiii.

Mahadeva B, Phillips LH II, Juel VC. Autoimmune disorders of neuromuscular transmission. *Semin Neurol*. 2008; 28(2):212–227.

Miller TM. Differential diagnosis of myotonic disorders. *Muscle Nerve*. 2008;37:293–299.

Mitsumoto H, Chad DA, Pioro EP. *Amyotrophic Lateral Sclerosis*. Philadelphia: FA Davis; 1998.

Norwood F, de Visser M, Eymard B, et al. EFNS guideline on diagnosis and management of limb girdle muscular dystrophies. *Eur J Neurol*. 2007;14:1305–1312.

Oskoui M, Kaufmann P. Spinal muscular atrophy. *Neurotherapeutics*. 2008;5:499–506.

Pourmand R. Metabolic myopathies. A diagnostic evaluation. *Neurol Clin*. 2000;18(1):1–13.

Saperstein DS. Muscle channelopathies. *Semin Neurol*. 2008;28:260–269.

Taylor RW, Schaefer AM, Barron MJ, et al. The diagnosis of mitochondrial muscle disease. *Neuromuscul Disord*. 2004;14:237–245.

Valdmanis PN, Rouleau GA. Genetics of familial amyotrophic lateral sclerosis. *Neurology*. 2008; 70:144–152.

Wolfe GI, Oh SJ. Clinical phenotype of muscle-specific tyrosine kinase-antibody-positive myasthenia gravis. *Ann N Y Acad Sci*. 2008;1132:71–75.

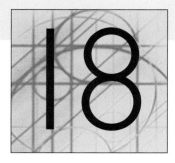

18 Peripheral Neuropathy

JOSHUA GORDON AND MORRIS A. FISHER

key points
- History and physical examination are the most important steps in determining the etiology of a peripheral neuropathy.
- Neuropathies can be categorized according to type of modalities involved (motor, sensory, or autonomic) and distribution (multifocal or diffuse).
- A distal symmetric pattern is the most common presentation of a polyneuropathy.
- Treatment of peripheral neuropathies is either directed at the underlying cause or is aimed at reducing the discomfort that is often associated with neuropathies.

CLINICAL FEATURES AND SCIENTIFIC BACKGROUND

The peripheral nervous system (PNS) starts as the pia arachnoid ends at the level of the intervertebral foramina and therefore encompasses those parts of the nervous system that lie outside the confines of the brain, brainstem, and spinal cord. It consists of those portions of the primary sensory neurons, lower motor neurons, and autonomic neurons that are outside the central nervous system (CNS). Therefore the PNS includes the cranial nerves, the spinal nerves with their roots and rami, the peripheral nerves, and those aspects of the autonomic nervous system that are outside the CNS. Because some disease processes preferentially involve the PNS, it is useful to consider this system as a nosologic entity.

All parts of the PNS are associated with Schwann cells or the comparable ganglionic cells, the satellite cells. This anatomic commonality may account for some of the pathologic aspects of the PNS. More significantly, the normal functions of all parts of the PNS are dependent on the proper functioning of the nerve cell bodies from which the motor and sensory axons originate. For example, the foot is supplied by nerve fibers whose cell bodies lie at the level of the lower thoracic/upper-lumbar vertebrae. A single neuron consists of the motoneuron and its associated motor axon innervating a foot muscle. The maintenance of this cell extending from the lower back to the foot is a complex process. There is constant anterograde transport system from the nerve cell bodies to their most distal axonal projections, and this system is necessary for maintaining normal nerve (and muscle) function. There is also retrograde transport so that the cell bodies are influenced by distal events. This system provides the conduit by which agents such as herpes virus may reach the nerve cell body. Given the complexity and length of the structures involved, it is not surprising that the normal functioning of the PNS frequently is disturbed.

ANATOMY

Except for the cranial nerves, peripheral nerves separate at the level of the roots. The dorsal roots contain sensory afferent (sensory) fibers that are located either preganglionic or postganglionic to the dorsal root ganglion on their way to the spinal cord. The ventral roots consist of efferent (motor) fibers that originate from the lower motor neurons. The ventral and dorsal roots joining shortly after exiting the spinal cord, and the resultant mixed (motor and sensory) nerves are the structures for providing information to and from the CNS. In the thoracic and upper-lumbar region, these nerves are joined by sympathetic fibers after these fibers have synapsed in the ganglionic chain adjacent to the vertebral column. The parasympathetic outflow originates either in the cranial region (cranial nerves III, VII, IX, and X) or in the sacral region passing distally as the pelvic splanchnic nerves (Fig. 18.1).

Individual muscles and areas of skin are supplied not only by particular nerves but also by fibers that originate in particular roots. The PNS distribution in the limbs is superficially complex because of the routing that occurs in the brachial plexus for the upper limb, and the lumbosacral plexus of the lower limb.

Individual nerves are composed of bundles of individual nerve fibers called fascicles, which, in turn, are surrounded by connective tissue. All of the motor fibers and many of the sensory fibers are surrounded by myelin. Myelin is formed by foldings of Schwann cell

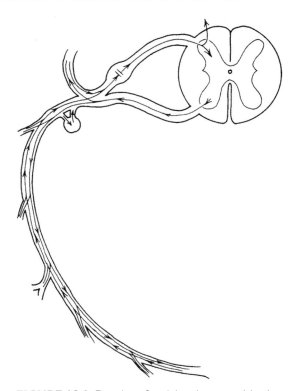

FIGURE 18.1 Drawing of peripheral nerve originating from (1) ventral root with cells of origin in the anterior horn of the spinal cord and (2) dorsal root with a dorsal root ganglion. The postganglionic dorsal root fibers pass to the dorsal horn or more superiorly in the spinal cord. The posterior primary ramus extends dorsally, whereas the anterior primary ramus is the main extension of the peripheral nerve. Sympathetic fibers join the peripheral nerve by way of the sympathetic ganglion.

membranes. These supporting cells are ubiquitous throughout the PNS. In myelinated fibers the gaps between myelin sheaths from two adjacent Schwann cells are referred to as nodes of Ranvier. Most sensory fibers and all autonomic fibers are either poorly myelinated or unmyelinated. Even unmyelinated nerve fibers, however, are ensheathed by Schwann cells.

Nutrient arteries that arise from adjacent blood vessels supply nerves. The arterial supply is richly collateralized both to and within the nerves themselves. The result is a system resistant to large-vessel ischemia.

INDICATIONS OF NEUROPATHIC INJURY

The symptoms and signs of neuropathic injury can be predicted from the preceding discussion. If nerves to muscles are disrupted, weakness may be present, and prominent atrophy of muscle fibers can occur. Cramping with fatigue is a common symptom. Reflexes may be decreased or absent if the afferent or efferent nerves that subserve the reflex are disturbed.

A wide range of sensory disturbances are found. With complete loss of innervation, there may be total loss of feeling-anesthesia. This rarely happens because of the considerable overlap of sensory nerve supply. More commonly, alterations in sensation are found. Unusual feelings such as "pins and needles" are called paresthesias, and unpleasant sensations such as burning are called dysesthesias. A decrease in sensation on examination is referred to as hypoesthesia; an increase is called hyperesthesia. Formication refers to the crawling feeling that some patients may experience. A decrease in perception of position and vibration indicates dysfunction in larger fibers, whereas diminished pinprick and temperature sensation indicates abnormalities in smaller fibers. Autonomic dysfunction can affect cardiac, vasomotor, gastrointestinal, sweating, and sexual functions. The skin may become smooth and glossy, hair may decrease (or occasionally increase), and the nails may become thickened. Because of loss of feeling, repeated injury and inadequate repair can result in permanent losses in limbs as well as of function of joints (Charcot joints).

ANATOMIC DISTRIBUTION

Motor and sensory changes caused by PNS disease occur in the distribution of nerve roots or the peripheral nerves themselves. Charts are readily available that show these distributions. The information has been obtained indirectly based on root or nerve injury. Although superficially complex, with practice the information becomes readily usable. There is some variability between different charts, and one should not attempt to fit each patient into a rigidly circumscribed view of normal. Patterns of root and nerve distribution in a broad sense are reliable, and it is important to try to identify these patterns clinically (Fig. 18.2).

The muscles of the shoulder girdle are innervated mainly by the C5 root, those of the arm by C5 and C6 (triceps brachii, C7), those of the forearm by C7 and C8, and those of the hand by C8 and T1. In the lower extremity, the thigh muscles are supplied by the L2, L3, and L4 roots. Those muscles of the anterior leg are innervated by L4 and L5 roots, those of the posterior leg by S1, and the small muscles of the foot by S1 and S2.

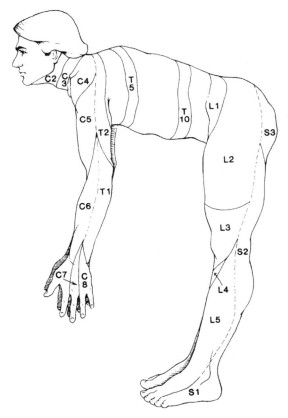

FIGURE 18.2 Sequential nature of the cutaneous root distribution as shown with the individual in the quadruped position.

The root sensory distribution can be visualized with the individual in the anatomic position. In general, C1-4 innervate the back of the head, the neck, and the shoulder region; C5 innervates the lateral aspect of the arm; C6 innervates the lateral portion of the forearm extending into the hand involving the thumb and index finger; C7 innervates the midportion of the hand and ring finger; and C8 innervates the more medial portion of the hand including the little finger. The posterior aspect of the upper extremity then is supplied by T1 and T2, and the torso is innervated sequentially by T2-L1, with T5 at about the level of the nipples and T10 at the umbilicus. The anterior thigh is supplied by L1, L2, and L3; the anterior leg and foot are supplied predominantly by L4 and L5; the posterior aspect of the lower extremity is supplied by S1 and S2; and the region of the anus is supplied by S3, S4, and S5.

The three main terminal nerves of the brachial plexus in the upper extremity are the radial, median, and ulnar nerves. The radial nerve innervates the extensor muscles and provides much of the cutaneous supply to the extensor surface of the arm, forearm, and hand. The median nerve is the predominant nerve innervating the forearm flexors as well as the muscles of the thenar eminence controlling thumb movement. The ulnar nerve innervates the remaining intrinsic hand muscles. The median and ulnar nerves supply the cutaneous sensibility to the hand. The ulnar territory characteristically encompasses the little finger, half of the ring finger, and the adjacent palmar surface, whereas the median nerve provides the remaining cutaneous innervation (Fig. 18.3). Variations, however, are frequently present.

In the lower extremity, the femoral nerve supplies the knee extensors in the thigh in addition to the cutaneous branches for the anterior thigh and medial aspect of the leg and foot (by way of the saphenous nerve). The posterior thigh muscles controlling knee flexion, as well as all the muscles of the leg and foot, are innervated by the sciatic nerve. The peroneal (anterior tibial) branch of the sciatic nerve supplies the anterior compartment of the leg—namely, those muscles that affect dorsiflexion of the ankle and toes as well as foot eversion. The tibial portion of the sciatic nerve innervates those muscles producing plantar flexion. The cutaneous distribution is comparable. Branches of the peroneal nerve supply the anterior leg and dorsum of the foot, whereas the posterior aspect of the leg and plantar aspect of the foot are innervated by branches

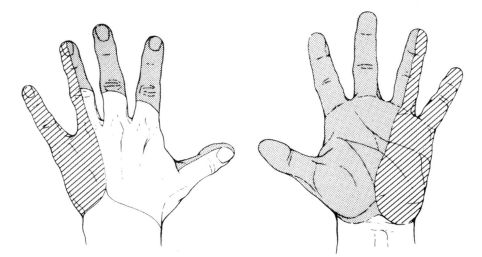

FIGURE 18.3 Cutaneous innervation of the hand by the radial (clear section), median (stippled section), and ulnar (diagonal lines) nerves.

of the tibial nerve. The medial plantar aspect of the foot and toes is supplied by the medial plantar nerve, whereas their more lateral aspect is supplied by the lateral plantar nerve. The medial and lateral plantar nerves are the terminal equivalents of the upper-extremity median and ulnar nerves, respectively.

Table 18.1 indicates selected muscle movements with their main innervation, and

Table 18.2 shows a schema of the cutaneous innervation of the limbs. These tables and the preceding discussion are designed to provide a framework for the clinical evaluation of peripheral nerve disorders. To do the examination well requires considerable experience. Obtaining the necessary information from the patients can be demanding, and the examination itself must be an active process looking for

---

TABLE 18.1

Selected Muscle Movements and Their Innervation

Joint Movement	Muscles[a]	Peripheral Nerves[a]	Spinal Segments[a]
	Upper	*Extremity*	
Shoulder abduction	Deltoid	Axillary	C5
Shoulder external rotation	Infraspinatus	Suprascapular	C5
Elbow flexion	Biceps brachii	Musculocutaneous	C5, C6
Elbow extensin	Triceps brachii	Radial	C7
Radial-ulnar supination	Biceps brachii	Musculocutaneous	C6
Pronation	Pronator teres	Median	C7
Wrist extension	Extensor carpi radialis	Radial	C7
Radial wrist flexion	Flexor carpi radialis	Median	C7
Ulnar wrist flexion	Flexor carpi ulnaris	Ulnar	C8
Thumb adduction	Interossei	Ulnar	T1
Thumb abduction	Abductor pollicis brevis	Median	C8
Thumb extension	Extensor pollicis	Radial	C7, C8
Thumb opposition	Opponens pollicis	Median	T1
Finger adduction	Palmar interossei	Ulnar	T1
Finger abduction	Dorsal interossei	Ulnar	T1
Finger extension	Extensor digitorum	Radial	C7, C8
Index finger extension	Extensor indicis	Radial	C8
	Lower	*Extremity*	
Hip flexion	Iliopsoas	Femoral	L2
Hip extension	Gluteus maximus	Inferior gluteal	S1, S2
Leg adduction	Adductor magnus	Obturator	L2, L3
Leg abduction	Gluteus medius	Superior gluteal	L4, L5
Knee extension	Quadriceps	Femoral	L3, L4
Knee flexion	Biceps femoris	Sciatic	S1
Ankle dorsiflexion	Tibialis anterior	Peroneal	L4
Plantar flexion	Gastrocnemius	Posterior tibial	S1, S2
Inversion	Tibialis posterior	Posterior tibial	L5
Eversion	Peroneus longus	Peroneal	L5
Large toe extension	Extensor hallucis longus	Peroneal	L5

[a]Only main controlling muscle, nerve, and roots listed.

Joint action listed because it can be easily tested and muscle, nerve, and root control are relatively simple.

Notes: Terminal divisions of the brachial plexus can be tested at the thumb. Hip action controlled by muscles innervated by L2–S2 roots.

TABLE 18.2	Schematic Cutaneous Innervation of the Limbs			
	Lateral	**Anterior**	**Medial**	**Posterior**
Arm	C5 axillary radial		Medial cutaneous nerve of arm T2	
Forearm	C6 musculocutaneous		Medial cutaneous nerve of forearm T1	
Hand and fingers	Thumb and index C6		Middle C7 Ring C8 Little C8	
Thigh	Lateral femoral cutaneous	Femoral L2, L3	Obturator	Posterior cutaneous nerve S2
Leg	Peroneal L5	Peroneal L5	Saphenous L4	Sural S1, S2
Foot		Peroneal L5		Plantar nerves S1

Portions of the posterior midline areas of the arm and forearm are supplied by branches of the radial nerve.
For cutaneous distribution, see Figures 18.2 and 18.3.

patterns of abnormality. As such, neurologic consultation for the evaluation of peripheral nerve disorders is frequently helpful.

PATTERNS OF ABNORMALITY

Derangements of motor, sensory, and autonomic function may be present with lesions at the level of the roots, plexuses, or peripheral nerves. Sensory loss, for example, involving the lateral aspect of the leg combined with weakness of dorsiflexion of the toes would be consistent with a lesion of the L5 root; motor and sensory changes in the distribution of both the axillary and radial nerves would be compatible with injury to the posterior cord of the brachial plexus; and weakness and atrophy of intrinsic hand muscles combined with sensory loss involving the medial aspect of the palmar surface of the hand, the little finger, and adjacent half of the middle finger would indicate an ulnar nerve lesion.

The most common pattern of PNS disease is a symmetric polyneuropathy. Sensory, usually more than motor, signs and symptoms are present in a more or less symmetric, predominantly distal distribution. The signs and symptoms start distally in the legs and progress proximally. Clinical findings in the legs and arms are related to the distance from the spinal cord (i.e., from C7 in the arms and T12-L1 in the legs). Sensory loss should extend to the midlegs, for example, before such findings are present in the arms. Diabetic polyneuropathy, uremia, and drug or toxic exposure are common examples. One possible cause for this distribution may be that longer nerve fibers are more vulnerable to disturbances in nutrient transport.

■ **SPECIAL CLINICAL POINT: In most distal symmetric polyneuropathies the portions of the nerve that are farthest from the spinal cord are affected first and symptoms progress proximally.**

Damage to a single nerve is called a mononeuropathy. An example would be the carpal tunnel syndrome (CTS) as a result of median nerve injury at the level of the wrist. Compressive injury is a frequent cause.

A mononeuropathy multiplex indicates dysfunction of multiple single peripheral nerves. This pattern is common in diabetes as well as vasculitides such as polyarteritis nodosa.

Plexopathies refer to injury at the level of the brachial, lumbar, or sacral plexuses. Idiopathic brachial neuritis, traumatic injury to the brachial plexus, and retroperitoneal or apical lung tumors are common causes. Radiculopathies are caused by injury to the roots. Sensory loss is in a dermatome rather than peripheral nerve distribution. Disc and vertebral bone disease are among the associated conditions.

An important clinical distinction is whether a process is diffuse or multifocal. In multifocal neuropathies, the length-dependent basis of nerve dysfunction in neuropathies is not necessarily present. Cranial nerves may be involved, the arms may be more affected than the legs, and there may be prominent differences in the degree of injury between similar nerves on the right or left or between nerves (e.g., tibial and peroneal) in comparable areas of a limb.

PATHOLOGY

Pathologic processes affecting nerves usually involve both myelin and axons, although at times the physiologic effects predominantly may reflect injury to one or the other of these structures. In demyelinating processes, myelin may be lost diffusely (e.g., inherited demyelinating neuropathies) as well as segmentally (e.g., acquired demyelinating neuropathies). There may be marked slowing and blocking of conduction. The axons may be relatively well preserved. As such, clinical recovery in the acquired demyelinating neuropathies such as the Guillain–Barré syndrome (GBS) can be both rapid and complete if remyelination occurs.

Prominent axonal degeneration is more common than primary demyelination. This is characteristic of neuropathies as a result of a large number of exogenous toxins and metabolic derangements. These processes may affect the nerve cell bodies as well as the axons and may be manifested as a dying back of the distal portion of the axon. Secondary demyelination occurs in those fibers with axonal damage. Recovery occurs by regeneration of axons, which often must then reinnervate denervated structures. As a result, recovery may be relatively slow and incomplete.

With physical injury to nerves, the injury may be limited to focal (paranodal) demyelination with associated conduction block and rapid recovery (neuropraxia). If axons are interrupted (axonotmesis), degeneration (Wallerian) of the axons and myelin may occur distal to the site of injury. If the Schwann cell basal lamina and endoneurial tissue remain intact, axonal regeneration commences promptly after injury. If both the axon and surrounding connective tissue are disrupted (neurotmesis), Wallerian degeneration is inevitable and axon regeneration may be disrupted by intervening connective tissue. Neuromas and aberrant regeneration may occur.

The potential pathologic processes that affect the PNS are similar to those that affect other systems. Metabolic or toxic derangements (e.g., vitamin deficiencies, uremia, alcoholism, heavy metals, industrial solvents, and certain medications) frequently result in nerve dysfunction. Vascular abnormalities affecting nerves usually involve the medium and small arteries, and these abnormalities may be found in rheumatoid arthritis, polyarteritis nodosa, and temporal arteritis. Diabetic mononeuropathies are probably vascular in origin, and the primary pathologic process in diabetic polyneuropathies may be a vascular-based ischemia. Idiopathic polyneuritis (Landry–Guillain–Barré syndrome) is representative of an inflammatory process. This probably has an immunologic basis, as do the neuropathies seen in paraproteinemias and paraneoplastic syndromes. Leprosy is a common infectious process affecting nerves, as are some of the neuropathies associated with human immunodeficiency virus (HIV) infection. A genetic basis for PNS dysfunction such as peroneal muscular atrophy (Charcot–Marie–Tooth disease) is also not uncommon. Schwannomas and neurofibromas are representative tumors. Trauma is a frequent cause of nerve injury. This includes entrapment neuropathies—namely, mononeuropathies resulting from vulnerability because of anatomic features of the nerves. CTS is the most common entrapment neuropathy, but other common injuries include the ulnar nerve at the elbow and the peroneal nerve at the fibula head.

Neuropathies are common. An approach to evaluating these problems is essential in all areas of medicine. Even under the best of circumstances, the cause for a neuropathy may not be established in about one-third of these patients. As in other areas of medicine, often the important thing for management to determine is what is not the cause as much as what is the cause.

■ **SPECIAL CLINICAL POINT: Even with a complete neurologic exam and appropriate diagnostic testing, up to one-third of neuropathies will not have an identifiable cause.**

DIAGNOSIS

The physical examination remains a powerful tool for the evaluation of disorders of the PNS. The examination need not be subtle, but it must be accurate. Motor and sensory distributions of a polyneuropathy, mononeuropathy, or radiculopathy often can be appreciated.

The action of individual muscles should be tested and rated as to strength. Strength may be normal (5), mildly decreased (4), moderately decreased (3) (movement against gravity only), markedly (1–2) decreased, or absent (0). This is a standard numerical system but has the limitation that the overwhelming majority of ratings are in the range of 3 to 5. Muscle strength testing should be concentrated in those areas that aid in the analysis of the particular problem.

The sensory examination need not be tedious, but it must be accurate. Again, concentration on areas relevant to the diagnostic question is important. The patient often can best outline a circumscribed area of sensory deficit. This area then can be analyzed in more detail for light touch and pain sensations using a finger and a sharp instrument such as a safety pin, respectively. (New and separate pins must be used for each patient to minimize risk of infection.)

A distal to proximal area of sensory change can be outlined in a similar fashion. Moving relevant joints can test position sense. Slight movements of distal joints should be appreciated accurately. A 128-cycles/sec (cps) tuning fork with the base placed on bony prominences is used for testing vibration. In neuropathies, vibration is characteristically more affected than position. The examination should start from the most distal area of abnormality. Then one should test vibration in more proximal locations only if the patient does not perceive the full duration of the vibration at the more distal site. A finger of the examiner touching the same bony region as the tuning fork helps evaluate the patient's sensitivity.

As mentioned previously, the sensory examination may be difficult and confusing. A primary care physician should have a low threshold for seeking consultation if it could be helpful.

The most valuable ancillary study for analysis of PNS disorders is electromyography (EMG). This is best viewed as an extension of the neurologic examination. Although an EMG is harmless, it does entail some discomfort. Reliable information obtained in an efficient fashion is crucial, and this, in turn, will depend on the experience and skill of the electromyographer.

Electromyography consists of two basic parts. The first is an evaluation of the conduction in nerves. The second part involves analysis of the electrical activity in muscles—the EMG per se. The data can define the location of a lesion and aid in understanding the pathophysiology.

Conduction in motor fibers is determined by stimulating nerves electrically and recording the resultant-evoked motor response. Muscle fiber contraction is associated with electrical activity caused by the movement of charged ions across membranes, and this electrical activity can be recorded. Latency refers to the time from the stimulus to the onset of the electrical activity. The latency will be shorter if the stimulus is closer to the muscle than if it is more distant. The time difference between a distal and a more proximal latency divided by the distance between the two stimulating points enables a conduction velocity (CV) to be determined—that is, distance/time = conduction velocity (CV). The time required for transmission in slow-conducting terminal fibers and across the neuromuscular junction is unknown. Therefore, when recording from muscle, a CV can be determined only if stimulation is performed in at least two points. The unknown time for transmission time is then "subtracted out" (Fig. 18.4).

Electrical responses from afferent (sensory) fibers also may be recorded. Because the amplitudes of these evoked afferent responses are several orders of magnitude less than the evoked motor responses, the sensory potentials are more difficult to record. At the same time, a meaningful CV can be obtained from a single latency because a CV may be calculated from the time taken to traverse a particular distance because there is no unknown time in the region of the neuromuscular junction.

The amplitude of evoked motor or sensory responses is a less accurate indicator of normality than is the latency. Amplitude may be affected by the site of the recording as well as by the amount of tissue between the electrical-activity generator in the muscle or nerve and the recording electrodes. Nevertheless, the amplitudes of the evoked efferent or afferent responses reflect the amount of electrical-activity-generating tissue. Decreased amplitude responses can be defined, and side-to-side comparisons of response amplitudes can be particularly helpful.

The different fibers in a particular nerve conduct impulses at different rates. There is a linear relation between fiber size and CV, with the largest fibers conducting at the fastest velocities. If activity in the largest fibers is lost, then conduction will be slowed. The maximum degree of slowing that may be present with axon loss alone, however, is considerably less than that which may be found with demyelination.

In addition to slowed conduction and decreased amplitude, nerve injury can produce altered configuration and dispersion of evoked

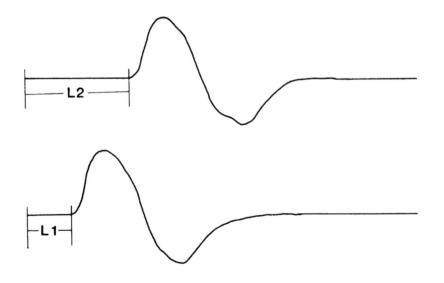

$$cv = d/L2-L1$$

FIGURE 18.4 Evoked motor responses with the shorter-latency L1 resulting from stimulation closer to the recording site, in comparison with the latency L2 resulting from stimulation of the nerve at a more proximal site. The conduction velocity (CV) in the nerve is determined by dividing the distance (*d*) between the stimulating sites by the latency differences.

responses. These changes in evoked responses can define the location of focal nerve dysfunction. Temporal dispersion is characteristic of demyelinating injury, as is conduction block. In the latter, the size of the response is meaningfully decreased or even absent during stimulation proximal to the block. The result may be a striking picture in which nerve function is lost but conduction studies distal to the region of conduction block are entirely normal because those portions of the nerve distal to the block may be normal.

Studies are available (i.e., H reflexes and F responses) that monitor conduction in nerve fibers to and from the spinal cord. These studies are important because proximal nerve injury may be present even in the absence of injury to the more distal nerves.

The electrical-activity generated by muscle contraction can be recorded from the muscle surface but is best evaluated by recording from a needle electrode inserted in the muscle itself. The resultant electrical activity then can be monitored, amplified, and displayed.

At rest, there is no electrical activity. Some activity usually is seen as a needle is moved through muscle (insertional activity), but these responses stop when needle movement stops. As muscle contracts, there is increasing activity. This consists of the firing of motor units. A motor unit is composed of a lower motor neuron in the anterior horn of the spinal cord, its motor axon, and the muscle fibers innervated by that axon. Increasing force of contraction results primarily from the recruitment of more units, although an increased rate of firing also contributes to the increase in muscle tension. This increased muscle activity with increasing force of muscle contraction is readily appreciated during routine EMG. More electrical activity is seen; the amount of visible baseline without motor unit activity decreases; and the audio amplification of the muscle activity becomes increasingly prominent (Fig. 18.5).

Each motor unit is composed of muscle fibers scattered widely throughout a particular muscle. The number of muscle fibers in a motor unit

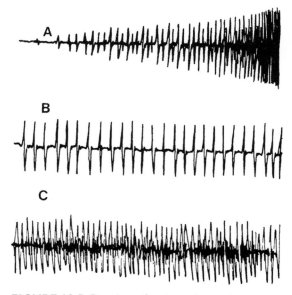

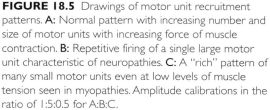

FIGURE 18.5 Drawings of motor unit recruitment patterns. A: Normal pattern with increasing number and size of motor units with increasing force of muscle contraction. B: Repetitive firing of a single large motor unit characteristic of neuropathies. C: A "rich" pattern of many small motor units even at low levels of muscle tension seen in myopathies. Amplitude calibrations in the ratio of 1:5:0.5 for A:B:C.

varies with the fineness of control required. For example, there may be only six muscle fibers per motor unit in the eye muscles but up to several thousand in some of the large postural muscles. The simultaneous contraction of all the muscle fibers in a motor unit results in the usual integrated smooth, triphasic electrical response (Fig. 18.6). Motor unit size varies not only between muscles but also within muscles. The larger motor units have more muscle fibers, and, therefore, with discharge they will generate more electrical activity than smaller units. Thus the larger units generally will be of larger amplitude. During normal reflex or voluntary recruitment, motor units are activated sequentially according to size, with the smaller units discharging first. As a muscle contracts, more, larger units are activated. The amplitude of a particular motor unit is, however, a relatively poor indicator of motor unit size because of

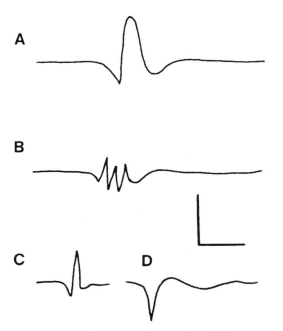

FIGURE 18.6 Tracings of **(A)**, normal triphasic motor unit potential; **(B)** polyphasic potential; **(C)** fibrillation; **(D)** positive sharp wave. Calibrations: vertical (microvolts)—**(A)** and **(B)**, 500; **(C)** and **(D)**, 50; horizontal (milliseconds)—**(A)** and **(B)**, 5; **(C)** and **(D)**, 2.

(a) the potential variation of muscle fiber organization within a particular motor unit and (b) the relation of the recording needle to those muscle fibers. Motor unit duration provides a better estimate of relative motor unit size because motor unit duration reflects the dispersion of the muscle fibers in an individual motor unit within a muscle; larger motor units have larger motor unit durations.

When there is a disruption of the normal connection between nerve and muscle (i.e., denervation), abnormalities appear at rest 1 to 3 weeks after injury, and EMG can detect them. Individual muscle fibers may discharge at rest, and this type of electrical activity is referred to as fibrillations or positive sharp waves. This activity is not visible clinically. Other types of abnormal spontaneous activity may be present, such as runs of complex potentials (complex repetitive discharges). Irregular

contractions of entire motor units may appear; these are called fasciculations. They are visible clinically and can be present in normal individuals, especially with fatigue. They also occur with axonal injury and are characteristic in disorders of the motor neuron such as amyotrophic lateral sclerosis (ALS).

Electromyography using special electrodes can record electrical activity from single muscle fibers. This technique is particularly useful for defining abnormalities of the neuromuscular junction such as myasthenia gravis. Similar abnormalities also may be seen in rapidly progressive neuropathic injury or with reinnervation.

In neuropathies, there is a loss of functioning axons. Fewer motor units than normal may be found on voluntary activation of a muscle. At its most extreme, only a single motor unit may be seen to discharge within the recording field of the electrode, even with maximum muscle contraction. In association with these changes, the motor units may be larger than normal. The muscle fibers that have been denervated may be reinnervated by the remaining viable axons of remaining motor units. As a result, these motor units may be larger than normal and also more complex in configuration. Small, complex (polyphasic)-appearing motor unit potentials, however, also may be found. Although these potentials are considered more characteristic of myopathies as a result of loss of functioning muscle fibers, they also are seen in neuropathic injury during reinnervation. As motor axons grow into muscle that has lost its innervation, new motor units are formed, and these new units initially will be small and polyphasic because they include a relatively limited number of muscle fibers. A reduced number of motor units, especially if they are large and associated with electrophysiologic evidence of denervation, would be characteristic of a neuropathic process.

These may be the only electrophysiologic findings in those neurogenic processes caused by loss of motoneurons such as ALS. More commonly in neuropathies, slowing of conduction is present and provides evidence of nerve dysfunction. Prominent slowing with no or relatively little denervation and preserved response amplitudes would be consistent with a demyelinating process. Borderline to mildly slowed conductions associated with clear and relatively diffuse axonal injury would indicate predominant axonal injury. Low-amplitude evoked responses are most characteristic of axonal dysfunction because of loss of functioning nerve or muscle tissue.

The patient's symptoms may not correlate with the degree of nerve injury found on EMG. The usual electrodiagnostic studies monitor function only in large fibers. Disabling dysesthesias as a result of small fiber dysfunction may occur with unremarkable or relatively minor EMG abnormalities. At the same time, severe, diffuse nerve abnormalities may be accompanied by few complaints because of preservation of sufficient, even if decreased, nerve fibers. In general, electrodiagnostic findings will correlate better with motor symptoms and signs (weakness) than sensory dysfunction. Electromyographic studies can provide information not only about the severity and duration of a neuropathic process but also about the prognosis of nerve injury.

Normal conduction and lack of denervation several weeks after the onset of nerve dysfunction could indicate a good prognosis because this pattern would be consistent with functional, but not necessarily structural, abnormalities of the nerve. This is a common clinical consideration, for example, in Bell palsy caused by disruption of facial nerve function.

At their best, electrodiagnostic studies should be considered not only for establishing the presence of a neuropathy—this is usually a clinical diagnosis—but primarily for establishing the pattern of abnormality. This includes not only whether a process is demyelinating or axonal; this distinction in fact is usually less easily established than one might think from reading the literature. Equally important is the degree of symmetry or asymmetry. If one can establish diffuse versus multifocal axonal or demyelinating patterns, the differential diagnosis

can be focused. For example, diffuse demyelinating patterns are characteristic of some inherited neuropathies; multifocal demyelinating patterns are characteristic of acquired neuropathies such as the GBS, diffuse axonal patterns suggest toxic neuropathies; and multifocal axonal patterns suggest vasculitic neuropathies such as those occur in collagen diseases.

■ SPECIAL CLINICAL POINT:

Electromyography is best viewed as an extension of the neurologic examination. Its primary utility is to identify patterns of abnormalities not observable during routine bedside testing.

Nerve biopsies can be performed. The sural or superficial peroneal nerve is biopsied most commonly. At times, the information may be pathognomonic, such as in infiltrative neuropathies (e.g., amyloidosis and metachromatic leukodystrophy). In other circumstances, the information may be important for patient management (e.g., defining the presence of chronic demyelinating inflammatory injury). "Teased" fiber preparations allow an examination of individual fibers and thereby more accurate analysis of the pathology of nerve injury. Immunologic staining can define the type of antibody and abnormal cells present in nerves. Nerve biopsy itself is performed under local anesthesia and is essentially a benign procedure, although there can be transient uncomfortable residua. Sophisticated judgment is required for determining when a nerve biopsy is indicated. As such, a nerve biopsy should probably only be performed in consultation with someone with expertise in neuromuscular disorders. Punch biopsy of the skin is also useful in the evaluation of certain neuropathies. It is particularly sensitive for small fiber neuropathies and is relatively noninvasive.

Antibody testing is increasingly being performed for evaluation of peripheral neuropathies. This stems from the increasing recognition that antibodies can be present in patients with neuropathies that may be pathogenetic for the neuropathies. This is particularly true for those antibodies against neural gangliosides. The anti-GQ1b antibody is present in about 95% of patients with a particular variant of the GBS (the Miller–Fisher syndrome). An immunoglobulin M (IgM) GM1 antibody is present in about 50% of patients with a variant of a chronic inflammatory demyelinating neuropathy (multifocal motor neuropathy), and a relatively specific neuropathic syndrome is present in those with an IgM monoclonal gammopathy and antibodies to myelin-associated glycoprotein. Nevertheless, the circumstances where these antibodies will be present and clinically useful are small. Given their expense and low yield, these studies are probably best ordered by one knowledgeable about their limitations and possible clinical usefulness.

Given the large number of causes for neuropathies, how one approaches the evaluation of neuropathies will depend on the patients being seen. If one works in an area with a large industrial base, the main concerns may be entrapment and toxic neuropathies. If one deals with an elderly population, the concerns would include diabetes, hypothyroidism, monoclonal gammopathies, and paraneoplastic neuropathies. B$_{12}$ deficiency may present in a subtle fashion and is worth evaluating in those with unexplained neuropathic sensory disturbances. A recent Practice Parameter evaluation of screening laboratory studies for neuropathies has emphasized the importance in distal symmetric sensory polyneuropathies of impaired glucose tolerance which can be documented by a glucose tolerance test.

Management

If the underlying cause of a neuropathy can be established, treatment of this cause can improve the neuropathy. The neuropathies associated with hypothyroidism, carcinoma, and vitamin deficiencies, for example, improve with treatment. Uremic neuropathies can resolve after transplantation, and nerve dysfunction related to drugs (vincristine, heavy metals [lead], and industrial solvents [n-hexane, acrylamide]) can improve by removing the offending agent. A representative list of systemic disorders and toxic causes associated with peripheral neuropathy is presented in Table 18.3. Disulfiram, dapsone, and vincristine all can cause peripheral neuropathies, but they are used to treat conditions in which peripheral neuropathy is a common presentation—alcoholism, leprosy, and carcinoma. Inherited neuropathies such as Charcot–Marie–Tooth disease are common. Two specific neuropathies and their management are discussed in the following sections—acquired inflammatory polyradicular neuropathies and diabetic neuropathies.

■ **SPECIAL CLINICAL POINT: Neuropathies that are due to metabolic derangements or vitamin deficiencies can improve with correction of these abnormalities.**

Treatment of neuropathies also may be symptomatic. Consultations with physiatrists and occupational therapists can be rewarding. Bracing, for example, may help a foot drop. Canes, walkers, and motorized wheelchairs can be helpful for those with gait problems. Useful implements can be made for those with limited finger and hand movement. Painful neuropathies are common, and pain is often the reason a patient with a neuropathy seeks medical attention. Neuropathic pain can be treated with medications. Common medications and their dosages are shown in Table 18.4. The tricyclic antidepressants commonly are used for aching discomfort. The exact mechanism by which these drugs alleviate pain is unknown. However, they must be given in high enough doses and for a long enough period (i.e., several months) to ascertain whether they will be effective.

The anticonvulsants are more commonly used for "positive" symptoms such as paresthesias and dysesthesias. The latter reflect abnormal discharges in diseased nerves, and anticonvulsants presumably help by decreasing these discharges. Opiates can be helpful. Given their potential for abuse, a program of opiates is probably best instituted in conjunction with neurologic consultation. The exception may be

TABLE 18.3 | **Disorders of the Peripheral Nervous System**

Systemic Diseases	Vitamin Deficiency	Exogenous Toxins
Diabetes mellitus	Thiamine	Alcohol
Hypothyroidism	Pyridoxine	Chloramphenicol
Renal failure	Niacin	Cis-platinum
HIV/AIDS	Riboflavin	Cyanide
Intestinal malabsorption	Folic acid	Dapsone
Acute intermittent porphyria	Vitamin B_{12}	Diphenylhydantoin
Amyloidosis		Disulfiram
Acromegaly		Ethionamide
Leprosy		Glutethimide
Diphtheria		Gold
Lyme disease		Hydralazine
Mycoplasma		Isoniazid
Rheumatoid arthritis		Lithium
Systemic lupus erythematosus		Metronidazole
Polyarteritis nodosa		Nitrofurantoin
Wegener granulomatosis		Nitrous oxide
Carcinoma		Paclitaxel (taxol)
Waldenström macroglobulinemia		Perhexiline maleate
Multiple myeloma		Pyridoxine (lack or excess)
POEMS (polyneuropathy, organomegaly, M protein, skin changes)		Thalidomide
		Vinca alkaloids
Cryoglobulinemia		*Heavy metals:*
Paraproteinemia (monoclonal gammopathy of uncertain significance—MGUS)		Lead
		Thallium
Sarcoidosis		*Industrial agents*
Whipple disease		Solvents:
Syphilis		*n*-Hexane
		Methyl-*n*-butyl-ketone
		2,5-Hexanedione
		Carbon disulfide
		Trichloroethylene
		Acrylamide
		Dimethylaminopropionitrile
		2,4-Dichlorophenoxyacetic acid
		Triorthocresyl phosphate
		Organophosphorus compound

tramadol because it has a relatively low potential for abuse. Nevertheless, it is important to be sensitive that tramadol is an opioid and has produced problems with addiction. The natural history for painful neuropathies is for improvement—either because of progression of the neuropathy and loss of pain fibers or because the neuropathies improve. Patients often are puzzled by the presence of pain and loss of feeling in the same area, such as the feet. This is common and reflects the differing effect of nerve injury on different nerve fibers.

TABLE 18.4

Drug Treatment of Painful Neuropathies

Drug	Suggested Starting Dose	Usual Maximum Dose
Antidepressants		
Amitriptyline	10–25 mg h.s.; inc. 10–25 mg q7 days	150–200 mg h.s.
Nortriptyline	10–25 mg h.s.; inc. 10–25 mg q7 days	100–150 mg h.s.
Duloxetine	60 mg q.d.	120 mg day
Anticonvulsants		
Carbamazepine	100–200 mg b.i.d.; inc. 100–200 mg q3–7d	1200 mg/d (given as t.i.d.)
Gabapentin	300–400 mg q.d.; inc. 300–400 mg q3–7d t.i.d.	3600 mg/d (given as t.i.d.)
Topiramate	50 mg qPM; inc. 50 mg q7d b.i.d.	200 mg/d (given as b.i.d.)
Pregabalin	50 mg t.i.d.	100 mg t.i.d.
Opioids		
Tramadol	50 mg q.d.; inc. 50 mg q3–4d q.i.d.	100 mg q.i.d.

GUILLAIN–BARRÉ SYNDROME

Of remitting polyneuropathies, acute inflammatory polyradiculoneuropathy, also known as the Guillain–Barré syndrome (GBS), is the most common, estimated to occur at a rate of 1.5 per 100,000 people. GBS occurs most commonly in young adulthood and early middle age, preceded in almost half of patients by an antecedent infectious illness (such as campylobacter) that usually clears before neurologic dysfunction begins. The etiology is thought to be immunologic. Of the patients, 20% to 30% have antiganglioside antibodies (GM1, GD1a) to neural antigens. The hallmarks of the syndrome are ascending progressive, often profound, weakness; complete tendon areflexia; high spinal fluid protein; possible cranial nerve and respiratory compromise; and substantial or complete spontaneous recovery. Weakness develops over hours to days but should not progress longer than 4 weeks. The severe motor compromise, short duration of progression, and elevated cerebrospinal fluid (CSF) protein with few (<10 mononuclear cells/mm^3) are features that distinguish this syndrome. Sensory loss may be mild but should be looked for carefully because abnormalities of sensation help differentiate this syndrome from other conditions that may appear similar, including hypokalemia, botulism, and poliomyelitis. Pathologically, there is widespread inflammatory segmental demyelination, most prominent proximally and presumably immunologically mediated. Prominent axonal injury and marked decrease in evoked motor response amplitudes argue for a slow recovery.

Although there are characteristic clinical features, the variability of clinical presentation in actual practice should be emphasized. These include the Miller–Fisher syndrome (ataxia, ophthalmoplegia, and hyporeflexia) as well as limited findings such as facial diplegia with cardiac arrhythmias indicative of focal injury to the facial and vagal nerves. The CSF protein may not be elevated initially, and repeated lumbar punctures may be necessary to demonstrate an increased protein with the associated characteristic dissociation between protein and cells. Autonomic instability may be a prominent feature and may result in morbidity and occasional mortality. EMG studies may reveal prominent slowing of nerve conduction, but evidence of conduction block associated with segmental demyelination and proximal conduction abnormalities may be the only findings. The EMG examination can have prognostic implications.

GBS is considered idiopathic in origin. Syndromes similar to GBS, however, may be found in conditions such as acute intermittent porphyria and Hodgkin disease and less commonly with other neoplasms, hepatitis, infectious mononucleosis, Lyme disease, and recently acquired HIV infection. Certain toxic neuropathies such as with thallium may be similar.

Although recovery may be slow, the characteristic history of GBS is one of almost complete improvement. As such, the most important treatment is symptomatic, particularly respiratory support and monitoring autonomic dysfunction. Steroids have been advocated, but they have not been beneficial and are possibly detrimental. Plasmapheresis or intravenous immunoglobulins (IVIG) can hasten recovery and appear particularly indicated for those with severe respiratory compromise and if used within 7 days of onset. A total of three to five courses of plasmapheresis usually is given every other day; the standard dose for IVIG is 0.4 g/kg/day for a total of 5 days. There is no proven benefit to combining both plasmapheresis and IVIG.

■ **SPECIAL CLINICAL POINT: Intravenous immunoglobulin and plasmapheresis are equally effective treatments for acute inflammatory polyradiculoneuropathy (Guillain–Barre syndrome).**

CHRONIC INFLAMMATORY DEMYELINATING POLYRADICULONEUROPATHY

A syndrome similar to GBS sometimes may occur in a chronic form termed chronic inflammatory demyelinating polyradiculoneuropathy (CIDP). In these patients, the symptoms progress for more than 4 weeks. In comparison to GBS, the onset is often more gradual; antecedent infections are less common; and sensory symptoms and signs are more frequent. As in GBS, the basic pathologic process is an inflammatory segmental demyelination, but there is also a loss of myelinated fibers. Onion bulbs are found as a result of repeated episodes of demyelination with remyelination. The CSF again shows high protein and relatively few cells at some stage in the illness, but it may be normal at the time of a particular examination. EMG studies characteristically show slowed conduction. Nerve biopsy may be helpful for the diagnosis. In contrast to GBS, steroids are thought helpful in CIDP. Immunosuppressive agents also have been used, and plasmapheresis and IVIG have produced a temporary improvement. The clinical presentation of patients with chronic acquired neuropathies can be quite variable; there are no firm diagnostic EMG criteria. The treatments are costly and can have serious side effects, such as with high-dose steroid therapy. As such, the diagnosis and management of this condition should be in conjunction with those experienced with these problems.

NEUROPATHIES ASSOCIATED WITH DIABETES MELLITUS

Diabetes mellitus is common and often is associated with nerve dysfunction. Diabetic neuropathies are probably now the most common neuropathies in the Western world. The reported incidence of neuropathic abnormalities in diabetes has varied widely, most likely as a result of differing criteria and techniques used to diagnose PNS injury in these patients. A balanced view probably would indicate a prevalence of 50% to 60% of some form of neuropathy in patients with diabetes. The prevalence increases with the duration of the disease, but diabetic nerve dysfunction may be the initial sign of diabetes. Given the various presentations and probable pathogenesis, it is best to think in terms of diabetic neuropathies rather than in terms of a single entity.

■ **SPECIAL CLINICAL POINT: Diabetes is one of the most common causes of neuropathy. Therefore, in patients with a consistent clinical presentation, appropriate screening includes a fasting blood glucose test and possibly a glucose tolerance test.**

Polyneuropathies, mononeuropathies, plexopathies, radiculopathies, and autonomic neuropathies all are found individually or in combination in diabetes, and diabetes therefore can be associated with abnormalities at any level of the PNS. Patients with asymptomatic diabetes may show decreased nerve conductions that can normalize with improved control of blood sugar. A distal sensory or sensorimotor polyneuropathy is the most common type of diabetic neuropathy. Although commonly described as "symmetric," careful examination of these patients frequently reveals some, even if limited, asymmetry. Describing the findings as "stocking glove" in distribution is actually somewhat misleading. The findings are related to the distance in the limbs from the spinal cord; sensory loss limited to the hands and feet would be consistent with spinal cord injury, not peripheral nerve. A loss of position, vibration, and light touch as well as decreased reflexes are prominent features of the "large fiber" pattern. Relatively pronounced loss of pain and temperature sensation, in association with pain, indicate predominant "small fiber" injury. The pain may have a dull, aching quality in the limbs and also a distal, burning discomfort most prominent at night. Rarely, there is a pattern of sensory ataxia, pain, and arthropathy (diabetic "pseudotabes"). The small fiber and pseudotabetic patterns may be associated with autonomic dysfunction, including an involvement of the gastrointestinal, cardiovascular, and genitourinary systems. Autonomic dysfunction also can occur without other evidence for a neuropathy. Postural hypotension, diarrhea, impotence, urinary retention, and increased sweating are examples of symptoms that may be caused by a diabetic autonomic neuropathy. The painful, asymmetric, proximal weakness of the legs found in diabetes (diabetic amyotrophy) is probably a result of the involvement of the lumbar plexus and frequently is found in the context of a history of weight loss. Clinical patterns of a polyradiculopathy may occur. Mononeuropathies can affect almost every major peripheral nerve as well as the cranial nerves, particularly the extraocular muscles. The onset of symptoms in mononeuropathies is characteristically abrupt and frequently painful. Diabetes may present as peroneal palsies.

The pathogenesis of diabetic neuropathies is complex. Metabolic derangements have been cited as the basis for the polyneuropathies. There is experimental evidence, however, that edema secondary to structural changes in endoneural blood vessels with associated ischemia may be the primary cause. This may account for the asymmetric clinical findings in patients with "symmetric" diabetic neuropathies. The abrupt onset of painful, focal lesions in the diabetic mononeuropathies is similar to that of other vascular neuropathies and has led to the concept that these neuropathies are the result of occlusion of the small, nutrient blood vessels supplying nerves. This finding, however, has not been confirmed pathologically.

The natural history of diabetic mononeuropathies, amyotrophies, and polyradiculopathies is one of improvement, even if slow. The course of diabetic polyneuropathies varies: some diabetic neuropathies improve, many plateau, and some steadily progress. A severe disability is the exception. The pseudotabetic variety is generally progressive and more disabling. Pain, particularly distal burning dysesthesias, can be a major problem. Although the manifestations of the autonomic neuropathy may be subclinical, they are not infrequently incapacitating. The prognosis for the autonomic neuropathy is among the worst of the diabetic neuropathies.

Good metabolic control is probably helpful for both preventing and ameliorating diabetic neuropathies, and good control of blood sugar therefore should be a goal in these patients. Exercise should be encouraged. Other therapies are symptomatic. An eye patch is helpful in patients with the self-limited diabetic ophthalmoplegia, and bracing may be helpful in those with peroneal palsy. Medications have been helpful in the painful sensory neuropathies (Table 18.4), and analgesics are reasonable for the acute pain associated with mononeuropathies. Trophic ulcers of the feet may require changes in shoe size, debridement, and antibiotics. Standard medical regimens should be tried for autonomic dysfunction. These regimens include codeine phosphate and diphenoxylate for diarrhea, support stockings and fludrocortisone or midodrine for postural hypotension, and regular voidings assisted ·by suprapubic pressure in those with bladder atony. Nighttime lights can assist walking in those patients with sensory loss by preserving visual cues.

FOCAL NEUROPATHIES

A patient complaining of numbness, weakness, or pain in a very specific distribution may be suffering from a focal neuropathy. Appropriate knowledge of peripheral neuroanatomy, key historical clues, and findings on clinical exam will often allow the clinician to identify a focal mononeuropathy.

Carpal Tunnel Syndrome

Carpal tunnel syndrome (CTS) is one of the most common peripheral nerve entrapment disorders. CTS results from compression of the median nerve as it passes through the carpal tunnel at the wrist. Symptoms typically include numbness and burning in the hand that may extend into the forearm and even the arm and neck. Patients often report symptoms to be worse at night and perceive relief with shaking of their hands. In most of the population sensory fibers of the median nerve that pass through the carpal tunnel travel into the hand to supply the volar portions of the thumb, index, middle, and the radial half of the ring finger. Typical findings on exam include decreased sensation in the distribution of the median nerve. A particularly useful finding is a clear decrease in sensation to pinprick in the radial half of the ring finger in comparison to the ulnar half. In more severe and long lasting cases there may be a flattening of the thenar eminence

and weakness of thumb abduction. Provocative maneuvers such as percussion of the wrist over the median nerve (Tinel's sign) or prolonged wrist flexion (Phalen's sign) may reproduce symptoms of paresthesias in the expected distribution. These findings are supportive of a diagnosis of CTS. Electrodiagnostic findings of prolonged distal motor latencies or relative slowing of median sensory conduction can also be used to support the diagnosis. Conservative treatment often begins with wrist splints that prevent excessive flexion particularly at night. Local glucocorticoid injections have been shown to provide modest and temporary relief of symptoms. Patients with severe CTS or those with moderate CTS who do not respond conservative therapy may be candidates for surgical decompression of the carpal tunnel.

Ulnar Neuropathy

The ulnar nerve is also susceptible to compression, particularly as it passes across the medial side of the elbow where the nerve is very superficial. The ulnar nerve supplies many of the intrinsic muscles of the hand and motor symptoms often predominate. They may include weakness of hand grip and pinch strength. More advanced cases will have associated atrophy of both the thenar and hypothenar eminence. There may be preferential weakness of the third dorsal interosseous which is responsible for adduction of 5th finger. The resulting posture is a relative abduction of the 5th finger, a posture referred to as the *Wartenburg sign*. Patients with this pattern of weakness may complain of catching their little finger when trying to put their hand in a pocket. The *Benediction posture* is another typical posture associated with advanced ulnar nerve lesions. It is the result of weakness of the finger adductors and a hyperextension at the metacarpal–phalangeal joints in combination with flexion at the proximal and distal interphalangeal joints of the ring and little fingers. Patients who have sensory complaints associated with ulnar nerve lesion will complain of pain or numbness in both the dorsal and volar distribution of the little and ulnar half of the ring finger. Percussion of the ulnar groove at the elbow may reproduce sensory symptoms. Although the elbow is the most common site of compression, the ulnar nerve is susceptible to compression along its entire course from the axilla to the wrist. Electrodiagnostic studies may help to localize the lesion by identifying areas of slowed CV or a significant drop in amplitude. Treatment is aimed at minimizing compression of the ulnar nerve. For ulnar neuropathy at the elbow initial conservative treatment measures include counseling to avoid prolonged flexion at the elbow, avoidance of positions that put external pressure on the ulnar nerve, and splints or elbow pads. Patients who fail to respond to conservative treatment may require surgery.

Peroneal Neuropathy

Peroneal neuropathy is the most common mononeuropathy of the lower extremity. This is because it is particularly susceptible to compression as it passes across the fibular head in the leg. Patients typically complain of inability to dorsiflex the foot, a condition often referred to as foot drop. Often times the presentation may be acute after the patient was in a prolonged position that allowed for compression of the common peroneal nerve such as a surgical procedure. Significant weight loss is also a proven risk factor for development of a peroneal nerve palsy. Other possible etiologies include trauma or less commonly a mass lesion. Physical examination will reveal weakness of foot dorsiflexion as well foot eversion. Importantly, in a pure peroneal lesion inversion of the foot will be normal. This finding helps to differentiate peroneal neuropathy from a L5 radiculopathy, another condition that commonly presents with foot drop. Sensation may be decreased along the lateral aspect of the leg and the dorsum of the foot. Electrodiagnostic studies help to confirm the area of damage. Management of peroneal nerve palsy depends on the underlying etiology.

FUTURE PERSPECTIVES

Our understanding of peripheral nerve disorders and their management remains unsatisfactory. There is the potential for an increased understanding of peripheral neuropathies. Newer techniques of histopathologic evaluation, including electron microscopy, teased fiber preparations, and morphometric analysis of nerves, already have added meaningfully to our understanding of both normal and abnormal nerves. Similarly, more sophisticated forms of electrophysiologic analysis should allow for a better evaluation of nerve dysfunction. These techniques include recording from single muscle fibers (single fiber EMG); computer analysis of motor unit firing, clinically applicable techniques for evaluating changes in ion conductances in nerves, and increasing routine study of a wider range of electrophysiologic responses and more sophisticated analysis in EMG studies. The recording of cortical responses evoked by peripheral nerve stimulation (somatosensory evoked responses) not only allows for a more detailed evaluation of certain peripheral nerve injuries but also provides a possible technique for evaluation at the interface between peripheral and CNS dysfunction. Immunologic studies are becoming increasingly important for understanding the pathogenesis of nerve disorders and for providing guides to therapy. Patients with a clinical picture similar to ALS but with conduction block on electrophysiologic examination and frequently elevated titers of anti-GM1 antibodies have been treated successfully with immunosuppressive agents. Finally, basic research in the physiology, biochemistry, immunobiology, and axonal transport of nerves provides a dynamism and makes an interest in peripheral nerves rewarding.

QUESTIONS AND DISCUSSION

1. A 64-year-old patient with a 10-year history of insulin-dependent diabetes mellitus complains of burning dysesthesias in the feet. Examination reveals a mild decrease in strength at the toes and ankles; absent Achilles reflexes; decreased pinprick to the knees and elbows; decreased vibration in the legs; and decreased position sense in the toes. Electrodiagnostic studies indicate slowed motor conduction velocities and absent sensory potentials in the legs with evidence of denervation distally in the lower extremities on needle EMG examination. Sensory conductions in the upper extremities are slowed. Which of the following is the most likely diagnosis at this time?
   A. Mononeuropathy
   B. Mononeuropathy multiplex
   C. Plexopathy
   D. Polyneuropathy
   E. Radiculopathy

The correct answer is D. This patient's clinical symptoms, signs, and electrophysiologic findings are most characteristic of a polyneuropathy. The clinical and electrodiagnostic examinations reveal a diffuse sensorimotor neuropathic process most prominent distally.

2. Four weeks later, the same patient as in question 1 develops weakness in the left leg associated with some pain in the region of the left knee. An examination 3 weeks after onset reveals relatively more prominent decreased pinprick and touch sensation in the lateral aspect of the left leg and dorsum of the left foot, as well as lack of dorsiflexion and eversion of the left ankle. EMG examination shows no evoked motor response stimulating at the fibula head and denervation in the left tibialis anterior, peronei, and extensor digitorum brevis muscles. Which of the following is the most likely diagnosis for the patient's new symptoms and signs?

A. Mononeuropathy
B. Mononeuropathy multiplex
C. Plexopathy
D. Polyneuropathy
E. Radiculopathy

The correct answer is A. This patient's current history and findings is most consistent with a mononeuropathy of the left peroneal (anterior tibial) nerve. Clinically, there is sensory loss, motor weakness, and EMG abnormalities in the distribution of that nerve.

Diabetes mellitus can produce both a polyneuropathy and a mononeuropathy, not infrequently in the same patient. The pathogenesis of his polyneuropathy is probably multifactorial, including metabolic derangements and ischemia, whereas the mononeuropathy may be secondary to vascular infarction of the peroneal nerve.

A diabetic polyneuropathy argues for good diabetic control. Diabetic mononeuropathies usually resolve with time because of the partial nature of the nerve injury secondary to the ischemic insult. A short leg brace to aid in dorsiflexion of the left ankle could be helpful for this patient during the recovery period.

3. A 50-year-old woman has a 6-month history of intermittent paresthesias and pain in her right hand. This pain awakens her at night, usually within several hours of falling asleep. She has noticed clumsiness in the use of that hand and complains of paresthesias radiating into the thumb and index fingers. Recently, she has noted some milder tingling in the left thumb and index finger. She was recently diagnosed with hypothyroidism. Examination shows paresthesias and pain radiating to the fingers on tapping the wrists bilaterally (positive Tinel signs); weakness of right thumb abduction (the right abductor pollicis brevis muscle); and numbness involving the right thumb, index finger, and middle finger as well as the adjacent one-half of the ring finger. There is also numbness involving the lateral half of the

palmar surface of the right hand. EMG examination reveals a prolongation of the median distal motor latencies and slowing of median sensory potentials bilaterally, more prominent on the right. Which of the following is the most likely diagnosis?

A. Brachial plexopathy
B. Carpal tunnel syndrome
C. Cervical radiculopathy
D. Cervical spinal cord compression
E. Polyneuropathy

The correct answer is E. This patient's symptoms, signs, and electrophysiologic findings are most compatible with a diagnosis of bilateral carpal tunnel syndrome (CTS), worse on the right. This syndrome is a mononeuropathy caused by "entrapment" of the median nerve as it passes through the carpal tunnel at the wrist. A positive Tinel sign is a common clinical finding in an area of partial nerve injury, and progression of this sign distally can be used to follow regeneration after a nerve has been severed. Characteristic electrodiagnostic findings in CTS are those that indicate median nerve dysfunction at the level of the wrist—that is, prolonged motor conduction stimulating the nerve at the wrist and recording from median-innervated thenar hand muscles as well as prolonged median sensory conductions with the level of injury at the wrist. The history would suggest a bilateral process—an assumption confirmed by the electrodiagnostic studies. Bilateral involvement in the CTS is present in approximately 25% of the cases. This syndrome is frequently part of several systemic illnesses including hypothyroidism. A CTS may be presenting complaint in a patient with abnormal thyroid function.

Initial treatment would consist of therapy for the hypothyroidism as well as splinting the wrists to limit movement. If these measures failed, the transverse carpal ligaments probably should be surgically sectioned. Steroid injections can produce symptomatic relief, but the long-term effectiveness and the possible harm of this therapy have been debated.

4. A 55-year-old man undergoing vincristine therapy for systemic lymphoma has developed progressive weakness over several weeks, resulting in an inability to walk. An examination reveals decreased vibration in the legs, decreased pin sensation to the upper legs and in the fingers, preserved position sense, absent reflexes in the legs, and moderate to marked weakness in the legs and mild-to-moderate weakness in the arms, most marked distally. Electrodiagnostic studies reveal borderline, slow motor conduction velocities with considerable evidence of denervation, again most prominent distally. Which of the following is most likely location of the nervous system lesion in this patient?

A. Brachial and lumbar plexus
B. Nerve roots
C. Peripheral nerve axons
D. Peripheral nerve myelin
E. Spinal cord

The correct answer is C (peripheral nerve axons). This patient's history and clinical and electrophysiologic findings would be typical for a polyneuropathy secondary to vincristine therapy. The prominent denervation indicates disruption of the normal connections between nerve and muscle. Combined with the borderline slowing of conduction velocities, the primary disease is of axons rather than of myelin—that is, an axonal type of neuropathy. The treatment is to stop the vincristine.

5. A 35-year-old man has a 6-month history of weakness in the hands that now involves the legs. An examination reveals atrophy and fasciculations in the intrinsic muscles of the hands, weakness that is more prominent distally in the upper than in the lower extremities, hyperactive reflexes, and extensor plantar responses bilaterally. Sensory testing is unremarkable. Electrodiagnostic examination reveals normal motor and sensory conduction studies in the presence of denervation and decreased activation of motor units in all

---

FLOW CHART FOR NEUROPATHY EVALUATION AND TREATMENT

Careful history with special attention to distribution and rate of progression of symptoms.

Thorough physical exam to determine if the neuropathy involves sensory, motor, or autonomic fibers and if it is diffuse or multifocal.

Ancillary testing which may include blood work, electromyography, nerve biopsy, and possibly genetic testing.

Address underlying cause if it is identifiable and treatable.

Treat neuropathic discomfort with agents proven to be effective (i.e., antiepileptics, antidepressants, or opioids).

Monitor for progression or improvement of the neuropathy with repeated physical examinations and symptom evaluations.

---

four extremities. Many of the motor units are both large and polyphasic. A cervical MRI is normal. Which of the following is the most likely diagnosis?
A. Amyotrophic lateral sclerosis (ALS)
B. Chronic inflammatory demyelinating polyneuropathy (CIDP)
C. Diabetic polyneuropathy
D. Guillain–Barré syndrome
E. Vasculitic neuropathy

The correct answer is A. The history and findings are consistent with a diagnosis of ALS. The extensor plantar responses and hyperactive reflexes would indicate some involvement of the long motor system tracts in the CNS, but the atrophy and fasciculations would be consistent with involvement of the lower motor neurons. This is confirmed by the electrodiagnostic studies, which indicate a chronic motor neuropathic process not readily explained by a process primarily affecting peripheral nerves, plexuses, or roots. The normal conduction velocities indicate preservation of at least some of the fast-conducting (i.e., largest) motor axons. Because the pathologic process involves strictly efferent (i.e., motor) fibers, a sural nerve biopsy would not be helpful. The sural is a sensory nerve and therefore contains only afferent fibers.

Nerve dysfunction may involve either motor or sensory fibers only. In ALS, the primary pathology is at the lower motor neuron level in the anterior horns of the spinal cord. It may be argued this is not an illness of the PNS. Conversely, because ALS involves the cell bodies of efferent fibers with resultant abnormalities in nerve and muscle, the illness might be considered a prototypical axonal neuropathy.

SUGGESTED READING

Aids to the Examination of the Peripheral Nervous System. Edinburgh: Saunders Publishers; 2000.

Blume G, Pestronk A, Goodnough LT. Anti-MAG antibody–associated polyneuropathies: improvement following immunotherapy with monthly plasma exchange and IV cyclophosphamide. *Neurology*. 1995;45:1577.

Brown WF, Bolton CF, Aminoff MJ, eds. *Neuromuscular Function and Disease: Basic, Clinical, and Electrodiagnostic Aspects*. Vols. 1 and 2. Philadelphia: WB Saunders; 2002.

Cros D, ed. *Peripheral Neuropathy: A Practical Approach to Diagnosis and Management*. Philadelphia: Lippincott Williams & Wilkins; 2001.

van Dijk JG. Too many solutions. *Muscle Nerve.* 2006;33(6):713–714.

Donofrio PD, Alber JW. Polyneuropathy: classification by nerve conduction studies and electromyography. *Muscle Nerve.* 1990;13:889.

Gibbons CH, Griffin JW, Polydefkis M, et al. The utility of skin biopsy for prediction of progression in suspected small fiber neuropathy. *Neurology.* 2006;66:256–258.

Kimura J. *Electrodiagnosis in Diseases of Nerve and Muscle.* Philadelphia: FA Davis; 2001.

Latov N. Pathogenesis and therapy of neuropathies associated with monoclonal gammopathies. *Ann Neurol.* 1995;37(suppl 1):S32.

Mendell JR, Kissel JT, Cornblath DR, eds. *Diagnosis and Management of Peripheral Nerve Disorders.* Oxford: Oxford University Press; 2001.

Parry JG. *Guillain-Barré Syndrome.* New York: Thieme; 1993.

Pestronk A. Motor neuropathies, motor neuron disorders, and antiglycolipid antibodies. *Muscle Nerve.* 1991;14:927.

Ropper AH, Gorson KC. Neuropathies associated with paraproteinemia. *N Engl J Med.* 1998; 338:1607.

Saperstein DS, Katz JS, Amato AA, et al. Clinical spectrum of chronic acquired demyelinating polyneuropathies. *Muscle Nerve.* 2001;24: 311–324.

Stalberg E, Trontelj JE. *Single Fiber Electromyography.* Old Woking, England: Miravalle Press; 1994.

Sumner CJ, Sheth S, Griffin JW, et al. The spectrum of neuropathy in diabetes and impaired glucose tolerance. *Neurology.* 2003;60(1):108–111

Tuck RR, Schmelzer JD, Low PA. Endoneurial blood flow and oxygen tension in the sciatic nerves of rats with experimental diabetic neuropathy. *Brain.* 1984;107:935.

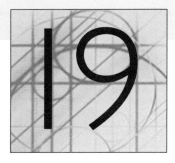

Neurologic Evaluation of Low Back Pain

MEGAN M. SHANKS

key points
- Most low back pain is from a nonspecific cause and will resolve with or without treatment in a few weeks.
- Some less common causes of low back pain should not be missed—these include cauda equina syndrome, neoplasm, infection, and unstable fracture.
- Evidence-based reviews of acute back pain increasingly recommend less initial imaging, less invasive treatment, and increased patient physical activity.

EPIDEMIOLOGY

A majority of doctors will encounter low back pain as a patient complaint. It comes second only to upper respiratory infections for sheer numbers of doctor visits and missed workdays. In young and middle-aged adults, it is the leading cause of activity-limiting illness. In Western countries, 50% to 80% of the adult population will have some level of back pain during their lifetime, and 15% to 30% within the past year. About 2% to 5% of low back pain patients will develop chronic low back pain (i.e., lasting more than 4 to 6 weeks), with psychosocial issues found as an even greater factor in these patients. The majority of patients recover within 4 to 6 weeks no matter what treatment they receive, but recurrence is also common. The neurologic approach to low back pain is emphasized here, especially for the 2% to 5% of low back pain patients with sciatica or radicular nerve pain that can radiate past the knee, and other disorders involving the lumbosacral nerves such as lumbosacral spinal stenosis and the cauda equina syndrome.

ANATOMY

Much about the mechanics of low back pain is not well understood. Other than the spinal cord and radicular nerves, structures that are known to possess nociceptive (pain) fibers include the outer annulus of the disc, the periosteum of the vertebral bodies, the blood vessel walls, the anterior dura, the posterior longitudinal ligament, the fibrous capsule of the facet joint, and the sacroiliac joint. Damage to or around these structures often, but not always, is a cause of pain. Approximately 85% of low back pain has no clear related injury to these structures and is known as nonspecific back pain. This is sometimes classified as nonspecific degenerative disease, myofascial pain, muscle spasm, or strain. The following details of spine anatomy may be a helpful reference in understanding the known causes and exam findings in more depth.

The low back consists of five lumbar vertebral bodies, and a single fused bony sacrum, with the coccyx (tailbone) below. The lumbar vertebrae are stabilized by various ligaments, as well as the surrounding musculature, and cushioned by intervertebral discs (Fig. 19.1). The dorsal vertebral spine makes up the protective neural arch, surrounding the spinal cord canal and descending nerve roots (Fig. 19.2). The adult spinal cord ends as the conus medullaris at L1-2, with the lumbosacral nerve roots descending through the spinal canal as the cauda equina. The descending five lumbar, five sacral, and single coccygeal nerve roots exit through their corresponding lateral neural foramina. Unlike the cervical nerve roots, the lumbar nerves descend for several levels before exiting *below* the corresponding numbered vertebral body (the L4 root between the L4 and L5 vertebrae, and so on). Thus, a far lateral L4-5 disc herniation will cause an L4 radiculopathy pattern. But more commonly the disc herniates posterolaterally within the neural canal, causing the more medially descending L5 root to be compressed (see Figs. 19.3 to 19.5). The most common disc herniation and root syndromes are the L4-5 (L5 root) and L5-S1 (S1 root). The joint between each lumbar vertebral body is the facet (zagopophyseal) joint. The pars articularis is the supportive bony bridge connecting the superior and inferior articular facets, and is prone to stress fracture (see *Spondylosis*).

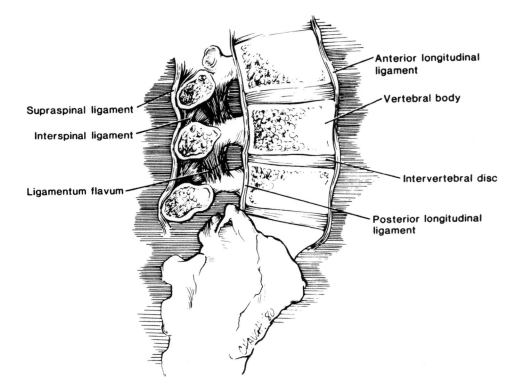

FIGURE 19.1 Anatomic landmarks of lumbosacral spine.

Supraspinal ligament

Interspinal ligament

Ligamentum flavum

Anterior longitudinal ligament

Vertebral body

Intervertebral disc

Posterior longitudinal ligament

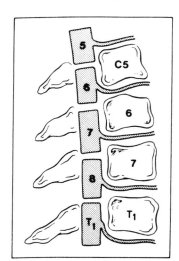

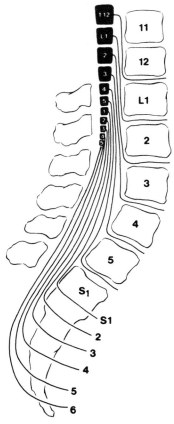

FIGURE 19.2 Cervical (upper right) and lumbosacral (lower left) spine, showing the emergence of spinal roots.

STRUCTURAL CAUSES

Muscle/Ligament Pain

Sprain or strain from minor trauma is the most common cause, although the etiology of pain from "spasm" is not well described. The onset is often related to unaccustomed physical activity or sudden unexpected movement. The pain limits movement and is painful with palpation of the back but without neurologic symptoms; that is, pain does not radiate into the legs, with no associated numbness, no weakness that is not related to pain, and no bowel or bladder symptoms.

Disc Herniation

Minor trauma is often an inciting factor, although it may be spontaneous. Disc bulging or dehydration can promote arthritic and

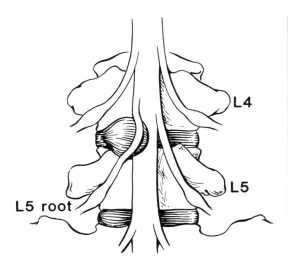

FIGURE 19.3 Herniated disc at L4-5 compressing the L5 rootlet.

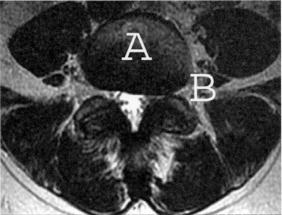

FIGURE 19.5 Axial spine MRI showing the same L4-5 disc (A), causing neural foraminal narrowing at the left nerve root exit (B). Note the normal appearance of the cauda equina nerve roots (black dots) floating within the spinal canal (the triangle of white cerebrospinal fluid).

ligamentous change. Discs may also be a site of infection, or discitis. Disc herniation without nerve impingement can cause a focal back pain without radiation down the legs past the knee, or be asymptomatic. Pain is typically worse with bending, coughing, or sneezing (see Neurogenic Pain, and Neurologic Exam below for symptoms found with specific nerve root impingements).

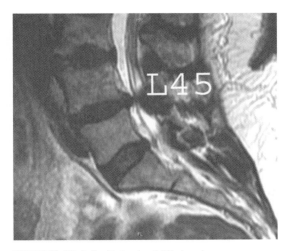

FIGURE 19.4 Sagittal spine MRI showing a posterolateral L4-5 disc herniation causing spinal canal narrowing.

Neurogenic Pain

This is called "sciatica" or radicular pain. Multiple etiologies can be the source of nerve impingement. Most commonly disc herniation causes nerves compression either in the spinal canal or neural foramen, but narrowing may also be caused by arthritic change, ligamentous hypertrophy, or often by a combination of all three. These areas may also be compromised by tumor, infection, or inflammatory disease. A typical presentation is that of a sharp shooting pain down the leg or legs, often with a tingling numbness, with a particular pattern of weakness if severe.

■ **SPECIAL CLINICAL POINT: It is often stated that radicular pain can be differentiated from other causes of radiating back pain by traveling below the knee; this may not be true for higher lumbar roots L1-3.**

Gradual narrowing of the spinal canal in the lumbosacral region can cause spinal stenosis around multiple nerve roots. Degenerative disease of bone, disc, and ligaments is the most common cause. This can cause a specific pattern of pain referred to as "neurogenic claudication." Like vascular claudication, exercise can bring on aching or cramping pain in the back, buttocks and legs, and sitting or standing still is needed to relieve the pain. Patients with neurogenic claudication may notice over time that the distance they can walk before they are stopped by pain becomes progressively shorter. Lumbar flexion may ease the pain. Low back pain is typically seen in neurogenic claudication, but may be absent.

Sudden simultaneous compression of multiple lumbosacral nerve roots causes the *cauda equina syndrome*. It can be caused by disc herniation, tumor, abscess, hemorrhage, spondylolisthesis (vertebral slippage), or fracture.

■ **SPECIAL CLINICAL POINT: Cauda equina syndrome is a neurologic emergency requiring immediate attention to prevent permanent neurologic damage. It should be suspected if the patient complains of sudden back and leg pain with leg weakness, loss of reflexes, saddle numbness, and bladder or bowel dysfunction with loss of anal tone.**

Spinal cord or conus medullaris compression have similar symptoms as cauda equina syndrome, but with the addition of upper motor signs such as hyperreflexia and spasticity. This will be found with lesions in the L1-2 region or above, as the cord ends at this level in adults.

Involvement of multiple nerve roots that can be rare causes of severe back pain include Guillain–Barré syndrome (acute inflammatory demyelinating polyneuropathy) with progressive weakness and areflexia, arachnoiditis (inflammatory clumping of the nerve roots), and carcinomatous meningitis. Low thoracic or high lumbar cord involvement may also cause low back pain, including transverse myelitis and spinal cord infarct. Cord infarct may spare the dorsal columns that carry joint position and vibration sense, but will affect pain and temperature as well as all strength below the level of infarct. Acute spinal shock from any cause (trauma, cord infarct, transverse myelitis) may cause initial flaccid paralysis and areflexia, but typically also has severe sensory loss.

Bony Spine Pain

Fracture or damage from trauma or osteopenia, neoplasm (metastases, primary bony tumors), infection or arthritis (inflammatory, degenerative, Paget disease) may affect the vertebral bodies, facet joints, pars articularis, or sacroiliac joints. Osteomyelitis of the spine may develop slowly with symptoms of focal, unrelenting back pain not relieved by rest. Fever and chills may also be present. This may lead to compressive neurologic symptoms by forming an epidural abscess. Compression fracture of the vertebral bodies after minor trauma may cause a constant focal tender region of the spine. Repetitive stress to the pars articularis may cause them to fracture, which is referred to as *spondylolysis*. This can be entirely asymptomatic, or cause focal back pain with flexion or extension. It is notable cause of low back pain in athletes. It predisposes patients to *spondylolisthesis*, which is the slipping forward of one vertebral body over the next. This may by itself cause unilateral or bilateral back pain, or cause root irritation with radiating leg pain. *Spondylosis* is arthritic change or bony spurring from the vertebral margins, and does not cause pain unless there is nerve impingement. Facet joint arthritis may cause a focal aching tenderness and pain with movement. Spinal deformities such as scoliosis or kyphosis can increase the risk of back pain. Sacroiliac joint pain may be due to arthritis or pregnancy, and causes an aching or sharp pain over the low back where the sacrum joins the pelvis. It is worse with standing or walking. Back pain may also be referred from the hip joints.

Referred Pain from Abdominal or Pelvic Structures

Pyelonephritis, kidney stones or urinary tract infection, pancreatitis, abdominal aortic aneurysm or dissection, gall bladder disease, peptic ulcer disease, prostatitis, endometriosis, and pelvic inflammatory disease can all potentially cause referred pain to the low back.

Psychosocial Factors

The levels of life stressors and emotional distress are key in predicting poor outcomes and chronic low back pain. This includes job dissatisfaction, depression, high levels of psychological distress regarding pain and disability, and medicolegal or compensation disputes. This is probably one of the most important factors in nonspecific back pain, but one that is more difficult to rate or treat.

■ **SPECIAL CLINICAL POINT: Most cases of low back pain have a benign course, but there are some less common causes of low back pain that should not be missed. These include cauda equina syndrome, neoplasm, infection, and unstable fracture.**

EXAM

As a general medical history can point toward the specific causes of low back pain, so too can the general exam. Fever is not always present in infections in or around the spine, but its presence with focal back pain is notable. Abdominal, pelvic, and hip exam may uncover referred sources of pain.

Percuss the spine for focal tenderness as can be seen in fracture, infection, or neoplasm. Palpate the back muscles for spasm and pain. Inspect the skin for signs of shingles or bruising. Investigate the curve and mobility of the back movements.

Neurologic Exam

■ **SPECIAL CLINICAL POINT: L5 radiculopathy is the most common radicular syndrome. The hallmarks are shooting pain into the leg, big toe dorsiflexion weakness, and trouble inverting the foot. The main differential diagnosis is peroneal palsy from a more distal lesion of the peroneal**

nerve, but this latter syndrome is not associated with shooting pain and the weakness is usually more pronounced (severe foot drop) than seen in L5 radiculopathy.

A distinction can be made between a drop foot from an L5 radiculopathy and that of a common peroneal neuropathy by checking for foot inversion (tibialis posterior). Peroneal palsies should spare foot inversion. Weakness of foot inversion suggests an L5 radiculopathy rather than a peroneal neuropathy.

A neurologic exam of the lower extremities is important in any low back pain patient to rule out nerve compromise, particularly if the clinical history suggests radiating pain or possible weakness or numbness.

Motor Strength (See also Table 19.1) Ask the patient to push against resistance. For L2-4, ask them to lift the leg at the hip and push the knees toward each other. For L5, have them push the knees apart, raise the foot at the ankle (this may also have some L4), flex at the knee (this may also have some S1), and tilt the foot inward and outward. For S1, have them push downward with the foot, or from a supine position have them try to keep the leg on the bed while the leg is raised. A straight leg raise (SLR) test may also be checked at this time with passive lifting of the leg to between 30 and 70 degrees to assess for painful radicular nerve stretch. SLR can also be tested from a sitting position, with gradual straightening of the leg. Patrick sign can be tested to check for referred pain from the hip or sacroiliac joint. Patrick sign is also referred to as FABER for flexion, abduction, and external rotation of the hip. Be aware that pain with certain movements may cause the so-called "give-way weakness" that will resolve when pain is controlled. Be sure to ask the patient whether any pain is occurring if weakness is found. Give-way can also be seen in a non-neurologic or diffuse pattern in embellishment or malingering. Check increased tone by lifting the legs at the knees gently to see if the heel drags along the bed or lifts up in a spastic bouncing fashion. A patient in pain may not be able to relax enough for this test to be done.

TABLE 19.1

Main Nerve Root Motor and Sensory Findings (Some Variations Possible)

Root	Muscle	Action	Reflex	Sensory Finding
L2-4	Quadriceps	Knee extension	Patellar	Anterior thigh
	Iliopsoas	Hip flexion		and medial calf
	Adductor magnus and longus	Hip adduction		
L5	Gluteus medius	Hip abduction	Hamstring	Lateral calf, medial
	Hamstrings	Knee flexion		foot and toes
	Extensor hallicus	Lift big toe		
S1	Gastrocnemius	Stand tiptoe, point foot	Ankle jerk	Posterior calf, and lateral foot
	Gluteus maximus	Extend leg back		and toes
	Toe flexors	Bend toes down		

Sensory Exam   Ask the patient if they have any numbness, then screen for the main dermatomes with light touch and pinprick (sometimes one modality may be more affected than another). Be sure to check the anterior and posterior thighs, lateral and medial calves, and lateral and medial foot. Check vibration sense in the toes with a tuning fork if available. Proprioception (joint position sense) in the toes and feet can be tested instead, but it is a less sensitive test than vibration sensation. Checking for a positive Romberg (swaying with eyes closed) is also a test for joint position sense. Peripheral nerve disease can cause this finding as well.

■ SPECIAL CLINICAL POINT: Check vibratory sensation (using a tuning fork) and joint proprioception to evaluate the spinal cord dorsal or posterior columns.

The vibratory exam can be extremely helpful in establishing any dorsal column spinal cord damage as can be seen with B_{12} deficiency, syphilis, or HIV. Alternately, complete loss of all function (motor and sensory) in the legs with the exception of vibration and proprioception is strongly suggestive of a spinal cord infarct. Acute spinal shock can occur early after cord infarct, however, and may be pan-sensory. Unlike the anterior spinal artery, the paired posterior spinal arteries have many collateral vessels and are

not prone to infarct, thus sparing the dorsal columns that carry joint position sense.

Reflexes   Knee reflex can be decreased or lost in L2, L3, or L4 radiculopathies, but may be maintained if only one root is affected. The ankle jerk is a good S1 indicator, but may also be lost in other conditions such as polyneuropathy, when it will be lost bilaterally. The hamstring reflex is rarely checked, as it is difficult to elicit. It is usually mediated by the L5 root, but occasionally also by the S1 root.

Rectal Exam   Rectal tone is a good indicator of sacral nerve involvement. This is important to check if spinal cord or cauda equina lesions are suspected. See Chapter 1 (The Neurologic Exam) for more details.

WORKUP

A recent argument is that the entity of acute low back pain is overly imaged. As mentioned earlier, nonspecific low back pain accounts for a majority of all back pain, and by definition, no structural cause may be found. There are certainly false negatives and false positives found by any diagnostic modality. For example, an MRI may reveal an unrelated right-sided bulging or herniated disc when the symptoms are clearly on the left or localizable to a different level. The abnormalities found may not relate to the current complaint. This can lead to unnecessary or ineffective invasive treatment, especially if the clinical history and exam is not kept firmly in mind when reviewing the diagnostic findings. In addition, it is important to realize that not every abnormality may be seen on diagnostic imaging or workup, even something presumably obvious like a slipped disc. With that in mind, the modalities discussed below are most helpful in specific structural causes, particularly those that are the main focus of this chapter, back pain with neurologic signs or symptoms.

Spine X-rays

These are most useful for fracture (traumatic or spontaneous), tumor (with bone metastasis, multiple myeloma, or primary bone tumors), osteoporosis, Paget disease, arthritic conditions with bony change (ankylosing spondylitis), spondylolisthesis or spondylolysis, and osteomyelitis. Limitations of this test include the following: the soft tissue is not visualized and changes from conditions such as osteomyelitis may take weeks to develop.

CT Spine

This modality provides good visualization of fractures, and is less affected by motion artifact, and cheaper, than MRI. CT of the spine is useful for patients where MRI is contraindicated (e.g., pacemakers, claustrophobia, over-size patient, and metal fragments). It has all the above advantages of spine x-ray with more details available. Limitations of CT of the spine include that soft tissue (and the spinal cord or nerve roots) are not well visualized.

CT Spine With IV Dye

The addition of intravenous contrast may add details for conditions of neoplastic, infectious,

or vascular cause. Limitations include the possibility of renal failure or allergic reaction.

CT Myelogram

This adds significant improvement of details regarding the CSF space surrounding the spinal cord, allowing further information regarding mass lesions, CSF leaks, and nerve root sleeves. Limitations: A lumbar puncture must be performed in order to introduce the dye. Post-LP postural headaches may occur. CT myelogram also has similar renal and dye allergy concerns as above, but it is also a rare cause of arachnoiditis (inflammation and pain with clumping of nerve roots).

MRI Spine Without Gadolinium Dye

This provides good identification of soft tissue and details of anatomy, and is the best modality for visualization of the spinal cord and nerve roots. MRI is also very good for diagnosis of tumor and infectious causes. MRI involves no radiation exposure and is safer in pregnancy. Limitations: MRI shows less bony detail so fractures are less clear. This cannot be done on patients with pacemakers, loose metal, claustrophobes, or over-sized patients. In addition, low back pain patients may find lying still for the extended time required for MRI to be intolerable. Open and upright MRI imagers are available but with some degradation of the image.

MRI Spine with Gadolinium

The addition of gadolinium contrast increases the information and yield of MRI in cases of neoplasm and infection. Gadolinium dye is not required for imaging of degenerative structural causes such as disc herniation or arthritic change. It can also be helpful in assessing postoperative scar formation. Limitation: Allergic reactions are less common than CT dye, but can occur. Patients with renal insufficiency are at risk for nephrogenic systemic fibrosis.

Radionuclide Bone Scan

This can be done if a condition such as bony metastatic disease, acute fractures, or osteomyelitis is suspected. Limitations: Findings from this modality are nonspecific, and there may be significant false negatives and positives.

■ **SPECIAL CLINICAL POINT:** If the patient has signs of spinal cord dysfunction (e.g. bilateral leg spasticity and hyperreflexia, with or without arm symptoms), a spine MRI should be done. The spinal cord does not usually go below L1-2 in adults, so a lumbosacral spine MRI will be less helpful than a cervical or thoracic spine MRI in patients with signs and symptoms of spinal cord dysfunction.

Electrodiagnostic Studies

Electromyogram/Nerve conduction studies (EMG/NCS): This is a study of the muscle and nerve, usually referred to as "EMG." EMG is helpful to evaluate lower motor neuron nerve damage, that is, damage of the motor nerve (to muscle) and below the sensory nerve cell bodies.

■ **SPECIAL CLINICAL POINT:** In typical radiculopathies, sensory nerve conduction studies will be normal despite a patient's symptoms of numbness, because the sensory cell body in the dorsal root ganglion is below the level of a typical disc herniation.

Limitations: EMG can be a painful study, motor nerve conductions can remain normal for 7 to 10 days following an injury, and needle studies of the muscle (which is the most helpful part of the test in determining radiculopathies with nerve root damage) can take 14 to 21 days to fully develop.

■ **SPECIAL CLINICAL POINT:** EMGs are best if done more than 3 weeks after onset of nerve damage.

Upper motor neuron cord lesions will not be apparent on EMG. Painful lumbar stenosis without weakness or numbness may not be apparent on EMG.

Labs

LDH (probably most sensitive but least specific in spinal infection) and also ESR and C-reactive protein (CRP) may be helpful. White blood cell count can be elevated or normal in spinal infections. Low platelets and increased PT/PTT may reflect bleeding risk and the possibility of epidural hematoma. Increased alkaline phosphatase, calcium, and serum and urine immunoelectropheresis may also suggest multiple myeloma. Alkaline phosphatase may also be increased in osteoporosis, hypoparathyroidism, and bony metastases. HLA-B27 is more common in inflammatory arthritis (ankylosing spondylitis). Limitations: These laboratory tests are low yield, playing less of a role in diagnosing most low back pain.

TREATMENT

There is wide variability in the treatment of low back pain, both between and even within specialties. Many treatments in common use may have little or no efficacy. Efforts are being made to perform systemic reviews of evidence-based data to correct this, and there are various guidelines put out by several groups and agencies available.

Treatment of Acute Low Back Pain (<4 to 6 weeks)

Emergent evaluation is required if the patient has signs of cauda equina compression (new onset of severe or progressive leg weakness or numbness, saddle numbness, or bowel or bladder dysfunction), or other "red flags" such as trauma, fever, or a suspicion for cancer (see Table 19.2). Surgical consultation should be considered. If evidence of cauda equina syndrome is found, the patient may require surgical decompression performed emergently. Similarly, any unstable fractures or spondylolisthesis must be surgically stabilized, and infections treated with antibiotics (after drainage if due to abscess). Tumors may require surgical removal or

TABLE 19.2	Indications for Possible Serious Underlying Causes of New-Onset Low Back Pain

Condition	Sign or Symptom
Cauda equina	New onset of severe or progressive leg weakness or numbness, saddle numbness, bowel or bladder dysfunction
Neoplasm	History of cancer, age >55, unexplained weight loss, constant pain not relieved by rest or change in position, progressive leg weakness or numbness
Infection	Fever, chills, pain unrelieved by rest, immune suppression, recent infection (e.g., UTI), IV drug use
Fracture	Recent trauma, osteoporosis
Guillain–Barré syndrome	Ascending leg weakness, areflexia, minimal numbness (pain is unusual)

nerve root decompression, steroids, chemotherapy, or radiation, depending on type and location. The reader is directed to surgery and oncology texts for more details. Although pain is unusual in Guillain–Barré cases (acute demyelinating polyneuritis), it can be associated with severe back pain. Guillain–Barré syndrome should be suspected with progressive, ascending weakness and areflexia, and negative spinal imaging. It can progress to respiratory arrest in hours or days. Neurologic consultation and a lumbar puncture should be considered for confirmation. Treatment consists of a course of plasma exchanges or IVIG (see Chapter 18).

Fortunately the emergent causes of low back pain are rare. Somewhat more common are the structural causes of acute low back pain with nerve involvement, which includes radiculopathies or "sciatica." If significant weakness is found in a root distribution, a more urgent MRI

should be scheduled, with a timely surgical consultation (neurosurgical or orthopedic) for compressive lesions. For mild motor deficits with acute radicular pain, an urgent spine MRI should also be considered, and an EMG considered if symptoms persist beyond 3 weeks. The patient may be reassured that most of these milder cases resolve without surgery. If severe radicular pain and/or sensory deficits are present, the usual conservative measures are used (see below), with the addition of a brief course of opioids if pain is intolerable. Although oral steroids are frequently recommended, there is no strong evidence that this is effective. There is some conflicting evidence that epidural steroids may hasten improvement in the first few weeks, and little data comparing it to other modalities of treatment. Conservative treatment should be used for all nonurgent forms of low back pain. The most common form of low back pain is non-neurologic, nonspecific low back pain. Conservative measures should be used as outlined below.

Conservative Treatment in Acute Low Back Pain

Reassure the patient that most low back pain resolves within a few weeks. They should avoid heavy lifting, twisting, or other aggravating movements, but otherwise stay as active as possible. Bed rest should be avoided if at all possible. Heat should be applied to the back. If needed, acetaminophen, paracetamol (outside the United Sates), NSAIDs (nonsteroidal anti-inflammatory drugs), and muscle relaxants can decrease pain levels. Stronger medications such as opioids, benzodiazepines, and tramadol can be effective, but should be avoided if possible due to side effects and dependency issues. Physical therapy and spinal manipulation may be helpful, although specific back strengthening exercises are probably not helpful in the acute period. Spinal manipulation is not recommended in those with radicular symptoms such as numbness or weakness. There is currently insufficient evidence to support massage or acupuncture, and no evidence to support traction, lumbar supports, or TENS (transcutaneous electrical nerve stimulation) in the acute low back pain patient.

Treatment of Chronic Low Back Pain (>4 to 6 weeks)

If conservative measures fail and back pain persists, a referral to a physician specializing in back pain may be required. Depending on presentation, this can include neurologists, physical medicine and rehabilitation specialists, rheumatologists, sports medicine specialists, anesthesia pain specialists, neurosurgeons, and orthopedic surgeons, among others. If milder, nonprogressive motor deficits, or disabling back or leg pain persists despite conservative treatment, imaging should be performed if not done already.

Conservative treatment measures may still be employed as in acute back pain, with increased concern over dependency and side-effect issues of stronger medications. Medications for chronic pain, including tricyclic antidepressants such as amitriptyline or nortriptyline may have some small benefit, although serotonin reuptake inhibitors (SSRIs) and trazadone have shown no benefit. There is conflicting data over the benefit of gabapentin or pregabalin for radicular nerve pain.

Physical therapy and spinal manipulation shows evidence of some benefit, as does exercise therapy, and possibly massage, acupuncture, and yoga. Cognitive-behavioral therapy, multidisciplinary rehabilitation, and back school (educating patients about back pain), may be helpful for chronic low back pain. Scant data suggests spinal manipulation is less effective in sciatica patients. TENS treatments and traction show no evidence of efficacy in the chronic low back pain patient. There is currently insufficient evidence to support the use of more invasive treatment for chronic low back pain, such as trigger point injections, epidural steroid injections, and facet joint injections.

Surgical procedures may be reconsidered. Pain with a clear structural cause seen on imaging has a much higher chance of good response to surgery. However, use of surgery is controversial given recent findings suggesting a more rapid recovery, but no long-term benefit over nonsurgical treatments. In radiculopathy (chronic sciatica), laminectomy (removal of the vertebral bony arch) with or without discectomy, partial facetectomy, or spinal fusion, are the decompressive spinal surgeries most commonly performed. A majority of patients have decreased pain symptoms after decompression for spinal stenosis. However, there is uncertain long-term benefit after several years, except in cases with acute onset. There is conflicting evidence for spinal fusion surgery in chronic low back pain with nonspecific degenerative spine disease. The reader is directed to neurosurgery or orthopedic surgical texts for more details on various surgical approaches.

Always Remember

- Severe or progressive neurologic deficits should be evaluated immediately.
- Cauda equina syndrome is a neurologic emergency requiring immediate attention to prevent permanent neurologic damage.
- Patient self-care with back pain education, avoiding bed rest, and application of heat are the first steps in the treatment of acute low back pain.
- Psychosocial factors play a major role in predicting poor outcomes and chronic low back pain.

QUESTIONS AND DISCUSSION

1. A 25-year-old woman presents to the office with 2 weeks of low back pain that began after moving some boxes. She describes a severe aching pain in the low back that is occasionally sharp with movement, but without radiation down the legs. On examination she has limited range of motion of her back, no

---

FLOW CHART: APPROACH TO ADULT LOW BACK PAIN

STEP 1: Assessment of Acute Low Back Pain (<4 to 6 weeks)
Evaluate history, general, and neurologic exam for serious underlying conditions:
a. Onset associated with trauma, suspected fracture, or fever and chills
b. History suggesting neoplasm, hemorrhage, immunosuppression, IV drug use, or recent systemic infection
c. Severe or progressive weakness, or bowel and bladder dysfunction
If any of the above red flags are present, immediate evaluation is required. Go to Step 2.
Otherwise, go to Step 4.

STEP 2: Emergent Care
a. Spine x-ray or CT spine if fractures suspected, if not, MRI is preferable
b. MRI lumbosacral spine, without gadolinium unless infection or tumor suspected
c. MRI with gadolinium and labs if infection or tumor suspected (ESR, LDH, CRP, CBC, alkaline phosphatase); bone scan if desired
d. MRI thoracic spine if focal lower extremity upper motor neuron signs present
e. If scans are normal and patient has areflexia, consider Guillain–Barré syndrome or acute spinal shock
If emergent or serious underlying cause found go to Step 3.
If no emergent cause found, go to Step 4.

STEP 3: Interventional Care
Consult or refer to a spine surgeon for decompression and stabilization, or a neurologist, oncologist, rheumatologist etc. as required to treat specific cause.

STEP 4: Acute Conservative Care
a. Education in self-care: Stay active but avoid aggravating movements. Use heat.
b. If needed use acetaminophen, NSAIDS, muscle relaxants
c. Consider physical therapy or spinal manipulation (unless radicular)
d. Re-evaluate patient in 4 to 6 weeks (Step 5)

STEP 5: Chronic Care (>4 to 6 weeks)
a. Re-evaluate history and exam for serious underlying causes (Step 1)
b. MRI spine without gadolinium if not already performed
c. EMG if radicular or spinal stenosis symptoms present
d. Return to Step 3 (Interventional Care) if indicated
e. Continue Step 4 (Conservative Care) measures with addition of gabapentin, pregabalin, or tricyclics for nerve pain if needed
f. Consider referral for physical therapy, spinal manipulation, exercise therapy, massage, acupuncture, yoga, cognitive-behavioral therapy, multidisciplinary rehabilitation, or back school. Consider referral to a neurologist when a radiculopathy is not responding to conservative measures, or when neurologic signs or symptoms such as weakness or numbness are present.

---

weakness, no sensory loss, and normal reflexes. She has a negative straight leg raise. Which of the following is the most appropriate management of this patient?

A. Strict bed rest for 2 weeks with codeine as needed, and then start physical therapy for back strengthening exercises.

B. Continue her usual physical activities as tolerated (except heavy lifting), with anti-inflammatories as needed.

C. Epidural steroid injections in the lumbar spine.

D. MRI of lumbar spine.

The correct answer is B. The patient has acute nonspecific back pain with onset of less than 4 to 6 weeks. There is no evidence by history or exam of a more serious underlying cause of low back pain, so back imaging is not indicated at this point. If symptoms do not respond in a reasonable time, a search for a structural abnormality of the spine would then be warranted.

This patient should be reassured that most low back pain resolves within a few weeks. She should avoid heavy lifting, twisting, or other aggravating movements, but otherwise stay as active as possible. Bed rest should be avoided if at all possible. Heat should be applied to the back. If needed, acetaminophen, paracetamol (outside the United States), NSAIDs (nonsteroidal anti-inflammatory drugs), and muscle relaxants can decrease pain levels. Stronger medications such as opioids, benzodiazepines, and tramadol can be effective, but should be avoided if possible due to side effects and dependency issues. Physical therapy and spinal manipulation may be helpful, although specific back strengthening exercises are probably not helpful in the acute period. Epidural steroids are not indicated for acute back pain.

2. A 40-year-old man has low back pain for 2 months, which began suddenly after playing basketball. It is not as bad as it was 2 months ago, but he complains of an occasional sharp pain radiating down his left leg and intermittent tingling in his foot. On examination he has limited range of motion of his back due to some pain, no weakness, no objective sensory loss, normal reflexes, and a positive straight leg raise on the left. MRI shows a small leftward herniated L5-S1 disc. Which of the following is the most appropriate treatment?
A. Strict bed rest for 2 weeks with codeine as needed.
B. Advise the patient to remain active, and refer to physical therapy.
C. Epidural steroid injections in the lumbar spine.
D. Surgery for the herniated disc seen on lumbosacral MRI.

The correct answer is B. The patient has chronic low back pain that is likely due to a lumbosacral radiculopathy, but without significant neurologic deficits. Many physicians would also consider answer C. This is controversial, as epidural steroid injections are considered by many to be standard care, but with variable results in formal studies. Epidural steroid injections are frequently used in nonsurgical radiculopathy cases, with many patients reporting pain relief after the injections. However, there is currently insufficient evidence to support epidural steroids as a treatment for chronic low back pain with radiculopathy symptoms. Back surgery is not usually indicated for a herniated disc without significant neurologic deficits (weakness, bowel and bladder dysfunction), although it is sometimes used in cases with severe unremitting radicular pain. Chronic opioid use should be avoided. As mentioned above, physical therapy shows some benefit, and complete bed rest has not been found to be helpful.

3. A 55-year-old man was in a fistfight 2 weeks ago, which caused skin abrasions, but no other injuries or pain. One week later he developed a constant low backache. Two weeks later he presents to the emergency department with new-onset bilateral leg weakness, numbness, constipation, and no urine output for 12 hours. On examination he has bilateral 3–4/5 leg weakness, patchy sensory loss in the legs and saddle region, decreased ankle reflexes, decreased rectal tone, and focal back pain to percussion in the low mid-back. Which of the following is the most appropriate emergency test at this time?
A. Radionuclide bone scan
B. Spine x-ray
C. EMG
D. Spine MRI

The correct answer is D. The patient appears to have cauda equina syndrome, possibly from an infectious source such as an epidural abscess. Cancer with bone metastases could have a similar presentation unrelated to his skin abrasions, so further history and examination relating to cancer should be sought. A CBC and LDH may be elevated with a focal infection, but are nonspecific. An x-ray would show fractures, and possibly osteomyelitis. However, plain radiographs can be normal in early osteomyelitis and will be normal with an acute epidural abscess, disc herniation, hematoma, or other nonbony abnormality. He had no back pain immediately after his fight to indicate an acute fracture at that time. An EMG will show evidence for polyradiculopathy in cauda equina syndrome in 2 to 3 weeks time, but will not be helpful in the acute setting. An emergent MRI of the spine will show the source of the cauda equina compression, and allow for immediate presurgical evaluation. To decrease the possibility of permanent neurologic deficits, surgical consultation should be called immediately, and not left until the next morning.

SUGGESTED READING

Available at: http://www.cochrane.iwh.on.ca/ for regularly updated evidence-based healthcare reviews of low back pain (Cochrane Review Back Review Group).

Chou R, Qaseem A, Snow V, et al. Clinical Efficacy Assessment Subcommittee, Diagnosis and treatment of low back pain: a joint clinical practice guideline from the American College of Physicians and the American Pain Society. *Ann Intern Med.* 2007;147:478–491.

Chou R, Huffman LH. Nonpharmacologic therapies for acute and chronic low back pain: a review of the evidence for an American Pain Society/American College of Physicians clinical practice guideline. *Ann Intern Med.* 2007;147:492–504.

Chou R, Huffman LH. Medications for acute and chronic low back pain: a review of the evidence for an American Pain Society/American College of Physicians clinical practice guideline. *Ann Intern Med.* 2007;147:505–514.

Weinstein JN, Tosteson TD, Lurie JD, et al. Surgical vs nonoperative treatment for lumbar disk Herniation. The spine patient outcomes research trial (SPORT): a randomized trial. *JAMA.* 2006;296:2441–2450.

Siemionow K, Steinmetz M, Bell G, et al. Identifying serious causes of back pain: cancer, infection, fracture. *Cleve Clin J Med.* 2008;75:557–566.

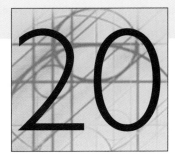

20 Dizziness and Vertigo

ROBERT K. SHIN AND JUDD M. JENSEN

key points

- Dizziness is a nonspecific term that may refer to presyncope, vertigo, or disequilibrium.

- Presyncope is primarily a cardiovascular problem rather than a purely neurologic disorder. Causes of presyncope include hypertension, orthostatic hypotension, vasovagal depression, and cardiac arrhythmia.

- Many causes of vertigo are benign (e.g., benign paroxysmal positional vertigo or Ménière disease), but acute or intermittent vertigo may be a sign of more serious disorders, such as vertebrobasilar disease.

- Disequilibrium may result from problems with sensation, vestibular function, central integration, or motor coordination.

Dizziness is a common complaint in the outpatient clinic and the emergency department, one that may be as anxiety-provoking for the physician as it is for the patient. Many causes of dizziness are benign, but dizziness can also be a symptom of cerebrovascular disease (transient ischemic attack [TIA] or stroke) or other disorders that may be potentially life-threatening. Clinicians should be familiar with the different causes of dizziness to assist in making an accurate diagnosis and should be able to recognize "red flags" that may signal potentially life-threatening causes of dizziness. Effective therapies for some dizziness syndromes have been developed, which the non-neurologist may find useful in clinical practice.

THREE TYPES OF DIZZINESS

Dizziness has traditionally been divided into three categories: *presyncope, vertigo,* and *disequilibrium*. Distinguishing between these different types of dizziness may help point to a particular diagnosis. Patients may have difficulty describing their dizziness in detail, however, and the clinician should keep in mind that some disorders, for example, cerebrovascular disease, can present with any form of dizziness.

Presyncope

Patients with presyncope may describe their dizziness as "lightheadedness" or "feeling like I'm going to faint." This sensation may be associated with generalized weakness, visual blurring or blackout, diaphoresis, pallor, shortness of breath, or palpitations. Presyncope is typically episodic and is caused by a transient reduction in global cerebral perfusion. Therefore, presyncope is usually a primary cardiovascular problem rather than a neurologic one.

Vertigo

Patients who have vertigo experience a false sensation of movement. Most commonly, they report that their environment is spinning around them; however, sensations of tilting, swaying, and being impelled forward, backward, or to either side are also vertiginous. Nausea, vomiting, and some degree of imbalance are common, as are autonomic signs such as diaphoresis, pallor, and tachycardia. Classically, patients with vertigo are thought to have a disorder of either the peripheral or central vestibular system, with peripheral vestibular disorders comprising approximately 90% of cases. Cerebellar lesions, however, may also cause vertigo and may mimic a peripheral vestibular problem.

Disequilibrium

Disequilibrium is a more complex category than the previous two. Whereas patients with presyncope and vertigo tend to have episodic symptoms or attacks, patients with disequilibrium typically have more continuous symptoms. Patients with disequilibrium are dizzy primarily when standing or walking and tend to improve when seated or supine. Disequilibrium may be difficult for patients to describe. Complains of "bad balance," "poor equilibrium," or "I'm just dizzy" are common. Disequilibrium is the result of dysfunction at one or more points in the complex system required for balance and ambulation.

■ **SPECIAL CLINICAL POINT: Distinguishing between these three types of dizziness can sometimes be difficult for the patient and, consequently, for the clinician. At times it may be more important to pay attention to the acuteness and pattern of the dizziness as well as associated neurologic signs and symptoms in order to arrive at the correct diagnosis.**

CAUSES OF PRESYNCOPE

Presyncope is characterized by lightheadedness, visual blurring or blackout, paresthesias, and/or generalized weakness that may result from a global reduction in cerebral perfusion from a decrease in systemic arterial pressure, failure of cardiac output, or diffuse cerebral vasoconstriction. Diaphoresis, palpitations, and nausea often are present as the autonomic nervous system attempts to restore cerebral perfusion. Presyncope may occur in a variety of clinical settings.

Hyperventilation Syndrome

Hyperventilation is a common cause of presyncope typically seen in anxious, pressured individuals. Patients with high-grade hyperventilation tend to have acute episodes of dizziness precipitated by stressful situations or panic attacks. They often are aware of breathing rapidly or feeling short of breath and may complain of visual blurring, paresthesias of the lips or fingers, and generalized weakness. Patients with low-grade hyperventilation have a more protracted and insidious form of dizziness in which symptoms tend to wax and wane over longer periods. Visual blurring, paresthesias, and generalized weakness are usually absent. Patients are almost never aware that they are overbreathing, and they may not feel short of breath.

Artificial hyperventilation can be useful in the evaluation of patients with dizziness. Hyperventilation results in a drop in arterial PCO_2 with subsequent cerebral arterial vasoconstriction and global reduction in cerebral blood flow. Hyperventilation can be induced by holding a tissue 12 inches in front of the patient's mouth and having the patient blow the tissue with rapid and deep breaths for up to 3 minutes. The tissue must be displaced significantly with each exhalation to ensure hyperventilation. If this procedure exactly reproduces the patient's dizziness, hyperventilation syndrome is suggested.

Both high-grade and low-grade hyperventilators tend to be very sensitive to even short periods of induced hyperventilation. Reassurance regarding the etiology and benign nature of their symptom complex is the most important aspect of treatment for these patients. The high-grade hyperventilator may be helped by placement of a paper or plastic bag over the mouth during the attacks. Supportive psychotherapy or counseling may be helpful in some patients. Anxiolytic medication may be appropriate in selected patients.

Orthostatic Hypotension

Orthostatic hypotension is another common cause of presyncope, particularly in the elderly. The symptoms almost always occur when the patient is standing and are frequently maximal just after the patient rises from the sitting or supine position. Gravity decreases venous return to the heart, resulting in a decline in left heart filling. The autonomic nervous system normally is able to adjust peripheral resistance, cardiac rate, and contractility so that cardiac output and blood pressure are maintained, but if patients are hypovolemic from fluid loss or diuretic therapy, if they have been pharmacologically vasodilated, or if their compensatory autonomic responses are blunted by medication or disease, cardiac output and blood pressure may fall sufficiently to produce presyncopal symptoms. In these patients, a significant drop in blood pressure usually can be demonstrated at the bedside and this procedure often will reproduce the patient's symptom complex.

To evaluate a patient for orthostatic hypotension, blood pressure should always be checked as the patient goes directly from the supine to the standing position. A drop of greater than 20/10 mm Hg 3 minutes after standing is considered abnormal. It is important to note that asymptomatic but demonstrable orthostatic blood pressure changes are common in the elderly. If the patient's history does not suggest orthostatic hypotension and orthostatic testing does not reproduce the symptoms, then the observed drop in blood pressure may not be the cause of the dizziness.

Diuretics and other antihypertensive medications are common causes of orthostasis. Other causes of this syndrome include autonomic neuropathy, primary orthostatic hypotension, and multiple system atrophy, also known as *Shy–Drager syndrome.*

Symptomatic orthostatic hypotension from antihypertensive medications should be treated by medication adjustments. Neurologic causes of chronic orthostatic hypotension have several possible treatments. Raising the head of the patient's bed by 10 to 15 degrees or recommending elastic stockings may be helpful. If these maneuvers do not provide adequate symptomatic relief, then sodium chloride tablets can be added judiciously if they are not contraindicated by hypertension, congestive heart failure, hepatic disease, or renal failure. The mineralocorticoid fludrocortisone acetate can be used in difficult cases, but blood pressure and serum electrolytes must be monitored closely. The alpha agonist midodrine also can be used in selected patients.

Vasovagal/Vasodepressor Presyncope

Vasovagal presyncope is probably more correctly called *neurocardiogenic presyncope.* The patient's history is usually diagnostic. Vasovagal dizziness may occur in a hot crowded room or in the setting of sudden pain or strong emotion. The patient is almost always standing and may have premonitory symptoms of yawning, diaphoresis, and pallor. In vasovagal syncope, reductions in blood pressure and cerebral blood flow are caused by sudden, reflux dilation of the resistance arterioles. This syndrome usually occurs in young, otherwise healthy adults but can occur in the elderly. Heat favors vasodilation and could produce symptomatic hypotension in an elderly patient with otherwise compensated mild orthostatic hypotension. The only treatments for this syndrome are reassurance and avoidance of the precipitating circumstances.

Cardiac Presyncope

Cardiac presyncope usually is caused by an arrhythmia that produces a sudden decrease in cardiac output and a subsequent decrease in cerebral perfusion. Common offending arrhythmias include sick sinus syndrome, paroxysmal supraventricular tachycardia, atrial fibrillation-flutter, complete heart block, and ventricular tachycardia. This diagnosis should be strongly considered in any patient whose presyncope occurs in the sitting or supine position. Workup includes an electrocardiogram and Holter monitoring, although it sometimes requires repeated or prolonged monitoring to document the arrhythmia.

Exercise-related presyncope may be caused by aortic stenosis or *idiopathic hypertrophic subaortic stenosis*. An echocardiogram is used for the diagnosis of these conditions. Paroxysmal episodes of lightheadedness and dizziness may sometimes be a manifestation of coronary ischemia, which should be considered in any patient with unexplained episodes of presyncope and the appropriate risk factors.

Carotid Sinus Hypersensitivity

Carotid sinus hypersensitivity is primarily a disorder of the elderly in which the carotid sinus in the neck becomes abnormally sensitive to pressure and produces episodes of bradycardia and reduced cardiac output. Classically, this syndrome was described in men who wore tight collars. Such a history, however, will not be present in most patients with this disease. It should be suspected in middle-aged or elderly patients with ongoing bouts of presyncope or syncope. The diagnosis is made by carotid massage under strictly controlled conditions (i.e., the presence of a crash cart and personnel skilled in cardiopulmonary resuscitation). The treatment is placement of a permanent pacemaker.

Hypoglycemia

Although this metabolic derangement does not cause a reduction in cerebral blood flow, its symptom complex is similar to that seen in presyncope. Thus, it should be considered in evaluating patients with episodic dizziness.

Most patients with symptomatic hypoglycemia are insulin-dependent diabetics who either did not consume an adequate caloric load for their insulin dose or took an excessive dose of insulin. Oral hypoglycemic agents are occasionally unpredictable in their action and can produce symptoms of hypoglycemia. Early diabetics who are not yet on therapy can have reactive hypoglycemia from surges of insulin. This typically occurs 2 to 5 hours after eating and is more often manifested by diaphoresis and palpitations than lightheadedness or other neurologic symptoms. The diagnosis is made by documenting serum hypoglycemia while the patient is symptomatic. In general, a serum glucose less than 50 mg/dL is necessary to produce neurologic symptoms. Rarely, insulin-secreting tumors may present with repeated episodes of hypoglycemia.

VERTIGO

Vertigo is the subjective sensation of movement or spinning when the head is actually stationary. Vertigo is generally a symptom of disease in the vestibular or cerebellar balance centers.

The peripheral vestibular apparatus includes the labyrinth, which is located in the petrous portion of the temporal bone, and the vestibular portion of the eighth cranial nerve, which connects the labyrinth to the brain stem and is located in the internal auditory canal and cerebellopontine angle. The labyrinth is divided into three semicircular canals that sense head rotation and the otolith organs (utricle and saccule) that sense head position relative to gravity.

The central vestibular apparatus consists of vestibular nuclei at the pontomedullary junction in the brainstem. These nuclei receive impulses from the eighth cranial nerve and have rich connections with cerebellum and the nuclei controlling eye movements.

Normally, the vestibular system sends balanced tonic impulses to the central nervous system (CNS) from the left and right inner ears regarding the position of the head and its movements. Vertigo occurs when a pathologic process acutely disrupts vestibular input on one side; the resulting discrepancy between right and left inputs produces the false sensation of movement—acute vertigo.

NYSTAGMUS

Vertigo is almost always accompanied by *nystagmus*, a rhythmic oscillation of the eyes. Although nystagmus may rarely be pendular, more commonly it is characterized by slow movement in one direction followed by quick movement in the other direction. This form of nystagmus (jerk nystagmus) is named for the direction of the quick phase, for example, "right-beating" or "down-beating." Two main forms of jerk nystagmus are *vestibular nystagmus* and *gaze-evoked nystagmus*.

Vestibular nystagmus, seen with central or peripheral lesions of the vestibular system, is primarily horizontal, but also has a rotatory or torsional component. Vestibular nystagmus is unidirectional—the fast component of the nystagmus always beats in the same direction, away from the vestibular lesion, no matter where the patient is looking. For example, with a left vestibular lesion, the quick phase of the nystagmus will be to the right ("right-beating") in all directions of gaze. Although unidirectional, vestibular nystagmus is greatest in amplitude when looking in the direction of the quick phase for example, a right-beating vestibular nystagmus will be greatest in right gaze (Alexander's law).

Nystagmus that changes direction depending on where the patient is looking is *gaze-evoked nystagmus*, and it generally signifies cerebellar dysfunction. Gaze-evoked nystagmus beats in the direction of gaze (e.g., right-beating in right gaze, left-beating in left gaze, up-beating in up gaze, etc.). Unlike vestibular nystagmus, which often has a torsional component, gaze-evoked nystagmus is usually purely horizontal (in left or right gaze) or purely vertical (in up or down gaze). Gaze-evoked nystagmus tends to be larger in amplitude and coarser than vestibular nystagmus.

■ **SPECIAL CLINICAL POINT: A mild form of gaze-evoked nystagmus may be observed normally in extreme gaze. This benign, physiologic "end point nystagmus" is symmetric and disappears when gaze is shifted slightly back toward midline. End point nystagmus is not associated with vertigo or dizziness.**

Central or Peripheral Vertigo?

Because peripheral causes of vertigo are typically benign while central causes of vertigo are usually more serious, emphasis has traditionally been placed on determining whether vertigo is of central or peripheral origin. The presence of associated signs and symptoms may be helpful in making this distinction (Table 20.1), but the

TABLE 20.1	**Distinguishing Peripheral and Central Vertigo**	
	Peripheral	**Central**
Brainstem signs or symptoms[a]	Never	Frequent
Alteration in consciousness	Never	Possible
Nystagmus	Vestibular	Vestibular or gaze-evoked
Positive head thrust test	Frequent	Rare
Gait ataxia	Rare (mild)	Possible (moderate to severe)
Limb ataxia	Rare	Possible
Hearing loss or tinnitus	Possible	Rare
Headache	Never	Rare (may suggest hemorrhage)

[a]Including double vision, blindness or blurred vision, homonymous hemianopia, slurred speech, trouble swallowing, Horner syndrome, hiccoughs, hoarseness, and weakness or numbness of the extremities or face.

clinician should keep in mind that in rare cases peripheral vertigo may be caused by stroke or TIA and that some causes of central vertigo are benign.

Hearing Loss and Tinnitus   Peripheral vestibular lesions are frequently associated with hearing loss and tinnitus. These occur in diseases affecting the cochlea, the middle ear, and the acoustic portion of the eighth cranial nerve. Processes that disrupt the vestibular portion of the eighth nerve in the cerebellopontine angle or in the internal auditory canal usually also affect the acoustic portion. Likewise, labyrinthine processes also may affect the cochlea or middle ear.

Unfortunately, the presence of hearing loss does not guarantee that the lesion is peripheral and benign. Rarely, central processes affecting the brainstem and cerebellum may be associated with hearing loss or tinnitus. Also, occlusion of the internal auditory artery may cause sudden, profound, unilateral hearing loss and vertigo indistinguishable from more benign causes of peripheral vestibulopathy.

Eighth cranial nerve and cerebellopontine angle mass lesions (e.g., acoustic neuroma) may present with progressive hearing loss or tinnitus associated with facial weakness, facial sensory loss, and/or a depressed corneal reflex, but rarely manifest as acute or recurrent vertigo. More commonly, they cause disequilibrium related to slow destruction of the vestibular portion of the eighth cranial nerve or pressure on the brainstem vestibular nuclei.

Brainstem and Cerebellar Signs   When vertigo is associated with brainstem or cerebellar symptoms and signs, the presence of such additional findings clearly identifies the vertigo as central in origin. The list of signs and symptoms that should raise "red flags" includes double vision, blindness or blurred vision, homonymous hemianopia, slurred speech, trouble swallowing, Horner syndrome, hiccoughs, hoarseness, and weakness or numbness of the extremities or face.

Ataxia may also be an important distinguishing feature in vertigo syndromes. Patients with peripheral vestibular syndromes usually can stand, although they typically complain of feeling unsteady and often will lean to one side when standing. Patients with central vestibular disorders often are unable to stand at all due to associated ataxia. In addition, prominent finger-to-nose or heel-to-shin dysmetria is suggestive of a cerebellar (and therefore central) process, possibly infarction or hemorrhage.

■ **SPECIAL CLINICAL POINT: Any patient with acute vertigo (dizziness) accompanied by ataxia (dysmetria), double vision (diplopia), slurred speech (dysarthria), hoarseness (dysphonia), trouble swallowing (dysphagia), or numbness of the extremities or face (dysesthesias) should be urgently evaluated for a possible brainstem or cerebellar stroke or hemorrhage.**

Head Thrust Test   The Halmagyi head thrust test distinguishes between vestibular and cerebellar disorders, and can be performed quickly and easily at the bedside. The patient should fixate on the examiner's nose and relax the neck while the examiner holds each side of the patient's head. The patient's head is turned slightly (about 10 degrees) to the right or left of midline, then quickly rotated back to the center.

Normally, the vestibulo-ocular reflex (VOR) will ensure that the patient's eyes remain fixed on the examiner's nose. In the setting of a vestibular lesion, however, the patient's eyes will move with the head, falling off target, and a corrective saccade to the examiner's nose will be observed after the head is snapped back to the primary position.

A quick saccade (toward the right) after the head is snapped to the left suggests a left vestibular lesion. A quick saccade (toward the left) after the head is snapped to the right suggests a right vestibular lesion.

In a patient with vertigo, a normal head thrust test (no corrective saccades noted) is suggestive of cerebellar disease, which by definition is central in origin. An abnormal head thrust test signifies a vestibular disturbance, which is usually peripheral, but may rarely be central.

PERIPHERAL CAUSES OF VERTIGO

Benign Paroxysmal Positional Vertigo

Benign paroxysmal positional vertigo (BPPV) is the most common cause of vertigo, particularly recurrent vertigo. Patients report the sudden onset of vertigo shortly after a change in position (often when reclining in bed). The vertigo typically lasts *15 to 30 seconds* and then resolves. The patients also may note that if they put their heads in the same position a second or a third time (within a relatively brief interval), the vertigo will be less intense each time. Key historical features of BPPV include the change in head position, the brief duration of the vertigo, a latency to onset of vertigo, and the fatigability of the vertigo with repeated trials.

BPPV can be reproduced in the office with the Dix–Hallpike maneuver (Fig. 20.1). This maneuver begins with the patient sitting on the examination table. The head is turned 45 degrees to the right, and then the patient is quickly put in the supine position with the head hanging over the edge of the table and extended approximately 30 degrees. If the vertigo does not begin within 30 seconds, the patient is returned to the sitting position, the head is turned 45 degrees to the left, and the patient is again made supine with the head extended. If vertigo is induced, it is associated with an up-beating torsional nystagmus that beats "toward the floor."

BPPV is usually idiopathic but can be seen after head trauma. The pathophysiology of this syndrome is thought to be an accumulation of calcium carbonate crystals (otoconia) within the labyrinth, usually in the posterior semicircular canal. With head movement, the debris drifts, resulting in movement of the endolymph, which in turn induces vertigo. The latency reflects the lag between the motion of the head and the drifting of the free-floating debris within the semicircular canal. With repeated head movement, the calcium carbonate crystals disperse temporarily resulting in fatiguing of the vertiginous effect.

Treatment of this syndrome is directed at moving the calcium carbonate crystals from the

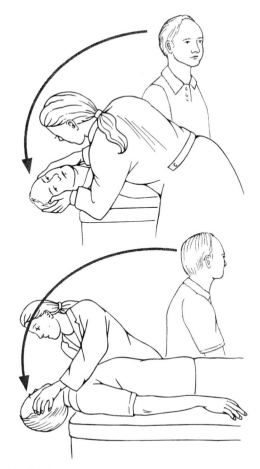

FIGURE 20.1 Dix–Hallpike positional test for benign positional nystagmus. Patient is moved rapidly from the sitting to the head-hanging position. (Redrawn from Baloh RW, Halmagyi GM, eds. *Disorders of the Vestibular System.* Copyright 1996 by Oxford University Press, Inc. Used by permission.)

posterior semicircular canal into the utricle using the modified Epley maneuver (Fig. 20.2). The Epley maneuver can be performed in the office setting and is highly effective in the majority of patients. The natural history of this disorder is typically a waxing and waning course over months to years. The treatments will put most patients into a "remission," but the symptoms may recur at some point. Patients can be taught to perform the Epley maneuver themselves at home in case of recurrence.

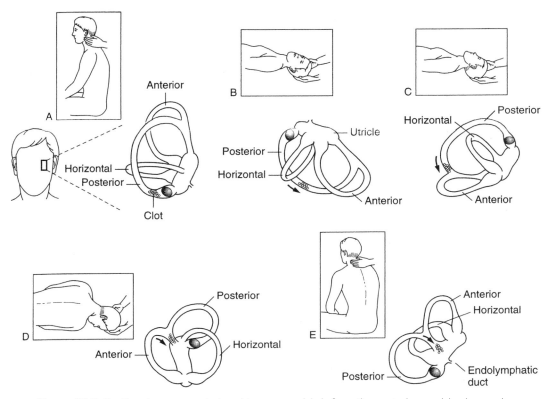

Figure 20.2 Positional maneuver designed to remove debris from the posterior semicircular canal (debris in left posterior semicircular canal depicted). **A:** In the sitting position, calcium carbonate crystals lie at the bottommost position within the posterior canal. **B:** Movement to the head-hanging position causes the crystals to move away from the cupula, producing an excitatory burst of activity in the ampullary nerve from the posterior canal (ampullofugal displacement of the cupula). **C:** Movement across to the other head-hanging position causes the crystals to move further around the canal. **D:** The patient then rolls onto the side facing the floor, causing the crystals to enter the common crus of the posterior and anterior semicircular canals. **E:** Finally, the patient sits up, and the crystals disperse in the utricle. The patient should not lie flat for 48 hours to prevent the debris from reentering the canal. (Redrawn from Epley JM. The canalith repositioning procedure: for treatment of benign paroxysmal positional vertigo. *Otolaryngol Head Surg.* 1992;107:399, with permission.)

In a classic case of BPPV (with characteristic head position, latency, and fatigability) with a normal neurologic examination and a positive Dix–Hallpike maneuver, no brain imaging is necessary. A screening audiogram is advised, however, to rule out significantly asymmetric sensorineural hearing loss, especially high tone loss.

■ **SPECIAL CLINICAL POINT: Episodes of BPPV should not be associated with hearing loss,** tinnitus, or other brainstem signs and should last for no more than a minute. The presence of any of these "red flags" should prompt an evaluation for an alternate diagnosis, which may include neurologic consultation and brain imaging.

Acute Peripheral Vestibulopathy

Acute peripheral vestibulopathy (vestibular neuritis or labyrinthitis) is the second most common cause of acute vertigo. Acute peripheral vestibulopathy is generally assumed to be benign, secondary to viral inflammation of the vestibular nerve or labyrinth, but it may rarely be cause by ischemia.

In typical acute peripheral vestibulopathy, vertigo is gradual in onset, peaking within *hours*, and resolving within *days*. The acute phase will be marked by a vestibular nystagmus beating away from the side of the lesion. Head thrust testing will be abnormal when the head is quickly turned toward the lesion. There may be mild gait ataxia, with the patient tending to veer to the side of the affected vestibular apparatus. Hearing loss may accompany labyrinthitis but is not a part of vestibular neuritis.

■ **SPECIAL CLINICAL POINT: Acute peripheral vestibulopathy may be accompanied by *mild* ataxia, but *prominent* gait ataxia, limb ataxia, or brainstem signs may signal a more serious central process (e.g., brainstem or cerebellar infarction or hemorrhage).**

Patients with peripheral vestibulopathy may be incapacitated acutely by associated nausea and vomiting, and they typically prefer to remain motionless during this time because head or body movements may exacerbate the vertigo.

Disequilibrium often follows the resolution of the vertigo and may persist for days, weeks, or even months, but eventually will resolve in the vast majority of patients. During this period of disequilibrium, the neurologic examination may be quite normal despite the patient's complains of persistent dizziness and imbalance.

A classic case of acute peripheral vestibulopathy in a young, healthy adult does not require brain imaging. Therapy for acute vertigo may include bed rest, intravenous fluids, phenothiazines, antihistamines, and benzodiazepines (Table 20.2). The use of corticosteroids and antiviral agents has been studied in patients with acute vestibular syndromes but no clear benefit has been found.

Ménière's Disease

Ménière's disease is characterized by recurrent attacks of vertigo, hearing loss, tinnitus, and aural fullness. Patients usually experience the entire symptom complex with each episode, but there are atypical cases of Ménière's disease that have only vestibular symptoms (i.e., vertigo) without cochlear symptoms (hearing loss and tinnitus) and others with cochlear symptoms and no vertigo.

TABLE 20.2   Pharmacologic Treatments for Acute Vertigo Syndromes

Drug	Starting Dose	Maintenance Dose	Potential Drug Interactions
Promethazine	25 mg IM/IV/PR/PO	12.5–50 mg q4–8h	Tranquilizers, antiparkinsonian medications
Prochlorperazine	10 mg IM/IV/PR/PO	5–20 mg q4–12h	Tranquilizers, antiparkinsonian medications
Dimenhydrinate	50 mg IM/IV/PO	25–100 mg q4–8h	Sedatives, tranquilizers, antidepressants
Meclizine	25 mg PO	12.5–50 mg q4–8h	Sedatives, tranquilizers, antidepressants
Diazepam	5 mg IM/IV/PO	2–10 mg q4–8h	Sedatives, antidepressants
Lorazepam	1 mg IM/IV/PO	0.5–2 mg q4–8h	Sedatives, antidepressants

IM, intramuscularly; IV, intravenously; PR, by rectum; PO, by mouth.
Note: All of these medications are useful for acute vertigo. However, they may exacerbate the chronic disequilibrium syndrome that often follows vertigo syndromes.

Attacks of vertigo can be as short as a few minutes or rarely may last longer than 4 or 5 hours. The hearing loss fluctuates and usually improves after the vertigo resolves, but over time there may be progressive loss of hearing. Symptoms typically begin in one ear but ultimately become bilateral in nearly 50% of patients. Approximately 80% of patients go into remission within 5 years, although most of these will be left with significant hearing loss. Some patients will develop chronic disequilibrium.

The pathologic findings associated with this syndrome are referred to as *endolymphatic hydrops*. It is possible, however, that multiple causes may lead to this common end point.

All patients suspected of having Ménière's disease should have an MRI of the posterior fossa to rule out a mass lesion. Serial audiograms are very helpful. As noted, fluctuating hearing loss is typical. Low-frequency hearing is lost first, but eventually there is a global loss of auditory function.

Salt restriction has been shown in some studies to reduce the frequency of the attacks of vertigo and hearing loss. This treatment should be initiated with a restriction of 1 to 2 g of sodium per day. If this level of restriction is ineffective, then sodium should be reduced to less than 1 g/day. Thiazide diuretics and acetazolamide also have been reported to be helpful in some patients. Smoking and consumption of caffeinated beverages exacerbate Ménière's disease and should be avoided.

Some patients have frequent, disabling attacks of vertigo that do not respond to medication. Chemical labyrinthectomy with intratympanic gentamicin or surgical labyrinthectomy or vestibular neurectomy, may be offered in such patients. Though destructive, these treatments help to prevent the recurring attacks of vertigo and may preserve some auditory function.

■ **SPECIAL CLINICAL NOTE:** Movement-related vertigo (MRV) can be a source of confusion and occasionally is misinterpreted as BPPV. In MRV, almost any head or body movement produces vertigo, with no latency or fatigability, distinguishing it from BPPV. In fact, head movement can worsen *any* form of vertigo (whether central or peripheral, vestibular or cerebellar), making MRV quite nonspecific.

Perilymph Fistula

Episodic vertigo, fluctuating hearing loss, tinnitus, or disequilibrium, triggered by Valsalva maneuver, exertion, or changes in barometric pressure, may suggest a *perilymph fistula*, an abnormal communication between the perilymphatic space of the inner ear and the pneumatized middle ear. Perilymph fistulae may be caused by trauma, including barotrauma, chronic ear infections, or as a result inner ear surgery. There is no completely satisfactory test for this disorder. Diagnosis, therefore, often depends on elicitation of a history of an appropriate inciting event (e.g., deep sea diving or stapedectomy) and the reproduction of symptoms with Valsalva maneuver. If conservative measures fail to result in improvement, then surgical repair may be considered.

■ **SPECIAL CLINICAL POINT:** All patients with suspected Ménière's disease should be seen by a neurologist or otolaryngologist with expertise in vestibular disorders. All patients whose history suggests the presence of a perilymph fistula should be evaluated by an otolaryngologist.

CENTRAL CAUSES OF VERTIGO

Vertigo may be caused by acute injury to the brainstem or cerebellum and, therefore, is a common symptom in posterior circulation syndromes, including stroke/TIA (vertebrobasilar insufficiency) and basilar migraine, cerebellar hemorrhage, and multiple sclerosis. A variety of brainstem signs and symptoms and ataxia commonly accompany central vertigo, but a central process may rarely cause isolated vertigo as well.

The most common cause of central vertigo is cerebrovascular disease (vertebrobasilar insufficiency), which should be considered in any patient with persistent vertigo who has risk factors for vascular disease (hypertension, diabetes mellitus, heart disease, hyperlipidemia, tobacco) or in older patients regardless of the presence of risk factors.

Specific central disorders associated with vertigo will be discussed here. General principles of diagnosis and management of vascular disease are discussed in Chapter 7, Cerebrovascular Disease.

■ **SPECIAL CLINICAL POINT: Any acutely vertiginous patient who has risk factors for vascular disease or is more than 50 years old should be evaluated for possible stroke or TIA by a neurologist. Vertigo from brainstem ischemia may also occur in younger patients in the setting of dissection of the vertebral or basilar arteries.**

Lateral Medullary Ischemia (Wallenberg Syndrome)

Occlusion of the posterior inferior cerebellar artery (PICA) or, more commonly, the vertebral artery may cause infarction of the lateral medulla. Lateral medullary infarction (Wallenberg syndrome) is the most common brainstem stroke syndrome and is associated with a wide variety of symptoms including dysarthria, dysphagia, hoarseness, hiccoughs, Horner syndrome, diplopia, facial pain or numbness, and gait and limb ataxia, in addition to vertigo.

In classic Wallenberg syndrome, pain and temperature sensation is decreased on the face ipsilateral to the infarction with loss of pain and temperature sensation on the contralateral side of the body. Vertigo, ataxia, nausea, and vomiting represent involvement of the inferior cerebellum. A small percentage of these patients develop significant edema in the area of cerebellar infarction with resultant brainstem compression. This group of patients, like those with cerebellar hemorrhage (see below), must be monitored closely as surgical decompression may be necessary.

Lateral Pontine Ischemia

The anterior inferior cerebellar artery (AICA) supplies the lateral pons, the vestibular and cochlear structures via a branch called the internal auditory artery, and the anterior inferior portion of the cerebellum. Occlusion of the distal portion of this vessel produces cerebellar symp-

toms similar to that seen in the PICA syndrome. Involvement of the more proximal portion of the AICA and the internal auditory artery produces lateral pontine infarction with ipsilateral facial weakness, resembling Bell's palsy, and sudden, profound hearing loss with severe vertigo.

Transient Ischemic Attack

Any ischemic stroke syndromes associated with vertigo may also present as transient ischemic attacks. An isolated TIA can be difficult to distinguish from a peripheral vestibular syndrome, especially if all symptoms have resolved, but as a general rule, any episode of vertigo lasting *minutes to hours* in a patient with risk factors for stroke should be considered a possible transient ischemic attack, especially when other central symptoms are reported. *Recurrence* of such episodes would also strongly suggest TIA over a more benign etiology.

Cerebellar Hemorrhage

Cerebellar hemorrhage is a life-threatening neurologic emergency. Patients with cerebellar hemorrhage may present with prominent headache, vertigo, nausea/vomiting, diplopia, imbalance, dysarthria, and/or an altered level of consciousness. When suspected, cerebellar hemorrhage can be quickly diagnosed with a noncontrast head CT. Patients with this disorder require an urgent neurosurgical evaluation and intensive care unit (ICU) monitoring as neurosurgical decompression is often required and may be life saving.

■ **SPECIAL CLINICAL POINT: Cerebellar hemorrhage must be considered in any patient with acute headache, vertigo, severe nausea/vomiting, and other brainstem or cerebellar signs or symptoms. Quick action, including an urgent noncontrast head CT and neurosurgical consultation, is essential and potentially life saving.**

Basilar Migraine

Because the vestibular nuclei in the brainstem are supplied by branches of the basilar artery, migrainous vasospasm of the basilar artery can produce vertigo. Hearing loss and tinnitus in addition to other neurologic symptoms such as scintillating scotoma, homonymous hemianopsia, cortical blindness, diplopia, dysarthria, ataxia, paresthesias, and quadriparesis may also occur.

These patients are usually young, and the history typically is dominated by the severe headache that follows the vertigo. In some patients, however, the headache may not be prominent, whereas in others the headache may not always follow the vasospastic component of the syndrome.

As in more common forms of migraine, the diagnosis of basilar migraine is a diagnosis of exclusion that should not be made until other cerebrovascular disorders, such as vertebrobasilar dissection, have been ruled out. The treatment of basilar migraine is similar to the treatment of other migraine syndromes (see Chapter 8, Headache Disorders).

Multiple Sclerosis

Vertigo may be a presenting symptom of multiple sclerosis, or may occur in a patient with an already established diagnosis. The clinical syndrome may mimic acute peripheral vestibulopathy. Hearing loss is rare but does occur. Previous neurologic symptoms may provide an important clue—isolated optic neuritis or transient tingling thought to be related to a pinched nerve in the past may hint at a relapsing CNS disorder. Brain MRI may not always demonstrate brainstem or cerebellar lesions, but periventricular white matter lesions usually are present. The diagnosis and treatment of multiple sclerosis is discussed in greater detail elsewhere (see Chapter 11, Multiple Sclerosis).

CAUSES OF DISEQUILIBRIUM

Disequilibrium is a common problem in the elderly but can be seen in younger patients after an acute vertigo syndrome or mild head trauma. The dizziness tends to be constant and is typically maximal with standing and ambulation. Patients with disequilibrium often complain of feeling off balance and are insecure when walking. They tend to reach for walls or furniture when ambulating at home or in the office. They may feel even more uncomfortable when outside.

Several coordinated elements are necessary to ensure proper maintenance of balance. Primary sensory input, including vision and proprioception, must be integrated with the vestibular system, and an appropriate motor response must be generated. Deficits in one or more of these physiologic functions result in imbalance or disequilibrium. There are, therefore, a number of etiologies of disequilibrium, and some patients have more than one contributing cause.

Visual Dysfunction

Whereas visual loss alone does not usually produce disequilibrium, visual distortion often does. Such distortion typically occurs when the visual input from one eye is significantly different from the other. Many patients with sudden ophthalmoplegia and resultant diplopia feel off balance during ambulation. Some corneal and retinal diseases that produce significant asymmetry of visual input also can produce disequilibrium.

Loss of Proprioception

Position sense or proprioception of the joints and muscles of the lower extremities is necessary for normal balance. Peripheral neuropathy can produce proprioceptive loss in the lower extremities and subsequent disequilibrium. This is most commonly seen with diabetic polyneuropathy but can result from any cause of peripheral neuropathy. Spinal cord disease, particularly when involving the posterior columns, as in vitamin B_{12} deficiency, can produce significant proprioceptive loss in the lower extremities and subsequent disequilibrium.

Vestibular Dysfunction

The vestibular system provides information regarding movement and the relationship of the head to the pull of gravity. Acute, unilateral vestibular disturbances produce vertigo, but slowly progressive, bilateral, or healing vestibular lesions may produce a disequilibrium syndrome.

Slow-growing neoplasms of the posterior fossa (e.g., *acoustic neuroma*) may produce a feeling of imbalance as well as hearing loss, facial numbness, and facial weakness. There are a variety of congenital and hereditary vestibular disorders that can produce progressive disequilibrium. Idiopathic degenerative vestibular dysfunction is a recognized cause of disequilibrium in elderly patients.

A number of drugs are known vestibulotoxins. Anticonvulsants and benzodiazepines may produce reversible vestibular dysfunction. Aminoglycoside antibiotics and cisplatin produce vestibular injury that is often irreversible. These drugs tend to produce bilateral vestibular dysfunction, resulting in a disequilibrium syndrome rather than acute vertigo.

Patients recovering from an acute peripheral vestibulopathy may have residual dizziness for as long as several weeks. Likewise, patients with recurrent peripheral vestibular dysfunction, as in Ménière's disease, may have persistent disequilibrium between their acute attacks of vertigo and hearing loss.

Abnormalities of Central Integration

Any process that produces a global impairment in CNS function can produce disequilibrium. Many patients complain of dizziness after minor head trauma, which may be the result of mild, diffuse cerebral dysfunction from the head injury. Medications, particularly those with sedative side effects, may impair central integration and result in disequilibrium. Similarly, patients with metabolic encephalopathy of any etiology may experience disequilibrium.

Abnormalities of Motor Response

There are three major elements in the human motor system: the pyramidal system, the extrapyramidal system, and the cerebellum. Disturbance in any one of these elements can produce a disequilibrium syndrome.

The pyramidal system can be involved at multiple levels. Hydrocephalus, neoplasms, or degenerative frontal lobe dysfunction can produce significant gait apraxia. Cervical spondylitic myelopathy is a common cause of lower-extremity stiffness and spasticity. Parkinson disease is associated with bradykinesia, rigidity, flexed posture, and loss of postural reflexes. The cerebellum is involved significantly in the coordination of gait and can be affected by a wide variety of disease processes, which would include primary and alcoholic degenerative syndromes, cerebellar neoplasms, paraneoplastic syndromes, cerebellar infarction, and demyelinating disease.

Always Remember

- Although defining the type of dizziness (presyncope, vertigo, or disequilibrium) may be helpful, the pattern of the dizziness and associated neurologic signs and symptoms may be more important.
- Presyncope may be benign (hyperventilation, vasovagal depression) or may be due to significant cardiac disease (arrhythmia, aortic or subaortic stenosis, coronary ischemia).
- Vertigo is often benign, but may be a symptom of a serious cerebrovascular disorder, especially when associated with brainstem or cerebellar signs and symptoms.
- Vertigo associated with headache, ataxia, vomiting, and other brainstem symptoms may signify a cerebellar hemorrhage, a neurologic emergency requiring emergent CT imaging and possibly neurosurgical intervention.
- Disequilibrium may be multifactorial and is often associated with more insidious vestibular or cerebral disorders.

QUESTIONS AND DISCUSSION

1. A 42-year-old man experienced the sudden onset of vertigo, nausea, vomiting, and ataxia 3 weeks ago. The vertigo, nausea,

and vomiting resolved in 48 hours, but the patient still complains bitterly of "dizziness" and states that he cannot go back to work because "I walk like a drunk." When questioned, he admits that his dizziness is present only when he is standing or walking and seems to resolve when he is sitting or supine. He denies hearing loss and tinnitus. There is no associated visual blurring, diaphoresis, or pallor. His neurologic examination is normal except that he tends to veer to the right when walking. How could this patient's current symptom of dizziness best be categorized?

A. Vertigo
B. Presyncope
C. Disequilibrium
D. Malingering
E. Not classifiable

The correct answer is C. The patient's syndrome began with vertigo, but has converted to a disequilibrium syndrome. Disequilibrium may follow any acute vestibulopathy, but it usually resolves over several weeks.

2. A 28-year-old woman complains of "everything spinning around" for 2 weeks. The episodes are precipitated by any movement in the horizontal or vertical plane. The vertigo begins immediately with each head movement. The patient denies hearing loss and tinnitus but does recall a 2-week episode of "numbness" below her waist about 3 months ago. When asked to follow the examiner's finger with her eyes, coarse horizontal nystagmus was present on lateral gaze bilaterally and vertical nystagmus was present on upgaze. Her neurologic examination was otherwise remarkable only for questionable bilateral Babinski signs. The most likely diagnosis is

A. Depression
B. Benign paroxysmal positional vertigo
C. Ménière disease
D. Multiple sclerosis
E. Perilymph fistula

The correct answer is D. This patient's symptoms are typical of movement-related vertigo, a nonspecific symptom that can be seen with any vestibular disorder. The gaze-evoked nystagmus suggests cerebellar involvement. The history of transient neurologic symptoms in the lower extremities would make multiple sclerosis a strong diagnostic consideration. The position-related vertigo of benign paroxysmal positional vertigo usually is produced by a specific head movement, with a latency of several seconds. Ménière's disease can be associated with movement-related vertigo, but is typically associated with a history of hearing loss and tinnitus.

3. A 69-year-old man complains of "dizzy spells." The patient describes 10 to 12 episodes in the last 6 weeks of sudden visual "blackout" and feeling "like I'm going to pass out." His wife notes that he breaks out in a cold sweat during the attacks and looks "glassy-eyed." The episodes last 30 to 60 seconds, and the patient feels "fine" afterward. There is no history of vertigo, hearing loss, tinnitus, or other focal neurologic symptoms. The spells are not related to body position or exercise and have occurred in many different situations including watching TV and eating in a restaurant. The patient's neurologic examination is normal. What is the most likely etiology of this patient's presyncope?

A. Hyperventilation syndrome
B. Vasovagal attacks
C. Orthostatic hypotension
D. Cardiac arrhythmia
E. Aortic stenosis

The correct answer is D. The diagnosis of hyperventilation syndrome is generally suggested by the situations of stress or anxiety in which it typically occurs. Vasovagal or vasodepressor attacks are also typically situational (i.e., hot, crowded room, or sudden emotion) and always occur when the patient is upright. Orthostatic hypotension typically occurs only when the patient is standing. Aortic stenosis is possible, but more commonly results in exercise-related presyncope. Cardiac arrhythmia may cause symptoms in any position or situation.

4. A 51-year-old woman complains of multiple episodes of isolated vertigo that have occurred over the past several weeks. She is not sure exactly how long the vertigo has lasted during each episode, "Thirty seconds? A few minutes, maybe?" The episodes may occur while she is lying down, sitting, or standing. She denies any hearing loss. What is the most likely cause of her recurrent vertigo?
   A. Transient ischemic attack (TIA)
   B. Vestibular neuritis
   C. Benign paroxysmal positional vertigo (BPPV)
   D. Cardiac arrhythmia
   E. Acoustic neuroma

The correct answer is A. Recurrent, unprovoked vertigo lasting for minutes to hours is suggestive of transient vertebrobasilar ischemia. Vestibular neuritis is unlikely to be recurrent or so brief in duration. BPPV may be recurrent, but episodes should not last for over a minute and are always provoked by changes in head position. A cardiac arrhythmia is more commonly associated with presyncope, though *very rarely* it may cause vertigo. A slow-growing mass lesion such as an acoustic neuroma more commonly results in disequilibrium than recurrent vertigo.

SUGGESTED READING

Baloh RW. Approach to the evaluation of the dizzy patient. *Otolaryngol Head Neck Surg.* 1995;112:3.

Baloh RW. Vestibular neuritis. *N Engl J Med.* 2003; 348:1027–1032.

Brandt T, Daroff RB. The multisensory physiological and pathological vertigo syndromes. *Ann Neurol.* 1980;7:195.

Epley JM. The canalith repositioning procedure for treatment of benign paroxysmal positional vertigo. *Otolaryngol Head Neck Surg.* 1992;107:399.

Furman JM, Cass SP. Benign paroxysmal positional vertigo. *N Engl J Med.* 1999;341:1590.

Hotson JR, Baloh RW. Acute vestibular syndrome. *N Engl J Med.* 1998;339:680.

Magnusson M, Karlberg M. Peripheral vestibular disorders with acute onset of vertigo. *Curr Opin Neurol.* 2002;15:5.

Newman-Toker DE, Guardabascio LM, Zee DS, et al. Taking the history from a dizzy patient: why "what do you mean by dizzy?" should not be the first question you ask. *Acad Emerg Med.* 2006;13:S79.

Newman-Toker DE, Cannon LM, Stofferahn ME, et al. Imprecision in patient reports of dizziness symptom quality: a cross-sectional study conducted in an acute care setting. *Mayo Clin Proc.* 2007;82:1329.

Newman-Toker DE, Kattah JC, Alvernia JE, et al. Normal head impulse test differentiates acute cerebellar strokes from vestibular neuritis. *Neurology.* 2008;70:2378.

Norrving B, Magnusson M, Holtas S. Isolated vertigo in the elderly: vestibular or vascular disease? *Acta Neurol Scand.* 1995;91:43.

Sloan PD, Coeytaux RR, Beck RS, et al. Dizziness: state of the science. *Ann Intern Med.* 2001;134:823.

Troost TB. Dizziness and vertigo in vertebrobasilar disease: peripheral and systemic causes of dizziness. *Stroke.* 1980;11:301.

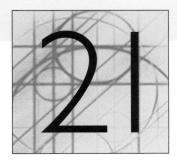

21 An Approach to the Falling Patient

KATHRYN A. CHUNG AND FAY B. HORAK

> key points
> - To diagnose the cause for falls, first determine whether falls are due to acute loss of brain activity/perfusion or to a balance problem.
> - Falls are often due to impairments in multiple physiologic systems affecting balance.
> - Damage to different systems underlying balance control results in different, context-specific instabilities.
> - Effective fall prevention requires an assessment of contributing intrinsic and extrinsic factors.
> - Refer patients to multidisciplinary resources early to prevent future falls.

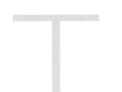he clinical problem of falls is complex and requires an especially thorough history and comprehensive physical examination of the patient. Although patients with neurologic disorders are particularly prone to injurious falls, many other diagnoses and environmental factors also contribute to falls. When a complaint of falling is presented, the clinician must be prepared to consider a broad differential diagnosis. This chapter will review epidemiologic factors about falls, present a practical approach to discover the correct diagnosis, and discuss how different underlying constraints on balance control can contribute to falls, even when patients have the same diagnosis. Treatment op-

tions to prevent future falls, including recommendations on when a referral should be made to a neurologist, will be highlighted.

DEFINITION

The World Health Organization defines a fall as "An event, which results in a person coming to rest inadvertently on the ground or other lower level." While this definition may seem so intuitive that defining it is redundant, Tinetti et al. (1997) offered an alternative definition that has become widely accepted because it acknowledges that many falls are secondary to other phenomena, not necessarily just a balance problem. Tinetti's definition of a fall is "A sudden, unintentional change in position causing an individual to land at a lower level, on an object, the floor or the ground, other than as a consequence of sudden onset of paralysis, epileptic seizure, or overwhelming external force." Illustrating this concept further, one can consider two broad categories of falls: (a) sudden loss of postural tone and/or consciousness (collapsing) and (b) loss of balance (falling like a tree), or failure to recover equilibrium. This distinction represents an important initial branch point in diagnosing pathologies related to falls, and it would be best to consider patients in these categories separately. Those who fall because of *loss of balance* will be the main focus of this chapter.

SCOPE OF THE PROBLEM

Falls are typically a problem that increases with aging. It is estimated that about 30% of community dwellers older than 65 fall at least once each year; for those in facilities, this number is even higher. As a consequence of falling, about 20% of falls result in medical attention for serious injury, approximately 10% resulting in a bony fracture. The economic cost of falling in the United States is estimated to be 19 billion dollars in total direct costs annually. In the year 2000, 10,300 falls resulted in a fatality in the United States, illustrating the seriousness of this highly prevalent problem. While it has been determined that the economic burden of falls is substantial, falls also lead to reduced quality of life, as immobility, loss of recreational activities, social isolation, and *fear of falling* are common after falling.

■ **SPECIAL CLINICAL POINT: Falls in patients with neurologic disorders are three to five times more common than in age-matched people without neurologic diagnoses.**

This statistic is not surprising, since balance control involves many parts of the nervous system, and impairments of balance control are a leading cause of falls. Some neurologic diagnoses are more associated with falls and fall injuries than other diagnoses, suggesting that they impair neural areas more critical for balance control. For example, Figure 21.1 shows the relative percentage of patients with falls in the previous 12 months for 489 inpatients admitted to a neurology ward. Patients with Parkinson disease (PD) showed the most falls, with syncope and peripheral neuropathy the next most common causes of falls.

Severity of neurologic disease is related to fall incidence, but not linearly. Early in neurologic

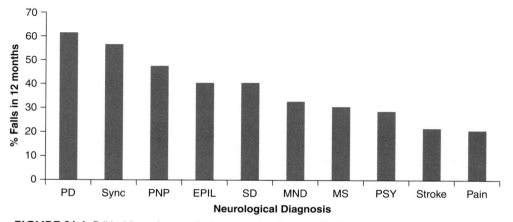

FIGURE 21.1 Fall incidence in neurologic patients by diagnosis. PD, Parkinson disease; Sync, syncope; PNP, peripheral neuropathy; EPIL, epilepsy; SD, spinal disorders; MND, motor neuron disease; MS, multiple sclerosis; PSY, psychogenic. (From Stolze H, Klebe S, Zechlin C, et al. Falls in frequent neurological diseases: prevalence, risk factors and aetiology. *J Neurol.* 2004;251:79–84, with permission.

disability, falls increase with the amount of neurologic damage. However, as the neurologic disability leads to immobility, patients who are confined to wheelchairs and beds fall less often. For example, patients with amyotrophic lateral sclerosis or severe stroke may not fall because they cannot stand or walk independently, whereas a person with mild PD who continues to ski may sustain a severe fracture from a fall. Thus, frequency of falls should always be considered in relationship to how mobile and active a patient engages in activities of daily living, sports, and outdoor activities.

RISK FACTORS

Many studies have examined risk factors leading to increased falling. It is useful to consider these factors as intrinsic or extrinsic. Examples of intrinsic factors include muscle weakness, balance dysfunction, cognitive impairment, orthostasis, gait abnormalities, mobility limitations, decreased functional status, and a history of previous falls in the last year. Increasing age, especially those 80 or older, use of an ambulatory device, such as a cane or walker, arthritis (especially of the feet), and depression are also associated risk factors. Table 21.1 summarizes how much various risk factors increase the chance of falling in a large cohort of older people.

Extrinsic factors are derived from the external environment, or risky behaviors.

■ **SPECIAL CLINICAL POINT:** An often overlooked extrinsic factor is polypharmacy, with five or more medications significantly increasing risk of falls in the elderly.

Psychotropic medications such as benzodiazepines, antipsychotics, antidepressants, as well as antihypertensives and anticonvulsants are especially associated with falling. Another important extrinsic risk factor is an unsafe environment, especially throw rugs, stairs, dark areas, and clutter or other obstacles. Behaviors, such as climbing ladders, working on roofs, and sports participation, especially skiing, also increase fall risk. The importance of a particu-

TABLE 21.1 Ratios of Increased Fall Risk Associated with Various Intrinsic and Extrinsic Factors in the Elderly

Risk Factors for Falls	Increased Risk of Falls Due to Factor
Weakness	4.4
Peripheral neuropathy	3.0
Balance impairment	2.9
Slow gait	2.9
Cane for impaired balance	2.6
Vision	2.5
Arthritis	2.4
Documented deficit in activities of daily living deficit	2.3
Depression	2.2
Cognitive decline	1.8
Ages >80	1.7
>5 Medications[a]	1.7

[a]Especially sedatives, antidepressants, pain medications.

lar extrinsic factor in increasing the risk for falling for individual patients will depend upon their specific type of balance problem. For example, a patient who shuffles when walking will be at particular risk of falling on throw rugs, a patient with leg weakness or knee joint impairments will be at particular risk on stairs, and a patient with multisensory deficits may be at particular risk of falling in the dark or on an unstable surface.

DIAGNOSING THE CAUSE OF FALLS

The complaint (often from family members) that the patient is falling should prompt investigation by clinicians, both neurologists and non-neurologists. The broad differential can be intimidating, and the following flowchart (Fig. 21.2) can help navigate the important branch points. While it is often suggested that determining if loss of consciousness has occurred in association with the fall is critical, this point may be unclear in the patient's mind and even by observers. While recognizing the limitations of this line of questioning, it can help to ask whether the falls

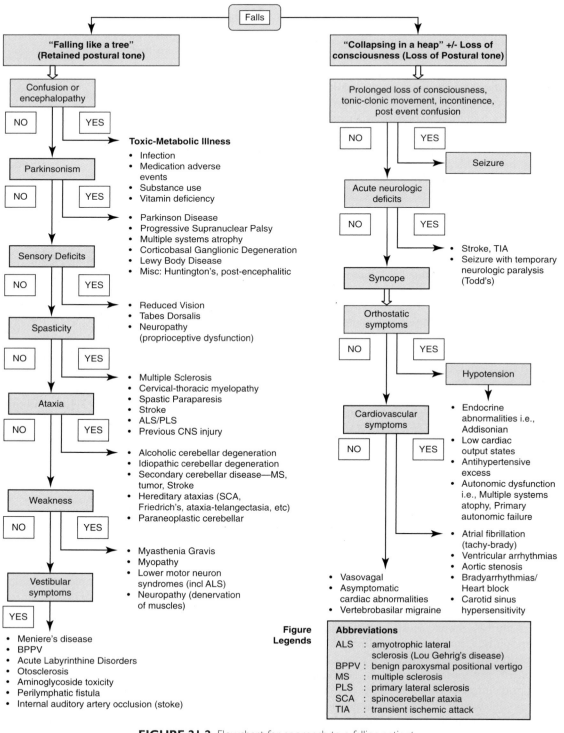

FIGURE 21.2 Flowchart for approach to a falling patient.

appear "collapsing" in nature or not. Often collapsing and impaired consciousness go together, and can indicate low cerebral blood perfusion or seizure, as shown in the right half of the flowchart.

If impairment of alertness appears to underlie a fall, further signs or historical points should be sought, including tonic–clonic or other rhythmic movements at the time of the fall, nystagmus, prolonged postevent confusion, or incontinence which could indicate seizure activity. If not, then stroke should be ruled out by assessing for new neurologic deficits, keeping in mind that occasionally a seizure can be accompanied by a temporary period of apparent weakness known as a Todd's paralysis. Once a stroke or seizure is ruled out, then syncope becomes the top consideration. If evidence of orthostasis is found by history or by examination, further investigation of blood pressure instability follows. Frequently, antihypertensive medication excess contributes to this problem, but endocrine deficiencies or autonomic dysfunction can also be causative. Autonomic dysfunction, for example, may result in postural hypotension that can lead to collapsing falls when patients attempt to quickly rise from sitting or lying positions. If no sign of orthostasis is evident, then cardiovascular causes of syncope need to be considered, which may require a cardiology specialty referral. At times, no cardiovascular causes can be identified, and rarer conditions including vertebrobasilar migraine may need to be considered. At this point, a neurologic consultation is warranted for the evaluation of these more unusual conditions.

Sometimes falls are a sign of underlying medical illness or an acute side effect of medications like sedative hypnotics, anticonvulsants, antihistamines/anticholinergics, or substances like alcohol. When falls are due to medication side effects, confusion or encephalopathy is a useful feature to recognize, and the expectation is that these falls will resolve when the illness has been treated or offending medication removed.

So far, this section has focused on the right half of the flowchart, which can be considered as the approach to acute global deficiencies of brain perfusion or electrical maintenance. The bulk of this chapter will now focus on the left half of the flowchart, which can be classified as the approach to falls due to balance maintenance problems. These types of falls are typically more chronic in their temporal course and often, though not always, associated with neurologic conditions. An examination focused on the neurologic system can help place the patient in broad categories that will lead to an accurate diagnosis and treatment plan.

Parkinsonism Examination findings of rest-predominant tremor, muscular rigidity, and slowness of movement (bradykinesia) signal parkinsonism, which is a manifestation of an abnormally functioning basal ganglia. Subjectively, patients experience parkinsonism as tremulousness, muscular stiffness, and slowness. Falling is associated with parkinsonism because rigidity and slowness of movement impair balance responses and because many important postural systems are directly affected. A number of diagnoses are characterized by parkinsonism. As the disease advances, cognitive deficits can also contribute to the accumulation of balance constraints.

The most common cause of parkinsonism is Parkinson disease. PD is clinically diagnosed and considered probable if two out of three cardinal signs are present. These signs include rest-predominant tremor, bradykinesia (slowness of movement), and rigidity during passive motion of the limbs or neck. Postural instability is also very common, though *not* at the beginning of the disease course. Indeed, postural stability deficits usually develop in the middle to later phases of the disease, occurring at least a few years after other parkinsonian symptoms develop.

■ **SPECIAL CLINICAL POINT: Early falls are considered a red flag indicating an alternate parkinsonian diagnosis.**

While PD accounts for the majority of cases of parkinsonism, the second most common cause is progressive supranuclear palsy (PSP). PSP is important in the context of this chapter because a hallmark feature of the disease is *early* falling and may be the main symptom presented to the medical provider's attention. Falls are typically backward in direction, as opposed to PD, where patients typically fall forward. Other symptoms include stiff axial musculature, restricted voluntary ocular excursions, particularly in the vertical downward direction, spastic–ataxic speech, dystonic facial features, and cognitive deficits that are frontal executive in nature.

Other less common conditions that may present with parkinsonism include multiple systems atrophy (MSA) and corticobasal ganglionic degeneration (CBGD). In MSA, combinations of parkinsonism, ataxia, autonomic dysfunction, and pyramidal tract findings can occur. In CBGD, apraxia, cortical sensory disturbance, dystonia, myoclonus, and rigidity present in a usually very asymmetric pattern of onset. Other conditions that also may be considered include fragile X premutation tremor–ataxia syndrome, drug-induced parkinsonism, normal pressure hydrocephalus, and Lewy body disease. If any type of parkinsonism is suspected, a referral to a neurologist or movement disorders specialist is highly recommended. It is important to recognize that several drugs prescribed by non-neurologists are dopamine receptor blockers and can cause drug-induced parkinsonism. These agents (see Chapter 12) include antipsychotic agents, reserpine, and metoclopramide.

Spasticity This problem occurs as a result of damage to the motor tracts originating anywhere from the motor cortex down to the spinal cord before the anterior horn cell (lower motor neuron of the spinal cord). Spasticity is the excessive tonic stretch reflex that is detected in a limb with velocity-dependent maneuvers and is sometimes described as having a "clasp-knife" character. Subjectively, it may be experienced as a stiffness or tightness in the involved muscles and can be associated with painful cramping. As a practical illustration, one may see this as the tightness of muscle tone greater in the extensor

and adductor muscles of the legs, causing foot inversion, toe pointing, and even curling in a patient with multiple sclerosis (MS).

Spasticity can lead to falls by a number of mechanisms. Simple reasons may include weakness of involved muscles because weakness often accompanies spasticity as part of an upper motor neuron syndrome (though not always). Another reason for falls with spasticity may be the abnormal posture of a foot, which results in a limited base of support for balance and leads to missteps and tripping while walking. Excessive muscle tone can interrupt the normal coordinated swing cycle of walking and results in weak postural responses and inflexible postural tone with delayed postural latencies. Acute spasms of muscles can add unpredictable instability during stance or gait.

Ataxia Ataxia is the result of hypermetric, poorly coordinated body movements with poor motor learning associated with abnormal cerebellar function. Ataxia can be inherited as a number of conditions, or can be acquired as a result of injury or damage to brain structures responsible for coordination. Clinicians may perceive ataxia in the common broad standing base that compensates for the effects of excessive involuntary body motions that disrupt equilibrium. Damage to the anterior lobe of the cerebellum results in excessive hip and trunk motion during stance and ataxic gait involving inconsistent variable positioning of the feet. When the cerebellar hemispheres are involved, ataxia includes the limbs with similar inaccurate, hypermetric, jerky, and poorly controlled purposeful movements. Ataxia leads to falls for many reasons: poor coordination of stepping, loss of righting mechanisms, hypermetric postural responses, and unstable gait with head motion. Depending on the cause of ataxia, somatosensory, visual, and/or vestibular disruptions may also contribute, as may executive deficits.

The inherited causes of ataxia include autosomal dominant, recessive, and X-linked conditions. Spinocerebellar ataxias are a group of genetically determined conditions that may have associated features such as neuropathy, cognitive dysfunction, parkinsonism, eye movement abnormalities, and other diverse neurologic signs. Other inherited ataxic syndromes have been identified and a thorough family history is important to explore, including mental retardation, as a recently described condition called fragile X tremor–ataxia syndrome especially affecting older males can be found in families where fragile X syndrome has been diagnosed. If an inherited cause is suspected, a referral to a neurologist or medical geneticist is warranted.

Acquired causes of ataxia can include toxic exposures like alcohol or anticonvulsants, paraneoplastic conditions accompanying cancers of the lung or gynecologic organs for example, structural abnormalities or infections, vitamin deficiencies, and autoimmune conditions such as MS. Idiopathic conditions like MSA or cerebellar degeneration may present with falls early in the course of the disease.

While cerebellar abnormalities can lead to ataxia, disruptions in sensory systems can also result in a similar appearance of ataxia. Neuropathy, especially when proprioceptive function is severely disturbed, or some vestibular disorders can result in unsteadiness of stance and gait that resemble ataxia and result in falls.

Vestibular System Disorders The vestibular system is a bilateral, reciprocal sensory system that contributes to balance control by sensing position and velocity of head motions, as well as gravity. It is useful to consider peripheral vestibular disorders in three broad groupings, those with (a) chronic unilateral or bilateral loss, (b) fluctuating or intermittent dysfunction, and (c) mechanically based vestibular dysfunction. Falls due to vestibular dysfunction can be due to any of the following components including unstable gait with head motion, asymmetric limits of stability, poor sense of the vertical, and loss of sensory feedback.

Examples of chronic or permanent loss of vestibular function include otosclerosis, stapedectomy, acoustic neuroma, aminoglycoside or other ototoxicity, vertebrobasilar stroke, or rarely a unilateral internal auditory artery occlusion leading to a stroke of the vestibular end organ. Ménière disease is a classic example of fluctuating vestibular dysfunction, though it may lead to a chronic pattern in later disease. Mechanically based dysfunction of the semicircular canals or otolith organs include benign paroxysmal positional vertigo (BPPV) in which otoconia become displaced from the otoliths and float in the canals, and perilymphatic fistulas or holes in the round or oval windows.

Patients with vestibular deficits may have very poor control of balance, complaints of dizziness, and abnormal eye movements, but not frequent falls. Falls can often be avoided in patients with vestibular injuries because they increase their dependence on vision and somatosensory function using central compensation processes. However, if patients with bilateral loss of vestibular function or with uncompensated unilateral loss of vestibular function find themselves in a dark environment standing on an unstable surface, they may fall "like a tree" without making automatic balance responses because of spatial disorientation from lack of sensory information about their body equilibrium. This "context-specific instability" is often missed when evaluating vestibular loss patients in a well-lit clinic on a firm surface.

Weakness While weakness is common when in conjunction with other neurologic findings such as spasticity in upper motor neuron syndromes, or atrophy of muscles associated with neuropathy, there are syndromes of lower motor neuron, pure muscle disorders, and neuromuscular junction dysfunction where weakness is singularly dominant. Muscle disease including endocrine, inflammatory or toxic myopathies, inclusion body myositis, or neuromuscular junction diseases such as myasthenia gravis can present with varying degrees of weakness and falls. Less common lower motor neuron diseases such as polio, or spinal muscular atrophy can lead to profound weakness especially of the lower extremities. Weakness of muscle activation causes falls because of inability to sustain strength against the pull of

TABLE 21.2

Examples for How Each Neurologic Disease is Associated with a Different Set of Constraints on Postural Control

Constraints on Balance Systems	PD	Spinal	Neurop	Spasticity	Ataxia	Vestibular	Cognitive Disorders
Weak postural responses	X	X		X			
High postural tone	X	X		X			
Delayed latencies		X	X	X			X
Small anticipatory adjustments	X						
Abnormal limits of stability	X					X	
Loss of sensory feedback			X		X	X	
Abnormal sensory weighting					X		X
Poor sense of vertical				X	X	X	
Unstable gait with head motion					X	X	
Executive deficits	X			X	X		X

PD, Parkinson disease; Neurop, somatosensory neuropathy; Vestib, bilateral vestibular loss; Spinal, spinal cord injury.

gravity and inability to generate adequate, quick increases in force between their feet and the ground to recover equilibrium with automatic balance responses.

Balance Constraints in Neurologic Patients

Since balance control is regulated throughout the nervous system, many very different neurologic diagnoses result in poor balance and falls.

■ **SPECIAL CLINICAL POINT: Each neurologic disease is associated with a different set of constraints on balance control, leading to balance problems for different reasons and, thus, risk for falling under different conditions.**

Each type of neurologic pathology can result in different types of balance deficits because many different neural circuits are responsible for different systems underlying postural control. Examples of constraints on balance systems are listed in Table 21.2.

BALANCE PROBLEMS LEAD TO FALLS IN NEUROLOGIC PATIENTS

As shown in Table 21.2, fall risk associated with motor problems such as weak postural responses, high postural tone, or late postural responses is

related to inability to recover equilibrium when it is disturbed from external perturbations. *Weak postural responses* result from any problem involving postural long-loop pathways from proprioceptors to the motor cortex and back to motoneuronal pools and muscles. *High postural tone* results in co-contraction and stiffness that limits synergic coordination of postural responses. *Delayed postural response latencies* from their normal 100 msec loop time result in ineffective responses to external perturbations like a push or trip.

Any motor deficits affecting the quick generation of muscle activation, such as PD, spinal cord lesions, or spasticity from stroke or MS, are likely to result in weak postural responses to external perturbations as well as weak self-generated postural movements. To effectively respond to postural perturbations such as slips or trips, subjects need to generate muscle force quickly. The amount of force needed to recover equilibrium is larger, the larger the individual and the stronger the perturbation. Despite high background muscle tone associated with rigidity or spasticity, studies show that these motor deficits are associated with a slowed rate-of-change of muscle activation for postural correction. Thus, neurologic patients with weak postural responses are likely to fall in response to external perturbations because they generate inadequate forces to recover equilibrium.

In contrast to deficits in postural response loops, *small anticipatory postural adjustments* prior to self-initiated movements, such as an arm raise or step, result in disequilibrium and falls during fast voluntary movements that require activation of postural muscles to compensate for self-induced perturbations. For example, patients with PD who show abnormal anticipatory postural adjustments may not be able to adequately unload a leg quickly to initiate a step. Patients with cerebellar ataxia may show such abnormally large anticipatory postural adjustments prior to each step, but in this situation, they accelerate the body too far laterally, requiring lateral protective steps to maintain equilibrium. Abnormal anticipatory postural adjustments prior to voluntary movements also lead to instability and falls when transitioning from sitting to standing or when attempting to lift a weighted object.

Asymmetrical limits of stability make it difficult to control position of the body over its base of support without changing the base of support with a step or grasp of a stable object. If patients do not accurately recognize their limits of stability, they may not make the postural adjustment necessary to maintain equilibrium. For example, patients with PD have particularly small limits of stability in the backward direction and patients with unilateral loss of vestibular inputs have asymmetrical limits of stability, at least acutely, before they compensate. Normal limits of stability while standing are about 8 degrees at the ankle forward and 4 degrees backward and can be due to central causes such as PD, to lack of sensory information such as in peripheral neuropathy, or vestibular loss, or to biomechanical limitations on strength or the base foot support. Reduced limits of stability are also common in patients who have fear of falling. Reduced limits of stability do not allow patients to balance over a large area, so the task of balancing becomes

more difficult and results in exaggerated postural responses.

Sensory deficits affecting sensory feedback or sensory weighting may result in falls either because of failure to generate a timely balance response or because an inappropriate balance response is generated. Falls from failure to generate a timely postural response are common in diseases affecting arrival of accurate somatosensory inputs to the nervous system such as peripheral neuropathy or damage to spinal pathways from MS or spinal stenosis. Delays in postural responses can also accompany central long-loop disruptions such as strokes or frontal lobe problems. A timely, but inappropriate, balance response can also result in falls. For example, when subjects with loss of vestibular information stand on a tilting surface with eyes closed, they fall because they actively use their somatosensory system to align their bodies to the moving support surface, rather than to gravity. Likewise, some peripheral and central vestibular patients fall as they respond to visual motion cues because of the inability to distinguish world motion from self-motion. *Loss of sensory feedback* from muscle proprioceptors is more likely to result in frequent falls than loss from vestibular or visual inputs because postural responses are triggered primarily by proprioceptors.

Abnormal sensory weighting results in falls when subjects change from one sensory environment to another. Healthy subjects rely primarily upon proprioceptive information from the surface for control of stance posture when sensory inputs from all three sensory systems are available. That is why healthy people sway more on an unstable surface such as compliant foam, than when they close their eyes. That is also why patients with neuropathy affecting somatosensory conduction, but not patients with blindness or vestibular loss are most likely to have large postural sway in stance and falls. However, healthy people decrease their reliance on proprioception and increase their reliance on vestibular or visual senses when standing on an unstable surface, such as soft sand or a boat. Some cerebellar or dementia patients who cannot quickly increase dependence on their intact vestibular or visual inputs and decrease dependence upon proprioception for balance control may be stable on a firm surface and only fall when attempting to balance on an unstable or tilted surface. Some patients with peripheral vestibular deficits may become overly dependent upon vision as an orientation reference, so they align their bodies with moving visual surround and become unstable or fall. Thus, either a central or peripheral sensory deficit often results in "context-specific" instability, in which patient can have excellent balance in one sensory context but very poor balance and falls in another sensory context. Context-specific instability explains why it may be difficult to identify a balance deficit in some neurologic patients in a well-lit clinic on a firm, flat floor surface, and then they fall when leaving the office to walk across the parking lot.

Poor verticality causes patients to lean and fall as they attempt to align their bodies with their inaccurate internal representation of vertical. For example, after a stroke resulting in hemineglect, it is common for patients to be unable to sit or stand upright because of strong leaning to the hemiplegic side. This leaning is not only due to inability to support the body with weak muscles but also because the patient may be attempting to align their bodies with laterally tilted sense of upright, vertical. Falls due to a tilted internal representation of vertical occur in the direction patients lean; for example, patients with peripheral neuropathy consistently fall backward and stroke patients with hemineglect fall to the side of neglect.

Unstable gait with head motion results in ataxic missteps and, potentially, falls when sensors in the head and neck are perturbed. Patients with cerebellar deficits and vestibular deficits are especially sensitive to imbalance and falls when they quickly move their heads while walking, even if they are relatively stable in walking with their heads facing straight ahead.

Executive cognitive deficits affecting attention, ability to change set quickly, navigation

memory, and body mapping can result in falls because of difficulty making quick decisions, affecting mobility in complex environments. Patients with Alzheimer disease and other cognitive deficits have higher rates of falls than age-matched controls, even when they do not have associated sensory or motor deficits. In addition, neurologic patients, such as patients with PD, who also show executive deficits are more likely to falls than patients without cognitive deficits.

One reason executive deficits are associated with increased fall risk is that balance control requires central attention. Although much of healthy control of balance and gait is "automatic," patients with balance disorders need to increase the amount of cognitive attention they devote to control of balance and gait. Patients with executive deficits may have reduced cognitive reserve, so they cannot increase their attention as needed for a difficulty postural task. One way to determine the extent to which a balance or gait task requires attention is to ask a patient to do a secondary cognitive task such as mental arithmetic or listing from a category while they are walking or performing another task involving balance control. The "Walk and Talk" task is particularly sensitive and useful when a stopwatch is used to time how long it takes to perform a Get Up and Go task with and without a cognitive task. Although a small amount of gait slowing is normal during a cognitive task, a large amount of slowing is associated with increased fall risk.

Although Table 21.2 differentiates how different neurologic diagnoses tend to be associated with a different set of postural constraints, even individuals with the same neurologic diagnosis may have a different set of constraints on these postural systems. For example, depending on which neural circuits are involved in MS or following a stroke, the root cause of a patient's balance problem, and therefore the nature of their individual fall risk, will vary. The specificity of type of balance problem in each neurologic patient demands treatments that are also specific to each patient's set of constraints, based upon a systematic assessment.

FALLS ARE MULTIFACTORIAL

■ **SPECIAL CLINICAL POINT: Most falls are a result of the complex interaction among many different intrinsic and extrinsic factors.**

A sudden onset of frequent falling may not necessarily be the result of a sudden, significant fall risk, but may be due to the addition of one more constraint on balance control to the previous set of constraints already present, but not yet bringing the subject to the threshold for falling. For example, a patient with PD may have impaired balance but not yet falling due to a combination of autonomic hypotension, weak postural responses, and high postural tone. When he suddenly is given a sleeping pill or changes prescription for his glasses, this new risk factor may put him over the threshold for falling, although this last factor is not the only reason for the fall. Figure 21.3 shows how the gradual addition of multiple constraints on balance control can bring a patient to the threshold for frequent falls.

The model shows the decline in mobility function in patients with a chronic, degenerative neurologic disease, such as PD. Superimposed upon the slow, degenerative decline in neural function that may affect mobility, such as bradykinesia and rigidity, are additional new constraints on balance control. Additional constraints, such as freezing, or impaired kinesthesia, may arise from continued progression of the same neurologic disease or from new constraints on balance control, such as arthritis or neuropathy from diabetes.

Each patient with multiple constraints may reach that falling threshold at different times for different reasons, like the proverbial "straw that broke the camel's back" (compare subject A and subject B). For example, if the threshold for falling is reached when freezing is added to the other constraints due to PD, patients are likely to fall forward onto their knees while attempting to start walking. In contrast, if the threshold for falling is reached due to the addition of neuropathy, falls are more likely to occur when standing on an unstable surface or in response to an external perturbation. This model can help explain how and why different individual patients with the same neurologic

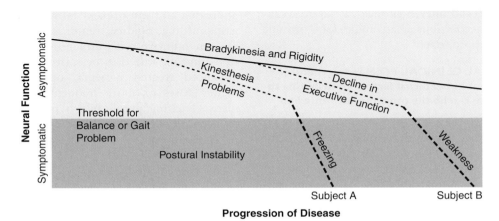

FIGURE 21.3 Model of how addition of multiple constraints on balance control eventually results in reaching the threshold for frequent falls.

disease can have different type of balance problems leading to different type of falls under different situations.

TREATMENT TO PREVENT FALLS IN NEUROLOGIC PATIENTS

Applying a useful treatment for falls is of course dependent on making the correct analysis of the fall risk problem. The practical approach begins with recognizing the predominant body system(s) impairment (see the flowchart). Once a patient is classified, it is then simpler to understand how balance is impaired by considering each individual's balance constraints (Table 21.2). The next steps are to identify reversible or treatable factors. For example, a new faller may be examined and found to have sensory deficits including poor proprioception with toe and ankle joint testing. A diagnosis of diabetes mellitus might be made after applicable testing, for example. By understanding that delayed sensory feedback results in failure to general timely postural responses, one understands the reason for falling better. Treatment (or prevention) of future falls will focus not only on trying to prevent ascension or worsening of the sensory deficit with good glucose control, but also on removing external hazards such as throw rugs, slippery footwear, and uneven surfaces. If severe weakness also contributes, an ankle–foot orthotic may be appropriate.

■ **SPECIAL CLINICAL POINT: In general, if the patient has external factors contributing to falls, these can be the most quickly remedied problems.**

Studies have shown that home visits by therapists or visiting nurses can alter home environments to reduce fall risk. Creative solutions can include offloading tasks such as cleaning gutters/washing windows to others, by preventing risky behaviors leading to falls.

Finding solutions for intrinsic causes for falling is usually more complicated, though simple solutions do exist for many problems.

Cataract surgery and improving nighttime lighting in the hallways and bathroom are examples of simpler solutions for those with visual impairments, for example. Conditions on the right side of the flowchart are often easily remedied by optimizing medications, placement of a pacemaker, or instituting antiseizure therapy, for example. Some conditions in the left half of the chart can be treated with a high degree of success. For example, if the problem is myasthenia gravis and late-day falls, then appropriate immunomodulating therapy will cause return of muscle strength and lessening of falls. On the other hand, some deficits cannot be fully treated and normal function may be not completely restored. In many cases, there are no significantly useful medical or surgical interventions. In these situations, the role of rehabilitation becomes paramount.

Medical Treatment of Neurologic Causes of Falls

Parkinsonism Although there is an array of symptomatic treatments for PD, the chronic progressive problem of postural instability remains a great source of disability especially in the later stages of the disease. While postural instability remains very difficult to treat, there are other complications in PD that should be addressed and can prevent falls. Freezing and gait shuffling, rigidity, tremor, and bradykinesia can improve with dopaminergic medications that may need to be started, or in more advanced treated patients, optimized with higher doses or more frequent dosing regimens. Treating autonomic hypotension may prevent falls when quickly rising from a sitting or supine position, but because these treatments are complex, referral to a neurologist or even a movement disorders neurologic specialist is recommended.

Occasionally, medications that boost dopamine production are useful in other conditions like MSA, though the effects are usually not as robust or as enduring as in PD. Avoiding dopamine receptor blockers such as antipsychotic drugs or metoclopramide will prevent potential worsening of parkinsonism and increased falling.

Spasticity A number of pharmacologic treatments for spasticity are in use including baclofen, tizanidine (imidazolines), and benzodiazepines. Botulinum toxin injections to affected muscles are another more recent treatment modality that can reduce tone with fewer side effects. A good example of the use of botulinum toxin might be injections to the gastrocnemius, soleus, and posterior tibial muscles to reduce spasticity associated with excessive foot plantar flexion and inversion in a patient with cerebral palsy, thereby decreasing falls from tripping.

Pharmacotherapy can help reduce spasticity in some patients, but in many others, the side effects of oral medications are a limiting problem. The development of alternate routes of delivery has helped many of these patients, such as intrathecal delivery mechanisms (baclofen pump). Sometimes orthopedic or neurosurgical treatments (rhizotomy) to relieve spasticity are needed.

In some cases, relieving spasticity does not provide a net benefit on balance, and in fact can lead to more falls, especially if the increased extensor leg tone helps compensate for weakness in a stroke patient, for example. Each individual case must be evaluated to determine the potential benefits, and it is not uncommon to decide upon no spasticity treatment.

Depending on the etiology, the role of disease modification cannot be underestimated. For example, prevention of MS exacerbations is possible with immunomodulating agents, or anticoagulation in atrial fibrillation to prevent stroke is obviously the best antispasmodic strategy.

Ataxia There are no known medical treatments that reliably reduce ataxia. It is important to prevent further disease progression if known toxic causes are identified. An example of this is the alcoholic who stops drinking. When neuropathy or "sensory ataxia" is iden-

tified due to diabetes, good glucose control can modify the incidence and rate of neuropathy progression, which should lead to less falling.

Vestibular Depending on whether the vestibular disturbance is "mechanical" or chronic versus intermittent will dictate the medical therapy instituted. It is common for vestibular quieting agents (antihistamines) like meclizine to be prescribed for vestibular-based dizziness, but this could be counterproductive for balance and falls since they suppress vestibular function and the ability of the central nervous system to compensate for chronic vestibular loss. Diuretics can improve certain vestibular disorders like Menière disease. Treatment of BPPV with canalith-repositioning techniques, which can be completed in a matter of minutes, shows great success in reducing positional dizziness. Surgical techniques for certain chronic labyrinthine disorders are occasionally utilized.

Weakness The differential diagnosis is broad and therefore the treatment options are also numerous. In general, myopathies due to toxic, inflammatory, or endocrine abnormalities have good chances for improvement using appropriate medical treatments. Neuromuscular junction impairment conditions like myasthenia gravis are chronic but usually well-treated conditions today. Conditions of lower motor neuron failure have dismally few medical treatment options.

Rehabilitation to Prevent Falls in Neurologic Patients

The main treatment to prevent falls in patients with neurologic disorders is physical therapy. Physical therapists should base their individualized treatment on a comprehensive assessment of the constraints on balance control for each individual patient.

Assessing Fall Risk Several clinical tools can be used to determine risk for a fall. For example, the Berg Balance Scale consists of a series of balance tasks, such as standing on one foot, reciprocal stepping onto a stool, and a 180-degree turn, which are related on a four-point scale from normal (4) to very abnormal (0). A total score on the Berg Balance Scale above 48 out of 56 has been shown to predict future falls in the elderly and in patients with PD. Tinetti's Balance and Gait Test was similarly designed to predict falls in the elderly but it also predicts falls in neurologic patients, such as those with PD. A quick and easy clinical test of mobility that is also related to falls in the elderly is the timed Get Up and Go test. Subjects are timed with a stopwatch for how long it takes them to rise of an armless chair, walk 3 m, turn and return to the chair and sit down. Frailty and falls can also be assessed with the Functional Performance Test, consisting of timing five times sit-to-stand, stance in tandem, and timed 2-minute walk. Although these functional balance tests are related to fall risk, they do not include tests of postural responses to external perturbations, balance under altered surface or visual conditions, or balance challenges during gait. These types of balance tests can determine whether neurologic patients need balance rehabilitation but not what type of rehabilitation is needed.

Balance Training   To design an effective exercise program for a neurologic patient with balance problems, therapists perform a comprehensive assessment to determine which systems are contributing to constraints on balance control. Using the Balance Evaluation Systems Test (BESTest), therapist can determine which of six systems underlying posture control are affected: biomechanical, verticality/limits of stability, anticipatory postural adjustments, automatic postural responses, sensory orientation, and stability during gait. If biomechanical constraints are found, such as muscle weakness or abnormal postural alignment, therapy will focus on strengthening, increasing range of motion, and improving postural alignment. Reduced limits of stability can be increased with practice using biofeedback. Practice unloading a leg prior to step initiation may improve anticipatory postural adjustments and practice re-sponding to external perturbations can improve automatic postural responses. Inability to use vestibular information for stance balance, in patients who have intact peripheral vestibular receptors, may be improved by practicing balancing with eyes closed on an unstable surface. Patients overly dependent upon vision for stance balance can practice balancing with "no-body" glasses or dark sun glasses that reduce viewing the body and the visual environment.

Patients who have balance deficits use more conscious attention to control their balance. Many aspects of balance and gait are automatic and require little conscious attention in healthy subjects. One way to determine how much attention is used by the nervous system to control balance is to ask patients to perform a secondary cognitive task while they simultaneously control their balance or gait. For example, in the BESTest, the timed Up and Go test is performed while performing mental arithmetic. The increase in time it takes to perform the test with versus without a cognitive task indicates how much attention is required for control of mobility. A secondary cognitive task, such as counting backward from 100 by threes or making a list from a category, can be added to almost any balance or gait task, such as one-foot standing, standing on foam with eyes closed, to determine how much it depends upon cognitive attention. Patients may improve doing a balance or gait task while concurrently doing a cognitive task with practice.

Strength Training   Weakness from a neurologic problem may be due to impaired central motor commands for voluntary movement from corticospinal damage, basal ganglia–related bradykinetic or slow movements with difficultly increasing or decreasing muscle force quickly, abnormal coordination of antagonists and synergists as in cerebellar impairment, and inability to recruit or unavailable large motoneurons in the spinal cord. Whatever the pathology responsible, if a neurologic patient presents with weakness, progressive resistance exercise focused on the weak muscles leading to postural instability can be helpful. The most important muscles for control of balance are the ankle muscles with tibialis anterior, in particular, important for preventing backward falls. Adequate strength in lateral hip abductor muscles is also important to prevent falls during gait and turns, and quadriceps strength is needed to prevent falls when transitioning from sit-to-stand or stand-to-sit posture. Even if isometric peak strength is within normal limits, the ability to generate joint torque quickly is important for adequate postural responses, so therapists need to focus on quick, dynamic strengthening exercises.

■ **SPECIAL CLINICAL POINT: In many cases, the most effective exercises for improving posture and balance may not be isolated muscle strengthening in well-supported conditions but strengthening exercises while practicing balancing tasks.**

For example, wearing a weighted vest while repeating sit-to-stand to strengthen quadriceps and pulling the upright body forward from leaning back against a wall to strengthen tibialis muscles.

Gait Training   Fall prevention by gait training involves identifying compensatory strategies and practicing with added balance challenges during gait. Normal gait is an efficient exchange of potential and kinetic energy in which subjects spend two thirds of the gait cycle in single leg support. Patients prone to falls, however, tend to slow gait, increase time in the double-support phase, increase variability of spatial–temporal gait parameters, and increase lateral body sway while walking.

Balance challenges can be added to gait training by increasing gait speed, decreasing the footfall width, adding changes in direction such as turns, sideways and backward walking: adding head motions, carrying and picking up objects, altering the surface or visual characteristics of the environment, and adding a secondary cognitive task. PD, stroke, or partial spinal lesion patients who fall because of inadequate toe clearance may also benefit from treadmill training focused on increasing toe clearance and stride length. However, when treadmill training is accompanied by hand or partial body weight support, the patient is not training their balance control system along with gait training.

Assistive Devices   The most effective assistive device to prevent a fall is use of a cane. Many studies have shown that appropriate use of a cane can prevent imbalance and falls in neurologic patients during gait and balancing tasks. A cane does not prevent falls by acting as a crutch to support body weight or to catch the person who is falling. Canes prevent falls by increasing the amount of accurate sensory information to the nervous system about where the body is with respect to earth reference. In fact, use of a cane is similar to use of light touch on a stable surface to prevent a fall since most neurologic patients do not place much support on a cane. Even light touch of less than 100 g, about the amount needed to read Braille, is sufficient to decrease postural sway in stance even more than opening the eyes to use vision. Patients who have loss of peripheral sensory feedback from the vestibular, proprioceptive, or visual systems show the most immediate improvement in balance, control, and stability during gait from use of a cane. Use of a cane or trekking pole also makes walking more energy efficient by decreasing the balance demands of gait. However, use of a cane requires sufficient sensory integration, strength, coordination, and executive control to be functional.

Some patients with central neurologic deficits do not benefit from a cane either because they cannot take advantage of the additional sensory information, because they cannot coordinate the use of a cane in a reciprocal gait pattern, or because their balance and strength constraints are too great for a cane alone. If a cane is insufficient for safe balance, then therapists can fit patients with appropriate walkers or wheelchairs. Large-wheel, swivel walkers with carrying baskets and seats can make walking safer and practical, although they make it more difficult to take a protective step for balance in response to an external perturbation.

It should be noted that an assistive device is only useful in preventing falls if it is appropriately fitted, tested, and trained for an individual patient by a licensed physical therapist. A cane should be the height of the greater trochanter from the floor and held in the hand opposite to the leg with the largest gait problem. A cane that is too tall or difficult to control can be more hazardous than no cane at all. Many patients need to be taught how to appropriately use a cane so they decrease, rather than increase, fall hazard. There are also an increasingly large variety of types of walkers, so a proper prescription by an experienced therapist is important.

Patients who continue to fall frequently, despite best efforts at rehabilitation, may benefit from padded clothing to prevent injuries. For example, padded hip protectors have been shown to be particularly useful in preventing hip fractures in older, osteoporotic patients with dementia. Kneepads may protect the legs in patients with PD who tend to fall forward while walking due to freezing episodes. Helmets can be worn in ambulatory patients who cannot protect themselves with their hands while falling.

WHEN TO REFER TO A SPECIALIST

Refer a falling patient to a neurologist once you have eliminated the probability that falling was due to loss of perfusion to the brain from a cardiovascular event, which may require referral to a cardiovascular specialist. Refer a falling patient to a neuro-otologist if they complain of spinning or positional vertigo, show abnormal nystagmus, or to rule out a bilateral, profound loss of vestibular function in patients without any vertigo or nystagmus. Refer to an ophthalmologist to determine if visual deficits or poor glasses prescription contribute to falling. Refer a falling patient to a physical therapist to remediate balance and gait impairments contributing to falls.

Always Remember

- To diagnose the cause for falls, always start by determining whether falls are due to acute loss of brain activity/perfusion or to a balance problem.
- A single deficit may not explain falling and a search for multiple, interlocking deficits must be pursued.
- The context of falls may be the most important clue to the cause, so detailed historical information is essential.
- Refer patients to multidisciplinary resources early to prevent future falls.

QUESTIONS AND DISCUSSION

1. A 72-year-old man presents with three falls in the last 6 months. He has a known history of atrial fibrillation, hypertension on two antihypertensive medications, and type II diabetes on a sulfonylurea. His wife, who witnessed two of the falls, reports one occurred while walking in the grocery store and appeared to be a sudden "crumple" with a very brief period of unresponsiveness, some confusion for a few minutes afterward, but recovery to his normal baseline. The second event occurred shortly after getting up from his recliner and walking to the kitchen. These falls can reasonably be explained by which of the following mechanisms?
A. Cardiac arrhythmia
B. Seizure
C. Hypoglycemia
D. Orthostasis
E. All of the above

The correct answer is E. The point here is to recognize that more history and physical is required to narrow this differential diagnosis, but the chances are high that a non-neurologic cause will be discovered because of the sudden collapsing nature without seizure-like accompaniments or residual neurologic deficits. While seizures are possible, it would be atypical with such short periods of postfall confusion, and without mention of repetitive motor activity (though not always present). Similarly for hypoglycemia, the short recovery time is less likely but can be investigated with random fingerstick glucose testing. Orthostasis can be investigated with questions about lightheadedness during other postural transitions or after meals and investigated with orthostatic vitals 3 minutes apart. As negative data accumulate, the likelihood of an arrhythmia becomes higher. In a patient with a known history of atrial fibrillation, the "collapsing" nature of the fall and probable brief loss of consciousness should make one suspicious of sudden loss of cerebral perfusion. In this case, long-term cardiac monitoring revealed bradycardic periods and pauses; the placement of a pacemaker resulted in no further falls.

2. An 84-year-old woman presents with a complaint of worsening balance and a nighttime fall for the first time. She has no history of coronary artery disease, diabetes, or seizures. She feels unsteady when she stands up and walks, but feels better when she touches the wall. Her medications include alendronate, calcium carbonate/ vitamin D, omeprazole, and hydrochlorothiazide. Which of the following is the most likely diagnosis?
   A. Orthostatic hypotension
   B. Multiple sensory deficits
   C. Anxiety
   D. Vertebrobasilar transient ischemic attack (TIA)
   E. Benign paroxysmal positional vertigo (BPPV)

The correct answer is B, multiple sensory deficits. The history is progressive worsening, and not episodic periods of disequilibrium; thus BPPV and TIA are not correct. Orthostasis is an important diagnosis to rule out, but touching the wall would not cause improvement.

3. A 72-year-old man who has had PD for 10 years presents to you for falls with injuries three times in the last 3 months. Prior to this he had a history of falling about once per year. Which potential constraints on balance control will you need to investigate to determine the reason for the increased risk of falls in this patient?
   A. New home environment
   B. Progression of disease with added new freezing or cognitive constraints
   C. Increase in lightheadedness after transitioning to upright positions
   D. Over-the-counter medication added to his antiparkinsonian medications
   E. All of the above

The correct answer is E. Both A and D are examples of extrinsic factors, which could be easily remedied by educating about medication interactions and by having a therapist or other visiting specialist evaluate the home for potentially hazardous features like abrupt surface transitions, loose carpets, etc. B and C are complications associated with advancing PD. These intrinsic factors can be improved with treatment of orthostasis with volume expanders or midodrine, adjusting the timing/dose of dopaminergic medications to reduce freezing, or adding an assistive device.

4. A 78-year-old woman comes to the office because of a year-long history of progressive worsening of gait and balance progressing to falls in the last few months. She feels "stiff-legged" and cannot walk quickly to answer a ringing telephone. Her bladder has become more urgent recently. Some of her examination findings include upgoing toes and sustained clonus at the ankles. You find no abnormalities above the waist, but you discover some loss of proprioception in the feet. Her gait is indeed stiff and slow in appearance, with the left leg appearing to be externally rotated. She admits to having a sore neck often and attributes it to arthritis. Which

of the following tests is the first priority in diagnosis of this patient?
A. MRI of the cervical spine
B. Nerve conduction studies of the lower extremities
C. Vitamin B_{12} level
D. Mammogram

The correct answer is A. Structural and treatable abnormalities in the cervical cord should be eliminated rapidly. In this case, MRI revealed central canal stenosis from a compressive disc protrusion, with abnormal signal in the spinal cord. A thoracic cord localization is also possible, though less common. In this case, the spinal cord subacute compression caused spastic gait abnormalities which led to falls. Surgical decompression followed by rehabilitation resulted in excellent improvement but not complete resolution of walking problems. Vitamin B_{12} deficiency is also possible and should be explored; however, a surgically treatable spinal cord lesion must be urgently ruled out.

5. A 35-year-old woman with MS presents due to a recent fall when attempting to walk down an incline, resulting in a skull injury. She had been walking by holding onto a spouse for support. She has unilateral ankle muscle weakness, delayed somatosensory conduction up the spinal cord, difficulty seeing to read, and complains of dizziness with head movements. A referral to which of the following professionals is most appropriate to prevent falls?
A. Physical therapy for strengthening, gait and balance training with a cane
B. Optometry for glasses
C. Neuro-otology to diagnose a potential vestibular disorder
D. All of the above

The correct answer is A. Her dizziness with head movements most likely reflects the damage due to a cerebellar lesion. Vision problems due to complications of MS often indicate optic nerve damage or problems with yoking of eye movements. These are usually not responsive to optometric treatment with simple glasses.

6. A 52-year-old woman stays indoors and fears walking in crowds or near moving traffic because of disorientation and fear of falling. How could this patient's complaints be categorized?
A. Malingering
B. Anxiety disorder with panic attacks
C. Presyncope
D. Visual motion sensitivity associated with vestibular disorder

The correct answer is D. Classically, those with visual motion sensitivity are bothered by complex movement as exemplified by rapidly moving traffic. Presyncope is usually more random in the setting it occurs, and malingering is quite unlikely without any evidence of a potential gain. Anxiety is possible, though fear of falling is more consistent with a history of actual falls and a physiologic etiology for disequilibrium.

REFERENCE

Tinetti ME, Baker DI, Dutcher J, et al. *Reducing the risk of falls among older adults in the community.* Berkeley, CA: Peaceable Kingdom Press; 1997.

SUGGESTED READING

Adkin AL, Frank JS, Carpenter MG, et al. Postural control is scaled to level of postural threat. *Gait Posture.* 2000;12:87–93.

Beidel DC, Horak FB. Behavior therapy for vestibular rehabilitation. *Anxiety Disord.* 2001;15:121–130.

Berg KO, Wood-Dauphinee SL, Williams JI, et al. Measuring balance in the elderly: validation of an instrument. *Physiotherapy Canada.* 1989;41(6):304–306.

Bloem BR, Grimbergen YA, Cramer M, et al. Prospective assessment of falls in Parkinson's disease. *J Neurol.* 2001;248(11):950–958.

Camicioli R, Howieson D, Lehman S. Talking while walking: the effect of a dual task in ageing and Alzheimer's disease. *Neurology.* 1997;48:955–958.

Frenklach A, Louie S, Miller M, et al. Excessive postural sway and the risk for falls at different stages of Parkinson's disease. *Mov Disord.* 2009;24(3):377–385.

Gillespie LD, Gillespie WJ, Cumming R, et al. Interventions for preventing falls in the elderly. *Cochrane Database Syst Rev.* 2003;(4):CD000340.

Grimbergen YA, Munneke M, Bloem BR. Falls in Parkinson's disease. *Curr Opin Neurol.* 2004;17(4): 405–415.

Horak F. Postural ataxia related to somatosensory loss. In: Ruzicka E, Hallett M, Jankovix J, eds. *Gait Disorders, Advances in Neurology.* Philadelphia: Lippincott Williams & Wilkins; 2001:173–181.

Horak FB. Postural orientation and equilibrium: what do we need to know about neural control of balance to prevent falls? *Age Ageing.* 2006;35-S2:ii7–ii11.

Horak FB, Frank JS, Nutt JG. Effects of dopamine on postural control in Parkinsonian subjects: scaling, set and tone. *J Neurophys.* 1996;75:2380–2396.

Horak FB, Macpherson JM. Postural orientation and equilibrium. In: Rowell LB, Shepard JT, eds. *Handbook of Physiology*: Section 12, Exercise Regulation and Integration of Multiple Systems. New York: Oxford University Press; 1996;255–292.

Horak FB, Shupert CL, eds. *Role of the Vestibular System in Postural Control. Vestibular Rehabilitation.* 2nd ed. Philadelphia: F.A. Davis; 1999.

Horak FB, Shupert CL, Mirka, A. Components of postural dyscontrol in the elderly: a review. *Neurobiol Ageing.* 1989;10:727–738.

Iyer S, Naganathan V, McLachlan AJ, et al. Medication withdrawal trials in people aged 65 years and older: a systematic review. *Drugs Aging.* 2008;25(12): 1021–1031.

Lord S, Sherrington C, Menz H, et al. *Falls in Older People: Risk Factors and Strategies for Prevention.*

2nd ed. New York: Cambridge University Press; 2007.

Lord SR, Ward JA, Williams P, et al. Physiological factors associated with falls in older community-dwelling women. *J Am Geriat Soc.* 1994;42:1110–1117.

Parker MJ, Gillespie LD, Gillespie WJ. Hip protectors for preventing hip fractures in the elderly. *Cochrane Database Syst Rev.* 2004;(3):CD001255.

Pickering RM, Grimbergen YAM, Rigney U, et al. A meta-analysis of six prospective studies of falling in Parkinson's disease. *Mov Disord.* 2007;22(13): 1892–1900.

Shupert CL, Horak FB. Adaptation of postural control in normal and pathologic ageing: implications for fall prevention programs. *J Appl Biomech.* 1999;15:64–74.

Stolze H, Klebe S, Zechlin C, et al. Falls in frequent neurologic diseases—prevalence, risk factors and aetiology. *J Neurol.* 2004;251(1):79–84.

Tinetti ME, Inouye SK, Gill TM, et al. Shared risk factors for falls, incontinence and functional dependence: unifying the approach to geriatric syndromes. *J Am Med Assoc.* 1995;273:1348–1353.

Tinetti ME, Speechley M, Ginter SF. Risk factors for falls among elderly persons living in the community. *N Engl J Med.* 1988;319:1701–1707.

Visser M, Marinus J, Bloem BR, et al. Clinical tests for the evaluation of postural instability in patients with Parkinson's disease. *Arch Phys Med Rehabil.* 2003;84(11):1669–1674.

Willemson MD, Grimbergen YAM, Slabbekoorn M, et al. Falling in Parkinson disease: more often due to postural instability than to environmental factors. *Ned Tijdschr Geneeskd.* 2000;144(48):2309–2314.

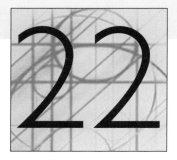

22

Neurotoxic Effects of Drugs Prescribed by Non-neurologists

KATIE KOMPOLITI

key points

- Careful assessment of the medication list should be part of the assessment of any new neurologic presentation.

- Drug-induced neurologic side effects do not always resolve immediately after discontinuation of the offending agent.

- Drug–drug interactions could be responsible for neurologic side effects by altering the offending agent's metabolism, and therefore its plasma concentrations.

- Neurotoxicity can occur even when levels of the offending agent are in the therapeutic range.

Neurotoxicology is a growing field of clinical interest, and physicians increasingly are required to evaluate and treat patients with numerous complications of toxic exposure. The usual compounds discussed in a chapter on neurotoxicology would include metals (e.g., lead, mercury, and arsenic), industrial toxins (e.g., organic solvents, gases, pesticides, and other environmental toxins), and biologic toxins (e.g., bacterial exotoxins, animal poisons, venoms, and botanical poisons). Syndromes associated with these toxins, however, are not frequently encountered by the non-neurologist. Yet many drugs that are commonly prescribed by treating physicians may precipitate neurotoxic signs or exacerbate the underlying neurologic disease. The neurologic complications of drugs commonly prescribed for the medical management of ambulatory adults are discussed in this chapter.

ANTIBIOTICS

Penicillins

Penicillin and related agents rarely cause nervous system toxic effects, although seizures and myoclonic jerks have been reported with high intravenous (IV) doses. Such effects appear more commonly in elderly patients with compromised renal function. Meningitic inflammation may enhance neurotoxic effects by promoting the penetration of these drugs into the central nervous system (CNS) and decreasing their egress. Polyneuritis, with paresthesias, paralysis, and loss of tendon reflexes, also has been reported.

Cephalosporins

Cephalosporins may cause a number of neurotoxic effects, especially in patients with renal dysfunction or in those receiving high doses. Symptoms can include confusion, coma, tremor, myoclonic jerks, asterixis, and hyperexcitability. Status epilepticus that did not respond to anticonvulsant therapy and subsequently resolved with discontinuation of cefepime has been described in two patients receiving this fourth-generation cephalosporin.

Aminoglycosides

The toxicities of all aminoglycoside antibiotics—neomycin, kanamycin, streptomycin, gentamycin, tobramycin, and amikacin—are similar. The two major adverse effects are (a) damage of the eighth cranial nerve and hearing apparatus and (b) a potentiation of neuromuscular blockade. Cochlear and vestibular damage is the result of direct toxicity of these drugs. Auditory toxicity is more common with the use of amikacin and kanamycin, whereas vestibular toxicity predominates following gentamycin and streptomycin therapy. Tobramycin is associated equally with vestibular and auditory damage. The incidence of clinical ototoxicity as a result of use of these drugs ranges from 5% to 25%, depending on

whether audiometry is used to detect hearing deficits. Aminoglycoside hearing loss is usually irreversible and may even progress after the discontinuation of drug therapy.

■ **SPECIAL CLINICAL POINT: A potentially fatal neurotoxic effect of all aminoglycosides is a neuromuscular blockade.**

The aminoglycosides act similarly to curare, blocking the neuromuscular junction. Aminoglycosides also possibly potentiate ether and other anesthetics during surgery. Sudden or prolonged respiratory paralysis resulting from aminoglycoside use may be reversed by the administration of calcium or neostigmine.

Antifungal Agents

The polymyxins are related closely to the aminoglycosides in structure and neurotoxicity. The incidence of neurotoxic reaction has been estimated at 7%, and syndromes other than neuromuscular blockade include paresthesias, peripheral neuropathy, dizziness, and seizures. Respiratory paralysis, however, is the most serious neurotoxic reaction. An underlying renal dysfunction predisposes to the neuromuscular blockade induced by this drug group. Signs of neuromuscular blockade include diplopia, dysphagia, and weakness.

Amphotericin B is widely used against systemic fungal infection. When the drug is used intrathecally, seizures, pain along the lumbar nerves, mononeuropathies (including foot drop), and chemical meningitis have occurred.

Antituberculous Drugs

Isoniazid (INH) has been associated with neurotoxic effects felt to be related to drug binding of pyridoxine and resultant excessive vitamin excretion. A prominent polyneuropathy is associated with chronic INH administration, and symptoms include paresthesias; diminished pain, touch, and temperature discrimination; and eventual weakness. Seizures, emotional irritability, euphoria, depression, headache, and psychosis rarely may occur. The neurotoxic reactions from INH use are dose related and are more common in "slow inactivators." In these patients, neurotoxic reactions can be prevented or diminished by the administration of pyridoxine at a dose of 50 mg daily. Patients who intentionally or inadvertently overdose acutely with INH may develop severe ataxia, generalized seizures, and coma. Supportive measures, anticonvulsants, and pyridoxine should be administered to these patients.

Rifamycin frequently is administered with INH. Neurologic side effects are uncommon but may include headache, dizziness, inability to concentrate, and confusion. Less commonly, signs of peripheral neuropathy may develop. Ethambutol precipitates a reversible optic neuritis as well as a more generalized peripheral neuropathy. A metallic taste in the oral cavity frequently is associated with ethambutol therapy and may be due to the result of an impairment of receptor activity.

Antiviral Drugs

The treatment of selected viral infections in individuals who are not positive for the human immunodeficiency virus (HIV) has become possible over the past few years. The neurologic complications of HIV and the drugs used to treat it will be discussed elsewhere.

Acyclovir can be administered either intravenously or orally. Acyclovir is used orally for the treatment of localized or ophthalmic varicella zoster, treatment of minor herpes simplex virus, and reducing the severity of varicella. It is used intravenously to treat herpes encephalitis. Neurologic side effects rarely are associated with oral acyclovir. However, seizures, encephalopathy, hallucinations, and coma have been described, as has tremor.

Amantadine has been used to prevent influenza A infections. This agent appears to have, in addition to its antiviral action, anticholinergic and dopaminergic effects, which has led to its use in mild Parkinson disease. The neurologic side effects associated with amantadine include, confusion, myoclonus, hallucinations, delirium, and seizures. As amantadine is excreted through the kidney, the presence of renal impairment may reduce its clearance, causing it to accumulate in the body and resulting in amantadine toxicity.

OTHER COMMONLY PRESCRIBED ANTIBIOTICS

Sulfonamide, pyrimethamine, and trimethoprim are used mainly in the treatment of urinary tract infections (UTIs). They generally are considered safe drugs and are not associated with marked neurotoxicity. They may cause headache, fatigue, tinnitus, and acute psychosis, however. Some signs may mimic meningitis. On the second or third day of therapy, patients may complain of difficulty in concentrating and impaired judgment. Nitrofurantoin also is used commonly in the treatment of UTIs. A polyneuropathy is the major toxic syndrome with this drug. Like the Guillain–Barré syndrome, this neuropathy is usually subacute and begins in the distal extremities, often with sensory complaints of paresthesias and numbness. The neuropathy ascends and involves the motor system, with progressive weakness and areflexia. Discontinuation of the drug is essential, and not all patients will recover. The prognosis appears to relate most significantly to the extent of the neuropathy at the time of drug withdrawal.

Tetracycline can be associated with pseudotumor cerebri or increased intracranial pressure. The syndrome is characterized by headache; papilledema; elevated spinal fluid pressure; and, in babies, bulging fontanels. Significant vestibular toxicity also has been associated with a tetracycline derivative, minocycline.

Erythromycin is probably the least toxic of the commonly used antibiotics from a neurologic perspective. An uncommon side effect is temporary hearing loss. Erythromycin interacts with carbamazepine; thus the anticonvulsant levels increase rapidly when erythromycin is introduced.

Azithromycin, a macrolide antibiotic, also has been reported to cause hearing loss. Clarithromycin has been reported to precipitate an acute psychotic episode.

Nitrofurantoin therapy has been associated with polyneuropathy. Generally seen with prolonged therapy, neuropathy can occur as early as the first week of treatment. It is usually subacute, begins in the distal extremities with paresthesias, and tends to progressively ascend to involve the motor system with weakness and areflexia. Although this polyneuropathy clinically resembles Guillain–Barré syndrome, the spinal fluid is usually normal, except that 25% of patients have a slight increase in protein without pleocytosis. When polyneuropathy is recognized, drug withdrawal is essential, although 10% to 15% of patients will not improve and 15% will have only partial recovery. The prognosis appears to correlate with the extent of the neuropathy at the time of drug withdrawal but not to the total dose exposure or the duration of therapy.

ANTIRETROVIRAL MEDICATIONS

Patients infected with HIV are living longer than before as the result of a better understanding of the disease process and newer pharmacologic agents often used in combination to control viral loads. The currently available classes of antiretrovirals for HIV infection include protease inhibitors, nucleoside reverse transcriptase inhibitors, nonnucleoside reverse transcriptase inhibitors, and fusion inhibitors. New drug regimens support the use of concomitant medications from each class in HIV-positive individuals to prevent the complications of AIDS. Most of these agents can have headache as a side effect.

The major neurologic side effects of nucleoside reverse transcriptase inhibitors include peripheral neuropathy. This is typically a distal symmetric predominantly sensory neuropathy and has been described with zalcitabine, didanosine, and stavudine. Electromyography demonstrates an axonal neuropathy. It may be difficult to determine the origin of the neuropathy because HIV infection also can cause a distal sensory neuropathy. The treatment includes removal of the offending agent. Myopathy of mitochondrial origin has been reported with both the nucleoside reverse transcriptase inhibitors and the nonnucleoside reverse transcriptase inhibitors. This is a proximal symmetric myopathy with a mitochondrial pattern of ragged-red fibers. Removal of the offending agent is the best treatment.

The major neurologic side effects of the nonnucleoside reverse transcriptase inhibitors include dizziness, somnolence, diminished concentration, and confusion. The patient also may experience psychiatric disturbances including agitation, depersonalization, hallucinations, insomnia, vivid dreams, depression, and euphoria. These symptoms are most severe at initiation of therapy. They typically resolve with elimination of the offending medication. Among the different nonnucleoside reverse transcriptase inhibitors, efavirenz has been commonly associated with neurotoxicity.

■ **SPECIAL CLINICAL POINT: People of African descent with a variant of hepatic enzyme CYP2B6 may experience slower clearance of nonnucleoside reverse transcriptase inhibitors and increased neurotoxicity.**

TRANSPLANT DRUGS

Cyclosporine

Neurotoxicity is a well-recognized sequela of cyclosporine, and the most common complications are tremor and altered mental status. Cyclosporine neurotoxicity can occur in 1 in 10 patients after liver transplantation. Behavioral signs include acute psychosis, restlessness, wide mood swings with inappropriate crying and laughing, cortical blindness, visual hallucinations, stupor, and akinetic mutism. Additionally, seizures, extrapyramidal symptoms, action myoclonus, and quadriparesis have been reported. In patients with neurologic signs, cyclosporine levels are usually outside the normal range, and after lowering the dose or withholding administration, neurotoxicity clears in most cases. MRI abnormalities are consistent with cortical or white matter high-signal changes with a predilection for the occipital lobes. The mechanism of cyclosporine neurotoxicity has not been fully elucidated. Both the clinical manifestations and the neuroimaging abnormalities of cyclosporine neurotoxicity usually resolve with a reduction or discontinuation of cyclosporine.

Other Transplant Immunosuppressives

Other transplant immunosuppressives include basiliximab, daclizumab, mycophenolate mofetil, sirolimus and tacrolimus. Typical neurologic effects of long-term immunosuppression include infections such as meningitis, encephalitis, and abscess formation and are similar with the newer agents as they were with the older ones. Direct neurologic toxicity is more common with tacrolimus, a calcineurin inhibitor–like cyclosporine, while the others exhibit toxicity that spares the nervous system.

Although tacrolimus may be a better immunosuppressant than cyclosporine, its neurologic effects may be worse. In a multicenter, randomized, parallel-group study of 545 patients undergoing primary liver transplantation, tacrolimus was associated with a higher incidence of neurologic symptoms than cyclosporine. The risk of tacrolimus-treated patients developing tremor was related to the initial IV dose, the rate of administration, and the total daily dose. Headache was significantly correlated with dose, while insomnia was not. Factors that may promote the development of serious complications include advanced liver failure, hypertension, hypocholesterolemia, elevated serum levels, hypomagnesemia, and methylprednisone. The symptoms may be reversed by reducing the dose of immunosuppressant or by discontinuation.

However, some patients have experienced permanent or even fatal neurologic damage even after discontinuation of tacrolimus. Occipital white matter appears to be uniquely susceptible to the neurotoxic effects of tacrolimus as is the case with cyclosporine. Magnetic resonance imaging has been reported to reveal bilateral symmetric regions of signal abnormality with abnormal contrast enhancement. The abnormal signal was more evident in FLAIR (fluid-attenuated inversion recovery) sequences. Epilepsy and cerebral hemorrhage have been reported to be associated with tacrolimus-induced neurotoxicity.

CARDIAC DRUGS

Glycosides

Digitalis and related agents are the mainstay of treatment for congestive heart failure. Neurologic complications of digitalis therapy have been recognized for almost 200 years and are characterized by nausea, vomiting, visual disturbances, seizures, and syncope. Adverse effects on the CNS reportedly occur in 40% to 50% of patients with clinical digitalis toxicity and may occur before, simultaneously with, or after the signs of cardiac toxicity develop.

The most frequent and often the first sign of clinical intoxication is nausea, which appears to be the result of central mechanisms rather than gastrointestinal irritation. The incidence of digitalis-related visual disturbances has been estimated at 40%, and although these symptoms may occur as an isolated symptom, they usually occur concomitantly with other toxic signs. Blurred vision, reversible scotomas, diplopia, defects of color vision, and total amaurosis represent the spectrum of optic side effects.

Seizures most commonly are seen in pediatric patients. The incidence of digitalis-related seizures is difficult to estimate because other seizure etiologies (e.g., arrhythmia) are so high in cardiac patients. Transient mental aberrations felt to be caused by intermittent cerebral hypoperfusion resemble transient global amnesia. Syncope, probably the result of conduction delay or hyperactivity of baroreceptors, also has occurred in digitalis toxicity. Other neurotoxic reactions include facial neuralgia, paresthesias, headache, weakness, and fatigue. Cerebral symptoms consisting of confusion, delirium, mania, and hallucinosis have been reported in as many as 15% of patients with digitalis toxicity. Although the mechanism for the symptoms is unknown, it is felt that they are not the result of altered cardiac function.

Antianginal Agents

Nitroglycerin and nitrate therapy frequently is associated with headache. According to currently proposed mechanisms, nitric oxide is the common mediator in experimental vascular headaches. Nitroglycerin produces a throbbing or pulsating sensation in many patients and an overt headache in many others. Often, the headaches attenuate or disappear with time, but 15% to 20% of patients will not be able to tolerate long-acting nitrates because of headache. Patients should be encouraged to use analgesics during the initial days or weeks of nitrate therapy and should be educated as to the nature of this problem and its probable resolution with time.

Nitroglycerin therapy can cause dose-related increases in intracranial pressure, which in rare cases can result in a clinically overt syndrome. Furthermore, the hypotensive effects of nitroglycerin can result in dizziness and light-headedness or even syncope.

Antiarrhythmics

Quinidine is used mainly to treat atrial fibrillation. Nervous system manifestations are usually not significant, but with overdosage or in susceptible individuals the following may occur: headache, nausea, vomiting, blurring of vision, ringing of the ears, flushing, palpitations, and even convulsions. A precipitous decrease in blood pressure related to vagal influences can cause syncope, vertigo, and respiratory arrest (on rare occasions).

Lidocaine-induced CNS toxicity occurs commonly and may relate to its rapid absorption across the blood–brain barrier. The syndrome appears to relate to a diffuse excitement of neuronal systems, with an early prodrome of altered behavior. Garrulousness and loss of inhibitions may be the prominent feature, as may agitation or psychosis. Circumoral numbness, diplopia, and tinnitus also may occur, with progressive muscle twitches and tremors. Generalized myoclonic seizures and finally CNS and respiratory depression are seen with higher doses. In both cardiac and surgical patients, hypoxia and acidosis develop rapidly if the lidocaine syndrome is not reversed. Treatment focuses on adequate oxygenation and support because the half-life of bolus lidocaine given acutely is 6 to 8 minutes. Because repeated injections change the kinetics of lidocaine and prolong its half-life to approximately 90 minutes, however, more long-lasting effects can be seen.

Procainamide may cause light-headedness and even syncope because of the hypotensive action. Additionally, a lupus erythematosus syndrome can develop in patients taking procainamide, and 80% of patients receiving the drug for 6 months have antinuclear antibodies; these antibodies clear with the withdrawal of the agent. During lupus-like syndrome, encephalopathy with confusion and agitation can develop. Procainamide also has a curare-like effect at the neuromuscular junction and hence can precipitate myasthenia gravis or exacerbate it.

Tocainide hydrochloride is an antiarrhythmic agent that is structurally and pharmacologically similar to lidocaine, except that it is well absorbed when given orally. Tocainide has been proven effective in managing various ventricular arrhythmias; however, because it crosses the blood–brain barrier, it frequently causes several neurologic side effects, which include light-headedness, dizziness, tremor, twitching, paresthesias, sweating, hot flashes, blurred vision, diplopia, and mood changes. Peak plasma concentrations of tocainide occur within 1 to 2 hours of ingestion; the plasma half-life is 12 to 15 hours in patients with unimpaired renal and hepatic systems. CNS side effects appear to be linearly related to the dose.

Bretylium is a parenteral antiarrhythmic drug used in the prophylaxis and treatment of ventricular fibrillation and life-threatening ventricular arrhythmias that do not respond to first-line agents such as lidocaine. The antiarrhythmic mechanisms of bretylium in humans are not clearly defined, but in animals it increases the ventricular fibrillatory threshold and also the action potential duration and effective refractory period. It induces a state of chemical sympathectomy.

The most significant side effect of this drug is severe supine and orthostatic hypotension. Patients report dizziness, light-headedness, vertigo, and faintness. Bretylium may also rarely cause flushing, hyperthermia, confusion, paranoid psychosis, mood changes, anxiety, lethargy, and nasal stuffiness.

Amiodarone is an orally effective antiarrhythmic drug that, like bretylium, slows repolarization in various myocardial fibers and raises the threshold for ventricular fibrillation. Early reports of adverse effects include corneal microdeposits, thyroid dysfunction, and cutaneous photosensitivity. However, toxic neurologic side effects now have been described, and in a series of 54 patients studied, these side effects were the most common reason for either altering or discontinuing amiodarone therapy.

A reversible syndrome of tremor, ataxia, and peripheral neuropathy without nystagmus, dizziness, encephalopathy, or long-tract signs developed in 54% of these patients. Tremor occurred earliest and most frequently (29%). The 6- to 10-Hz flexion–extension movements in the fingers, wrists, and elbows were indistinguishable from essential tremor. Of the patients, 37% reported ataxia associated with falls, staggering, and difficulty in dressing the lower limbs. The ability to walk was seriously impaired in 18% of the patients. None of these patients had preexisting gait problems, and

none had sensory or long-tract abnormalities on examination. Peripheral neuropathy associated with this drug was first reported in 1974 and continues to account for a significant portion of the neurologic toxicity reported today. The neuropathy is sensorimotor in type and generally causes numbness and tingling of all four extremities. Proximal weakness occasionally accompanies the paresthesias. Sural nerve biopsies have been examined and have revealed demyelination with mild axonal loss in some cases. Lamellated inclusions of lysosomal origin were found in all cell types in the nerves and are a characteristic finding of this neuropathy.

Diuretics

Diuretics are divided into three principal groups: thiazide, loop, and potassium sparing. Diuretics most frequently cause extracardiac side effects as a direct result of the electrolytes lost or retained in the renal system. Each group, however, can cause adverse effects that are linked indirectly to electrolyte and water balance.

The thiazide diuretics have been reported to cause syncope, acute muscle cramps and pain, hyporeflexia, weakness, flaccid paralysis, and epileptiform movements. The deterioration of mental function, including the development of coma, can be precipitated with thiazide administration in patients being treated for cirrhosis. Thiazides given concomitantly with triamterene and amantadine can increase the likelihood of neurotoxicity from the amantadine.

If loop diuretics, particularly furosemide, are given quickly and in high doses, they can cause deafness and paresthesias. If they are given to a patient who also is receiving lithium chronically, loop diuretics can alter the renal clearance of lithium and increase the risk of lithium toxicity and fluid electrolyte abnormalities. Loop diuretics also potentially can increase the success with which succinylcholine blocks the neuromuscular junction in anesthetized patients.

Potassium-sparing diuretics, including spironolactone and triamterene, have been reported to cause confusion, drowsiness, muscle weakness, paresthesias, dizziness (although this may be a result of cardiac rhythm changes), and headache.

Sympatholytics

Clonidine is an alpha 2-noradrenergic agonist, and some have suggested that this drug induces an overall decrease in norepinephrine release, possibly through a presynaptic mechanism. Sedation is the most common adverse neurologic effect of clonidine. Other less common neurotoxic reactions include depression, nightmares, and reversible dementia syndrome.

Neuropsychiatric symptoms occur frequently during treatment with beta blockers. The pharmacology of CNS side effects is unclear, although presynaptic and postsynaptic adrenergic inhibition has been implicated, as has serotonergic antagonism. Nonselective beta blockers seem to cause CNS-related side effects to a greater extent than beta 1-selective blockers. It is unclear to what degree lipophilicity is responsible for this kind of side effect. Lassitude or insomnia and depression are the most common reactions, although vivid dreams, nightmares, hypnagogic hallucinations, and psychotic behavior have been reported with high doses (more than 500 mg/day of propranolol). Preexisting major psychiatric illness and hyperthyroidism may predispose to the previously mentioned symptoms.

Prazosin competitively blocks the vascular postsynaptic alpha-adrenergic receptors and is the first of a class of similar antagonists derived from quinazoline. The selective affinity of prazosin for alpha-receptors allows it to block the contractile response of vascular smooth muscle to norepinephrine, consequently lowering mean arterial pressure and peripheral resistance. Like other antihypertensives that cause vasodilatation, prazosin causes hypotension; dizziness and faintness have been reported in up to 50% of patients receiving this drug. These are most pronounced after the first dose(s) or in patients who have had a hiatus from the drug and are reinstituting treatment. Hypotension can be minimized if the initial dose is small and is given at bedtime. Other CNS side effects include headache, dry mouth, nasal stuffiness, lassitude, hallucinations, depression, paresthesias, nervousness, and priapism.

Vasodilators

Hydralazine is the only direct-acting vasodilator generally available for the treatment of chronic hypertension. The neurologic side effects of hydralazine are few and uncommon in clinical practice. Peripheral neuropathy characterized by diffuse numbness and tingling is the only consistent neurotoxic reaction and is felt to be the result of a direct toxic effect of the drug.

Calcium channel blockers, particularly flunarizine and cinnarizine, have been associated with dystonia, parkinsonism, akathisia, and tardive dyskinesia (TD). Theoretic explanations for these events include the inhibition of calcium influx into striatal cells and direct dopaminergic antagonistic properties. Evidence also suggests that inhibition of proton pumping and catecholamine uptake are possible mechanisms. In addition, the chemical structures of flunarizine and cinnarizine, which are related to neuroleptics, may explain the greater incidence of such side effects with these agents compared with those of calcium channel blockers available in the United States. Suggested risk factors appear to be advanced age and a family history of tremors or Parkinson disease, or both. The onset and type of presentation are unpredictable. The long-term evolution was assessed in a prospective follow-up study of 32 patients with diagnoses of calcium channel blocker–induced parkinsonism. Eighteen months following discontinuation of the offending agent, 44% of the patients had depression, 88% had tremor, and 33% still had criteria for diagnosis of parkinsonism.

Angiotensin-Converting Enzyme Inhibitors

Angiotensin-converting enzyme inhibitors have been used in the United States to treat moderate to severe hypertension, based on its effect on the renin–angiotensin–aldosterone (RAA) axis. This cascading hormonal axis simultaneously maintains systemic arterial pressure and sodium balance by detecting and correcting even small changes in renal perfusion. Alongside the increased understanding of the RAA axis has come the discovery of drugs that specifically and selectively inhibit the RAA cascade.

Few neurologic side effects have been reported; however, in a large multinational study, 5% of the participating patients reported symptoms of hypotension, including dizziness, light-headedness, and vertigo. These symptoms were generally transient and mild and most frequently occurred in patients who were sodium or water depleted. Dysgeusia occurred in 2% to 4% of patients participating in this small trial. The incidence of taste change or loss increased in patients with impaired renal function.

Cholesterol-Lowering Agents

Clofibrate, an aromatic monocarboxylic acid, is capable of inducing myotonia in humans and experimental animals and is clinically significant because it is widely used to reduce serum triglyceride levels. The mechanism by which it induces myotonia is believed to be through a decrease in chloride conductance.

HMG-CoA reductase inhibitors or statins have been implicated in causing toxic myopathy. Statin myotoxicity ranges from asymptomatic creatine kinase elevations or myalgias to muscles necrosis and fatal rhabdomyolysis. Statins may also cause an autoimmune myopathy requiring immunosuppressive treatment. The mechanisms of statin myotoxicity are unclear. If unrecognized in its early manifestations, complications from continued statin therapy may lead to rhabdomyolysis and death. Risk factors for myotoxicity are concomitant medication use and medical conditions that alter statin metabolism as well as the patient's underlying genetic constitution. According to findings from 21 clinical trials providing 180,000 person-years of follow-up in patients treated with statin or placebo, myopathy (defined as muscle symptoms plus creatine kinase [CK] >10 times the upper limit of normal) occurs in 5 patients per 100,000 person-years and rhabdomyolysis in 1.6 patients per 100,000 person-years (placebo corrected). The most common muscle side effects remain myalgia (i.e., muscle pain or soreness), weakness, and/or cramps without CK elevations. These symptoms are most often tolerable, but occasionally can be intolerable and debilitating, requiring the statin to be withdrawn. Muscle symptoms have been reported in clinical trials to occur in 1.5% to 3.0% of patients receiving statin therapy, most often without an elevation in the CK level, and at an equivalent rate in patients given placebo. The incidence of muscle complaints among patients being treated in a practice setting ranges from 0.3% to 33% (Bays, 2006). The higher rate may occur partly because statin-intolerant patients and those with risk factors for muscle toxicity are more likely to be excluded from clinical trials.

■ **SPECIAL CLINICAL POINT: The potential of different statins for myotoxicity may be altered by concomitant medications that alter their metabolism.**

GASTROINTESTINAL AGENTS

Common gastrointestinal problems include the hypermotility disorders with vomiting and/or diarrhea; hypomotility disorders, with constipation; or excessive acid secretion leading to "heartburn" or ulcerations. A wide variety of drugs commonly are recommended for these disorders. Fortunately, neurologic complications from these frequently prescribed agents are infrequent.

Laxatives

There are only a few neurologic complications associated with the drugs used to treat constipation. Docusate sodium (Colace) is a stool softener that occasionally causes nausea or a bitter taste. The long-term use of nonprescription laxatives may cause neurologic complications arising secondary to depletion of electrolytes. Profound muscle weakness may occur from the potassium depletion following chronic laxative intake. The irritant purgatives, such as cascara, may damage the myenteric plexus of the colon, leading to a reduction of intestinal motility and a worsening of constipation.

Antiemetics

Of the antiemetic drugs, several commonly prescribed agents act as dopamine receptor blockers in a similar fashion to the neuroleptic drugs described later. Metoclopramide (Reglan), prochlorperazine (Compazine), and promethazine (Phenergan) are three widely used antiemetics with neuroleptic properties. Sedation may occur as an early complaint with the introduction of these agents. In addition, acute dystonia, with distressing involuntary spasms of head, neck, eyes, facial, and trunk muscles, may occur, particularly in children treated with prochlorperazine. If not recognized by the clinician, these acute, sometimes bizarre, symptoms may be inaccurately thought to have a psychogenic etiology. The treatment of the acute dystonia from the dopamine receptor–blocking antiemetics is the administration of anticholinergic agents.

In addition to acute dystonia, these dopamine receptor antagonist, antiemetic agents may cause a parkinsonian syndrome, clinically indistinguishable from idiopathic Parkinson disease. Those of more advanced age appear to be more susceptible to this neurologic complication and may even be treated with antidopaminergic agents if the symptoms are not recognized as being associated with the medication. Akathisia also may occur as a side effect of these medications. If these agents are used on a long-term

basis, as in the treatment of chronic esophageal reflux, the potentially irreversible symptoms of TD even may occur.

■ **SPECIAL CLINICAL POINT:**
Metoclopramide (Reglan), prochlorperazine (Compazine), and promethazine (Phenergan) induced parkinsonism may take up to 6 months to reverse after discontinuation of the medication.

A different type of agent with predominantly anticholinergic effect, scopolamine, is prescribed for the treatment of motion-induced nausea and vomiting. Scopolamine has become available in a long-acting, transdermal patch preparation. The neurologic side effects of scopolamine are those associated with blockade of muscarinic receptors. The most frequent is xerostomia. The reduction in saliva production, if severe, can lead to mucosal ulcerations and dental problems. Other peripheral effects of scopolamine include blurred near vision resulting from alterations in accommodation, reduced sweating, and urinary retention from effects on bladder muscles. A potentially irreversible effect of the anticholinergic agents is the exacerbation of closed-angle glaucoma with the potential for causing blindness.

The CNS side effects of these drugs include sedation and confusion. Losses in recent and immediate memory can occur at high doses. Finally, with toxicity, delirium and hallucinations have been described.

Antidiarrheals

Drugs used to symptomatically alleviate diarrhea frequently contain morphine or morphine derivatives. These compounds act to reduce the propulsive contractions of the small bowel and colon. The neurologic adverse effects from these agents include sedation, respiratory depression, and coma, typically with pupillary constriction.

Anticholinergic agents also have been used to treat symptoms of diarrhea. Diphenoxylate–atropine (Lomotil) is a widely prescribed antidiarrheal agent. Overdoses of this agent most frequently cause a predominantly opioid intoxication.

Some antidiarrheal compounds (e.g., Donnatal) are combinations of morphine derivatives and from one to three different anticholinergic agents. Donnatal contains phenobarbital, hyoscyamine, atropine, and scopolamine. Although each component is present only in small amounts, patients taking several tablets a day or elderly persons may experience significant side effects.

Bismuth compounds, as found in the nonprescription bismuth subsalicylate (Pepto-Bismol), have been recommended for the treatment of "traveler's diarrhea." The neurologic sequelae of these agents are rare. There have been reports of an acute reversible psychotic reaction following excessive use of these compounds as a result of acute bismuth toxicity. More commonly, tinnitus is noted with large doses, arising from the salicylate component in this compound.

Antiacidity Agents

The magnesium and aluminum antacids, if taken in large quantities or with renal impairment, may cause neurologic symptoms secondary to alteration in electrolytes. Sucralfate is an aluminum compound that coats the gastric mucosa. Although little of this agent is absorbed directly, sucralfate may reduce the absorption of phenytoin and, in those taking this anticonvulsant, may result in a drop in phenytoin levels below the therapeutic range.

The H_2 receptor antagonists inhibit acid secretion from the parietal cells. Currently, four H_2 receptor antagonists are approved for use in the United States. Cimetidine (Tagamet) was the first to be developed. More recently developed H_2 receptor antagonists include ranitidine (Zantac), nizatidine (Axid), and famotidine (Pepcid). The neurologic complications of these medications include lethargy, confusion, depression, hallucinations, and headache. Individuals treated with these drugs who develop unexplained encephalopathic symptoms may improve with the discontinuation of these agents. Additionally, the effect of cimetidine—and, to a lesser degree, the other H_2 blockers—on the cytochrome P450 enzymes in the liver may alter the pharmacokinetic profile of other drugs undergoing hepatic degradation, including warfarin and phenytoin.

RESPIRATORY AGENTS

Adrenergic Drugs

Of the three types of adrenergic receptors (alpha, B1, B2), it is the B2 receptor that mediates bronchodilation. The first sympathomimetics available for the treatment of asthma were not B2 selective (metaproterenol, isoproterenol, epinephrine, ephedrine); therefore, in addition to dilating the bronchioli, they also produced significant cardiac and CNS effects. The introduction of B2-selective agents (albuterol, terbutaline) resulted in a reduction in the number of adverse effects. These agents are administered most efficiently by inhalation, resulting in benefit with minimal side effects. When these agents are administered parenterally, there may be nausea, vomiting, headache, and a variable-amplitude postural and action tremor associated with these agents.

Xanthine Bronchodilators

The xanthine compounds include aminophylline and theophylline. These agents now are prescribed only for those patients suffering with chronic rather than intermittent symptoms of bronchoconstriction. Theophylline is metabolized primarily in the liver, and drugs that affect hepatic enzymes, including tobacco, may alter the metabolism of theophylline. Liver disease, heart failure, and pulmonary disease tend to slow the metabolism of theophylline, sometimes resulting in toxicity even at low dosages. The therapeutic serum concentration of theophylline is 10 to 20 mg/mL. The side effects from theophylline tend to be dose related. However, even in the therapeutic range, neurologic side effects may occur. These include nausea, nervousness, insomnia, and headache. Although usually associated with toxic levels of theophylline, seizures also may occur in the high therapeutic range, particularly in the elderly or those with a history of previous brain injury. This latter group is likely to develop prolonged seizures with a poor outcome. The mechanism of theophylline-induced seizures is not clearly understood. In otherwise healthy asthmatics, the seizures are typically short lived with a good outcome. A recently described neurologic side effect observed in children is the occurrence of acquired stuttering, which resolves with the discontinuation of this drug.

PSYCHIATRIC DRUGS

Neuroleptic Agents

The neuroleptic agents or major tranquilizers exert their antipsychotic activity by blocking dopaminergic receptors at the level of the limbic system, forebrain, and basal ganglia. They also have antihistaminergic, anticholinergic, and anti–alpha 1-adrenergic properties. The newer, so-called atypical agents include clozapine, olanzapine, quetiapine, and risperidone. Many newer agents have some affinity for 5-HT$_2$ serotonin receptors as well (clozapine, risperidone). The atypical neuroleptic agents have become favored because of their lower extrapyramidal side effect profile. Many newer agents have some affinity for 5-HT$_2$ serotonin receptors as well (clozapine, risperidone). Neuroleptics, as a class, are associated with a variety of important neurologic complications. These can be classified as acute, subacute, and chronic side effects (Fig. 22.1).

Neuroleptics may cause a toxic confusional state, especially in the elderly, and confusion occurs more frequently with the low-potency, high-anticholinergic activity subclass (chlorpromazine, thioridazine, mesoridazine). These drugs also can produce profound sedation, especially with initiation of therapy.

Neuroleptics also lower the seizure threshold and have been associated with exacerbation of preexisting epilepsy as well as the de novo appearance of seizures. Clozapine

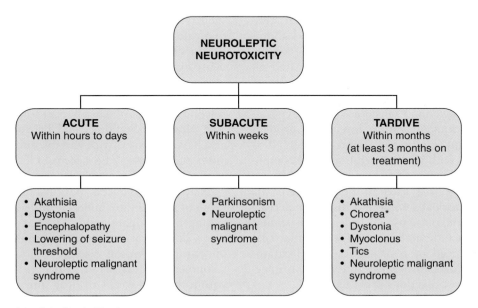

*classic tardive dyskinesia.

FIGURE 22.1 Acute, subacute, and chronic side effects of neuroleptic agents.

has been associated with generalized and myoclonic seizures. Seizures were present during the titration phase at low dosages (<300 mg/day) and at high dosages during the maintenance phase (600 mg/day).

Neuroleptic malignant syndrome (NMS) is associated with neuroleptic use. The pathogenesis of NMS is not completely understood. Alterations in dopaminergic transmission, changes in sympathetic outflow, alterations in central serotonin metabolism, and abnormalities in muscle membrane function have been implicated. NMS has been associated with all groups of neuroleptics, although high-potency agents, specifically haloperidol and fluphenazine, have been cited most frequently. NMS has been described with the atypical neuroleptic medications, clozapine, risperidone, and olanzapine. NMS tends to occur with the initiation of treatment or increases in dose and is more common with depot forms of neuroleptics. Affective disorder, concomitant lithium carbonate administration, psychomotor agitation, dehydration, exhaustion, and mild hyperthermia seem to increase susceptibility toward this condition. The principal features of NMS are hyperthermia, muscle rigidity, autonomic dysfunction, and mental status changes. Laboratory findings include elevated creatine kinase; polymorphonuclear leukocytosis; elevated aldolase, alkaline phosphatase, lactic dehydrogenase (LDH), alanine aminotransferase (ALT), and aspartate aminotransferase (AST); hypocalcemia; hypomagnesemia; low iron; proteinuria; and myoglobinuria. Approximately 40% of patients with NMS develop medical complications that may be life threatening. NMS is a clinical diagnosis based on the presence of the proper historical setting and the characteristic constellation of signs. Disorders with similar features include malignant hyperthermia; heat stroke induced by neuroleptics; lethal catatonia; other drug reactions; and vascular, infectious, or postinfectious brain damage.

NMS is a potentially fatal disease, and a high index of suspicion is required for early recognition and intervention. Treatment includes ceasing of the offending agent, providing supportive measures, and administering dantrolene or bromocriptine or a combination of the two.

Acute neuroleptic-induced dystonia can be seen early in the course of neuroleptic therapy or with dose increases. It often is seen following a single parenteral dose of neuroleptics. The manifestations can be diverse, although the most typical clinical signs involve oculogyric crises and opisthotonic posturing. Risk factors include young age, male gender, and use of high-potency neuroleptics. Acute dystonic reactions are self-limited, and if they are left untreated, they usually subside within 24 hours. Parenteral administration of anticholinergics, such as benztropine or diphenhydramine, offers immediate relief in the majority of cases, but oral anticholinergics should be continued for a few days until the causative neuroleptic is cleared.

Akathisia is a severe form of restlessness associated with the need to move. Typically, the patient paces incessantly in place and cannot sit down without continual volitional movement of the legs or feet. The pathophysiology of the syndrome is not well understood but may relate to the development of acute imbalance between the dopaminergic and cholinergic systems. This neuroleptic side effect usually occurs within the first days of therapy or with dose increases, and it resolves with withdrawal of the neuroleptic agent. Anticholinergics, amantadine, beta blockers, clonidine, and benzodiazepines also have been used with variable success. Late-onset akathisia may be a form of TD and may be more difficult to treat.

Neuroleptic-induced parkinsonism is the result of striatal dopaminergic underactivity resulting from dopaminergic D_2 receptor blockade. Clinically, it cannot be distinguished from idiopathic Parkinson disease, although its development occurs as a subacute syndrome within the first weeks of drug introduction or drug dosage increase. Parkinsonian symptoms resolve over a few weeks to 6 months after stopping the causative agent or with the use of antiparkinsonian drugs. Proposed risk factors for development of neuroleptic-induced parkinsonism are female gender, older age, and the use of high-potency agents. Treatment consists of discontinuing or reducing the dose of the offending agent. A lower-potency neuroleptic or one of several novel neuroleptics that lack prominent striatal receptor blockade, such as clozapine, can be substituted. Anticholinergics, amantadine, and electroconvulsive therapy are also possible treatments.

TD usually appears after several months or years of treatment with antipsychotic medications and almost never before 3 months. No consistent neuropathologic changes have been seen in patients with TD, and the predominant hypothesis for its genesis is denervation supersensitivity of the striatal dopamine receptors following chronic blockade. Risk factors for the development of TD include old age; female gender; presence of affective disorders; history of neuroleptic-induced parkinsonism; presence of organic brain disease; high-potency neuroleptics use; sufficient duration of treatment with neuroleptics; and possibly the use of anticholinergic medications, previous electroconvulsive treatment, and drug holidays.

In addition to the well-known oral–buccal–lingual masticatory movements and generalized chorea, dystonia, akathisia, tics, and myoclonus have been described. Once TD has appeared, its peak severity is reached rapidly and often is maintained. Following neuroleptic withdrawal, TD may transiently worsen, but this exacerbation is short lived. TD resolves in up to 33% of patients within 2 years after discontinuation of the offending agent. A prospective study comparing risperidone and haloperidol in 350 neuroleptic-naive patients, however, showed that each drug had a similar incidence of dystonia, parkinsonism, akithisia, and dyskinesia.

At present, prevention is the treatment of choice for TD. Therefore, neuroleptic agents should be used only when specifically needed and at the lowest possible doses. Once TD develops, the causative agent should be discontin-

ued, if possible. Alternatively, the patient should be switched to an atypical neuroleptic such as clozapine, which not only does not regularly cause TD but may even improve its symptoms. If neurologic impairment, disfigurement, or discomfort exists, treatment with the dopamine depleters reserpine or tetrabenazine should be considered. Noradrenergic antagonists (propranolol, clonidine); gamma-aminobutyric acid (GABA) agonists (clonazepam, diazepam, valproate, baclofen); botulinum toxin injections; and to a lesser degree, vitamin E, buspirone, and calcium channel blockers have been used with variable success.

Anxiolytics

Benzodiazepines are commonly prescribed anxiolytic agents. The therapeutic index of these agents is 10 to 30 times that of the barbiturates and, hence, their absolute toxicity is less. However, because these agents are so widely used, adverse reactions frequently are reported. The predominant toxic symptom is drowsiness or paradoxical excitation. Withdrawal seizures also have been reported. Dry mouth, tachycardia, dilated pupils, and depressed bowel sounds may occur early after the introduction of benzodiazepines because of possible anticholinergic effects. Withdrawal symptoms include excessive apprehension, anorexia, nausea, postural tremulousness, insomnia, and confusion. Withdrawal symptoms are best handled in the hospital, and barbiturates usually are substituted.

Antidepressant Agents

Tricyclic antidepressants (TCAs) induce an acute encephalopathy that is characterized by agitation, confusion, mydriasis, and sometimes convulsions. Tremor and myoclonus may be prominent motor features of this syndrome. Medical complications of these drugs include complex cardiac arrhythmias and heart block. Generalized support measures should be instituted for the patient who takes an overdose of

TCAs. Physostigmine, a centrally active cholinesterase inhibitor, 1 to 2 mg given IV, often will awaken a patient from coma. This finding suggests that much of the toxic mental alteration relates directly to central anticholinergic toxicity.

TCAs also may precipitate a more chronic neurotoxic syndrome in which tremor and sedation or insomnia are the prominent features. The tremor is usually postural or intentional and resembles that seen with amphetamine intoxication or use of lithium. Currently, most TCAs can be monitored with plasma levels, so that intoxication can be detected at early stages.

Newer-generation TCAs have been developed to be more selective for the noradrenergic or serotonergic systems. Many of these agents (e.g., trimipramine, amoxapine, or maprotiline), however, still have significant anticholinergic side effects, including blurred vision, urinary retention, and confusion. Trazodone can cause priapism.

Selective serotonin reuptake inhibitors (SSRIs) are potent and selective inhibitors of serotonin reuptake at the presynaptic terminal. They currently are considered first-line therapy for depression because of their prescribing ease and superior side effect/safety profile. SSRI-induced side effects are usually transient and rarely result in discontinuation of the medication. In addition, they appear to be safer than TCAs in overdose.

The major CNS side effects of the SSRIs include nausea, headache, dry mouth, insomnia/somnolence, agitation, nervousness, sweating, dizziness, tremor, myoclonus, and sexual dysfunction. Fluoxetine often is associated with anxiety, nervousness, insomnia, and anorexia. Paroxetine, fluvoxamine, and nefazodone are associated with sedation. Sexual dysfunction manifests itself as ejaculatory delay in men and anorgasmia in women. There have been reports suggesting that fluoxetine can induce or exacerbate suicidal tendencies, and several mechanisms have been proposed. However, because suicide is an important feature of depression, it is difficult to draw conclusions; however, it is difficult to exclude the possibility that suicidal ideation occurs as a rare adverse reaction with some drugs.

SSRIs have been shown in vitro and in vivo to inhibit the P450 system and therefore to result in increased levels of drugs that are substrates of P450 as well (e.g., TCAs). There has been debate over whether the combination of SSRIs and monoamine oxidase (MAO) inhibitors or TCAs can lead to the serotonin syndrome characterized by hyperpyrexia, myoclonus, rigidity, hyperreflexia, shivering, confusion, agitation, restlessness, coma, autonomic instability, nausea, diarrhea, diaphoresis, flushing, and (rarely) rhabdomyolysis and death. This occurrence is probably very uncommon but should be watched for and handled immediately with supportive care and drug withdrawal if it occurs. Several case reports in the literature suggest that SSRIs can produce extrapyramidal symptoms in the form of akathisia, dyskinesia, acute dystonia, and deterioration in Parkinson disease, but controlled clinical studies are needed to determine the validity of these observations.

MAO inhibitors are drugs that have been used for decades in the treatment of depression. The characteristic of acute MAO inhibitor intoxication is hyperpyrexia, with fevers as high as 108°F. Coma, tachycardia, tachypnea, dilated pupils, and profuse sweating occur. Rapid recovery after hemodialysis suggests that this means of therapy is effective. A second cataclysmic syndrome is the hypertensive crisis associated with combined use of MAO inhibitors and tyramine products or other centrally active agents. Cheese, chicken livers, chocolate, wine, and some forms of herring have been associated with this syndrome in patients ingesting MAO inhibitors. Much less dramatic and also more common are mild side effects, such as mild dizziness, a generalized weakness, dysarthria, and confusion, which can occur in patients receiving therapeutic doses of these agents.

Lithium carbonate is well established as an effective agent in the treatment of manic-depressive illness. Neurotoxic effects are not rare, and the most common and annoying effect is a fine postural intention tremor, which may be seen even in therapeutic doses. A reduction of the dosage usually either will eliminate the tremor or significantly reduce its intensity. The beta-adrenergic blocker propranolol may prove beneficial. Toxic confusional states also may occur with lithium, and, if this develops, lithium blood levels should be checked. Ataxia, seizures, and coma can occur at high doses (serum levels exceeding 2.0 mEq/L). There is no specific antidote for severe lithium intoxication. After severe intoxication, residual symptoms including ataxia, nystagmus, choreoathetoid movements, and hyperactive deep tendon reflexes have been reported.

■ **SPECIAL CLINICAL POINT: Lithium-induced tremor does not necessarily present on toxic levels of the medication and can be seen with therapeutic doses.**

Hypnosedative and Other Agents

Barbiturates usually are used to manage seizure disorders but still are used to calm patients and facilitate sleep. Drowsiness is a common complaint associated with their use, and ataxia (often without nystagmus) can develop when the plasma level rises above 50 mg/mL. At higher doses, severe ataxia, nausea, vomiting, and nystagmus predominate. A second encephalopathic syndrome occurs in children taking phenobarbital and is highly distinctive. Instead of somnolence, these children develop remarkable agitation and hyperactivity. This can give the picture of attentional deficit disorder (ADD), or childhood hyperactivity. Patients with chronic toxic exposure to barbiturates show ataxic gait, slurred speech, and periods of intermittent agitation. Tremors and confusion, as well as diplopia and nystagmus, are characteristic.

Methaqualone may induce transient and persistent paresthesias and other signs of peripheral neuropathy. Paradoxic restlessness and anxiety instead of sedation and sleep also are reported with this drug. As with many of the drugs already mentioned, methaqualone with alcohol may have addictive sedating effects. Other drug interactions include enhanced effect of MAO inhibitors and TCAs. Delirium and marked myoclonus also may occur in patients who acutely overdose with these drugs.

Disulfiram is used in the rehabilitation of alcoholics because high levels of acetaldehyde accumulate when alcohol is ingested with the drug. Chronic disulfiram therapy is associated with two distinct neurotoxic syndromes, an encephalopathy and a neuropathy. The encephalopathy is usually acute or subacute in onset, characterized by delirium and paranoid and psychotic behavior, and it often is confused with the diagnosis of schizophrenic reaction. The behavioral response to neuroleptics or other psychotropic drugs is generally not marked, a finding that should suggest a toxic cause; withdrawal of disulfiram and mild sedation with supportive care (but without neuroleptic therapy) are recommended in the treatment of disulfiram encephalopathy.

Disulfiram also is associated with a rare axonal distal sensory/motor polyneuropathy. The recovery after drug withdrawal both clinically and pathologically suggests a dying-back or distal axonopathy rather than new degeneration secondary to the loss of nerve cells. It is not known whether disulfiram is the responsible agent or whether a toxic metabolite induces the neuropathy. Disulfiram possibly is metabolized to carbon disulfide, a compound capable of causing an axonal neuropathy in humans and animals.

ANTIINFLAMMATORY AGENTS

Salicylate Compounds

Because of their ready availability in most households, salicylates represent a common source of intoxication, accounting for the largest yearly number of serious childhood poisonings. In acute intoxication, the prominent neurologic and respiratory signs may immediately suggest the correct diagnosis and direct prompt and appropriate intervention. The neurologic manifestations of salicylate toxicity include a rapid and dramatic alteration in consciousness and global function with convulsions and coma. Confusion and restlessness are seen early, leading within a few hours to excitability, tremor, incoherent speech, and often delirium or hallucinosis. This phase has been referred to as a "salicylate jag" to indicate its similarity to alcoholic inebriation, although euphoria and elation are conspicuously absent with salicylates. After this phase, a gradual depression in the level of consciousness occurs with a rapid lapse into coma. Seizures are especially common in children and are usually generalized. The pathophysiology of the convulsions appears to relate to combined effects of metabolic and respiratory disturbances. In infants, salicylate intoxication induces a marked hypoglycemia, and seizure activity is especially hazardous in this young age group. Diplopia, dizziness, and decreased visual acuity also can be seen with salicylate intoxication. Involvement of the audiovestibular (eighth cranial) nerve can lead to tinnitus, vertigo, and complete deafness. This complication is more common with chronic salicylate intoxication and is seen especially in elderly patients treated for arthritic or headache conditions where aspirin or salicylate compounds are ingested daily. The treatment of salicylate toxicity involves minimizing drug absorption, hastening drug elimination, correcting acid–base disturbance, and treating existing neurologic or medical complications. Induced emesis in the awake patient is the most effective means of emptying the stomach. Enhanced elimination is affected by alkalinization of the urine or by peritoneal dialysis or hemodialysis. Careful fluid and electrolyte management is tantamount and depends on the age of the patient and the stage of intoxication. The complications of hypoglycemia in infants must be anticipated and thereby prevented. Seizures usually are treated with phenytoin and phenobarbital.

There is a poor correlation between the serum salicylate levels and the clinical severity of intoxication. Despite apparently adequate treatment and progressive lowering of toxic plasma salicylate levels, sudden and unexplained deaths are not rare.

Steroids

Steroids induce three neurotoxic syndromes: increased intracranial pressure (pseudomotor cerebri), toxic encephalopathy, and myopathy. Infants are more likely than adults to develop steroid-related increased intracranial pressure, hydrocephalus, and papilledema. This syndrome may occur while patients are receiving steroids or after withdrawal. The pathophysiology of this syndrome is unknown, although it may relate to water intoxication. When it occurs, patients have been treated for weeks or months with steroid compounds.

In contrast, steroid-induced toxic encephalopathy may occur within days of steroid introduction. The behavior is varied and fluctuant, ranging over 24 hours from momentary euphoria to depression to fully developed psychosis. Depersonalization and motor retardation may make these patients difficult to manage during the intoxication phase. Paranoia with visual and auditory hallucination and markedly delusional thinking may predominate. Although this syndrome typically occurs early in the course of steroid therapy, cases exist where mental decline developed after more than 3 months of treatment. Doses of medication do not clearly correlate with symptoms, although the encephalopathy is generally more frequent in high-dose treatment groups. Patients with a prior history of psychiatric care or depression may be at higher risk for encephalopathy than other patients. Suicides have occurred, making this encephalopathy a significant source of potential morbidity. Treatment focuses on withdrawal of the steroid and medical and psychiatric support. Steroids sometimes can be reintroduced later without the reappearance of the problem.

Steroid myopathy, characterized by proximal weakness and atrophy, appears unrelated to the actual duration of drug treatment, and type II fibers appear to be selectively affected. Patients complain of progressive weakness that focuses primarily on the proximal muscles (shoulders and thighs).

Rapid withdrawal of steroids induces the behavioral manifestations seen clinically in Addison disease. These manifestations are secondary phenomena and are not related directly to drug neurotoxicity.

Nonsteroidal Agents

The nonsteroidal anti-inflammatory agents (NSAIDs) account for approximately 4% of the prescription market. There are a variety of types currently available, and ibuprofen is available in low doses as a nonprescription drug. Despite widespread use, these agents infrequently cause significant neurologic adverse effects. The most common neurologic side effect is headache. Other rare but serious central disturbances include confusion, hallucinations, and overt psychosis. Although these agents have not been evaluated well in controlled studies, it has been suggested that there may be subtle associated cognitive and memory changes, particularly in more elderly patients. Another infrequent yet important side effect described is the occurrence of aseptic meningitis. Initially reported in 1978, there have been subsequent case reports in which ibuprofen was the most commonly associated drug, although sulindac, naproxen, and tolmetin also have been implicated. From these case reports, it appears that young women with connective tissue disorders are the most likely to develop this side effect. The clinical picture is that of aseptic meningitis, with fever, chills, and meningismus. The cerebrospinal fluid has an elevated protein content, a pleocytosis of granulocytes, and a normal or reduced glucose level. The underlying mechanism for this syndrome is felt to be a hypersensitivity reaction to the drugs. Although an infectious source for meningitis must be sought, no communicable agent has been isolated. The meningeal syndrome resolves with the discontinuation of the nonsteroidal agent, only to recur, sometimes more rapidly and severely, if treatment is reinitiated.

Indomethacin has proved to be a potent anti-inflammatory drug but appears less efficacious than salicylates in the treatment of arthritis and rheumatoid variants. Its mode of action is still uncertain, but it may act by way of inhibition of prostaglandin synthesis. CNS toxicity is one of the most frequent dose-limiting factors, precluding the use of indomethacin in 30% to 50% of patients. Neurotoxic effects consist of headaches, depression, agitation, and (rarely) hallucinations. Ataxia, clumsiness, and impaired postural reflexes also may occur, although slow increases in dosage may prevent their development.

Naproxen has been associated with adverse neurologic reactions in approximately 8% of patients. These effects include headache, drowsiness, vertigo, inability to concentrate, and depression. Because of its protein-binding affinity, naproxen can be associated with phenytoin toxicity in seizure patients. By displacing phenytoin from proteins, naproxen causes higher levels of unbound phenytoin to circulate, so that toxic signs develop, although the total serum phenytoin level remains in the therapeutic range.

Hormones

Female hormones in the form of oral contraceptives or postmenopausal replacement therapy have become widely prescribed. It is clear that oral contraceptives increase by three to eight times the risk of stroke in women taking them. Oral contraceptive–associated strokes can occur in any vascular distribution. Factors predisposing to cerebrovascular disease in women taking birth control pills include the use of compounds containing high levels of estrogen, multiparity, and a change in migraine headache pattern. Of probable but less certain importance are previous thrombotic or embolic disease and hypertension. Inherited resistance to activated protein C, which is caused by a single factor V gene mutation, is a frequent risk factor for thrombosis. Activated protein C resistance was found to be highly prevalent in women with a history of thromboembolic complications during pregnancy or use of oral contraceptives. The gene defect is common in the general population, and the question is raised as to whether it would be reasonable to perform general screening for activated protein C resistance early during pregnancy or before prescription of oral contraceptives. Progesterone-only contraceptives do not increase the risk of stroke. Hormone replacement therapy with estrogen alone or combined with progesterone increases the risk of ischemic stroke with no effect on hemorrhagic stroke. Stroke risk increases with the dose of estrogen. The time between menopause and the initiation of hormone replacement therapy does not influence ischemic stroke risk.

■ **SPECIAL CLINICAL POINT: Progesterone-only contraceptives are preferable in women with cerebrovascular disease or risk factors for cerebrovascular disease.**

Chorea is another serious problem related to oral contraceptives. The involuntary movements appear days or weeks after starting birth control pills and may be more frequent in patients with a prior history of Sydenham's chorea. The chorea starts abruptly and may involve only one side of the body. A similar phenomenon occasionally occurs during pregnancy when a woman develops severe involuntary movements that spontaneously resolve when the pregnancy ends (chorea gravidarum). Birth control chorea may disappear within 48 hours of cessation of the medication, although the abatement can take longer.

Whereas pseudotumor cerebri can occur in patients taking oral contraceptives, another cause of blurring of the optic disc is papilledema related to venous sinus obstruction. Vascular headaches also may appear for the first time or suddenly change in pattern when oral contraceptives are started. Common mi-graine may become classic migraine, with patients experiencing symptoms or signs of focal cerebral dysfunction at the onset of the headache. In cases in which migraines either appear for the first time, increase in frequency, or become focal, cessation of oral contraceptives is suggested. However, a subgroup of patients with headache find relief of headache pain while taking oral contraceptives. These headaches may have a close relationship with menstruation, and while taking the oral contraceptives, the patient has minimal pain.

Various other neurologic disorders occasionally are associated with the use of oral contraceptives. Seizures may change in pattern of frequency. Carpal tunnel syndrome of median nerve neuropathy or other pressure neuropathies may occur related to the increased fluid retention associated with oral contraceptives. Drug-induced and reversible myasthenia gravis also has been reported but rarely.

Vitamins and Additives

Caffeine and other xanthine derivatives, including aminophylline, are CNS stimulants that excite all levels of the CNS, the cortex being the most sensitive. Caffeine increases energy metabolism throughout the brain but decreases cerebral blood flow, inducing a relative brain hypoperfusion. The drug activates noradrenaline neurons and may act as a second messenger at dopamine receptors to affect the local release of dopamine. Mobilization of intracellular calcium and inhibition of specific phosphodiesterases occur at high, nonphysiologic concentrations of caffeine. The most likely mechanism of action of methylxanthine is the antagonism at the level of adenosine receptors.

Caffeine's psychostimulant action on humans is often subtle and difficult to detect. Its effects on learning, memory, performance, and coordination are related to methylxanthine-induced arousal, vigilance, and fatigue. An increased awareness of the environment or hyperesthesia may be an unpleasant experience for some patients. The patient becomes loquacious and restless and often complains of ringing in the ears and giddiness. At high doses, xanthines affect the spinal cord, resulting in increased reflex excitability, tremulous extremities, and tense muscles. Caffeine clearly alters sleep patterns, and if taken within 1 hour of attempted sleep, it increases sleep latency, decreases total sleep time, and worsens the subject's estimate of sleep quality. Less time is spent in stages 3 and 4 and more in stage 2. Xanthine-associated seizures are seen as a complication of aminophylline therapy, especially when the drug is administered intravenously. They usually are generalized but can be focal. Cessation of the use of products containing caffeine can cause a withdrawal syndrome of headaches; drowsiness; fatigue; decreased performance; and, in some instances, nausea and vomiting. These symptoms begin within 12 to 24 hours after the last use, peak at 20 to 48 hours, and last approximately 1 week.

Nicotine increases circulating levels of norepinephrine and epinephrine and stimulates the release of striatal dopamine. It exerts stimulant effects through specific nicotinic receptors, whose activation may facilitate dopaminergic transmission centrally. Nicotine has been reported to affect a number of neurologic diseases, such as spinocerebellar degeneration, multiple system atrophy, multiple sclerosis, tic disorders, parkinsonism, and myoclonic epilepsy.

Nicotine, despite being a powerful stimulant, has no major therapeutic application. Its high toxicity and presence in tobacco smoke give nicotine a considerable medical importance, however. Clinically, tremors and convulsions are major neurologic signs of nicotine intoxication. Respiration is stimulated, and vomiting is induced. Nicotine also has marked antidiuretic activity resulting from direct hypothalamic stimulation. If acutely ingested, nicotine can be fatal at a level of approximately 60 mg of the base product. Autonomic overactivity with dilated pupils, irregular pulse, sweating, and muscle twitching are characteristic signs of nicotine toxicity. Coma may rapidly supervene, although convulsions are usually not present. If death occurs, it is caused by paralysis of respiratory muscles. Cardiac arrhythmias are significant and are other potential sources for demise. Chronic intoxication as a result of nicotine occurs among tobacco pickers, or "croppers," consisting of nausea, vomiting, dizziness, and prostration. The illness is intermittent and lasts between 12 and 14 hours; it then clears, only to recur with return to work. There are no mortalities or long-term sequelae, however. During the 1973 harvesting season, an estimated 9% of the 60,000 tobacco growers in North Carolina reported illnesses.

Vitamins are vital trace substances, and neurologic syndromes generally are associated with deficiency syndromes. However, because health enthusiasm has reached passionate proportions for many individuals, especially Americans, clinicians are encountering neurotoxic syndromes associated with these seemingly safe agents. Of the fat-soluble vitamins, vitamin A is directly associated with neurotoxicity, and vitamin D can alter bone and renal metabolism, causing secondary neurologic dysfunction. Of the water-soluble vitamins, only pyridoxine (B_6) is established to provoke neurologic complications.

Vitamin A, required for normal growth, vision, reproduction, and maintenance of epithelium, in high doses accumulates and can induce the syndrome of increased intracranial pressure (pseudotumor cerebri). Foods high in vitamin A include broccoli, cabbage, and liver, although dietary hypervitaminosis A is most unusual. Medically, vitamin A is used in the treatment of acne vulgaris and other dermatologic illnesses. Whereas the generally recommended daily allowance is 5,000 IU, individual capsules can contain five times that value, with subjects often ingesting 100,000 IU daily. At these doses, intoxication will develop over several months; at 200,000 IU daily, intoxication may develop within weeks. Publicity about putative cancer preventive properties of vitamin A may increase the number of people who expose themselves to this product.

Early signs of increased intracranial pressure include headaches, blurred vision, transient obscuration of vision, and sixth cranial nerve paresis. On funduscopic examination, gradual papilledema develops without further signs of focal neurologic deficit. No neurologic clue exists to establish the etiology, but the skin changes, organomegaly, and history of vitamin ingestion will establish the diagnosis. Because vitamin zealots are often "antimedication," these patients must be questioned specifically about vitamins.

Vitamin D, when given in massive amounts, mobilizes bone calcium and phosphorus. When there is bone demineralization and degeneration, nerve root and spinal cord compression can occur. Alterations in the calcium balance can produce generalized weakness, muscle aches, cramps, and mild metabolic encephalopathy. Meningeal symptoms and trigeminal neuralgia are two additional reported findings without clear pathogenesis. The latter may relate to bony foraminal alterations. When renal impairment occurs, progressive secondary encephalopathy, not directly related to the vitamin, develops, and coma may result.

Pyridoxine, or vitamin B_6, has been implicated in a highly selective toxic syndrome provoking a sensory ataxia and dorsal root ganglia dysfunction. Widely used, especially by women to treat premenstrual tension and edema, pyridoxine induces this neurotoxic syndrome in occasional patients consuming chronic daily doses of 2 g or more. Gradually, the patient notes difficulty walking, with lightning-like dysesthesias in the back. Numbness of the extremities occurs, and, importantly, facial dysesthesias, so uncommon with most toxic neuropathies other than trichloroethane, quickly develop. Areflexia, stocking-glove sensory loss, and profound sensory ataxia with preserved strength are typical. On electromyography, marked slowing of the sensory nerve conduction is seen with normal motor conduction.

Tryptophan is an amino acid that has become popular for management of insomnia and behavioral changes related to the menstrual cycle (premenstrual syndrome). Myalgia and eosinophilia have been reported in numerous patients, as well as a progressive neuropathy affecting primarily the lower extremities with aching weakness. In some instances, patients are so disabled that they are wheelchair bound and need ventilatory assistance. Cessation of exposure to tryptophan and plasma exchange have been associated with clinical improvement in some cases.

Always Remember

- Drug-induced neurologic symptoms can be diagnosed with careful history and vigilance of the examining physician.
- The physician should be careful to inquire about the use of supplements and vitamins as the patients do not always volunteer their use.
- Polypharmacy can alter drug levels and increase the potential for neurotoxicity.
- Some side effects appear after a while following the initiation of the offending medication and in a similar manner can take a while before they resolve.

QUESTIONS AND DISCUSSION

1. Which one of the following medications can cause visual disturbance in as many as 40% of patients?
   A. Propranolol
   B. Digitalis
   C. Alpha-methyldopa
   D. Lidocaine

The correct answer is B. Digitalis has prominent visual side effects, and patients often complain of halos around everything. Propranolol and other beta-antagonists can cause depression and impotency that can be obscured in the rehabilitative setting after a myocardial infarction or surgery. Alpha-methyldopa can cause or aggravate parkinsonism, and lidocaine often is associated with a bizarre and alarming change in behavior.

2. The factor(s) that contribute(s) to the acid–base abnormality of salicylate intoxication include the following?
   A. Salicylates initially depress medullary breathing activation.
   B. Salicylates are acids that displace bicarbonate and also can lead to ketosis.
   C. Myoglobinuria usually precipitates renal shutdown and metabolic acidosis.
   D. All of the above.

The correct answer is B. Salicylates initially activate the medullary breathing center and cause respiratory alkalosis. Later, at high doses, the medullary breathing center can be inhibited. In addition, salicylates induce and enhance the chemosensitive response and are acids. The net response is a metabolic acidosis with either a respiratory acidosis or alkalosis. Myoglobinuria is not a feature of salicylate intoxication.

3. In regards to neurologic disability associated with birth control pills:
   A. Peripheral neuropathy of the axonal type can mimic multiple sclerosis.
   B. Cerebrovascular accidents usually relate to cardiac valvular vegetations.
   C. Chorea often resolves within days or weeks of drug cessation and is rarely a permanent sequela of oral contraceptive ingestion.
   D. Papilledema, when it occurs, is caused by steroid-induced hypervitaminosis A.

The correct answer is C. Birth control pills are not associated with a peripheral neuropathy; instead, their toxicity relates predominantly to a CNS function. Cerebrovascular accidents are an alarming complication of these drugs in young women and may be of embolic or thrombotic origin. They do not relate specifically to valvular vegetations. Chorea often occurs within days of the first ingestion of birth control pills and may stop promptly after drug cessation. Only in rare instances (usually a hemiballistic syndrome) will the chorea be longstanding after drug cessation. In such cases, a static cerebrovascular accident is hypothesized to underlie the chorea as opposed to the transient chorea, which probably relates to a hormonally induced functional alteration in dopaminergic sensitivity at the striatum. Papilledema, when it occurs in patients taking birth control pills, may have multiple etiologies, including venous thrombosis and pseudotumor cerebri. It does not appear to relate to hypervitaminosis A.

4. Which one of the five neurologic complications of neuroleptic therapy listed can occur as a subacute event, occurring days, weeks, or a few months after starting the drug?
   A. Dystonia
   B. Parkinsonism
   C. Chorea
   D. Akathisia
   E. Oculogyric crises

The correct answer is B. The subacute problem associated with neuroleptic medications is parkinsonism, which may include any of the following: tremor, bradykinesia, rigidity, or postural reflex compromise. The acute neurologic side effects related to neuroleptic drugs are dystonia and akathisia. The contorted posture of dystonia is frightening to see or experience. An oculogyric crisis, with the eyes thrown back and the neck usually hyperextended, is only one example of a dystonic complication of neuroleptics. A late-onset dystonia has been described as within the realm of tardive dyskinesia, but this is probably uncommon. Tardive dyskinesia is mainly a choreic or stereotypic disorder but may be dystonic and is the major chronic side effect of neuroleptic drugs.

5. Which statement is true regarding antiemetic drugs and neurologic use or adverse effects?
   A. Metoclopramide is particularly useful in patients with Parkinson disease with nausea secondary to their dopaminergic medication.
   B. Children receiving prochlorperazine for gastrointestinal distress are less likely

than adults to have neurologic complications.

C. In a patient using a scopolamine patch who reports acute right eye pain, an emergency visit to an ophthalmologist and removal of the patch should be recommended.

D. Scopolamine may cause drug-induced parkinsonism by a mechanism similar to that of neuroleptics.

The correct answer is C. Scopolamine is an anticholinergic agent that may exacerbate narrow-angle glaucoma, with painful symptoms in the eyes. If not recognized and treated emergently, this may result in blindness. Both metoclopramide and prochlorperazine are dopamine receptor blockers, similar to the neuroleptics. Hence, both agents may cause drug-induced parkinsonism or worsen preexisting Parkinson disease. Children treated with these drugs are at more risk for developing acute dystonic reactions. In contrast, scopolamine, being an anticholinergic agent, does not cause drug-induced parkinsonism.

6. In patients receiving theophylline, which of the following is true?

A. Seizures occur only if serum levels are in the toxic range.

B. Theophylline is a useful agent in an elderly patient with congestive heart failure and a previous stroke with a history of intermittent asthma.

C. A child receiving IV infusions of theophylline is at increased risk for developing acute dystonic reactions.

D. The pharmacokinetics of drugs metabolized in the liver may affect the metabolism and serum levels of theophylline.

The correct answer is D. Theophylline is metabolized by the hepatic enzymes. Other drugs metabolized in the liver may alter theophylline metabolism, affecting the serum levels. The seizures associated with theophylline may occur in the therapeutic range. In particular, patients with previous brain injury are at

increased risk. Congestive heart failure may increase theophylline levels even when the drug is administered at recommended doses. Theophylline is a xanthine compound without dopamine receptor activity, and it is not known to cause acute dystonic reactions.

7. Which of the following antibiotics is associated with a high incidence of neurotoxicity?

A. Penicillin

B. Trimethoprim

C. Minocycline

D. Erythromycin

The correct answer is C. Minocycline provokes ototoxicity, and women are more susceptible to these effects than men. The remaining agents are associated with neurotoxic syndromes only on occasion, unless they are given by unusual routes or in unusual doses.

8. Which condition is associated with vitamin excess?

A. Clinical findings of Guillain–Barré syndrome

B. Increased intracranial pressure

C. Myasthenia gravis

D. Wernicke–Korsakoff syndrome

The correct answer is B. Excess vitamin A and B_6 are known to cause neurotoxic syndrome. B_6 provokes a sensory neuropathy with loss of reflexes, but it should not be confused with Guillain–Barré, which predominantly affects the motor system. Vitamin A causes the syndrome of pseudotumor cerebri, with increased intracranial pressure, often associated with headache and other nonfocal neurologic findings. (Sixth-nerve paresis, unlike other cranial neuropathies, is a "false-localizing" sign. Because of the long trajectory of the nerve along bony surfaces, a sixth-nerve paresis does not locate the level or side of neurologic damage.) Vitamin D, when given in high doses chronically, affects calcium and phosphorus balance, which may clinically provoke global weakness. The classical neuromuscular fatigue typical of myasthenia and the response to edrophonium are not seen. Wernicke–Korsakoff syndrome is related to vitamin deprivation and not to intoxication.

SUGGESTED READING

Bahls FH, Ma KK, Bird TD. Theophylline-associated seizures with "therapeutic" or low toxic serum concentrations: risk factors for serious outcome in adults. *Neurology.* 1991;41:1309.

Bays H. Statin safety: an overview and assessment of the data—2005. *Am J Cardiol.* 2006;97(suppl 8A):6C–26C.

Carbone JR. The neuroleptic malignant and serotonin syndromes. *Emerg Med Clin North Am.* 2000;18(2): 317–325.

Davis PH. Use of oral contraceptives and postmenopausal hormone replacement: evidence on risk of stroke. *Curr Treat Options Neurol.* 2008;10:468–474.

Giménez-Roldàn S, Mateo D. Cinnarizine-induced parkinsonism. *Clin Neuropharmacol.* 1991;14:156.

Goetz CG. *Neurotoxins in Clinical Practice.* New York: SP Medical and Scientific Books; 1985.

Goetz CG, Kompoliti K, Washburn KR. Neurotoxic agents. In: Joynt RJ, Griggs RC, eds. *Clinical Neurology.* Philadelphia: Lippincott–Raven; 2002:1.

Heiman-Patterson TD, Bird SJ, Parry GJ, et al. Peripheral neuropathy associated with eosinophilia–myalgia syndrome. *Ann Neurol.* 1991;28:522.

Hoppmann RA, Peden JG, Ober SK. Central nervous system side effects of nonsteroidal anti-inflammatory drugs. *Arch Intern Med.* 1991;151:1309.

Kompoliti K, Horn SS. Drug-induced and iatrogenic neurological disorders. In: Goetz CG, ed. *Textbook of Clinical Neurology.* Philadelphia: Saunders Elsevier; 2007:1285–1318.

Law M, Rudnicka AR. Statin safety: a systematic review. *Am J Cardiol.* 2006;97:52C–60C.

Lipsy RJ, Fennerty B, Fagan TC. Clinical review of the histamine-2 receptor antagonists. *Arch Intern Med.* 1990;150:745.

Miller LG, Jankovic J. Persistent dystonia possibly induced by flecainide. *Mov Disord.* 1992;7:62.

Neuhaus P, McMaster P, Calne R, et al. Neurological complications in the European multicentre study of FK 506 and cyclosporin in primary liver transplantation. *Transpl Int.* 1994;7(suppl 1):S27–S31.

Pappert EJ. Neuroleptic-induced movement disorders: acute and subacute syndromes. In: de Wolff FA, ed. *Intoxication of the Nervous System, Part II.* Amsterdam: Elsevier Science BV; 1994.

Sacristan JA, Soto JA, de Cos MA. Erythromycin-induced hypoacusis: 11 new cases and literature review. *Ann Pharmacother.* 1993;27:950.

Silverstein A, ed. *Neurological Complications of Therapy: Selected Topics.* Mt. Kisco, NY: Futura; 1982.

Spencer PS, Schaumburg HH, eds. *Experimental and Clinical Neurotoxicology.* Baltimore: Williams & Wilkins; 1980.

Stenzel MS, Carpenter CC. The management of the clinical complications of antiretroviral therapy. *Infect Dis Clin North Am.* 2000;14(4):851–878.

Subbaraman R, Chaguturu SK, Mayer KH, et al. Adverse effects of highly active antiretroviral therapy in developing countries. *Clin Infect Dis.* 2007;45:1093–1101.

Vinken PJ, Bruyn GW, Cohen MM, et al., eds. *Intoxications of the Nervous System. Handbook of Clinical Neurology.* Vols 36 and 37. Amsterdam: North Holland; 1979.

Wald JJ. The effects of toxins on muscle. *Neurol Clin.* 2000;18(3):695–718.

Warnke D, Barreto J, Temesgen Z. Antiretroviral drugs. *J Clin Pharmacol.* 2007;47:1570–1579.

Yokota T, Kagamihara Y, Hayashi H, et al. Nicotine-sensitive paresis. *Neurology.* 1992;42:382.

23 Neurologic Complications of Alcoholism

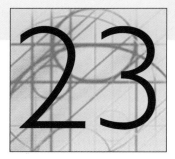

ALLISON L. WEATHERS

key points

- The potential neurologic consequences of chronic alcoholism are wide ranging with potential involvement of both the central nervous system and peripheral nervous system.

- Wernicke encephalopathy is a neurologic emergency, whose diagnosis and the decision to treat should be based on the clinical picture alone. This diagnosis should be considered in all high-risk patients.

- In addition to the more commonly occurring neurologic complications of alcoholism such as hepatic encephalopathy and Wernicke encephalopathy, more rare manifestations such as pancreatic encephalopathy, pellagra encephalopathy, and Marchiafava–Bignami disease may occur and should be considered in the differential of an alcoholic patient with mental status changes.

thanol is one of the most commonly abused substances in the United States. Chronic alcoholism results in substantial health consequences for those who suffer from this disease and overall impacts our medical resources to a significant degree. The potential neurologic complications of chronic alcoholism are broad, with both the central nervous system (CNS) and peripheral nervous system (PNS) possible targets of the adverse effects of chronic alcohol abuse. This chapter will cover these potential complications ranging from those that may be considered acute neurologic emergencies, such as Wernicke encephalopathy, to more chronic, insidious processes such as alcoholic neuropathy. Internists, family medicine practitioners, and emergency department physicians are usually well versed in the potential neurologic complications of acute alcohol intoxication and withdrawal and their management, often more so than neurologists. Therefore, this chapter will focus solely on the neurologic manifestations of chronic alcohol abuse.

WERNICKE ENCEPHALOPATHY

Though Wernicke encephalopathy is not one of the most common neurologic manifestations of alcoholism, its potential for devastating neurologic consequences and ultimately death if unrecognized and untreated makes it one of the most significant possible complications of alcohol abuse. It is now recognized that a number of clinical scenarios may result in Wernicke encephalopathy; however, chronic alcohol use remains one of the most common causes of thiamine deficiency and therefore is still the underlying cause in the majority of cases. In this patient population, the onset of Wernicke encephalopathy is especially likely to occur during concurrent febrile illnesses, during or following treatment of delirium tremens, during detoxification, with the administration of glucose (often as a component of intravenous fluids), or during refeeding after prolonged starvation. The unifying feature of all of these circumstances is that they result in increased metabolic demand or stress. Physicians who care for alcoholic patients need to be cognizant of these inciting factors and aware of the wide range of clinical features of this illness.

Although the triad of mental status changes, ophthalmoplegia, and ataxia is well-recognized as the classic clinical picture of Wernicke encephalopathy, in actuality the full triad occurs in relatively few patients. Mental status and personality changes, including insomnia, lethargy, anxiety, apprehension, apathy, confusion, memory loss, and difficulty with concentration, are frequently the initial symptoms. Ocular symptoms, including wavering of vision, double vision (diplopia), and photophobia, may precede the mental status changes, and nystagmus may be the initial neurologic finding on exam. Lateral rectus palsies, conjugate gaze palsy, complete ophthalmoplegia, pupillary abnormalities, and ptosis are not as frequently seen. Ataxia may also be a presenting sign, but occurs less commonly than mental status changes and eye signs. If untreated, the neurologic symptoms and signs will progress with increasingly severe confusion, confabulation, hallucinations, and ultimately coma and death are possible outcomes. Though rare, patients may present in coma without focal neurologic signs, mimicking other metabolic encephalopathies, and patients may also present with systemic signs including hypotension, hypothermia, and tachycardia.

Although controversy exists surrounding the pathophysiology of many of the neurologic complications of alcoholism, specifically whether they are due to the direct toxic effects of alcohol and its metabolites or to superimposed nutritional and vitamin deficiencies. Wernicke encephalopathy is known to be the result of thiamine deficiency. Thiamine deficiency is common in this population for a number of reasons including decreased gastrointestinal (GI) absorption of thiamine both by chronic alcohol use and by the concurrent use of alcohol with thiamine administration, decreased thiamine storage in the liver, impaired transformation of thiamine into its active form, and independently decreased absorption due to malnutrition. Thiamine deficiency can occur within weeks without continued dietary (or supplemental) intake, and symptoms can start within a few weeks of the onset of the deficient state.

The active form of thiamine, thiamine diphosphate, plays a critical role in three different enzyme pathways, which in turn are vital to a number of biologic functions, such as the synthesis of neurotransmitters, the maintenance of myelin sheaths, the production of energy through lipid and glucose metabolism, and branched-chain amino acid production. As a consequence, thiamine deficiency results in cerebral energy deficits, focal lactic acidosis, glutamate-mediated excitotoxicity, blood–brain barrier breakdown, and free radical formation, which in turn are thought to result in the pathologic changes seen in Wernicke encephalopathy, and therefore the clinical picture.

It is possible to measure thiamine levels, as well as to assess thiamine status through the measurement of red blood cell transketolase; however, these studies, though they may identify at-risk patients, are not diagnostic, may not be available emergently, and should not be relied on to make treatment decisions. This holds true for other adjunctive studies such as magnetic resonance imaging (MRI) and lumbar puncture. Although MRI may show signal abnormalities, usually in the medial thalami, mammillary bodies, and certain regions of the midbrain in acute cases, these findings will not be seen in all patients. Cerebrospinal fluid (CSF) studies are often normal.

■ **SPECIAL CLINICAL POINT:** Wernicke encephalopathy is a neurologic emergency, whose diagnosis, and therefore the decision to treat, should be based on the clinical picture alone.

Although the need for thiamine replacement in these patients is clear, exact treatment recommendations cannot be made on the basis of the literature. Treatment should be given in parental form in all cases due to the known decreased absorption from the GI tract in alcoholic patients, and alcoholic patients require higher doses than do those with other underlying etiologies for the same reasons that this population is more often deficient. Alcoholic patients may require several hundred milligrams of parental thiamine given up to twice daily for several days. Magnesium is a required cofactor in the metabolism of thiamine and is frequently a codeficiency in alcoholics. It should be replenished as well in deficient patients to ensure response to treatment. Although parenteral thiamine is thought to have a good safety profile, anaphylaxis is a possible reaction and treatment should only be given in a setting where cardiopulmonary resuscitation and epinephrine are available emergently.

Generally, the response to adequate treatment is fairly rapid, with the eye movement abnormalities improving first and resolving within days, followed by the cognitive deficits and ataxia within weeks to months. A potential consequence of inadequate and of course a complete lack of treatment is Wernicke–Korsakoff syndrome. Patients with this chronic amnestic condition will have severe anterograde amnesia with retrograde amnesia for the months to years prior to the onset of the illness. Confabulation is a common associated finding in patients with this severe amnestic syndrome.

Given the potential for a devastating neurologic outcome, Wernicke encephalopathy is a neurologic emergency and treatment should not be delayed.

■ **SPECIAL CLINICAL POINT:** As treatment is generally well tolerated and the risk of missing the diagnosis is so great, the diagnosis of Wernicke encephalopathy should be considered in all high-risk patients, including those with hepatic encephalopathy, those with encephalopathy secondary to head trauma, and those with any one of the possible presenting clinical symptoms, particularly when the patient presents acutely intoxicated.

PELLAGRA ENCEPHALOPATHY

As with Wernicke encephalopathy, although a number of medical conditions may predispose patients to pellagra, chronic alcoholism has long been known to be the chief underlying condition; both for cases in nonendemic areas at the height of the epidemic in the mid-20th century and today, despite the enrichment of bread and flour by niacin. Although vitamin enrichment did greatly reduce the incidence of this disease, it still persists, especially in malnourished, indigent alcoholics, and therefore pellagra encephalopathy should still be considered a potential neurologic complication of alcoholism.

In addition to being associated strongly with chronic alcoholism and the result of a vitamin deficiency, pellagra shares other characteristics with Wernicke encephalopathy, including the fact that the diagnosis is coupled to a classic triad of clinical symptoms that does not actually occur in the majority of patients. In this case, the triad is dermatitis, diarrhea, and dementia, also known as "the three Ds" of pellagra. "Dementia" is often a late characteristic with mild cognitive and personality changes occurring early in the disease course. These include fatigue, insomnia, anorexia, apprehension, anxiety, depression, mania, apathy, and mood lability. Headache, mild memory loss, and vertigo may also be early neurologic manifestations of this illness. With disease progression, both the psychiatric and neurologic symptoms and signs will often increase in severity. Patients may develop acute psychosis, paranoid delusions, and hallucinations, and most will develop confusion with disorientation and fluctuations in their level of consciousness. Neurologic examination may reveal spastic weakness, extrapyramidal signs, hyperreflexia, Babinski sign, myoclonus, gait abnormalities, gegenhalten tone, tremor, dysphagia, and bowel and bladder incontinence. Seizures may occur. The neuropsychiatric manifestations of pellagra may occur in isolation, often making it hard to distinguish pellagra encephalopathy from other encephalopathies seen in alcoholic patients, such as delirium tremens.

The "dermatitis" of pellagra is classically a symmetric, sharply demarcated, erythematous, photosensitive rash that occurs is sun-exposed areas in the spring and summer, including the face, dorsal surfaces of the hands and arms, and the front of the neck. Other dermatologic manifestations of this disease may occur, including desquamation of the skin, thickening, mild hyperpigmentation, and eczema-like lesions. The classic rash may not develop in patients who are not exposed to sunlight. The potential GI manifestations are also broad, and in addition to diarrhea include abdominal pain, nausea and vomiting, steatorrhea, and constipation. Stomatitis and glossitis are common clinical features.

Pellagra is the result of niacin deficiency or of a deficiency of tryptophan, the essential amino acid that is the precursor of niacin. Niacin, through the enzymes nicotinamide adenine dinucleotide (NAD) and nicotinamide adenine dinucleotide phosphate (NADP), plays a crucial role in multiple oxidation–reduction reactions in the body, including glycolysis and fat synthesis. Multiple other vitamins are essential for the synthesis of niacin from tryptophan, including thiamine, riboflavin, and pyridoxine, and a codeficiency of protein or of one of these other vitamins is likely needed for the development of the disease. As chronic alcoholics often will be overall malnourished with deficiencies in more than one vitamin, this population is especially predisposed to the development of pellagra.

Niacin deficiency can be assessed in the laboratory, both by the direct blood levels of niacin and tryptophan and by the urinary metabolites of niacin-dependent pathways, but these tests are not routinely available or have low specificity or poor reliability.

■ **SPECIAL CLINICAL POINT: As with Wernicke encephalopathy, pellagra encephalopathy remains a clinical diagnosis that can be confirmed by clinical improvement with replacement therapy.**

Pellagra differs from Wernicke encephalopathy in that large oral doses of niacin and a diet enriched in niacin and protein is sufficient for treatment. Niacinamide is frequently used due to its improved adverse effect profile compared to niacin, including less GI effects and less vasoactive properties (less flushing); however, both are U.S. Food and Drug Administration (FDA) approved for the treatment of pellagra. Adequate replacement of the other B vitamins is necessary due to both the frequently associated codeficiencies of these vitamins and to the requirements for them in niacin metabolism. Magnesium may be required, if found to be deficient.

Though relatively rare, pellagra did not disappear with the end of the epidemic in the mid-20th century. Pellagra encephalopathy often responds rapidly and completely to treatment, especially when treatment is started early in the course of the illness, and has a very high mortality rate when untreated. For all of these reasons, it must be considered in the differential diagnosis of the encephalopathic alcoholic patient and the diagnosis should not be discarded on the basis of the absence of GI and dermatologic manifestations.

METABOLIC ENCEPHALOPATHIES

Hepatic Encephalopathy

Alcohol abuse is a very common cause of cirrhosis and therefore a common etiology of hepatic encephalopathy associated with cirrhosis with portal hypertension or portosystemic shunts. The potential clinical findings of hepatic encephalopathy are broad and may range from the subtle personality changes and cognitive deficits detectable only on formal neuropsychiatric testing found in minimal hepatic encephalopathy, to coma. The degree of severity of the encephalopathy is characterized by the level of consciousness, intellectual function, and the extent of personality and behavioral changes. With progression of the disease course, patients will usually have worsening of all of these individual components.

The impairment in level of consciousness will advance from mild fatigue or insomnia to lethargy to somnolence and then on to coma. Diminished attention span may progress to mild disorientation, amnesia, and mild confusion, and then further to marked cognitive impairment. Mild irritability and depression will evolve to clear personality changes with inappropriate behavior, followed by paranoid ideations and hallucinations. Finally, while a slight tremor or incoordination may be the only motor findings in the early stage of hepatic encephalopathy, examination will often evolve to show dysarthria, hyporeflexia, and ataxia, and in later stages hyperreflexia, weakness, nystagmus, Babinski sign, clonus, and rigidity are all possible. In late-stage hepatic encephalopathy, opisthotonus and posturing may be associated with the comatose state. Asterixis, a well-recognized feature of hepatic encephalopathy, is a prominent feature of the middle stages of the disease process. Although this is the usual course of disease progression, patients may have swift progression between stages, with rapid evolution to coma. Though not an absolute, patients often demonstrate other findings consistent with liver disease, such as ascites, jaundice, and spider angiomas.

Hepatic encephalopathy is a clinical diagnosis based on the history and physical examination; however, adjunctive studies may be helpful as supportive evidence. Serum ammonia levels do not clearly correspond to the level of severity of the encephalopathy, though a normal level is not consistent with this diagnosis. Electroencephalogram is useful to rule out underlying seizures, such as in nonconvulsive status epilepticus, a potential mimicker of hepatic (and other) encephalopathies. It will often be abnormal with potential findings including diffuse slowing and triphasic waves. Neuroimaging with computer tomography (CT) or MRI is useful to rule out a structural lesion, but will not confirm the diagnosis. MRI will often show high signal on the T1 images in the globus pallidus, likely due to manganese deposition, but this finding is seen in patients with chronic liver disease and is not in itself specific for the clinical diagnosis of hepatic encephalopathy.

■ **SPECIAL CLINICAL POINT: A triggering clinical event superimposed on chronic underlying liver disease is often responsible for the development of hepatic encephalopathy.**

These events include dehydration, GI bleeding, infections, intake of excessive dietary protein, electrolyte abnormalities, surgery, transjugular intrahepatic portosystemic shunt placement, and additional hepatic insults.

■ **SPECIAL CLINICAL POINT: As a result, treatment of hepatic encephalopathy starts with a search for and correction of any triggering factors.**

After this initial step, pharmacologic treatment consists of administration of the nonabsorbable disaccharide lactulose and the oral antibiotic rifaximin, which may be administered in combination. Both act by inhibiting absorption and production of ammonia. Although there is controversy regarding the efficacy of lactulose and it is often not well tolerated by patients given its unavoidable GI effects, its use remains widespread. Rifaximin has improved tolerance over other antibiotics.

Although not as common in chronic alcoholics as hepatic encephalopathy secondary to cirrhosis with portal hypertension or portosystemic shunts, encephalopathy due to fulminant, acute liver failure may occur, most likely due to an acute hepatic insult superimposed on chronic liver disease. This type of hepatic encephalopathy is considered a neurologic emergency due to the frequent occurrence of cerebral edema, which results in increased intracranial pressure. Emergent neurosurgical consultation is indicated in the management of these cases for the placement of an intracranial pressure transducer, as head CT may be unremarkable. Aggressive treatment of this potential complication is necessary.

Acquired Hepatocerebral Degeneration

Acquired (or "non-Wilsonian" to distinguish it from the classic genetic form) hepatocerebral degeneration (AHCD) is a neurodegenerative disease comprising chronic neurologic and psychiatric impairment that occurs as a complication of chronic liver failure and that is unrelated to the underlying cause of liver disease. Its incidence is less than that of hepatic encephalopathy, but it does appear to be an associated process as its onset seems to be related to repeated episodes of hepatic encephalopathy, and especially of hepatic coma. However, this is not an absolute and overt episodes of hepatic encephalopathy do not always precede this illness. There may also be a correlation between the onset of this syndrome with the degree of portosystemic shunting and the ammonia level.

The majority of neurologic symptoms and signs may be classified as extrapyramidal (i.e.,

secondary to dysfunction of the basal ganglia) including choreoathetosis, tremor, myoclonus of the face and limbs, dystonia, rigidity, and dysarthria. Of the above, tremor, which is often coarse, postural, and kinetic; myoclonus; and mild gait unsteadiness are often the presenting symptoms. Frank ataxia, pyramidal tract signs, and dementia are later signs. A parkinsonian form of AHCD is characterized by the relatively rapid onset of symmetric akinesia, cogwheeling rigidity, and resting tremor in association with a gait disorder, postural instability, and less frequently, focal dystonia. Hepatic myelopathy, also known as portosystemic or postshunt myelopathy, presents with a progressive spastic paraparesis with associated hyperreflexia and minimal sensory involvement.

AHCD differs from Wilson disease by the later age of onset, absence of Kayser–Fleischer rings, and normal copper metabolism. However, a diagnosis of Wilson disease should always be excluded when a diagnosis of AHCD is entertained. Clinical features of cirrhosis including ascites, spider angiomata, palmar erythema, and hypoalbuminemia are often present.

As with hepatic encephalopathy, neuroimaging in patients with AHCD will often reveal hyperintense signal abnormalities on the T1-weighted imaging sequences in the lenticular nuclei, particularly the globus pallidus. These changes correspond to the underlying chronic liver disease and occur regardless of the existence of clinical neurologic impairment consistent with a diagnosis of AHCD.

While the pathophysiology of AHCD remains not fully understood, the predominance of extrapyramidal symptoms may be due to the loss of dopamine D_2 receptors in the lentiform nuclei of AHCD patients. It is unknown if the reduction in dopamine receptors is a direct effect of the abnormal manganese deposition in the basal ganglia that is thought to be the culprit of the T1 signal changes seen on MRI. Other metabolic derangements such as reduced glucose consumption in the basal ganglia may also contribute to the clinical picture. Chronic exposure to toxic nitrogenous substances that are not being metabolized by the liver and cumulative damage from multiple episodes of hepatic encephalopathy are also likely responsible in some way.

AHCD is a chronic condition; patients do not generally respond to pharmacologic measures used in the treatment of hepatic encephalopathy. There may, however, be improvement in both the cognitive deficits and the extrapyramidal signs following liver transplant.

Pancreatic Encephalopathy

Alcoholism is one of the most frequent underlying etiologies of acute pancreatitis and though not as common as hepatic encephalopathy, pancreatic encephalopathy is a well-recognized neurologic complication of this common medical illness. There are no neurologic findings that are specific to this form of encephalopathy. Confusion with disorientation, fluctuating alterations of consciousness, agitation, paranoid ideations, and hallucinations are common manifestations. Less frequently, depressed mood, seizures, tremor, aphasia, weakness, frontal release signs, meningismus, ataxia, nystagmus, akinetic mutism, and coma may occur. The onset of the encephalopathy is usually within 2 weeks of the onset of the underlying pancreatitis, often within the first week. Though more unusual, patients may have neurologic symptoms develop within the first day of their GI symptoms. There does not seem to be a clear correlation between the severity of the pancreatitis and the occurrence of encephalopathy.

■ **SPECIAL CLINICAL POINT: As with the ammonia level for hepatic encephalopathy, the degree of elevation of the amylase level does not correlate with the presence or severity of the pancreatic encephalopathy; however, this is a useful adjunctive laboratory study in an encephalopathic patient with severe abdominal pain associated with other GI symptoms.**

EEG is often abnormal with diffuse slowing, though again these findings are not specific to this diagnosis. CT and MRI of the brain may

be normal or may show scattered areas of signal abnormality on the T2, FLAIR (fluid-attenuated inversion recovery), and diffusion-weighted images. As none of these studies, even when positive, have findings specific to this diagnosis, they are more useful to exclude the differential diagnoses such as infection, mass lesion, and status epilepticus.

In addition to the above differential which is common to all encephalopathic patients, patients with pancreatitis are also at increased risk for electrolyte and calcium abnormalities, pH disturbances, superimposed infections, other metabolic derangements, and secondary liver injury. Though rare, osmotic demyelination and pancreatitis-induced disseminated intravascular coagulation syndrome may complicate acute pancreatitis and all of these may result in an encephalopathy. This patient population is also at especially high risk for Wernicke encephalopathy, owing to the frequent clinical features of hyperemesis and anorexia and management with "pancreatic rest" with holding of oral feedings and administration of total parenteral nutrition, in the absence of adequate vitamin supplementation. Therefore, pancreatic encephalopathy is a diagnosis that the physician should feel comfortable with only once all of these other possibilities have been excluded. Making this diagnosis even more complicated in alcoholic patients is the fact that pancreatic encephalopathy may be strikingly similar in presentation to delirium tremens.

Several pathophysiologic mechanisms are thought to be responsible for pancreatic encephalopathy including the activation of phospholipase A, which causes a chain of events that ultimately result in demyelination, encephalomalacia, hemorrhage, mitochondrial injury, diminished acetylcholine release, and edema due to alterations in vascular permeability. Acute pancreatitis may be complicated by fat necrosis with fat embolism. Both hypoxia due to pulmonary fat embolism and the direct effects of cerebral fat embolism may underlie pancreatic encephalopathy.

There are no directed treatments based on these mechanisms, with treatment instead consisting only of supportive and symptomatic therapy. Early and aggressive management of the acute pancreatitis is recommended. Neurologic improvement usually mirrors that of the underlying pancreatitis, though it may be delayed, following the resolution of the GI symptoms. Mortality is high, occurring in approximately half the cases, and residual neurologic impairment without full recovery may occur.

CENTRAL PONTINE MYELINOLYSIS

Central pontine myelinolysis (CPM) is a rare condition most commonly associated with the rapid correction of hyponatremia, where it occurs due to the extracellular sodium concentration increasing faster than the intracellular uptake of electrolytes and organic osmolytes. As a result, water will shift from the intracellular to the extracellular compartment, which causes cell injury and demyelination. CPM is now more accurately called osmotic demyelination syndrome, as these changes are not restricted to the pons. Although classically associated with the clinical scenario described above, other causes of serum hyperosmolality may result in CPM, and it may occur even with slow correction of hyponatremia. Patients will often have a chronic underlying predisposing condition and chronic alcoholism is one of the most frequent.

Clinically, CPM often presents as an acute decline in the patient's neurologic status with an acute confusional state. In cases due to rapid correction of hyponatremia, this decline often follows an initial brief improvement in the encephalopathy due to the hyponatremia itself. Patients may develop a pseudobulbar affect (inappropriate laughing and crying), and motor manifestations may be a prominent feature and may include flaccid quadriparesis with progression to spasticity, dysarthria, dysphagia, and a complete locked-in syndrome. With progression of the disease process, stupor and coma may occur. Cognitive and psychiatric symptoms may also be more subtle, such as restlessness, emotional lability, apathy, akinetic mutism, agitation, insomnia, paranoia, delusions, and disinhibited and aggressive behavior. MRI may show findings supportive of the clinical diagnosis with hyperintensities seen on the T2-weighted and FLAIR images in the pons and other extrapontine locations.

■ **SPECIAL CLINICAL POINT: Treatment of central pontine myelinolysis is mainly limited to supportive measures, with an important component being correction of all other underlying possible etiologies of encephalopathy (such as other electrolyte or metabolic disorders) and management of comorbidities such as aspiration pneumonia.**

Patients will often have some degree of neurologic improvement with supportive therapy followed by rehabilitation, but this is not always complete.

MARCHIAFAVA–BIGNAMI DISEASE

Once thought to be an extremely rare and uniformly fatal disease seen only in chronic male drinkers of Italian red wine, Marchiafava–Bignami disease (MBD), although still rare and still most commonly encountered in chronic alcoholics, is now known to be a survivable illness that can occur in either gender no matter what type of ethanol-containing product is chronically abused. Though it may also be seen in patients who are chronically malnourished from diseases other than alcoholism, it is still most frequently encountered in male, middle-aged, malnourished alcoholics. MBD is characterized by demyelination and necrosis of the corpus callosum and was initially a diagnosis that required pathologic confirmation. As neuroimaging techniques, especially MRI, have improved and became more helpful in revealing the classic corpus callosum lesions, the historical description provided above has been expanded.

There are now known to be three clinical variations of MBD. The acute form is manifested by rapid alteration of consciousness and seizures, with swift progression to coma and then frequently death within a matter of days.

This variant is often associated with diffuse hypertonia and rigidity, dysphagia, and muteness. The subacute form is similar, with hypertonia and dysarthria also frequent features, as well as facial grimacing and opisthotonus. However, as the name suggests, it differs in its time course, with patients presenting with a dementia of rapid onset which then evolves into a vegetative state. Death may occur within months. In the chronic form, the neurologic symptoms and signs may persist for months to years, but may then resolve and a wide range of clinical manifestations are possible. An interhemispheric disconnection syndrome manifested by limb apraxia, agraphia, and alexia is common, and a gait disorder, urinary incontinence, hemiparesis, aphasia, disorientation, and memory loss may occur. Patients with the acute and subacute form may also present with an interhemispheric disconnection syndrome.

MRI will usually reveal areas of low signal intensity on the T1-weighted images, with analogous areas of high signal intensity on the T2 and FLAIR images, in a portion of the corpus callosum; the entire corpus callosum is usually not involved. Extracallosal lesions may occur in the adjacent white matter, hemispheric white matter, and middle cerebellar peduncles. Callosal atrophy may be seen in chronic cases. Cortical lesions are not inconsistent with this diagnosis, but are seen more frequently on pathologic studies at autopsy than on neuroimaging.

Although the exact pathophysiologic mechanism of MBD is not known, vitamin B complex deficiencies and vascular injury have been proposed as possible underlying etiologies. On the basis of the former possible mechanism, patients may respond to treatment with high-dose vitamin B complex supplementation. Corticosteroids are sometimes administered as well.

ALCOHOLIC CEREBELLAR DEGENERATION

Unlike some of the other neurologic complications discussed, alcoholic cerebellar degeneration (ACD) is not a rare neurologic manifestation of

longstanding alcohol abuse, occurring more frequently than Wernicke encephalopathy. Alcoholism is a frequent etiology of acquired cerebellar impairment. The clinical manifestations are usually subacutely progressive over months, but may occur more rapidly, or more chronically over years.

■ **SPECIAL CLINICAL POINT: The classic clinical picture of alcoholic cerebellar degeneration is that of a very ataxic gait (wide based, unsteady, with shortened steps) and stance with only minimal to mild cerebellar findings in the upper extremities.**

Cerebellar abnormalities involving speech and ocular movements are not usually seen. The pathologic findings correspond to the clinical manifestations of ACD, with either the degenerative changes restricted to the anterior and superior portions of the cerebellar vermis, or in some cases, with these regions being affected earlier and more severely than adjacent areas. Focal atrophy of the vermis may be seen in chronic alcoholics on the T1-weighted sagittal MRI images, even in the absence of clinical signs.

Although this is a neurologic complication most often seen in longstanding alcoholics, an exact relationship between the amount of alcohol consumption and the onset of cerebellar symptoms has not been clearly delineated. In addition to the direct neurotoxic effects of alcohol and its metabolites such as acetaldehyde, thiamine deficiency and overall nutritional status are also thought to be contributing factors to the development of ACD; however, the degree to which each of these is responsible is not known. Environmental and genetic variables and age are thought to play a role as well. Clinical improvement may occur with abstinence.

ALCOHOLIC DEMENTIA

In addition to cerebellar atrophy, chronic alcoholics also develop diffuse atrophy that may be evident on neuroimaging by the presence of enlarged ventricles and sulcal widening. The atrophy is attributed mainly to a decrease in the cerebral white matter and while it is widespread, there is disproportionate involvement of the frontal and frontoparietotemporal regions. Chronic alcoholics frequently have cognitive deficits, especially apparent on formal neuropsychological testing, that are not limited to one domain and may be seen on tests of memory, attention, visual and verbal learning, visuospatial abilities, psychomotor speed, and executive functions. The presence or degree of cognitive manifestations of chronic alcoholism does not clearly correspond to the neuroimaging findings of atrophy. It is unclear if alcoholics truly have deficits in these individual modalities or have an overall deficit of higher-order processes.

Patients may develop cognitive impairment and neuroimaging findings consistent with atrophy without previous episodes of Wernicke encephalopathy and therefore independently from a diagnosis of Wernicke–Korsakoff syndrome. This supports a pathophysiologic mechanism other than thiamine deficiency as the etiology of alcoholic dementia. These changes are therefore considered to be due to the toxic effects of ethanol and its metabolites, with the exact mechanism of this toxicity not yet fully elucidated. Likely contributing to the cognitive impairment in many patients is the high comorbidity of head trauma and other coexisting encephalopathies. Patients may have improvement in their cognitive impairment and atrophy with abstinence, with recovery occurring in as early as a few weeks and as late as several years after stopping drinking.

PERIPHERAL NERVOUS SYSTEM MANIFESTATIONS OF CHRONIC ALCOHOLISM

Although much of the emphasis of this chapter has been placed on the potential CNS manifestations of chronic alcoholism, complications of the PNS, namely neuropathy and myopathy, are well described. The onset of these manifestations tends to be insidious and therefore, they may go undiagnosed. This, in turn, has considerable clinical implications, because unlike many of the above discussed CNS complications, there is great potential for significant improvement with alcohol cessation alone.

Alcoholic Neuropathy

Alcoholic neuropathy is a distal axonal sensorimotor polyneuropathy. A wide incidence has been cited in the literature, with an even greater number of chronic alcoholics found to have evidence for neuropathy when electrodiagnostic testing is utilized. Like many other peripheral polyneuropathies, such as that due to diabetes, a patient's initial symptom is usually distal paresthesias involving the feet, often with associated numbness, which gradually progress in a proximal distribution. Over time, symptoms will progress in intensity, becoming more painful, and spread to include the fingers. The pain may become so severe that the patient's activities of daily living are adversely impacted. Motor manifestations, including weakness and atrophy, develop after the sensory symptoms, but do not usually reach the degree of the sensory involvement. Autonomic involvement manifested by constipation, urinary retention, impotence, impaired sweating, gastroparesis, orthostatic hypotension, and cardiovascular autonomic dysfunction may occur. The autonomic symptoms are usually not as frequent and are often more mild than the sensory and motor findings. Cranial nerve involvement is rare.

Neurologic examination reveals early loss of nociception, with loss of all sensory modalities being seen in more advanced cases. With loss of proprioception, patients may have a resultant sensory ataxia with gait instability, and Romberg sign may be present on examination. Loss of the Achilles reflex is a common sign. Chronic findings may include the development of Charcot joints and distal hair loss. The diagnosis of alcoholic neuropathy may be supported by other findings on examination consistent with chronic alcoholism, such as those findings seen in cirrhotic patients discussed previously.

Electromyography and nerve conduction studies will confirm the presence of an axonal polyneuropathy. Further invasive studies, such as nerve biopsy or nerve fiber density, are not indicated for the routine diagnosis of alcoholic neuropathy. It is critical, however, to consider, and rule out as appropriate, other underlying etiologies of a painful peripheral neuropathy, such as diabetes, amyloidosis, cryoglobulinemia, HIV, and Fabry disease.

Thiamine deficiency is known to result in a peripheral polyneuropathy, and neuropathy is a frequently associated finding in patients with Wernicke encephalopathy. Therefore, alcoholic neuropathy was initially thought to be a direct result of alcoholism-induced thiamine deficiency. The pathophysiology of alcoholic neuropathy is now known to not be this straightforward. This is supported by the presence of alcoholic neuropathy in patients without thiamine deficiency, the distinct clinical presentation and pathologic findings of pure thiamine deficiency neuropathy, and by the finding of a dose-dependent relationship between the presence and severity of alcoholic neuropathy and total lifetime dose of alcohol. Alcoholic neuropathy is now thought to be, at least in large part, a result of the toxic effects of ethanol or its metabolites on the PNS. The superimposed presence of thiamine deficiency may result in variation of the clinical picture of the classic alcoholic neuropathy described above.

Prognosis is often poor in patients who continue to drink heavily, with further progression of their alcoholic neuropathy resulting in worsening pain and gait instability. Patients may also stabilize with no further deterioration, despite continued drinking. The reverse is also true, and patients with severe alcoholic neuropathy may have a good prognosis with improvement of their symptoms and resolution of the abnormalities found on neurologic examination and electrodiagnostic

studies with sustained abstinence. Patients with mild to moderate neuropathies tend to recover more fully. Patients who significantly decrease their alcohol intake, without complete abstention, may also recover. The lack of efficacy of vitamin supplementation in patients who continue to drink further supports a direct toxic effect of ethanol and its metabolites as the underlying pathophysiology of pure alcoholic neuropathy. Concomitantly occurring diseases such as diabetes will adversely impact prognosis.

In addition to alcohol cessation, patients may have some improvement of their painful paresthesias with symptomatic therapies such as gabapentin and pregabalin. Topical treatments, such as the lidocaine patch, may also provide some pain relief. In patients with a sensory ataxia, physical therapy with gait and balance training may result in improved patient safety.

In addition to the commonly encountered variant of alcoholic neuropathy, alcoholics with alcoholic neuropathy are also at increased risk for superimposed compression neuropathies. A common site of compression is the radial nerve at the spiral groove, known as the "Saturday night palsy," which results from falling asleep in a sitting position with their upper extremities dangling over the arms of a chair, then awakening with a wrist drop. Other common sites susceptible to compression injury include the peroneal nerve at the fibular head and the ulnar nerve at the elbow. Very rarely, alcohol neuropathy will present with an acute or subacute course. In these cases, the main differential diagnosis is Guillain–Barré syndrome, which may be distinguished from an acute alcoholic neuropathy by normal CSF protein and evidence of an axonal, not demyelinating, process on electrodiagnostic studies.

Alcoholic Myopathy

Although alcoholic myopathy often occurs concurrently with alcoholic neuropathy, it is a distinct phenomenon with the clinical picture the result of a unique pathologic process. As with alcoholic neuropathy, there is an acute and chronic form, and although the chronic form is much more common than the acute form, the acute form does occur with more regularity than the rare cases reported of acute alcoholic neuropathy. The clinical syndrome of acute alcoholic myopathy consists of usually proximal myalgias (cramping and pain) in association with muscle tenderness, swollen muscles, and weakness. Calf involvement is not rare. The onset of symptoms is usually over hours to days, and patients will often have associated myoglobinuria due to rhabdomyolysis, with markedly elevated serum creatine phosphokinase (CK). Myoglobinuria results in acute tubular necrosis and, in turn, renal impairment. This risk for acute renal failure is the most clinically significant aspect of this condition. Patients may have bulbar and respiratory muscular involvement, especially in the acute diffuse necrotizing form. Acute alcoholic myopathy usually is triggered by a severe alcoholic binge, especially in malnourished chronic alcoholics or in those who binge after a long period of abstinence, and has a male gender predominance. There is a wide spectrum of disease; while patients may have a severe course with acute renal failure, many are asymptomatic or experience only mild myalgias and a milder transient rise in CK.

In addition to serum CK levels, serum and urine myoglobin may support the diagnosis. Also, evidence for an acute myopathic process may be seen on electrodiagnostic studies, although these changes may not be apparent until approximately 2 weeks after the onset of symptoms. On pathologic studies (not indicated in the routine diagnosis of this illness), there is necrosis and phagocytosis of both the red and white muscle fibers.

Muscle injury is thought to be due to a toxic effect of ethanol, either through direct injury or through impairment of metabolic processes. Electrolyte derangements such as hypokalemia and hypophosphatemia may contribute to this process, but acute alcoholic myopathy occurs in the absence of electrolyte abnormalities and therefore this is not a sufficient explanation on its own. However, due to the potential to exacerbate the acute illness, nutritional, vitamin, and electrolyte deficiencies and disturbances should be actively sought out and corrected. Adequate intravenous fluid replacement and maintenance of a high urine pH may protect against the renal complications. Neurologic prognosis is often good with patients able to recover full strength within days to weeks with avoidance of alcohol, even following repeated episodes; overall prognosis is dependent on how well patients recover from the associated renal failure.

Chronic alcoholic myopathy is estimated to be one of the most common causes of muscle disease, occurring much more frequently than genetic muscular disorders. It is also one of the most frequent neurologic complications of alcoholism. Chronic alcoholic myopathy differs greatly from the acute variant in its clinical presentation, not just its time course. Progressive proximal muscle weakness (mainly involving the shoulder and pelvic girdles) occurs over many weeks to months with minimal to no associated myalgias. Although this is the usual pattern of muscle involvement, patients may have more widespread involvement, with generalized muscle weakness sometimes seen. A subclinical form also exists in which patients are not symptomatic, but mild weakness and atrophy may be detected by physical examination.

Chronic alcoholic myopathy occurs equally in both sexes, most commonly in patients who have been drinking heavily for over 10 years. It naturally follows that patients will often have other manifestations of chronic alcohol abuse such as cirrhosis, peripheral neuropathy, and cardiomyopathy due to cardiac muscle involvement.

Neurologic examination of patients with chronic alcoholic myopathy will usually reveal atrophy in addition to the proximal muscle weakness. Fasciculations may be seen. Serum CK levels are frequently normal or only mildly elevated and patients do not have myoglobulinuria. In a chronic alcoholic with this clinical picture and without any other underlying etiologies of a myopathy, muscle biopsy revealing atrophy of primarily the type II muscle fibers and myocyte necrosis is considered diagnostic. These biopsy findings are not specific to chronic alcoholic myopathy and it is the presence of all of these criteria and not the biopsy alone that allows for the diagnosis to be made. Rarely, however, in clinical practice is biopsy necessary, with the diagnosis usually made based on the history, examination findings, and supporting laboratory and electrodiagnostic data.

Like acute alcoholic myopathy, chronic alcoholic myopathy is the result of the direct toxic effects of alcohol on striated muscle and its pathogenesis is not related to nutritional, electrolyte, or vitamin derangements or to the frequently concurrent liver dysfunction. Multiple theories exist for how ethanol results in muscle disease, including the production of free radicals, alterations of protein and glycogen metabolism, and impairment of mitochondrial function. Likely, a combination of multiple different alcohol-induced mechanisms results in the final clinical picture. Patient-specific variables such as gender, nutritional status, and the presence of other disease processes may make a patient more susceptible to these toxic effects.

As with the acute variant, treatment consists mainly of abstinence; however, correction of electrolyte, vitamin, and other nutritional deficiencies, such as inadequate calorie or protein intake, may hasten and result in a more complete recovery. Ethanol toxicity on muscle is known to be dose dependent and this applies to recovery as well. Patients who are truly abstinent will have improvement or at least stabilization of their disease and patients who continue to drink heavily will have further progression of their myopathy. Patients who are not fully abstinent but significantly reduce their alcohol intake will usually also have improvement. With cessation of ethanol use, most patients will undergo significant gradual recovery. Patients may benefit greatly from physiotherapy during the recovery period to improve muscle bulk and motor function.

WHEN TO REFER PATIENTS TO A NEUROLOGIST

The spectrum of potential neurologic complications of chronic alcoholism is broad, ranging from commonly encountered manifestations, such as hepatic encephalopathy and cerebellar degeneration, to the more rare manifestations, such as MBD. Further complicating the diagnosis and, in turn, the management of these patients is that they often do not present with "classic" clinical presentations such as the full triad of Wernicke encephalopathy, and patients suffering from chronic alcoholism will often not have a singular complication, but rather multiple ones superimposed on each other, involving both the PNS and CNS. Although the only treatment for many of the possible neurologic complications of alcoholism is alcohol cessation, some, such as Wernicke and pellagra encephalopathy, constitute neurologic emergencies and therefore need to be recognized promptly. Therefore, practitioners who care for this patient population must have a high index of suspicion for some of the rarer, yet treatable complications of chronic alcoholism.

A neurologist may be consulted whenever the primary physician is uncomfortable with the diagnosis or management of the patient, or the patient does not respond to therapy in the expected manner for the presumed diagnosis. A neurologist may be consulted prior to the ordering of diagnostic studies such as electrodiagnostic testing or MRI as this testing may not be necessary and is not always helpful in confirming the neurologic diagnosis. The evaluation and treatment of acutely ill patients, such as those in whom Wernicke encephalopathy or superimposed CNS infection or hemorrhage is suspected, should never be delayed in order to obtain a neurologic consultation.

Always Remember

- Wernicke encephalopathy is a neurologic emergency, whose diagnosis, and therefore the decision to treat, should be based on the clinical picture alone.
- As treatment is generally well tolerated and the risk of missing the diagnosis is so great, Wernicke encephalopathy should be considered in all high-risk patients.
- Pellagra encephalopathy is a clinical diagnosis that can be confirmed by clinical improvement with replacement therapy.
- A triggering clinical event superimposed on chronic underlying liver disease is often responsible for the development of hepatic encephalopathy. As a result, treatment of hepatic encephalopathy starts with a search for and correction of any triggering factors.
- The classic clinical picture of alcoholic cerebellar degeneration is that of a very ataxic gait and stance, with only minimal to mild cerebellar findings seen in the upper extremities. If there are prominent upper extremity symptoms, another diagnosis should be strongly considered and searched for (such as a cerebellar infarct or hemorrhage).
- When diagnosing alcoholic neuropathy, it is critical to rule out other underlying etiologies of a painful peripheral neuropathy.

QUESTIONS AND DISCUSSION

1. A 56-year-old man who has been a recovering alcoholic for a number of years relapses at a party. He then goes on to drink multiple bottles of hard liquor over the next several days. Two days later, he presents to the emergency room reporting severe cramping and muscle pain of his proximal lower extremities which has progressed over the past day, and an episode of "cola-colored" urine. On examination, he has exquisite muscle tenderness to palpation and mild proximal weakness. CK is 850 IU/L. Electrolyte levels are normal. What is the most appropriate initial management of this patient?
   A. Transfer from the emergency room to an inpatient alcohol rehabilitation program
   B. Discharge home with a nonsteroidal anti-inflammatory agent
   C. Intravenous fluid replacement and maintenance of a high urine pH
   D. Phosphorus supplementation
   E. EMG and nerve conduction studies

The correct answer is C. This patient's clinical history and his clinical symptoms and signs are most compatible with an acute alcoholic myopathy. Intravenous fluid replacement and maintenance of a high urine pH may protect against the renal complications of this condition. Electrodiagnostic studies may ultimately be helpful but are not necessary immediately. The overall prognosis in this condition is dependent on how well patients recover from the associated renal impairment of acute alcoholic myopathy.

2. A man is brought to the emergency room after being found in the street by the police. He appears to be in his mid-forties and severely malnourished, smells of alcohol, and has a laceration on his forehead with dried blood. He is mildly lethargic, oriented only to person, and is dysarthric. CT scan of the head without contrast does not reveal any acute intracranial pathology. What diagnostic studies should be performed prior to administering the appropriate treatment in this patient?
   A. Administration of 1 mg of IV thiamine to ensure that the patient does not have an anaphylactic reaction prior to administering the full dose
   B. Lumbar puncture to assess the CSF thiamine level
   C. No studies are indicated prior to treatment

D. Red blood cell transketolase levels in serum

E. Serum thiamine level

The correct answer is C. Wernicke encephalopathy is a neurologic emergency, whose diagnosis, and therefore the decision to treat, should be based on the clinical picture alone. As treatment is generally well tolerated and the risk of missing the diagnosis is so great, this diagnosis should be considered in all high-risk patients, particularly when the patient presents acutely intoxicated. Measures of thiamine status, including thiamine levels and red blood cell transketolase, are not diagnostic, may not be available emergently, and should not be relied on to make treatment decisions.

3. A 60-year-old woman with longstanding alcoholic cirrhosis is brought by her children to her hepatologist's office for several days of progressive lethargy, mild confusion, and mild tremor and incoordination, mainly noticed during meals. She is afebrile and normotensive. On examination, she is disoriented to place and time. There is no papilledema. Strength is normal in the extremities and she has a mild postural tremor in the arms. Reflexes are mildly brisk and no Babinski signs are present. Gait is mildly wide based and unsteady. Which of the following is the most appropriate first-line evaluation and treatment of this patient?
A. Admission to the hospital for careful investigation for a triggering clinical event such as superimposed infection or GI bleeding
B. Neurosurgical consultation for possible intracranial pressure monitoring
C. Emergent MRI of the brain to assess for the presence of high signal in the basal ganglia on the T1-weighted images.
D. Outpatient initiation of treatment with lactulose in combination with rifaximin with close clinical follow-up in 1 week's time

E. Outpatient initiation of treatment with rifaximin alone

The correct answer is A. A triggering clinical event superimposed on chronic underlying liver disease is often responsible for the development of hepatic encephalopathy. As a result, treatment of hepatic encephalopathy starts with a search for and correction of any triggering factors. MRI will often show high signal on the T1 images in the globus pallidus, but this finding is seen in many patients with chronic liver disease and is not in itself specific for the clinical diagnosis of hepatic encephalopathy.

4. A 70-year-old woman presents with 6 months of progressively painful paresthesias that began in the feet and have spread up to the ankles. She denies any other known medical problems, but does admit to 25 years of drinking a half a pint of whiskey daily. Neurologic examination reveals marked decrease to pinprick in the distal lower extremities and severely decreased vibration sense over the great toes. Strength is normal. Routine laboratory studies including CBC, fasting blood sugar, liver and kidney function tests, and electrolytes are normal. Which of the following is the most appropriate next step in the investigation of this patient?
A. Glucose 2-hour tolerance test
B. MRI of the lumbar spine to rule out lumbar stenosis mimicking a peripheral polyneuropathy
C. No further workup is indicated given the patient's clear history of alcohol abuse
D. Serum thiamine levels
E. Sural nerve biopsy

The correct answer is A. In patients with suspected alcohol neuropathy, it is critical to rule out other underlying etiologies of a painful peripheral polyneuropathy, such as diabetes, amyloidosis, cryoglobulinemia, and HIV. Therefore, in this case, extensive laboratory testing, including further assessment for diabetes, should be performed. Nerve biopsy and nerve fiber density are not indicated for the routine diagnosis of alcoholic neuropathy.

SUGGESTED READING

Bartha P, Shifrin E, Levy Y. Pancreatic encephalopathy—a rare complication of a common disease. *Eur J Intern Med*. 2006;17:382.

Burkhard PR, Delavelle J, Du Pasquier R, Spahr L. Chronic parkinsonism associated with cirrhosis: a distinct subset of acquired hepatocerebral degeneration. *Arch Neurol*. 2003;60:521–528.

Delgado-Sanchez L, Godkar D, Niranjan S. Pellagra: rekindling of an old flame. *Am J Ther*. 2008;15: 173–175.

Fitzpatrick LE, Jackson M, Crowe SF. The relationship between alcoholic cerebellar degeneration and cognitive and emotional functioning. *Neurosci Biobehav Rev*. 2008;32(3):466–485.

Kleinschmidt-DeMasters BK, Rojiani AM, Filley CM. Central and extrapontine myelinolysis: then . . . and now. *J Neuropath Exp Neurol*. 2006;65(1):1–11.

Kohler CG, Ances BM, Coleman AR, et al. Marchiafava–Bignami disease: literature review and case report. *Neuropsychiatry Neuropsychol Behav Neurol*. 2000;13(1):67–76.

Koike H, Sobue G. Alcoholic neuropathy. *Curr Opin Neurol*. 2006;19:481–486.

Lockwood AH. Hepatic encephalopathy. In: Aminoff MJ, ed. *Neurology and General Medicine*. 4th ed. Philadelphia, PA: Churchill Livingstone; 2008:265–279.

Ménégon P, Sibon I, Pachai C. Marchiafava–Bignami disease: diffusion-weighted MRI in corpus callosum and cortical lesions. *Neurology*. 2005;65(3):475–477.

Menza MA, Murray GB. Pancreatic encephalopathy. *Biol Psychiatry*. 1989;25:781–784.

Munoz SJ. Hepatic encephalopathy. *Med Clin North Am*. 2008;92:795–812.

Pearce JMS. Wernicke–Korsakoff encephalopathy. *Eur Neurol*. 2008;59:101–104.

Preedy VR, Adachi J, Ueno Y, et al. Alcoholic skeletal muscle myopathy: definitions, features, contribution of neuropathy, impact and diagnosis. *Eur J Neurol*. 2001;8(6):677–687.

Sechi GP, Serra A. Wernicke's encephalopathy: new clinical settings and recent advances in diagnosis and management. *Lancet Neurol*. 2007;6:442–455.

Thomson AD, Cook CCH, Guerrini I, et al. Wernicke's encephalopathy: 'Plus ca change, plus C'Est a mem chose'. *Alcohol Alcohol*. 2008;43(2):180–186.

Urbano-Márquez A, Fernández-Solá J. Effects of alcohol on skeletal and cardiac muscle. *Muscle Nerve*. 2004;30(6):689–707.

van der Helm van Mil AHM, van Vugt JPP, Lammers GJ, Harinck HIJ. Hypernatremia from a hunger strike as a cause of osmotic myelinosis. *Neurology*. 2005;64(1):574–575.

Victor M, Adams RD, Collins GH. *The Wernicke–Korsakoff Syndrome and Related Neurologic Disorders Due to Alcoholism and Malnutrition*. 2nd ed. Philadelphia, PA: FA Davis Company; 1989.

Wijdicks EFM, Wiesner RH. Acquired (non-Wilsonian) hepatocerebral degeneration: complex management decisions. *Liver Transpl*. 2003;9(9):993–994.

Yokota O, Tsuchiya K, Terada S. Frequency and clinicopathological characteristics of alcoholic cerebellar degeneration in Japan: a cross-sectional study of 1509 postmortems. *Acta Neuropathol*. 2006;112:43–51.

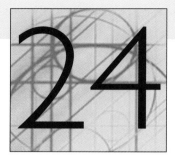

24

Central Nervous System Infections

LARRY E. DAVIS

key points

- Meningitis may be viral, bacterial, or fungal. These different types of meningitis differ in terms of time course, severity, and recommended treatments.

- Encephalitis is usually viral. Herpes encephalitis in particular should be treated with acyclovir.

- Brain abscesses are usually bacterial and may cause significant symptoms based on mass effect.

- Prion diseases (e.g., Creutzfeldt–Jakob) are characterized by rapidly progressive dementia.

entral nervous system (CNS) infections can be caused by viruses, bacteria, fungi, parasites, and prions, but bacteria and viruses are the most common causes. All but one class of human infectious agents (called prions) possess nucleic acid (DNA, RNA, or both) surrounded by a variety of proteins and lipids to create a particle, single cell, or complex cellular organism. Infectious agents enter the body by way of the gastrointestinal tract or respiratory tract or following skin inoculation (animal or insect bite) and set up the initial site of replication in these tissues.

■ **SPECIAL CLINICAL POINT: The majority of organisms then reach the CNS by way of the bloodstream, but occasional organisms reach the brain by way of peripheral nerves or by direct entry through adjacent bone following open skull fracture or from infected mastoid or air sinuses.**

Despite the many infections we develop during our lifetimes, organisms rarely reach the brain. For example, transient bacteremias are common following vigorously brushing teeth, yet the bacteria do not cause meningitis. Important protective systems include the reticuloendothelial system (which efficiently removes bacteria and viruses from blood), cellular and humoral immune responses (which destroy organisms from the blood and primary site of infection), and the blood–brain barrier (which prevents entry of organisms into the brain or cerebrospinal fluid [CSF]). Organisms that do enter the brain or CSF from blood do so by infecting endothelial cells of the cerebral blood vessels (many encephalitis viruses), penetrating the blood–CSF barrier in the meninges or choroid plexus (many bacteria) or occluding small cerebral blood vessels with infected emboli from the blood (brain abscess organisms). Once the invasion has occurred, the brain and CSF have less immune protection than the rest of the body. Normal CSF has about 1/500th the amount of antibody as blood and has few white blood cells (WBCs). Thus, individuals who develop a brain or meningeal bacterial or fungal infection usually die without antimicrobial intervention.

Inflammation of the meninges or brain is the hallmark of CNS infection. Inflammatory cells may be present in the meninges, in perivascular spaces, or within brain parenchyma such as around an abscess or with encephalitis. The inflammatory monocytes show specific immune activity against the infectious agent.

■ **SPECIAL CLINICAL POINT:** The signs and symptoms of a CNS infection depend on the site of the infection—not the organism. The organism determines mainly the time course and severity of the infection.

In general, the time course to develop CNS signs depends on the microorganism class: viruses (hours to 1 day); aerobic bacteria (hours to a few days); anaerobic bacteria, tuberculosis, and fungi (a few days to weeks); parasites and *Treponema pallidum* (syphilis) (weeks to years).

MENINGITIS

A variety of viral, bacterial, fungal, parasitic, chemical, and neoplastic agents may cause inflammation of the meninges. These patients all have common clinical features:

- Early features: Prodromal illness, fever, headache, stiff neck, relative preservation of mental status, no focal neurologic signs, no papilledema.
- Later features: Seizures, stupor and coma, cranial nerve palsies, deafness, focal neurologic signs may develop if the etiology is other than viral.

■ **SPECIAL CLINICAL POINT:** The time course of the meningitis may give clues as to its etiology. Viral and bacterial meningitis are acute illnesses with symptoms developing over hours to 1 day. Patients with fungal meningitis or tuberculous meningitis develop symptoms over days to 2 weeks.

Common Laboratory Findings

The WBC in blood usually is elevated, as is the erythrocyte sedimentation rate. The CSF examination is the key to the diagnosis of meningitis with ascertainment of the type of infecting agent, establishment of the etiologic agent, and determination of antimicrobial sensitivities (Fig. 24.1). Viral, bacterial, tuberculous, and fungal infections of the meninges have differing CSF profiles (Table 24.1). CSF culture determines the etiology of the infection as well as antimicrobial sensitivities. In general, cultures for bacteria take 1 to 3 days, virus cultures take days to 3 weeks, and tuberculosis and fungi cultures take 1 to 6 weeks. Rapid diagnosis of bacteria can be made by Gram stain of CSF sediment and by testing CSF for common bacterial antigens. The Gram stain will detect bacteria in CSF sediment in more than three fourths of patients with acute bacterial meningitis and often gives clues for initial antibiotic treatment. Latex agglutination antigen tests are commercially available to detect *Haemophilus influenzae*, *Streptococcus pneumoniae*, *Neisseria meningitidis*, and group A beta-hemolytic streptococci. Antigen tests have about the same sensitivity as the Gram stain and may be useful if the patient is already receiving antibiotics. The polymerase chain reaction (PCR) diagnostic test is readily available to rapidly diagnose *Mycobacterium tuberculosis*, enteroviruses, and herpes simplex virus. Many others are available on a research basis. PCR detects tiny amounts of nucleic acids of these infectious agents in CSF. Advantages of the PCR assay is that it can be performed within hours and can detect nucleic acid from organisms that may be very difficult

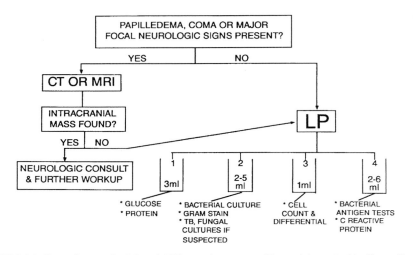

FIGURE 24.1 Flow diagram for LP and CSF tests in suspected bacterial meningitis. (From Davis LE. Acute bacterial meningitis. In: Weiner WJ, ed. *Emergent and urgent neurology.* Philadelphia: JB Lippincott, 1992:139, with permission.)

to culture. However, the PCR does not give information regarding antimicrobial sensitivities. Thus, the best diagnostic test is still to culture the CSF and blood for an infectious agent and use the isolate to determine antimicrobial sensitivities.

Viral Meningitis

Enteroviruses (echoviruses and Coxsackie viruses) are the most common cause of viral meningitis. Less common viruses include herpes simplex virus type 2, mumps virus, lymphocytic choriomeningitis, and human immunodeficiency

TABLE 24.1

Spinal Fluid Profiles in CNS Infections

	Opening Pressure	White Blood Cells	Protein	Glucose	Bacterial or Fungal Culture
Epidural abscess	N or sl ↑	0–20 (lymphs)	N or sl ↑	N	Negative
Subdural empyema	↑	10–1000 (polys)	sl ↑	N	Negative
Viral meningitis	N or sl ↑	20–1000 (lymphs)[a]	sl ↑	N	Negative
Bacterial meningitis	↑	50–5000 (polys)	↑	Low	Positive
Fungal or tuberculous meningitis	↑	50–5000 (polys and lymphs)	↑	Low	Positive
Meningovascular syphilis	N or sl ↑	10–1000 (lymphs)	↑	N	Negative
Brain abscess	↑	0–10 (lymphs and polys)	N	N	Negative
Viral encephalitis	sl ↑	10–200 (lymphs)	N or sl ↑	N	Negative

[a]CSF may show poly predominance during the first day.
N, normal; sl ↑, slight increase; ↑, increased.

virus. Typically in viral meningitis, the CSF contains a pleocytosis with predominately lymphocytes, mildly elevated protein, normal glucose, and negative Gram stain of sediment. However, in the first day of the meningitis, there may be a predominance of neutrophils in the CSF. Viruses often can be isolated from CSF early in the meningitis, and PCR analysis of CSF rapidly diagnoses enteroviruses and herpes simplex type 2 viruses. Treatment of most viral meningitis is usually symptomatic and may include analgesics for the headache and antiemetics for nausea and vomiting. In sexually active adults, genital herpes simplex may develop accompanied by meningitis, which can recur for years. If herpes simplex virus is identified in CSF or in herpetic vesicles, use of high-dose acyclovir may shorten the duration of the meningitis.

■ **SPECIAL CLINICAL POINT: Hospitalization for viral meningitis may not be required if the diagnosis is certain, but the patient should be observed at home by a responsible individual. The prognosis of viral meningitis is excellent, and most patients fully recover within 1 to 2 weeks.**

Acute Bacterial Meningitis

Both gram-positive and gram-negative aerobic bacteria cause meningitis. *S. pneumoniae* is the most common bacterium affecting all ages followed by *N. meningitidis* and *H. influenzae*. Since the introduction of *H. influenzae* type B and pneumococcal vaccines to children, the incidence of meningitis in children has decreased dramatically.

■ **SPECIAL CLINICAL POINT: Unlike viral meningitis, patients with bacterial meningitis will progress to death if untreated with antibiotics. Therefore, prompt diagnosis and treatment are essential.**

If bacterial meningitis is suspected, the lumbar puncture (LP) becomes an emergency procedure (Fig. 24.1). Although increased intracranial pressure is common in bacterial meningitis, it rarely poses a risk of brain herniation that would prevent an LP. Thus, it seldom is necessary to perform a computed tomography (CT) or a magnetic resonance imaging (MRI) scan before the LP unless the patient is immunosuppressed; is elderly; or presents with coma, focal neurologic signs, or papilledema that places them at increased risk for a focal CNS mass. If there is to be a significant delay before the neuroimaging can be obtained, broad-spectrum antibiotics should be given before the LP. However, one always should obtain a blood culture before administrating the antibiotics. A blood culture is positive in 60% of patients with bacterial meningitis and thus could yield antibiotic sensitivities.

The key to treatment of acute bacterial meningitis is the prompt administration of appropriate antibiotics. General principles involved in the use of antibiotics include the following: (a) the antibiotic should be given early in the clinical course; (b) the bacteria must be sensitive to the antibiotic; (c) the antibiotic must cross the blood–brain barrier and achieve sufficient CSF concentrations to kill the bacteria. Once the diagnosis of bacterial meningitis is made, one should begin treatment with broad-spectrum antibiotics, which later can be modified when antibiotic sensitivities become available. The choice of an antibiotic for initial treatment depends on several factors: age, immune status, and predisposing medical conditions of the patient; results of CSF Gram stain and bacterial antigen tests; knowledge of the types of drug-resistant bacteria in the community; and whether the patient is allergic to any antibiotic. Table 24.2 gives common initial antibiotic regimens, but one should check references such as the *Medical Letter* for the latest recommendations.

Neurologic injury in bacterial meningitis occurs in up to 20% of patients. Mechanisms of cerebral injury include meningeal vasculitis causing spasm or thrombosis of meningeal arteries, arterioles, veins, or venules. The consequence is ischemia to the underlying brain resulting in infarctions. Second, a variety of toxins are produced within the CSF by the bacteria and inflammatory cells such as endotoxin, reactive oxidizing chemicals from neutrophil granule

TABLE 24.2 | **Initial Antibiotic Therapy While Awaiting Identification of Infecting Organisms**

Setting	Therapy
Preterm and newborn	Ampicillin plus cefotaxime, or ampicillin plus aminoglycoside
2 months to adulthood	Ceftriaxone or cefotaxime plus vancomycin, usually with ampicillin; vancomycin and ampicillin can be stopped if the bacteria are sensitive to cephalosporins; ampicillin is given if *Listeria monocytogenes* is suspected
Cranial trauma, recent neurosurgery, or CSF shunt	Vancomycin, cefepime, ceftazidime, or meropenem

One should always check with references such as the *Medical Letter* for the latest recommendations because resistance patterns are changing.

release, and cytokines released from mononuclear cells that cross the pial barrier to reach cerebral gray matter causing neuronal necrosis. The third mechanism develops from inadequate cerebral arterial perfusion producing global cerebral ischemia. Cerebral perfusion pressure results from systemic blood pressure minus intracranial pressure. Increased intracranial pressure can result from increased brain water from the first two mechanisms, increased CSF pressure due to obstructive hydrocephalus and from increased cerebral blood from dilated meningeal arteries and veins responding to the inflammation. Systemic hypotension can develop from shock, hypovolemia, dehydration secondary to fever and vomiting, and inadequate fluid replacement in the hospital. Meningeal bacteria do not readily penetrate the pia mater and invade the brain. However, interactions between meningeal bacteria and host result in meningeal inflammation; vascular injury; disruption of the blood–brain barrier; vasogenic, interstitial, and cytotoxic edema; and disruption of normal CSF flow. At present, corticosteroids have been shown to have a modest benefit in preventing neurologic morbidity in children and adults. Dexamethasone (0.15 mg/kg intravenously in children every 6 hours and 10 mg in adults every 6 hours for 2 to 4 days) commonly is administered as early as possible. To minimize risks from administering corticosteroids, dexamethasone should be given only when the illness and CSF findings are highly suggestive of community acquired bacterial meningitis in an immunocompetent patient without contraindications for steroid administration such as a recent GI bleed.

In general, the CSF becomes sterile within 1 day after antibiotic treatment. The fever usually disappears within a few days but may persist for up to 2 weeks. CSF abnormalities rapidly return toward normal, but the pleocytosis and elevated protein may persist for several weeks. Dead bacteria may be seen on Gram stain of CSF for several days as are PCR assays for the offending bacteria.

Even if the patient is treated promptly with appropriate antibiotics and steroids, serious complications still may develop. Seizures develop in about one third of patients, occur usually during the acute phase of the meningitis, and seldom recur after the hospitalization. Causes of seizures in meningitis include cerebral cortex irritation from bacterial toxins or meningeal inflammation, CNS vasculitis, brain infarction, high fever, and hyponatremia from the syndrome of inappropriate antidiuretic hormone coupled with excess fluid administration. Treatment of the seizures is usually with intravenous phosphenytoin or levetiracetam until hospital discharge. Focal neurologic sequelae include cranial nerve palsies, especially cranial nerves VIII (deafness) and VI and III (diplopia), cerebellar ataxia, and hemiparesis. In surviving children and adults, 15% have language disorders and 10% have cognitive problems. CT or MRI of the head is often helpful in the evaluation of these complications and may demonstrate cerebral or cerebellar infarction, brain necrosis, subdural hygromas, or mild ventricular dilatation. Hydrocephalus, subdural empyema, and brain abscess occur but are uncommon. Patients with focal neurologic damage benefit from rehabilitation following acute antibiotic therapy, especially if deafness is identified. Mortality from bacterial meningitis ranges from 5% to 20%, depending on the strain of infecting bacteria, the age group, and predisposing illnesses in the patient.

Some bacterial meningitis requires chemoprophylaxis of immediate family members and close contacts because of their increased risk of developing meningitis. In *N. meningitidis* meningitis, treatment of all close contacts is indicated. Rifampin (600 mg for adults or 10 mg/kg for children twice daily orally for 2 days) or ciprofloxacin (single oral dose of 500 mg for adults) may be given. If the patient has *H. influenzae* type B meningitis, chemoprophylaxis is indicated for children younger than 4 years of age who have been in close contact with the patient and not previously vaccinated with the *H. influenzae* type B vaccine. Rifampin (10 mg/kg twice daily orally for 4 days) usually is given. All close contacts should be observed carefully for the next week.

Many cases of bacterial meningitis can be prevented by immunizing infants and small children with *H. influenzae* type B and pneumococcal vaccines and by immunizing high-risk populations such as college students and military recruits with the meningococcal vaccine.

Spirochete Meningitis

Spirochetes produce chronic bacterial meningitis. *Borrelia burgdorferi* (CNS Lyme disease) and *T. pallidum* (neurosyphilis) both cause acute and occasionally chronic meningitis. Patients develop headaches, cranial nerve palsies (especially the Bell palsy in CNS Lyme disease), and occasionally brain infarctions from thrombosis of cortical blood vessels (meningovascular syphilis). Years later, the spirochetes occasionally invade the brain causing a low-grade encephalitis (general paresis or CNS Lyme disease). The CSF contains a lymphocytic pleocytosis, elevated protein, and usually normal glucose level. Spirochetes seldom are isolated from CSF, and the diagnosis is made by serologic tests (CSF-Venereal Disease Research Laboratory or Lyme antibody titers). Workup for subacute meningitis is given in Table 24.3. Treatment is with high-dose penicillin or ceftriaxone for several weeks.

Tuberculous and Fungal Meningitis

Patients with tuberculous and fungal meningitis usually develop subacute meningitis with the onset of CNS signs developing over days to weeks. These infections occur most often in individuals who are malnourished, debilitated, or immunosuppressed and have been exposed to others with pulmonary tuberculosis. Although initial entry is usually by way of the lungs, less than 50% will have an active pulmonary infection at the time of the meningitis. The best methods to establish the etiology are by (a) culture of the CSF, (b) identification by PCR infectious agents such as *M. tuberculosis*, (c) QuantiFERON–TB Gold test (white blood test to detect cells sensitive to TB antigens), (d) antigen detection for *Cryptococcus neoformans*, and (e) serologic tests for several fungi. Because tuberculous or fungal organisms may be in low concentrations in the CSF, one should culture a concentrate of 5 to 15 mL of CSF on several occasions.

Treatment of tuberculous meningitis usually requires administration of four drugs (rifampin, isoniazid, pyrazinamide, and streptomycin or ethambutol) for 2 months followed by rifampin and isoniazid for another 7 months, depending on the antibiotic sensitivities of the *M. tuberculosis* isolate. Of

TABLE 24.3

Evaluation of Subacute Meningitis

CSF studies: Opening pressure, cell count with differential, glucose, protein, IgG, Gram stain, acid-fast stain, and cytology; CSF serology includes CSF-VDRL, *Coccidioides immitis, Histoplasma capsulatum* antibody titers, and *Cryptococcus neoformans* antigen titer; PCR assays for *M. tuberculosis* and other fungi as available; QuantiFERON–TB Gold test for *M. tuberculosis*

Skin tests: Intermediate purified protein derivative tuberculin test and anergy skin tests

Serum antibody tests: Brucella, syphilis, toxoplasmosis, *Coccidioides immitis,* other fungi, Lyme disease, and human immunodeficiency virus

Cultures for bacteria, M. tuberculosis, and fungi: CSF cultures repeated three times; blood, urine, sputum, or gastric aspirate; bone marrow biopsy; and skin lesion biopsy

Magnetic resonance image or computed tomograph of head with contrast

Chest x-ray and computed tomograph of abdomen, if indicated

IgG, immunoglobulin G; VDRL, Venereal Disease Research Laboratory.

note, multidrug-resistant tuberculous strains are beginning to cause TB meningitis, especially in individuals from developing countries. Their treatment is complex and difficult. Dexamethasone often is added if the patient is comatose or has severe neurologic deficits. Patients with fungal meningitis are treated either with broad-spectrum triazoles such as fluconazole, itraconazole, voriconazole, or posaconazole or with liposomal amphotericin B such as AmBisome for weeks to months. Fluconazole has been shown to be nearly as efficacious as liposomal amphotericin B in the treatment of cryptococcal and coccidioidal meningitis. The triazoles have the advantage that they can be given orally and have less renal and hematopoietic toxicity. In immunosuppressed or AIDS patients with fungal meningitis in remission, continued use of fluconazole in a lower dosage may prevent recurrence. Complications are similar to those seen in acute bacterial meningitis. Mortality rates range from 20% to 50% depending on the organism and predisposing factors. Survivors may be left with neurologic sequelae similar to those seen in acute bacterial meningitis.

ENCEPHALITIS

The majority of infectious agents that cause encephalitis are viruses that reach the brain by way of a hematogenous route. Once the virus reaches brain parenchyma, a widely disseminated infection of neurons and glia ensues. Neuronal necrosis and lysis of glial cells result in secondary cerebral edema. The inflammatory response includes perivascular cuffing with inflammatory cells and infiltration of lymphocytes and macrophages into the adjacent brain parenchyma. The invading immune response often terminates the infection, but the patient may be left with permanent neurologic sequelae.

Viruses cause more than 90% of cases. Worldwide, arboviruses (togaviruses) are the most common cause. In the United States, West Nile virus is the most common etiology. Because arboviruses require a vector (mosquito or tick), arbovirus encephalitis often occurs in clusters or epidemics in late spring to early fall. Herpes simplex type 1 virus is the most common sporadic cause of encephalitis. Herpes simplex virus is a latent infection in most individuals, following a primary stomatitis infection in childhood. Years later the latent virus can reactivate to cause encephalitis that occurs year round. Other causes of encephalitis are the result of spirochetes (*T. pallidum, B. burgdorferi*), parasites (toxoplasmosis or falciparum malaria), and other viruses (cytomegalovirus, varicella-zoster, adenovirus).

Clinical Features

■ **SPECIAL CLINICAL POINT: Acute encephalitis is a febrile illness characterized by the abrupt onset of headache and mental obtundation.**

Other common features include seizures, which may be generalized or focal; hyperreflexia; spasticity; and Babinski signs. Some patients develop hemiparesis, aphasia, ataxia, limb tremors, and cortical blindness. Patients with West Nile neuroinvasive disease usually develop the typical clinical picture of encephalitis, but 10% also develop a myelitis that is similar to paralytic poliomyelitis. Patients often have a prodromal illness, which varies with the infectious agent and can include parotitis (mumps virus), fever, malaise, and myalgias (arbovirus). Encephalitis differs from meningitis primarily because patients with encephalitis develop prominent mental changes and a minimal or absent stiff neck.

Laboratory Findings

The electroencephalogram (EEG) is always abnormal and usually shows diffuse bilateral slowing with occasional seizure activity. An LP in a patient with early encephalitis will have an opening pressure that is normal or slightly elevated. The CSF contains five to several hundred WBC/mm^3 (predominantly lymphocytes). CSF glucose is normal, whereas CSF protein is elevated. Viral cultures are usually sterile. Early in the course of encephalitis, the CT scan may be normal, whereas the T2-weighted MRI scan often shows areas of hyperintensity as a result of edema from cerebral vascular permeability. Later, both scans may demonstrate areas of necrosis or hemorrhage. The presence

of T2, diffusion-weighted images, or FLAIR lesions on MRI that are located mainly in the medial aspect of the temporal lobe is suggestive of herpes simplex encephalitis.

The diagnosis of viral encephalitis usually is made by serologic tests or PCR assays. Because most arboviruses rarely infect humans in the United States and produce a systemic viral infection before producing the viral encephalitis, immunoglobulin M (IgM) antibodies to the virus often are present early in the encephalitis. The IgM-antibody-capture enzyme-linked immunoabsorbent assay (Mac ELISA) can be used to detect arbovirus antibodies in serum and CSF during the first few days of the encephalitis. Acute and convalescent serum titers can be determined for many viruses with a fourfold increase in antibody titer being diagnostic. Serologic tests are not useful in establishing the diagnosis of herpes simplex encephalitis, but the diagnosis can be made by detection of herpes simplex viral DNA in CSF by PCR. Although herpes simplex virus is almost never cultured from CSF, enough viral DNA leaks into the CSF from the brain infection to be detected by PCR. The CSF PCR test is quite sensitive even during the first few days of the encephalitis.

Management and Prognosis

All patients require excellent symptomatic care to minimize complications. If seizures develop, anticonvulsant medications are indicated. If increased intracranial pressure develops from vascular engorgement and cerebral edema, treatment may require hyperventilation or the administration of mannitol. Use of corticosteroids is controversial. In patients with herpes simplex encephalitis, treatment with acyclovir significantly improves outcome. Acyclovir should be administered early in the encephalitis course. Current recommendations are to give 30 mg/kg/day of acyclovir that is divided into three doses per day for 14 to 21 days. The drug should be delivered intravenously slowly over 1 hour to prevent renal toxicity. Drug complications include transient renal failure, thrombophlebitis, and elevations of serum liver enzymes. For most RNA viruses such as arboviruses, no antiviral treatment is available.

Prognosis of encephalitis depends on the infectious agent. Patients with mumps meningoencephalitis and Venezuelan equine encephalitis have an excellent prognosis. Patients with West Nile, western equine, St. Louis, and California encephalitis usually have a reasonable prognosis (2% to 15% mortality), but up to 25% of patients are left with dementia, seizures, or focal neurologic deficits. Patients with eastern equine, Japanese B, and Murray Valley encephalitis have mortality rates from 20% to 40%. Patients with herpes simplex encephalitis who are treated with acyclovir have a 20% mortality rate, and 55% are left with some neurologic sequelae. Rabies encephalitis is fatal. Patients with cognitive impairment or focal neurologic signs benefit from rehabilitation that may take weeks.

BRAIN ABSCESS

Although viruses tend to cause diffuse brain infections, most bacteria, fungi, and parasites cause localized brain disease. Brain abscesses may arise by direct extension from other foci of infection within the cranial cavity (mastoiditis and sinusitis) and from infections following skull fracture or craniotomy, or as metastasis carried by the blood from infections elsewhere in the body. The infection usually begins as a localized encephalitis with focal softening, necrosis, and inflammation. As the process continues, fibroblasts proliferate at the edges, forming a capsule wall. A variable amount of cerebral edema surrounds the lesion. If the etiology is bacterial or fungal, the space-occupying lesion slowly expands. If untreated, the brain mass is lethal. Patients with neurocysticercosis develop cysts that usually stop growing after they reach about 10 to 15 mm in size.

Anaerobic bacteria are found in more than one half of brain abscesses. Anaerobic streptococci and *Bacteroides fragilis* are common

organisms. Occasionally, multiple bacteria are found in abscesses. Brain abscesses following head trauma or neurosurgery may contain *Staphylococcus aureus*.

Clinical Features

■ **SPECIAL CLINICAL POINT: Symptoms from localized brain infections typically are subacute in onset and produce symptoms from increased intracranial pressure and their location in the brain.**

Early symptoms include headaches, lethargy, intermittent fever, and focal or generalized seizures. Focal neurologic signs may develop depending on the lesion site. Thus, lesions in the frontal cortex may produce hemiparesis, whereas lesions in the occipital cortex cause homonymous visual defects. As the mass expands, increased intracranial pressure becomes more pronounced. Psychomotor slowing, lethargy, and confusion increase in severity. Papilledema and horizontal diplopia from a sixth-nerve palsy may be seen. Focal neurologic signs become more prominent. Eventually, the abscess expands to cause brain herniation or ruptures into the ventricle-producing ventriculitis. Both usually result in death.

Laboratory Findings

CT and MRI scans are extremely helpful in diagnosing brain abscesses. The CT scan with contrast usually demonstrates a lesion with a low-density necrotic center, a well-developed contrast-enhancing capsule, and surrounding cerebral edema (Fig. 24.2). A somewhat similar picture is seen on MRI scan, and administration of gadolinium causes the capsule wall to enhance. The EEG is often abnormal, usually producing localized slowing in the region of the abscess. An LP, rarely helpful in establishing the diagnosis, is potentially dangerous because it increases the risk of brain herniation if the intracranial pressure is markedly elevated.

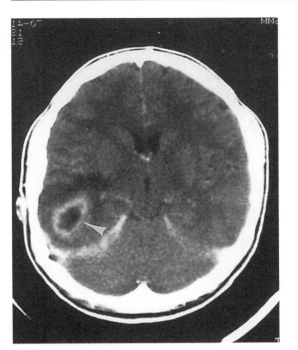

FIGURE 24.2 CT scan with contrast demonstrating a brain abscess in the posterior temporal lobe. *Arrow* shows the enhancing capsule with necrotic center. There is some low-density surrounding edema.

Management and Prognosis

Treatment of brain abscesses usually entails appropriate antibiotic therapy and surgical drainage. Broad-spectrum antibiotics, started as soon as the clinical diagnosis is made, are selected for their effectiveness against all likely pathogens as well as their ability to penetrate brain abscesses and surrounding brain parenchyma. Broad-spectrum antibiotic coverage should be efficacious against both common anaerobic (especially *Streptococcus intermedius* and *B. fragilis*) and aerobic bacteria. Possible combinations include the use of cefotaxime or ceftriaxone plus metronidazole or chloramphenicol. If staphylococci are suspected or isolated, antistaphylococcal drugs should be given. Once the bacteria are isolated, therapy should be directed by their antibiotic sensitivities. Intravenous antibiotics should be administered for 6 to 8 weeks.

Because the most immediate threat from brain abscesses is the mass effect, surgical aspiration of pus often reduces the increased intracranial pressure. The simplest method is aspiration of the pus using a CT-guided stereotactic technique. The received fluid should be Gram stained and cultured for anaerobic and aerobic bacteria, fungi, and tuberculosis. If the brain abscesses are multiple and small or deep involving the basal ganglia and brainstem, they occasionally can be treated only with broad-spectrum antimicrobial agents. However, careful clinical observations and repeated CT scans are needed to determine whether the abscess continues to expand.

Mannitol or corticosteroids may be necessary initially to control cerebral edema. However, corticosteroids should be used cautiously and tapered rapidly because they may interfere with capsule formation and host defenses against the organism.

Mortality from brain abscesses ranges from 30% to 65%, with the lower rates for patients who receive combined therapy with antibiotics and surgery. About 50% of survivors have neurologic sequelae, including seizures and focal neurologic deficits. These patients require rehabilitation.

PRION DISEASES (CREUTZFELDT–JAKOB DISEASE)

Prion disease of the CNS can be divided into clinical categories: Creutzfeldt–Jakob disease (CJD the most common form, with incidence of 1/1,000,000 per year); Gerstmann–Sträussler syndrome; fatal familial insomnia; and Kuru. This class of CNS infections breaks all the rules for conventional infections of the CNS. First, no nucleic agent has been identified in the infectious particle. The infectious agent is a protein normally made by neurons that is somehow misfolded into an abnormal infectious molecule. Second, patients with the illness do not present with typical signs of an infection. They lack fever and an elevated WBC and have CSF that appears normal on standard tests because an immune response is not made by the host against the infectious particle. Third, the infectious particle is not killed by formalin, ethanol, or boiling (methods that normally destroy infectious agents) but can be destroyed by autoclaving. Fourth, most patients present with a subacute to chronic progressive dementia that is fatal over 6 months to 2 years.

The prion infectious agent is present in CSF, brain, pituitary, and peripheral nerves that innervate cornea and dura. The infectious agent does not appear to be present in saliva, urine, sweat, or stool so isolation of the patient is not necessary. Blood should be considered infectious, but no documented human cases of the sporadic disease have occurred from blood transfusions.

■ **SPECIAL CLINICAL POINT: Transmission of a prion infectious disease may occur through inoculation via infected human cornea, dura, pituitary, or surgical instruments, or it may be hereditary as in familial CJD, Gerstmann–Straüssler syndrome, and fatal familial insomnia.**

In the United Kingdom, rare cases of a variant of CJD (vCJD) appear to be transmitted from infected cattle with bovine spongiform encephalopathy (mad cow disease). Fortunately the incidence of vCJD continues to fall since changes were made to the feed of cattle. However, most cases of CJD appear to be sporadic without a known source of the transmission.

Diagnosis may be difficult because there is no simple diagnostic test. CJD should be suspected in an adult with rapidly progressive dementia, myoclonic jerks, and normal CSF. In many patients with CJD, the CSF demonstrates abnormal 14-3-3 proteins on electrophoresis. An EEG may show characteristic abnormalities. MRI shows progressive brain atrophy often with abnormal gadolinium enhancement of the anterior basal ganglia. Pathologically, the brain shows a characteristic spongiform encephalopathy without inflammation. Currently, there is no available treatment to stop disease progression. Patients suspected of having this disease should not donate blood or autopsy organs.

Always Remember

Follow these steps to diagnose and treat CNS infections:

1. Determine the site of infection based on history, exam, CSF and blood findings, and neuroimaging.
2. Obtain appropriate CSF, blood, or tissue specimens for culture and serology to determine the type of organism (e.g., bacteria, virus, fungus) and antimicrobial sensitivities.
3. Begin initial broad-spectrum antimicrobial treatment.
4. Determine specific etiology and antimicrobial sensitivities, and modify treatment if necessary.
5. Watch for and treat complications.

QUESTIONS AND DISCUSSION

1. Herpes simplex encephalitis
   A. Is best diagnosed by isolation of herpes simplex virus from CSF
   B. Is accompanied by a herpetic blister on the lip
   C. Is best treated with acyclovir administered early in the disease
   D. Isolation is necessary as the patient is infectious to others
   E. Has characteristic clinical features

The correct answer is A. Untreated herpes simplex encephalitis (HSE) carries a 70% mortality rate but early administration of high-dose acyclovir reduces the mortality rate to about 25%. Patients with HSE do not present with any characteristic history on exam and do not occur in clusters like arbovirus encephalitis. The diagnosis is best made by detection of herpes virus DNA in CSF by PCR assay. The presence of herpes lesions on the lip or virus isolation from the mouth does not help in establishing the diagnosis.

2. West Nile viral encephalitis
   A. Occurs sporadically all year
   B. Is contagious to others
   C. Is best diagnosed by virus isolation from CSF
   D. Produces widespread but intermittent death of neurons
   E. Is best treated with acyclovir

The correct answer is D. West Nile encephalitis virus in the brain and spinal cord mainly infects neurons in a widespread fashion, often resulting in their death. West Nile virus is an arbovirus that is transmitted to humans from the bite of infected mosquitoes during the summer and early fall. West Nile virus is not present in urine, saliva, or stool so the patient is not contagious and does not need isolation. The diagnosis is usually made by detection of IgM antibodies to West Nile virus in serum or CSF as the virus is difficult to isolate from CSF. Acyclovir offers no benefit to RNA virus like West Nile virus. Thus, current treatment is symptomatic and the prevention of severe increased intracranial pressure.

3. In a brain abscess, the best way to establish the etiology is to
   A. Isolate bacteria from CSF
   B. Detect specific bacterial antigen in CSF
   C. Identify bacteria in CSF by Gram stain
   D. Isolate bacteria from abscess pus
   E. Isolate bacteria from blood or urine

The correct answer is D. In a brain abscess, the bacteria are surrounded by a capsule and confined to the pus. Therefore, the CSF does not contain any bacteria or bacterial products. In a few patients, the blood may contain the bacteria if the organism reached the brain from a bacteremia. The only certain method of isolating the bacteria causing the abscess is to culture the pus. This can be done by stereotactic aspiration of the pus or from a craniotomy and direct surgical aspiration or drainage. The pus should be cultured for anaerobic and aerobic bacteria, fungi, and M. tuberculosis.

4. Enterovirus meningitis
   A. Is transmitted by a bite of an infected mosquito
   B. Is the most common cause of aseptic meningitis
   C. Follows a prodrome of an upper respiratory tract infection
   D. Causes cranial nerve palsies in 30% of patients
   E. Is best treated with acyclovir

The correct answer is B. In the United States, enterovirus causes about 75% of cases of viral meningitis and the majority of aseptic meningitis cases. The virus is transmitted to the gastrointestinal tract from infected water or oral spread from infected feces. Most patients develop an asymptomatic gastrointestinal infection. In a few patients a viremia occurs that spreads virus to the meninges. No antiviral drugs are available for treatment, but the clinical course is benign, with more than 99% of patients making a complete recovery.

SUGGESTED READING

Bernardini GL. Diagnosis and management of brain abscess and subdural empyema. *Curr Neurol Neurosci Rep*. 2004;4:448–456.

Davis LE. Subacute and chronic meningitis. *Continuum*. 2006;12:27–57.

Davis LE, Beckham JD, Tyler KL. North American encephalitic arboviruses. *Neurol Clin*. 2008;26:727–757.

Davis LE, Kennedy PGE, eds. *Infectious Diseases of the Nervous System*. Oxford: Butterworth-Heinemann; 2000.

Irani DN. Aseptic meningitis and viral myelitis. *Neurol Clin*. 2008;26:635–655.

Kastenbauer S, Pfister HW. Pneumococcal meningitis in adults: spectrum of complications and prognostic factors in a series of 87 cases. *Brain*. 2003;126:1015–1025.

Kent ME, Romanelli F. Reexamining syphilis: an update on epidemiology, clinical manifestations and management. *Ann Pharmacother*. 2008;42:226–236.

Knight R. Creutzfeldt-Jakob Disease: a rare disease of dementia in elderly persons. *Clin Infect Dis*. 2006;43:340–346.

Lu C-H, Chang WN, Lin YC, et al. Bacterial brain abscess: microbiological features, epidemiological trends and therapeutic outcomes. *Q J Med.* 2002;95:501–509.

Thompson RB Jr, Bertram H. Laboratory diagnosis of central nervous system infections. *Infect Dis Clin North Am.* 2001;15:1047–1071.

Tunkel AR, Hartman BJ, Kaplan SL, et al. Practice guidelines for the management of bacterial meningitis. *Clin Infect Dis.* 2004;39:1267–1284.

Tyler KL. Update on herpes simplex encephalitis. *Rev Neurol Dis.* 2004;1:169–178.

Whitley RJ, Kimberlin DW. Herpes simplex: encephalitis children and adolescents. *Semin Pediatr Infect Dis.* 2005;16:17–23.

Ziai WC, Lewin JJ. Update in the diagnosis and management of central nervous system infections. *Neurol Clin.* 2008;26:427–468.

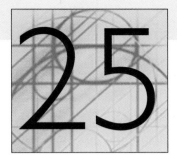

25 Neurologic Aspects of Cancer

DEBORAH OLIN HEROS

key points
- Primary central nervous system (CNS) tumors include gliomas (astrocytomas, oligodendrogliomas, and ependymomas), meningiomas, and primary CNS lymphomas.
- Systemic cancers may affect the CNS via intracranial, leptomeningeal, or spinal metastases.
- Nonmetastatic cancer effects may include cerebrovascular complications, metabolic and nutritional complications, and paraneoplastic syndromes.
- Cancer treatment with radiotherapy may be associated with significant neurologic complications.

ancer is the second leading cause of death in the United States, with an incidence of more than 1 million cases of cancer each year and resulting in more than 1 million cancer-related deaths per year. More than 20,500 new cases of primary brain tumors were diagnosed in 2007 in the United States. Primary central nervous system (CNS) tumors occur in people of all ages; they are the third leading cause of cancer deaths between the ages of 15 and 34 years. Statistical data suggest that the incidence of primary CNS tumors is increasing.

Autopsy studies identify metastatic tumors to the brain in 24% of patients with systemic cancer, the majority of which are symptomatic. Furthermore, systemic cancer may affect the peripheral and central nervous systems as a result of metastatic involvement of the dura and leptomeninges, bony metastases resulting in epidural spinal cord compression, and peripheral involvement to the brachial and lumbosacral plexuses.

Cancer also may result in nonmetastatic complications to the CNS, including various vascular disorders, metabolic and nutritional disorders, infection, and neurologic complications from cancer treatment. Indirect, or paraneoplastic, syndromes have been recognized as the result of systemic cancer. More than 80% of cancer patients will develop neurologic complications, and the resultant impact on their quality of life and survival is significant.

Identification and treatment of neurologic complications may improve the quality of life and survival of the cancer patient. It is, therefore, very important for any clinician involved in the care of cancer patients to be aware of the neurologic aspects of cancer.

PRIMARY CENTRAL NERVOUS SYSTEM TUMORS

Primary CNS tumors are classified by the cell of origin. The incidence of primary intracranial tumors is between 2 and 19 per 100,000 persons per year and is dependent on age. In adults, supratentorial tumors are more common, whereas the majority of primary intracranial tumors of childhood occur in the posterior fossa. The most common primary brain tumors are glial in origin and include astrocytomas, oligodendrogliomas, and ependymomas.

Astrocytoma

The most common glial tumor is the astrocytoma, which stains positive for glial fibrillary acidic protein (GFAP) and is classified or graded according to histologic characteristics reflecting aggressiveness and survival. The traditional classification system is the Kernohan grading system of astrocytoma, based on the pathologic characteristics of cellularity, pleomorphism, proliferation, and necrosis. Kernohan grades I and II represent "low-grade" or "well-differentiated" astrocytoma, Kernohan grade III represents the intermediate or anaplastic astrocytoma, and grade IV astrocytoma is synonymous with a glioblastoma multiforme. In an attempt to improve the correlation between prognosis and grade of the tumor, the World Health Organization (WHO) in 1993 suggested a descriptive, three-tier system that includes the well-differentiated astrocytoma, anaplastic astrocytoma, and glioblastoma multiforme. Because there is a slight difference between the pathologic characteristics described by the two systems, the clinician must know which system is being used.

Clinical Presentation   The clinical presentation of astrocytoma is determined by tumor location, pathology, and age of the patient. The majority of astrocytomas in adults occur in the supratentorial compartment. Presenting symptoms may include headache, seizure, focal neurologic deficits, and personality change. The increasing availability of neuroimaging studies with improved resolution has resulted in earlier discovery of brain tumors.

■ **SPECIAL CLINICAL POINT: Unexplained first seizures in adults, unusual neurologic symptoms, or an unexplained change in personality or mood should be investigated by either computed tomography (CT) or magnetic resonance imaging (MRI).**

Contrast for the appropriate neuroimaging studies is important if a primary brain tumor is in the differential diagnosis (see Chapter 4, Fundamentals of Neuroradiology). Brainstem gliomas are less common and may present with sensorimotor abnormalities, coordination difficulties, or cranial nerve dysfunction. The tumor grade correlates somewhat with the abnormalities on the neuroimaging study. Low-grade tumors usually do not enhance, and they appear hypodense on a computed tomography (CT) scan and have abnormalities on magnetic resonance imaging (MRI) fluid-attenuated inversion recovery (FLAIR) and T2-weighted images. Increasing tumor grade results in increasing contrast enhancement. Central necrosis, with surrounding enhancement and peritumoral edema, is suggestive of a glioblastoma.

The most important factors that determine the prognosis of a patient with an astrocytoma include histology, age of the patient, and the level of disability or performance status. Patients with low-grade tumors have the best prognosis. Patients with an anaplastic astrocytoma have a significantly better prognosis than patients with a glioblastoma. Younger patients and patients with less disability do better than their older, more disabled counterparts. Less significant prognostic factors may include a long duration of symptoms prior to diagnosis, presence of seizures, location of tumor, and degree of surgical resection. As our understanding of the genetic abnormalities of specific tumors increases, the presence or absence of chromosomal abnormalities may provide prognostic and therapeutic information.

Treatment   Treatment options for astrocytoma are determined by pathology, location, clinical presentation, and age of the patient. Often, the patient is clinically symptomatic from cerebral edema; therefore, corticosteroids (usually dexamethasone) are started prior to surgery, and they often improve symptoms. Caution should be used if a primary CNS lymphoma (PCNSL) is in the differential diagnosis because the use of corticosteroid therapy prior to biopsy may decrease the chance of obtaining a positive biopsy. An anticonvulsant to prevent seizures for supratentorial lesions is also often started prior to surgery.

A definitive diagnosis is obtained by pathologic examination of brain tissue. Surgical debulking is preferred over a biopsy, when possible, to reduce the tumor burden, provide an adequate pathology specimen, and improve symptomatic relief from mass effect. Theoretically, tumor debulking also may improve the chance to respond to adjuvant therapy. Stereotactic biopsy is most often reserved for patients whose poor medical condition precludes a craniotomy and for those with deep-seated lesions or lesions in neurologically eloquent locations.

■ **SPECIAL CLINICAL POINT: The primary goals of tumor surgery for astrocytoma are (a) to determine pathology, (b) to identify tumor grade, (c) to identify any subtype of glioma that may affect prognosis and treatment options, and (d) to directly reduce mass effect.**

The use of neuronavigational systems and intraoperative neuroimaging studies have improved the ability of the neurosurgeon to attain maximal resection with minimal morbidity. Survival benefit has been correlated with good tumor resection, but the infiltrative nature of astrocytomas generally prohibits a complete resection.

Postoperative radiation therapy increases the median survival of patients with an anaplastic astrocytoma and glioblastoma. Limited-field brain irradiation with a "radiation boost" to the most active central portion of the tumor is performed over a course of 5 to 6 weeks. Additional techniques to deliver radiation therapy to astrocytomas include radiosurgery, three-dimensional conformal radiation therapy, boron neutron capture therapy, and the use of radiosensitizers. The role of these techniques for the treatment of high-grade astrocytomas has yet to be defined. Stereotactic radiosurgery, when added to fractionated radiotherapy, does not improve clinical outcome.

The role of radiation therapy for low-grade astrocytomas is even less clear. Statistically, patients with low-grade astrocytomas who have received radiation therapy have improved survival over those patients not so treated. However, the timing is controversial. It is not clear whether radiation therapy should be administered at the time of diagnosis (e.g., when the neoplasm has been identified after a single seizure or perhaps as an incidental finding by a neuroimaging study) or delayed until the tumor is more symptomatic from tumor transformation. Studies suggest that the timing is not a major prognostic determinant.

Historically, chemotherapy has not been a primary treatment for malignant astrocytomas, but the recognition that some subtypes of glial tumors (e.g., anaplastic astrocytomas in younger patients) are chemosensitive has increased enthusiasm for chemotherapy for primary brain tumors. The preferred combination of therapeutic agents for anaplastic astrocytomas has been procarbazine, CCNU, and vincristine (PCV regimen). Carmustine had previously been the most widely used single agent for glioblastoma, but temozolomide, a recently developed oral alkylating agent, has demonstrated significant activity against malignant gliomas. Temozolomide used concurrently with radiotherapy and then continued as adjuvant treatment has significantly improved the survival outcome for patients with high-grade gliomas.

Glioblastoma multiforme is a highly vascular tumor and demonstrates elevated production of vascular endothelial growth factor (VEGF). Targeted therapy using angiogenesis inhibitors such as bevacizumab, a monoclonal antibody to VEGF, has shown efficacy in the treatment of recurrent malignant gliomas. Clinical studies are being conducted using bevacizumab with radiotherapy and temozolomide as initial therapy in newly diagnosed glioblastoma. Preliminary results are encouraging. Other angiogenic inhibitors are also under investigation.

■ **SPECIAL CLINICAL POINT: Ethical decisions involving the appropriateness of participation in experimental treatment protocols for astrocytomas are challenging because patients and families are often desperate or frightened, potentially compromising informed consent. Furthermore, investigational treatments are potentially hazardous and full understanding of risk–benefit ratios is often unclear. Given the poor prognosis for patients with high-grade gliomas, however, it is important for the clinician caring for these patients to be aware of the clinical protocols available and to make an appropriate referral for patients interested in investigational treatment.**

In a national survey, less than 8% of patients with astrocytoma were enrolled in treatment protocols. As participation in investigational protocols by patients with other malignancies has resulted in improved treatment modalities, it is important to encourage participation.

Oligodendroglioma

The oligodendroglioma is a type of glial tumor derived from the oligodendrocyte, the myelin-producing cell within the CNS. Histologically, this tumor is identified by its characteristic "fried-egg" appearance and a positive stain for myelin basic protein. The tumor tends to be slow growing; therefore, it is most often considered to be a low-grade tumor. However, varying degrees of

anaplasia, and therefore aggressiveness, do occur. Most often, the tumor presents as a nonenhancing hypodense lesion on CT scan or a hypointense T1-lesion on MRI scan. Calcifications may be present. Enhancement may suggest a more aggressive tumor or the presence of a mixed oligoastrocytoma. Occasionally, symptom onset may be abrupt as the result of hemorrhage.

Management of the oligodendroglioma depends on location, clinical presentation, and neuroimaging appearance. Surgical resection generally is attempted if possible. The oligodendroglioma has been identified as a chemosensitive tumor; therefore, chemotherapy has played a major role in its treatment in recent years. The use of chemotherapy for low-grade oligodendroglioma is being studied. Approximately 60% of oligodendrogliomas demonstrate genetic deletions or "loss of heterozygosity" (LOH) of 1p and 19q chromosomes. The presence of LOH of 1p and 19q is an indicator of chemosensitivity and favorable prognosis (greater than 90% response rate to chemotherapy and improved overall survival). Testing for these genetic abnormalities has become more readily available and an important part of the neuropathology report for oligodendroglioma. The chemotherapy most commonly used for this tumor has been the PCV regimen, but temozolomide is increasingly replacing PCV as first-line therapy. Although radiation therapy has been shown to improve survival of patients with oligodendroglioma, the role of radiation therapy remains controversial, especially if total resection has been accomplished. However, if subtotal resection or a limited biopsy has been performed, radiation therapy may offer some survival advantage.

Ependymoma

The ependymoma is a glial tumor arising from the ependymal cells lining the ventricles and the cerebrospinal fluid (CSF)–filled spaces. This tumor usually occurs during childhood in the posterior fossa arising from the floor of the fourth ventricle, but it may present in the spinal cord or in the cerebral hemispheres along the lining of the lateral ventricles. When an ependymoma occurs in the posterior fossa, it usually presents with symptoms of increased intracranial pressure, including headache, nausea, and vomiting, and it often causes obstructive hydrocephalus. The treatment of choice is surgical resection, and the prognosis depends on the degree of resection. A 45% overall 5-year survival is reported in the literature, with an increased chance of long-term survival after complete resection. This tumor lines the CSF pathways and may seed the neuraxis, although the majority of tumor recurrence is local within the posterior fossa. Local radiation therapy usually is recommended for supratentorial and spinal lesions. Local or craniospinal radiation therapy may be appropriate for ependymomas of the posterior fossa. Chemotherapy has been of limited benefit in the treatment of ependymoma.

Meningioma

Meningiomas are tumors derived from the arachnoid lining of the nervous system and, therefore, are extrinsic to the neuraxis. The tumors are most often histologically benign and are found more frequently with increasing age as the result of the slow growth rate.

■ **SPECIAL CLINICAL POINT: Meningiomas may be found incidentally, and observation may be appropriate, especially when asymptomatic or when found in an elderly patient.**

The incidence increases with age starting in the sixth decade. Women are affected two to three times more than men. Symptoms are dependent on location, size, and rate of growth. Symptoms may include seizures from cortical irritation over the convexity of the cerebral hemisphere, headache from pressure within the cranium, or symptoms of cranial nerve or brainstem dysfunction from direct compression of neural structures.

Meningiomas typically demonstrate homogenous enhancement on CT or MRI studies following administration of contrast. Often a dural attachment or "dural tail" can be seen radiologically, which helps to identify the tumor as a meningioma. Significant edema surrounding the mass is not typically seen, and its presence should raise the suspicion for either an atypical, malignant meningioma or another type of tumor such as a metastatic tumor, especially from a breast or prostate primary. Meningiomas are also more common in women with breast cancer.

The treatment for meningioma is most often surgical resection with the goal of complete removal because the risk of recurrence is directly related to the completeness of the resection. This in turn mainly is determined by the location of the tumor; tumors that are not amenable to complete resection have a much greater risk for recurrence. For example, tumors over the cerebral convexities are more accessible surgically as compared to tumors at the base of the skull, and therefore cerebral convexity tumors are less likely to recur.

Radiotherapy by conventional fractionated radiation, stereotactic radiosurgery, or fractionated radiosurgery may play an important role for incompletely resected or recurrent tumors.

The role of traditional chemotherapy is limited, but agents such as hydroxyurea and interferon alpha-2b have been described as having some activity. Meningiomas may contain progesterone and, less frequently, estrogen receptors. Consequently, meningiomas may enlarge during periods of elevated hormonal levels such as pregnancy. Treatment with antiestrogen or antiprogesterone agents such as tamoxifen or mifepristone (RU-486), respectively, has been used.

Although the majority of meningiomas are histologically benign, infrequently atypical or malignant variants with more aggressive behavior may occur. A subtype of meningeal tumor, the hemangiopericytoma, may present similarly, but it has a high rate of recurrence and a propensity to seed the leptomeninges and metastasize outside of the CNS.

Primary CNS Lymphoma (PCNSL)

PCNSL is a non-Hodgkin lymphoma, usually of B-cell origin, that arises within the brain, spinal cord, or leptomeninges. This tumor may occur in otherwise healthy patients with normal immune systems, usually in older men, but it more often occurs in patients with a compromised immune system. It has been seen with increasing frequency as a result of the growing population with human immunodeficiency virus (HIV). This tumor does not tend to metastasize systemically and is a separate entity from systemic lymphoma with CNS metastasis. Patients with inherited, acquired, or iatrogenically induced immunodeficient states, particularly transplant patients, are at an increased risk for developing this tumor, and it may occur in up to 10% of patients with acquired immunodeficiency syndrome (AIDS). The clinical presentation may include headache, personality changes, seizures, and focal neurologic symptoms. Often the lesions are multifocal, frequently involving deep midline structures with contrast enhancement and minimal surrounding edema on neuroimaging studies. The diagnosis usually is established by biopsy, but surgical resection is usually not an option. The use of corticosteroid therapy prior to biopsy may decrease the opportunity to obtain an accurate pathologic diagnosis.

The presentation of PCNSL in an immune-compromised patient may resemble CNS toxoplasmosis clinically. It is therefore common to treat a patient with a known immunodeficiency empirically for toxoplasmosis for a limited period with clinical and radiologic follow-up. If the lesions improve, the assumption is that the patient has toxoplasmosis, whereas if the lesions progress or do not improve, then the possibility of CNS lymphoma increases and a biopsy may be performed. Occasionally, an immune-compromised patient may have simultaneous toxoplasmosis and CNS lymphoma, complicating the interpretation of the empiric trial. A lumbar puncture with cytologic examination may be helpful if the tumor is in the midline or if the leptomeninges are involved. CSF cytology may help to distinguish between a neoplastic monoclonal lymphocytosis and an inflammatory process. Intraocular involvement can occur, and a slit lamp examination or vitreous biopsy may be helpful in establishing the diagnosis. A systemic evaluation including a bone marrow biopsy may help to exclude the possibility of systemic lymphoma or other small-cell malignancies. Most often, a brain biopsy is indicated, however.

Once the diagnosis of PCNSL has been established, corticosteroid therapy may offer improvement of neurologic symptoms. For many years, radiation therapy has been the mainstay of treatment, but the prognosis was limited. The median survival of immunocompetent patients with PCNSL is approximately 14 months, and it is much less in patients with immunodeficiency. Combined treatment with chemotherapy and radiation therapy has resulted in improved survival. Unfortunately, relapse remains common, and late neurologic toxicity from combined therapy is a significant complication resulting in a progressive dementing leukoencephalopathy.

Chemotherapy has generally not been used in patients with CNS lymphoma associated with immunodeficiency because of the overall poor prognosis and response rate. PCNSL has been associated with the presence of Epstein–Barr virus in patients with AIDS. As a result of this observation, antiviral therapy has been suggested for treatment of PCNSL. Recently, rituximab, a monoclonal antibody that targets CD20, has shown some promise as well.

METASTATIC COMPLICATIONS OF SYSTEMIC CANCER

Intracranial Metastases

Systemic cancer may spread to the CNS to involve the skull, dura, parenchyma, or leptomeninges. Specific tumors may metastasize in predictable patterns, and understanding these trends is important to correctly diagnose metastases in order to offer palliative therapy.

■ **SPECIAL CLINICAL POINT: Breast cancer, prostate cancer, lung cancer, malignant melanoma, and cancers of the head and neck frequently metastasize to the skull.**

Neurologic symptoms are most common if the tumor involves the base of the skull, resulting in localized pain, headache, or cranial nerve dysfunction (Fig. 25.1). Special views on a CT or an MRI scan may be necessary to identify skull base metastases. Standard screening studies may not image this region well, giving the false impression of a negative study; thus, the opportunity to offer effective palliative therapy may be missed. The nuclear bone scan is not a very sensitive study (despite the fact that the symptoms are the result of bony metastases) because of the overlapping nuclear isotope uptake by the venous sinuses in this region. Localized radiation often offers effective palliation of symptoms, especially pain.

Intraparenchymal brain metastases occur in nearly 25% of patients with systemic cancer.

■ **SPECIAL CLINICAL POINT: Breast cancer, lung cancer, and malignant melanoma frequently metastasize to the brain. Less commonly, tumors of the gastrointestinal tract, kidney, or genitourinary system may do so as well.**

The majority of tumors metastasize to the cerebral hemispheres and less commonly to the brainstem and cerebellum in the posterior fossa. Metastases to the pituitary region, often from tumors of breast origin, have been described.

The risk of developing brain metastases from lung cancer varies with the pathology of the primary lung tumor. Small-cell lung cancer has the highest risk (60%), adenocarcinoma has an intermediate risk (40%), and squamous cell carcinoma is the least likely to spread to the brain (20%). From 25% to 30% of patients may present with neurologic symptoms without a known primary cancer. Nearly one-half of these patients will subsequently be found to have some form of lung cancer. Although brain

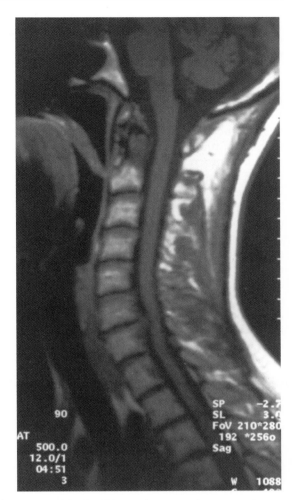

FIGURE 25.1 MRI scan demonstrating metastatic cancer to the upper cervical spine in a man with lung cancer and severe, localized occipital pain. Metastasis to the base of the skull was clinically suspected from the location of the pain. However, it is interesting that the pain was aggravated by neck movement.

metastases occur with high frequency in both lung and breast tumors, brain metastases often occur early in lung cancer (within months), whereas brain metastases are more likely to occur much later in breast cancer (within years). Although malignant melanoma is a relatively uncommon tumor, it has a very high propensity (up to 80% at autopsy) to spread to the CNS, often with multiple metastases.

Brain metastases originate from hematogenous spread, and therefore the majority of patients develop multiple lesions. Approximately 20% to 30% of patients have a single metastatic tumor. Treatment options often are determined by whether the lesion is single or multiple.

The signs and symptoms are determined by the size, number, and location of the tumors. Metastatic tumors of the cerebral hemispheres may cause progressive hemiparesis, language disturbance, confusion, seizures, sensory symptoms, visual field abnormalities, or personality changes. The development of depression in a patient with cancer could be a sign of brain metastases, particularly if he has never previously been prone to depression. Tumors in the cerebellum may result in dizziness, unsteadiness of gait, dysarthria, clumsiness of an extremity, or headaches from obstructive hydrocephalus. Cranial nerve dysfunction, motor and sensory signs, unsteadiness, and incoordination result from brainstem involvement. Hemorrhage into a metastasis may result in the abrupt onset of neurologic symptoms.

■ **SPECIAL CLINICAL POINT: Metastatic tumors with a tendency to bleed include melanoma, renal cell carcinoma, choriocarcinoma, and some forms of lung cancer.**

The diagnosis of metastatic brain tumor is established by a neuroimaging study, either CT or MRI "(see Chapter 4, Fundamentals of Neuroradiology). When a patient presents with brain metastases without a known primary tumor, diagnostic studies are performed to identify the primary tumor, with special attention to imaging of the chest, since approximately one-half of these patients will be found to have a primary lung cancer.

Treatment Corticosteroids, usually dexamethasone, are very effective in treating patients with symptoms that result from vasogenic edema. The appropriate dosing is determined by the number, size, and location of lesions and by the severity of the symptoms. The most common initial dosage of dexamethasone is 4 mg four times daily. It often is used in conjunction with an H2-receptor antagonist to reduce the risk of gastric complications from the corticosteroid therapy.

An anticonvulsant medication is indicated if the patient has experienced a seizure. The role of prophylactic use of an anticonvulsant is less clear, and many neurologists prefer to avoid the risk of side effects from the medication in patients who have not experienced a seizure. It may be prudent, however, to consider the use of a prophylactic anticonvulsant medication for lesions in potentially epileptogenic areas of the cerebral hemispheres such as near the motor cortex. Serum drug levels should be monitored appropriately.

Conventional treatment of brain metastases includes whole brain radiation therapy (3000 cGy over 10 or 15 fractions). The whole brain is treated because of the high likelihood of multiple lesions and the chance of multiple microscopic foci of metastatic tumor from hematogenous dissemination. Advances in neuroimaging and neurosurgical techniques and the development of radiosurgery have increased the options for treatment of metastatic tumors. The current trend is to use radiosurgery (a) to boost the effect of whole brain radiation therapy or (b) to treat recurrences of metastatic tumors after whole brain radiation therapy. Some clinicians are using radiosurgery alone for the treatment of metastatic tumors. The maximal number of tumors that may be treated with radiosurgery is under investigation.

In general, surgery is reserved for removal of a single lesion in a surgically accessible area (e.g., a tumor in the posterior fossa causing hydrocephalus or a large tumor in the cerebral hemispheres) (Fig. 25.2). Shunting also is considered for treatment of hydrocephalus if the cause of the hydrocephalus cannot be surgically excised. Stereotactic biopsy may be considered in patients presenting with neurologic symptoms without a known primary tumor or in patients in whom the specific tumor type cannot be established otherwise.

The experience of using chemotherapy for brain metastases is limited as a result of

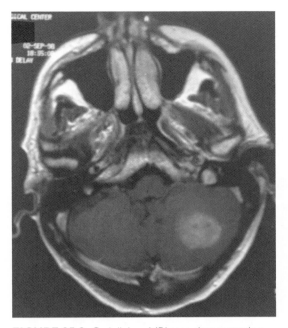

FIGURE 25.2 Gadolinium MRI scan demonstrating contrast-enhancing single metastasis of the cerebellum in a patient with gastric carcinoma. His headaches, nausea, and unsteadiness improved after surgical resection.

the inability for most chemotherapeutic agents to penetrate the blood–brain barrier. Temozolomide, an oral alkylating agent that readily crosses the blood–brain barrier and is used for treatment of primary brain tumors, may also be helpful in treating metastatic brain tumors when used in combination with radiotherapy.

If untreated, the median survival for patients with brain metastases is 4 to 6 weeks. Appropriate therapy offers an improved quality of life and prolongation of survival. The overall median survival of patients treated for metastatic brain tumors is 6 months. Long-term survival usually is described in patients treated with surgery. The cause of death in patients with brain metastases is most often progression of systemic disease.

Leptomeningeal Metastases

Systemic tumors may diffusely seed the leptomeninges, resulting in a condition known as *neoplastic meningitis*. Other terms used to describe this condition include *carcinomatous meningitis* and *meningeal carcinomatosis*, or *lymphomatous meningitis*, depending on the tumor of origin. The incidence of this serious complication is thought to be increasing as control of systemic disease improves.

The leptomeninges serve as a sanctuary site from systemic therapy as a result of the blood–brain barrier. Neoplastic meningitis may occur in isolation or in combination with other sites of CNS involvement, such as intraparenchymal brain metastases. Most commonly, neoplastic meningitis is caused by tumors of the breast and lung and malignant melanoma. Less commonly, tumors of the gastrointestinal tract, ovary, prostate, uterus, and bladder spread to the leptomeninges. Various types of lymphoma and leukemia also have a tendency for leptomeningeal spread.

The clinical presentation of neoplastic meningitis is variable and often subtle. Symptoms and signs reflect the diffuse involvement of the neuraxis at three levels: (a) the cerebral cortex, resulting in confusion, headache, and seizures; (b) cranial nerves, resulting in diplopia, facial numbness, hearing loss, visual loss, and tongue weakness; and (c) spinal and nerve roots, with a propensity for the lumbosacral spine region, resulting in low back pain, leg numbness and weakness, and sphincter dysfunction. Communicating hydrocephalus develops in 15% to 20% of patients with neoplastic meningitis. The diagnosis should be suspected in a patient with cancer with neurologic symptoms and signs at various levels of the neuraxis. Often the findings on clinical examination are multiple and out of proportion to the symptoms described by the patient.

The diagnosis of neoplastic meningitis is established by positive cytology of the CSF. Repeated CSF examinations may be necessary to establish the diagnosis. The CSF examination also may demonstrate elevation of opening pressure, lymphocytic pleocytosis, a depressed glucose level, or protein elevation. Elevated biochemical markers may be used to diagnose the condition as well as to follow the response of treatment. Such markers include *carcinoembryonic antigen*, *beta human chorionic gonadotropin*, and *alpha-fetoprotein*. If a sufficient number of lymphocytes are present, specific immunohistochemical studies may help differentiate reactive inflammatory lymphocytes from neoplastic lymphocytes in patients with lymphoma and leukemia.

Gadolinium MRI of the brain and spinal cord may demonstrate leptomeningeal enhancement, and helps to exclude the possibility of intracranial brain metastases that might contraindicate a lumbar puncture. Bulky disease that may be treated with localized radiation therapy also may be identified. In general, MRI with gadolinium is more sensitive than CT with contrast (Figs. 25.3 and 25.4).

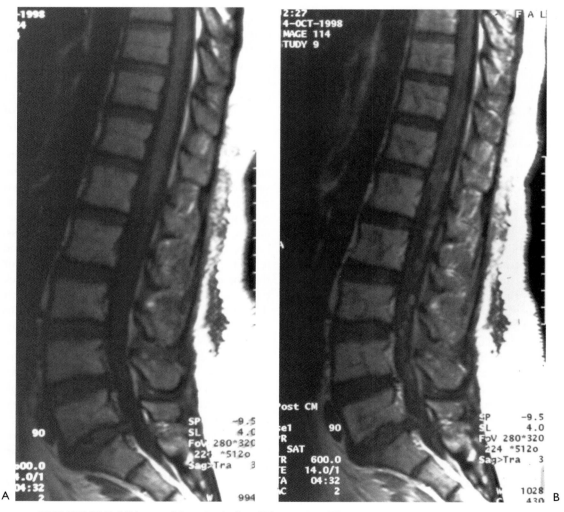

FIGURE 25.3 MRI scan of the spine before **(A)** and after **(B)** gadolinium, demonstrating enhancing nodular defects in the leptomeninges of a woman with metastatic breast cancer, who presented with paraparesis and urinary retention. Cerebrospinal fluid examination from an Ommaya reservoir confirmed the diagnosis of neoplastic meningitis.

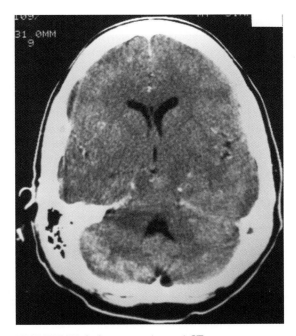

FIGURE 25.4 Contrast-enhanced CT scan demonstrating multiple metastatic tumors in the woman (with metastatic breast cancer) seen in Fig. 25.3. The patient required focal radiotherapy to the cauda equina, whole brain radiotherapy, and intrathecal chemotherapy.

Treatment   Treatment of neoplastic meningitis includes the use of intrathecal chemotherapy by lumbar puncture or through an Ommaya reservoir into the lateral ventricles. A limited number of chemotherapeutic agents are available for intrathecal use, including methotrexate, cytosine arabinoside, and thioTEPA. Liposome-encased cytarabine arabinoside administered intrathecally allows for treatment every 2 weeks, in contrast to twice weekly with standard chemotherapy, and has been beneficial for lymphoma and some solid tumors causing neoplastic meningitis. Systemic chemotherapy is not thought to be effective in neoplastic meningitis, and radiotherapy is reserved for localized treatment of bulky disease. Patients with sphincter dysfunction may benefit from local radiotherapy to the conus medullaris and cauda equina.

In patients with cranial nerve dysfunction, radiotherapy to the basal cisterns may be beneficial. Dexamethasone may improve symptoms.

If untreated, the median survival of neoplastic meningitis is 6 weeks. The overall median survival with treatment is 4 to 6 months. A chance for longer survival in select patients has been described in patients with chemosensitive tumors such as lymphoma and breast cancer. Patients with neoplastic meningitis from malignant melanoma have a particularly poor prognosis. Often, a patient with neoplastic meningitis will have concomitant progression of systemic cancer.

Spinal Metastases

Spinal cord dysfunction from metastatic cancer may be the result of tumor metastasis to vertebral bodies, extension of a paravertebral mass, or intramedullary metastases from hematogenous spread to the spinal cord (5%). The most common cause of spinal cord compression is metastasis to the vertebral body from tumors with a tendency to spread to bone, such as multiple myeloma and tumors of breast, lung, or prostate origin.

Pain is present in the majority of patients, and may be localized or radicular, often directing the clinician to the appropriate spinal level.

■ **SPECIAL CLINICAL POINT: The presence of back or neck pain in a patient with known cancer should raise the suspicion of a spinal metastasis and prompt appropriate investigation.**

The absence of pain in a patient with spinal cord dysfunction should raise the possibility of a different etiology for the patient's symptoms such as radiation myelopathy, intramedullary spinal cord metastases, or a paraneoplastic syndrome.

The neurologic examination is very important to determine the level of spinal cord involvement "(see Chapter 5, Neurologic Emergencies). Symptoms may include motor and sensory abnormalities and sphincter dysfunction. The neurologic examination may demonstrate hyperreflexia and dorsal column signs, with impairment of position sense and vibration. Spinothalamic dysfunction may result in abnormalities of pain and temperature sensitivities.

■ SPECIAL CLINICAL POINT: Spinal cord compression from metastatic tumor is a true neurologic emergency in the patient with cancer. The rate of progression is variable, and failure to diagnose and treat spinal cord compression may result in irreversible neurologic injury, thus limiting the quality of life as well as potentially the survival of the patient with cancer.

In general, the neurologic outcome in spinal cord compression is determined by the neurologic status at the time treatment is initiated. A patient who is ambulatory at the time of treatment has a good chance of remaining ambulatory, whereas it is unlikely that the nonambulatory patient will regain significant function. Sphincter involvement is considered to be a poor prognostic sign and often occurs later in spinal cord compression; early involvement should alert the clinician to consider conus medullaris or cauda equina involvement.

Total spine MRI (cervical, thoracic, and lumbar) with gadolinium is the neuroimaging study of choice for evaluation of spinal cord dysfunction because 15% to 30% of patients with spinal cord compression may have involvement at multiple levels. Imaging the entire length of the spine is also useful for optimal planning of radiotherapy. A gadolinium-enhanced spine MRI also may identify leptomeningeal involvement or intramedullary metastasis.

Treatment   Corticosteroids, usually dexamethasone, are administered when the diagnosis of spinal cord compression is made. Initial doses range between 20 and 100 mg. The subsequent dosing is determined on symptoms, rate of progression, and extent of disease. Radiotherapy and surgery are the main therapeutic options. Radiotherapy usually is initiated urgently in a patient with known cancer. Surgery is appropriate for patients without a known cancer or in the setting of deterioration despite radiotherapy. Newer approaches to surgical decompression using anterior and anterolateral approaches address the location of tumor involvement and may be preferred to the more traditional posterior surgical decompression. However, often the cancer patient in this situation has extensive systemic disease with a limited life expectancy and surgery is not well tolerated.

NONMETASTATIC COMPLICATIONS

Cerebrovascular Complications

Patients with cancer are at increased risk for a variety of cerebrovascular complications resulting either from the effects of malignancy or from treatment. The cerebrovascular complications may be either ischemic or hemorrhagic.

Accelerated atheromatous disease resulting in thrombotic strokes may occur following radiation therapy to the head and neck region. Systemic cancer may cause a hypercoagulable state, resulting in arterial or venous sinus occlusion. Patients with mucin-producing adenocarcinomas, in particular, have been described to be at risk for the development of a hypercoagulable state and suffer subsequent cerebral infarction. Mucin deposits have been found in the venous walls at the sight of the infarct.

Bacterial endocarditis may occur as a complication of tumor therapy, because of neutropenia, and it may cause septic emboli resulting in stroke. Less commonly, a mycotic aneurysm may develop with the risk of subarachnoid hemorrhage. Nonbacterial thrombotic endocarditis is a well-recognized complication of cancer and may result in cerebral embolism.

Thrombocytopenia, either as a direct result of the malignancy (usually one of a hematologic origin) or a consequence of tumor therapy, may cause hemorrhagic complications including subdural hematoma, spinal epidural hematoma, or intracerebral hemorrhage.

Chemotherapeutic drugs including bevacizumab and cisplatin have been associated with a reversible posterior leukoencephalopathy syndrome also known as *posterior reversible encephalopathy syndrome* (PRES). The clinical presentation includes headache, visual disturbances, confusion, and alteration of consciousness. Seizures may also occur. This disorder is thought to be the result of endothelial dysfunction and impaired autoregulation of the posterior intracranial circulation. PRES has been associated with several other causes including severe acute hypertension, preeclampsia, and exposure to immunosuppressive therapy used in organ transplantation. Neuroimaging demonstrates symmetric, predominantly occipital, white matter changes. Diffusion-weighted imaging can help differentiate PRES from ischemia. Recovery is possible with appropriate management.

Metabolic and Nutritional Complications

Metabolic abnormalities may develop as a direct result of systemic cancer or may be secondary to cancer treatment, and can affect both the peripheral and central nervous systems.

■ **SPECIAL CLINICAL POINT: Metabolic derangements in cancer patients may cause an encephalopathy, resulting in generalized confusion, personality changes, alteration of alertness, seizures, and coma. These symptoms may fluctuate or be associated with physical and neurologic exam findings that may include tremor, myoclonus, or asterixis.**

The cancer patient often takes multiple medications, including narcotics for pain management. A thorough review of the medication list is essential in evaluating the cancer patient with neurologic symptoms. Although narcotics and pain medications most commonly cause neurologic symptoms in the cancer patient, the clinician needs to be aware of the potential neurologic side effects of all medications the patient is receiving.

TABLE 25.1	Complications of Corticosteroids

Medical
    Weight gain, striae
    Diabetes mellitus
    Skin fragility
    Insomnia
    Infection susceptibility
    Candidiasis (oral thrush, esophagitis)

Neurologic
    Anxiety, emotional lability
    Psychosis, confusion
    Proximal myopathy
    Spinal lipomatosis (rare)

Corticosteroids are used for a variety of reasons in the patient with cancer. Systemic and neurologic complications are common (Table 25.1). Anxiety, insomnia, and emotional lability, also common, may be managed either by altering the schedule (e.g., to avoid a late-night dose that causes insomnia) or by the administration of an antianxiety medication such as a benzodiazepine. Chemotherapeutic agents can affect the peripheral and central nervous systems in a variety of ways (Table 25.2). Toxicity depends on the age, specific agent, drug dosage, and associated therapies. It is imperative that the clinician caring for a patient with cancer be aware of the neurotoxicity associated with each chemotherapeutic regimen.

Nutritional status, often poor in the patient with cancer, should be addressed if there are neurologic symptoms. Neurologic syndromes from deficiencies of thiamine and B_{12} are well-recognized.

Paraneoplastic Syndromes

Several distinct syndromes have been recognized in patients with systemic cancer that are not related directly to metastatic disease or treatment toxicity. These syndromes are considered to be remote effects of the cancer and are known as paraneoplastic syndromes. The paraneoplastic syndromes are of clinical significance for two reasons:

1. The neurologic symptoms may cause significant morbidity and therefore have

---

TABLE 25.2 Neurotoxicity of Chemotherapy

Cerebral Hemispheres
    Acute encephalopathy
    Procarbazine
    Interferon
    Interleukin-1,2
    Ifosfamide
    Methotrexate (high-dose intravenous or intrathecal)
    Asparaginase
    Vincristine
    Bevacizumab (PRES)
    Cisplatin (PRES)
    Chronic encephalopathy
    Methotrexate (high-dose intravenous or intrathecal)
    Fludarabine
    Leukoencephalopathy
    Methotrexate
    5-Fluorouracil + levamisole
    Carmustine (intra-arterial)

Cerebellum
    5-fluorouracil
    Cytarabine

Visual System
    Tamoxifen (reversible retinopathy)
    Fludarabine (cortical blindness)
    Cisplatin (cortical blindness)
    Intra-arterial chemotherapy (optic neuropathy)

Myelopathy
    Methotrexate (intrathecal)
    Cytarabine (intrathecal)
    ThioTEPA (intrathecal)

Peripheral Nerves
    Vincristine
    Cisplatin
    Paclitaxel
    Suramin
    Etoposide

---

a significant impact on the quality and survival of life of the cancer patient.

2. The neurologic symptoms may develop prior to the actual diagnosis of the systemic cancer; therefore, if the clinician is familiar with the various paraneoplastic syndromes, an earlier diagnosis of the systemic malignancy is potentially possible.

The disorders are thought to be related to an autoimmune process, and various specific antineuronal antibodies have been identified (Table 25.3).

COMPLICATIONS FROM RADIATION THERAPY

Complications from radiation therapy may mimic tumor progression or recurrence. In general, radiation therapy is initially well tolerated. An acute encephalopathy may develop, however, particularly if large radiation fractions are delivered to a large volume of brain in patients with increased intracranial pressure. The patients may complain of increased headaches, somnolence, lethargy, nausea, or worsening of focal neurologic symptoms. The symptoms of acute radiation toxicity are the result of disruption of the blood–brain barrier resulting in cerebral edema, and usually improve with corticosteroid therapy. If the symptoms are not responsive to corticosteroid therapy, the radiation therapy may need to be postponed temporarily.

Subacute or "early delayed" complications from radiation therapy usually begin within 2 weeks of completing radiation therapy and may persist up to 4 months after completion of radiation therapy. This disorder is thought to be a reversible injury to the oligodendroglial cells resulting in demyelination, and it is responsive to corticosteroid therapy. During this phase, neuroimaging studies may demonstrate an increased mass effect and increased contrast enhancement, suggesting tumor progression. However, symptoms may be controlled with dexamethasone, and the clinical situation may stabilize over time. This phase of radiation

TABLE 25.3

Paraneoplastic Syndromes

Syndrome Associated	Autoantibodies	Associated Tumors
Cerebellar degeneration	Anti-Yo (Anti-Purkinje cell)	Ovarian, breast
Encephalomyelitis	Anti-Hu	Lung
Opsoclonus-myoclonus	Anti-Ri	Breast, bladder, and lung
Sensory neuronopathy	Anti-Hu	Lung
Lambert–Eaton syndrome	Anti-VGCC (antisynaptotagmin)	Lung (small-cell)

injury often is mistaken for tumor progression. Pseudoprogression is a term applied to a delay in improvement or apparent worsening of the neuroimaging in patients with gliomas treated with concurrent radiotherapy and temozolomide. The MRI study may demonstrate worsening up to several months after completion of the combined therapy. Functional MRI is being investigated as a means to differentiate pseudoprogression from early tumor progression.

A possible late or "delayed" effect of radiation therapy is *radiation necrosis*. This process may be indistinguishable from tumor recurrence using contrast-enhanced CT or MRI studies. Attempts have been made to differentiate between the two processes by various metabolic neuroimaging studies, such as positron emission tomography (PET) and single photon emission computed tomography (SPECT). (Radiation necrosis should be hypometabolic, whereas recurrent tumor is expected to be hypermetabolic.) Often, both radiation necrosis and recurrent tumor are present simultaneously. If treatment options are available, a biopsy may be necessary. Reoperation with attempted resection and debulking may reduce chronic corticosteroid needs and improve neurologic symptoms but is usually only considered when additional treatment modalities are available. Reoperation alone offers very limited benefit.

Late effects of radiation therapy also may result in a diffuse *leukoencephalopathy*, manifested by gait disturbance, urinary incontinence, and dementia. Although the ventricles may appear large on neuroimaging, symptoms of leukoencephalopathy do not improve with shunting. Central endocrinopathies including central hypothyroidism, adrenal insufficiency, and decreased sex hormones also may occur as a late complication of radiation therapy. An elevated prolactin level may be seen as the result of radiation injury to the hypothalamus.

SPECIAL CHALLENGES FOR HOSPITALIZED PATIENTS

The general oncology patient may require intermittent hospitalization during the course of illness as a result of severe nausea and vomiting, dehydration, sepsis, pain, or new neurologic symptoms. The various medical problems often cause secondary somnolence, weakness, and alternation of mental status. The oncology patient often is receiving multiple medications that may cause somnolence, confusion, or weakness. Clinicians need to be alert and sensitive to metabolic abnormalities, nutritional and hydration needs, the possibility of infection, and unusual medication schedules that may contribute to any of these problems. The toxicity profile of cancer therapy, including radiotherapy and chemotherapy, also needs to be considered.

The patient with a brain tumor may require hospitalization for management of seizures, increased intracranial pressure, or neurologic deterioration with disease progression.

Always Remember

- Neurologic symptoms may develop in a patient with known cancer or may be the presenting symptoms in a patient with no previous diagnosis of cancer.
- Neurologic symptoms may be the direct or indirect result of the malignancy itself or may develop as a result of treatment for the cancer.
- Any patient with a known malignancy who develops unexplained neurologic symptoms, lethargy, depression, or personality changes should be referred to a neurologist.

QUESTIONS AND DISCUSSION

1. A 50-year-old woman has an unexplained episode of loss of consciousness while home alone. Upon awakening, she was aware of being incontinent of urine and complained of a very sore tongue. You determine that she probably had a seizure. The patient's MRI with gadolinium demonstrates multiple ring-enhancing lesions in various parts of the cerebral hemispheres. Infection is ruled out. Which of the following is the most likely diagnosis?
   A. Glioblastoma multiforme
   B. Meningioma
   C. Oligodendroglioma
   D. Metastases

The correct answer is D. Most primary brain tumors present as solitary lesions. Multiple ring-enhancing lesions are suggestive of metastases and should prompt a workup to identify the primary tumor.

2. The chest CT scan of the patient in Question 1 is abnormal, and a diagnosis of adenocarcinoma of the lung is confirmed histologically by bronchoscopy. The patient is treated with high-dose steroids, whole brain radiation therapy, and radiotherapy to the lung tumor. Four months later, the patient returns with back pain, urinary frequency, and bilateral leg weakness. Which of the following is the most likely cause for this patient's new symptoms?
   A. Radiation myelopathy secondary to the chest radiotherapy
   B. Bony metastases to the spine or epidural cord compression
   C. Steroid myopathy
   D. Urinary tract infection secondary to chronic immunosuppression

The correct answer is B. The major clinical concerns are epidural spinal cord compression from bony metastases. MRI of the spine should be performed with gadolinium using the clinical examination to guide localization. Steroid myopathy does not cause urinary frequency. Radiation-induced myelopathy is a rare diagnosis usually occurring later, and it should be considered only if the other direct metastatic complications have been excluded.

3. A 62-year-old man complains of a 2-month history of burning numbness in his legs and feet. He has lost 10 pounds and describes decreased appetite. He has normal cognition. Strength in the extremities is full, and coordination is normal. Electrodiagnostic studies (EMG/NCS) reveal a pure sensory neuropathy. The paraneoplastic syndrome that would best fit this clinical picture is
   A. Anti-Hu
   B. Anti-Yo
   C. Anti-Ri
   D. Anti-VGCC

The correct answer is A. Anti-Hu antibodies in the setting of lung cancer may be associated with either limbic encephalitis or a subacute sensory neuropathy. Anti-Yo is associated with cerebellar degeneration. Anti-Ri may cause opsoclonus-myoclonus. Anti-VGCC is associated with Lambert–Eaton myasthenic syndrome.

4. A 52-year-old man is receiving bevacizumab for adenocarcinoma of the lung.

The following day after an infusion he became confused, complained of inability to see clearly, and then became agitated. On the way to the hospital, he experienced a seizure. Which of the following complications of chemotherapy is most likely to be present in this patient?

A. Peripheral neuropathy
B. Toxic optic neuropathy
C. Posterior reversible encephalopathy syndrome (PRES)
D. Myelopathy

The correct answer is C. The symptoms suggest acute dysfunction of the posterior cerebral hemispheres. Bevacizumab may cause either thrombosis or hemorrhage, but has also been associated with PRES syndrome. Peripheral neuropathies, optic neuropathies, and myelopathies can result as complications of chemotherapy but would not be expected to cause seizures or altered mental status.

SUGGESTED READING

Bindal AK, Bindal RK, Hess KR, et al. Surgery versus radiosurgery in the treatment of brain metastasis. *J Neurosurg.* 1996;84:748.

Cairncross JG, MacDonald DR, Ramsay DA. Aggressive oligodendroglioma: a chemosensitive tumor. *Neurosurgery.* 1992;31:78.

Chamberlain MC. Current concepts in leptomeningeal metastasis. *Curr Opin Oncol.* 1992;4:533.

Glusker P, Recht L, Lane B. Reversible posterior leukoencephalopathy syndrome and bevacizumab. *N Engl J Med.* 2007;354:980.

Heros DO. Neuro-oncology. In: Weiner WJ, Shulman LM, eds. *Emergent and Urgent Neurology.* New York: Lippincott Williams & Wilkins; 1999.

Hochberg FH, Miller DC. Primary central nervous system lymphoma. *J Neurosurg.* 1988;68:835.

Hwu WJ, Raizer J, Panageas KS, et al. Treatment of metastatic melanoma in the brain with temozolomide and thalidomide. *Lancet Oncol.* 2001;2:634–635.

Kori SH, Foley KM, Posner JB. Brachial plexus lesions in patients with cancer: 100 cases. *Neurology.* 1985;35:8.

Moll JWB, Antoine JC, Brashear HR, et al. Guidelines on the detection of paraneoplastic anti-neuronal-specific antibodies. *Neurology.* 1995;45:1937.

Patchell RA, Tibbs PA, Walsh JW, et al. Surgery versus radiosurgery in the treatment of brain metastasis. *J Neurosurg.* 1996;84:748.

Perrin RG, McBroom RJ. Metastatic tumors of the spine. In: Rengachary SS, Wilkins RH, eds. *Principles of Neurology.* St. Louis: Wolfe; 1994.

Posner JB. *Neurologic Complications of Cancer.* Philadelphia, PA: FA Davis; 1995.

Raez L, Cabral L, Cai JP, et al. Treatment of AIDS-related primary central nervous system lymphoma with zidovudine, ganciclovir, and interleukin 2. *AIDS Res Hum Retroviruses.* 1999;15:713–719.

Smalley SR, Laws ER, O'Fallon JR, et al. Resection for solitary brain metastasis: role of adjuvant radiation and prognostic variables in 229 patients. *J Neurosurg.* 1992;77:531.

Stupp R, Dietrich PY, Ostermann Kraljevic S, et al. Promising survival for patients with newly diagnosed glioblastoma multiforme treated with concomitant radiation plus temozolomide followed by adjuvant temozolomide. *J Clin Oncol.* 2002;20:1375–1382.

Thomas JE, Cascino TL, Earie JD. Differential diagnosis between radiation and tumor plexopathy of the pelvis. *Neurology.* 1985;35:1.

Vredenburgh JJ, Desjardins A, Herndon JE, et al. Phase II trial of bevacizumab and irinotecan in recurrent malignant glioma. *Clin Cancer Res.* 2007;13:1253–1261.

Westphal M, Hilt DC, Bortey E, et al. A phase 3 trial of local chemotherapy with biodegradable carmustine (BCNU) wafers (Gliadel wafers) in patients with primary malignant glioma. *Neuro-oncol.* 2003;5(2):79–88.

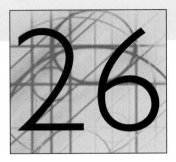

26 Eye Signs in Neurologic Diagnosis

ROBERT K. SHIN AND JAMES A. GOODWIN

key points

- Specific patterns of vision loss correlate with specific lesions along the visual pathway from the eye to primary visual cortex.

- Distinct higher-order visual processing disorders (e.g., visuospatial neglect or an inability to recognize faces) are associated with specific cortical regions.

- The pupils are under autonomic control. Afferent (sensory) lesions cause poorly reactive pupils while parasympathetic and sympathetic efferent (motor) lesions cause anisocoria (unequal pupils).

- Eye movement abnormalities may be conjugate (eyes remain aligned) or disconjugate (the eyes are no longer aligned). Disconjugate eye movement abnormalities are associated with diplopia (double vision).

- Nystagmus (rhythmic, conjugate eye movements) are associated with vertigo (subjective feeling of movement) and oscillopsia (shaking of the visual field). Different forms of nystagmus suggest specific disorders of the brainstem or cerebellum.

umans are highly visual animals. In order to fully scan the environment, our two spherical, lensed eyes synchronously rotate in three spatial dimensions under the control of 12 extraocular muscles, guided by the parietal lobes, frontal lobes, cerebellum, midbrain, and pons. More than half of our cranial nerves are involved in coordinating, directing, and protecting these delicate visual organs, which can move faster than any other part of the human body. Over a million retinal ganglion cells carry information from over 100 million photoreceptors from each exquisitely formed eye to multiple brainstem and subcortical nuclei, from which myriad neuronal axons splay out into the temporal and parietal lobes and down as far as the thoracic spinal cord to connect these nuclei to a network of autonomic structures and to primary visual cortex. Visual information radiates from the occipital lobe in concentric, widening circles across the neocortex, approximately one third of which is involved in higher-order visual processing, providing us with real-time, full-color, panoramic, stereoscopic views of the world around us.

Because this elegant but complex system involves every lobe of the brain, multiple subcortical structures, multiple brainstem nuclei, multiple peripheral and cranial nerves, the autonomic nervous system, and even the spinal cord, it is not surprising that many different neurologic problems (stroke, migraine, seizures, multiple sclerosis, movement disorders, dementia, traumatic brain injury, neuromuscular disorders, alcoholism, CNS infections, and cancer) affect the visual system in some way, leading to a wide variety of neuro-ophthalmologic disorders.

This chapter is a survey of a number of visual signs and symptoms that are useful in localization and diagnosis in neurologic disease. Broad categories of neuro-ophthalmologic complaints that neurologists and non-neurologists may encounter include: *vision loss* (blindess or blurred vision), *higher-order visual processing disorders* (cognitive disorders), *pupillary abnormalities* (poorly reactive or unequal pupils), *eye movement problems* (gaze palsies and double vision), and *nystagmus* (shaking eye movements). Each of these broad categories is organized into smaller subsections, with each subsection focusing on a limited number of related neuro-ophthalmologic disorders.

VISION LOSS

Vision loss may range from mild blurred vision to complete blindness and may involve one or both eyes. When approaching a patient who complains of blurred vision or vision loss, the first step is to make sure that the patient has been evaluated by an eye doctor (ophthalmologist or optometrist) to rule out an ocular disorder (a problem with the cornea, lens, vitreous, or retina). Once disorders such as refractive error, glaucoma, cataract, vitreous hemorrhage, retinal artery or vein occulusion, and retinal detachment have been ruled out, a neurologic evaluation can begin.

■ **SPECIAL CLINICAL POINT: Every patient with vision loss should be evaluated by an eye doctor to rule out ocular problems before the neurologic evaluation begins.**

Evaluation of Vision Loss

The evaluation of vision loss involves tests of *visual acuity* and *color vision*, the *swinging flashlight test*, an evaluation of the *optic disc appearance*, and testing for *visual field defects*. The information gleaned from these tests must be combined in order to accurately localize and diagnose the source of the vision loss.

Visual Acuity   Visual acuity, tested with handheld or wall-mounted Snellen eye charts, is the most basic part of the visual examination. The best corrected visual acuity possible is desired (patients should wear their glasses or contact lenses). A pinhole may be used to minimize refractive error if lenses are not available.

Color Vision   Color perception is an extremely sensitive, although subjective, measure of optic nerve dysfunction. If specialized color plates are not available, present a fairly large bright red object and ask the patient if there is any apparent difference in the redness of the object between the two eyes. Patients may report a subjective loss of color intensity (*color desaturation*) in one eye compared to the other. Reds may be shifted to a darker amber color or bleached toward a lighter, pinkish, or yellowish color. Patients can be asked to subjectively quantitate the degree of color

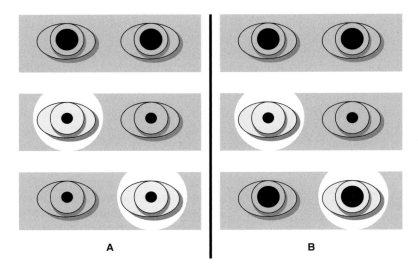

A   **B**

FIGURE 26.1 Swinging flashlight test. In the darkness (top) both pupils dilate. **A:** Under normal conditions, when light shines is either eye, both pupils constrict equally. **B:** In the setting of injury to the left optic nerve, both pupils constrict when light shines in the right eye but dilate when light shines in the left eye.

desaturation—"If this (covering one eye) is a dollar's worth of red, how much is this (covering the other eye) red worth?"

Swinging Flashlight Test   Damage to the anterior light pathway (optic nerves, optic chiasm, and optic tract) can be detected by illuminating each eye separately with a focal light source. Swinging the flashlight back and forth provides a sensitive means of comparing the afferent function of the two eyes (Fig. 26.1).

Normally, the amount of pupillary constriction will be the same regardless of which eye is being stimulated by the flashlight. In the setting of an afferent defect, however, both pupils may dilate when the light is swung to the affected eye, with both pupils constricting when the flashlight is swung to the normal eye. (Remember that even if only the eye illuminated by the flashlight can be seen, the unseen fellow eye is undergoing the same consensual pupillary constriction and dilation that is observed in the illuminated eye.) This asymmetry is the *relative afferent pupillary defect (RAPD)* or Marcus Gunn pupil (see section Relative Afferent Pupillary Defect).

If a patient has decreased visual acuity in one eye with normal visual acuity and a full visual field in the other eye, but has no RAPD, the possibility of refractive error, cataract, or other media opacity should be considered. If the ocular examination is normal, the absence of a RAPD could suggest that the monocular vision loss is functional (nonorganic).

■ **SPECIAL CLINICAL POINT: Cataracts and other opacities do *not* produce a significant RAPD even with major visual loss. This is because such opacities diffuse light within the eye and blur the visual image but do not significantly reduce the total quantity of light that reaches the retina.**

Optic Disc Appearance

Ophthalmoscopy, though a challenging skill to master, is an essential part of any evaluation for vision loss (see Chapter 1). At a minimum, clinicians should be able to distinguish between a normal optic disc, optic disc pallor, and optic disc swelling with a handheld direct ophthalmoscope (Fig. 26.2).

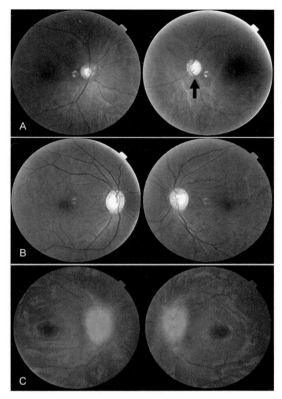

FIGURE 26.2 Fundus photographs. Photos are displayed as though looking at the patient (right eye on the left, left eye on the right). Veins (thicker lines) and arteries (thinner lines) radiate to and from the optic disc, which lies nasal to the macula (visible as a pigmented spot). **A:** Unilateral optic disc pallor following a left ischemic optic neuropathy (black arrow). **B:** Bilateral disc pallor in a patient with multiple sclerosis. **C:** Bilateral disc swelling in a young patient with idiopathic intracranial hypertension (pseudotumor cerebri).

Normal Optic Disc   When decreased vision is accompanied by other signs of optic neuropathy (decreased color vision, RAPD, field loss) but the optic disc is normal, consider the possibility of *acute optic neuritis* or a *posterior ischemic optic neuropathy*, both of which may present without disc pallor or swelling. Retinal disorders may also be associated with a normal optic disc, but rarely present with decreased color vision or a RAPD.

Optic Disc Pallor   Damage to the optic nerve is associated with *optic disc pallor* (a loss of color). Optic disc pallor generally takes time to develop, and may be associated with a history of prior optic neuropathy. Gradually progressive vision loss accompanied by optic disc pallor is concerning for a *compressive optic neuropathy* from an aneurysm or tumor. An optic disc that is both pale and swollen is concerning for *ischemic optic neuropathy*, particularly arteritic ischemic optic neuropathy caused by giant cell arteritis.

Optic Disc Swelling   Swelling or edema of the optic disc may be unilateral or bilateral. Ischemic, inflammatory, and demyelinating optic neuropathies may cause disc swelling, as can increased intracranial pressure. The key to distinguishing between disc swelling from optic neuropathy and disc swelling from increased intracranial pressure (*papilledema*) is comparing the visual function of the nerve to its appearance.

Disc swelling due to optic neuropathy will be associated with decreased visual acuity, decreased color vision, a RAPD (if unilateral or asymmetric), and characteristic optic nerve visual field defects (see section Visual Pathway and Visual Field Defects). Disc swelling due to optic neuropathy may be unilateral or bilateral depending on its etiology.

Papilledema (which refers specifically to optic disc swelling due to increased intracranial pressure) is typically associated with relatively little visual dysfunction, especially early on. Visual acuity and color vision are often normal or only mildly affected. No RAPD is usually seen unless significant nerve damage has occurred. Visual fields may show enlargement of the blind spot or nonspecific constriction. Although papilledema is usually bilateral, it is often asymmetric (see section Papilledema).

The combination of a pale optic disc on one side and optic disc swelling on the other is the *Foster Kennedy syndrome*, signifying a mass lesion (e.g., olfactory groove meningioma) that compresses one optic nerve (causing disc pallor) and raising intracranial pressure (causing papilledema of the opposite nerve). More commonly seen is the *pseudo-Foster Kennedy* syndrome in which sequential optic neuropathies (e.g., optic neuritis or ischemic optic neuropathy) result in a pale optic disc on one side (due to an old optic nerve injury) and a swollen optic disc on the other (due to an acute optic neuropathy).

Visual Pathway and Visual Field Defects

Each eye has its own visual field. These visual fields are slightly different from each other, but overlap substantially. The retina does not directly project to the occipital lobe. Instead, visual information travels along a six-part visual pathway (Fig. 26.3).

- Retinal ganglion cell (RGC) axons converge to form the *optic nerves*, which "punch through" the back of the eye nasal (medial) to the macula, forming the optic disc. Because there are no photoreceptors on the optic disc itself and due to the optics of the eye (images are reversed and upside-down), a blind spot is created temporal (lateral) to central fixation in each eye.
- Both optic nerves cross, forming the *optic chiasm*. Within the chiasm are RGC fibers from both eyes, some of which cross, others of which remain uncrossed.
- Beyond the chiasm, crossing and uncrossed RGC fibers join to form the *optic tracts*. Unlike an optic nerve, which carries information from a single eye, each optic tract carries binocular information from the opposite (left or right) visual hemifield.
- RGC axons (having formed the optic nerves, chiasm, and tracts) finally project onto the *lateral geniculate nucleus (LGN)* of the thalamus.
- Axons from each LGN spread out and separate into the *optic radiations*. Visual information from the upper half of the visual hemifield travels through the inferior or temporal radiations (Meyer's loop); visual information from the lower half of the visual hemifield travels through the superior or parietal radiations.
- The radiations converge on the *visual cortex*, where higher-order visual processing begins.

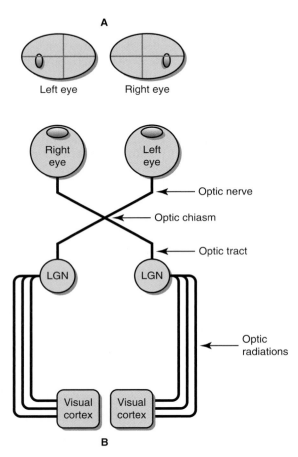

FIGURE 26.3 Visual fields and the visual pathway. **A:** Visual fields are always depicted from the patient's point of view (right eye on the right, left eye on the left). Note that the temporal field of each eye is larger than the nasal field. A blind spot lies temporal and slightly inferior to the central fixation point in each eye. **B:** The visual pathway runs from the retina to the occipital lobe. (The diagram is oriented "radiologically" with the eyes toward the top of the page and the left eye toward the right side of the page.) Retinal ganglion cell axons project to the lateral geniculate nucleus (LGN) of the thalamus via the optic nerve, optic chiasm, and optic tract. Axons from the LGN project to the visual cortex via the superior (parietal) and inferior (temporal) optic radiations.

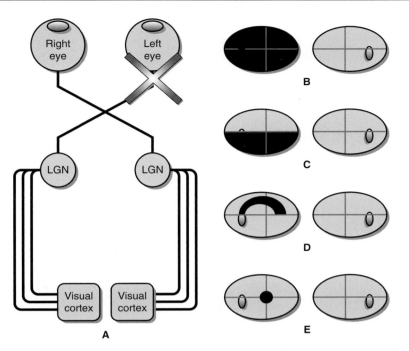

FIGURE 26.4 Optic nerve visual field defects. **A:** A lesion of the left optic nerve may result in a variety of visual field defects. **B:** Monocular blindness. **C:** Inferior altitudinal defect. **D:** Superior arcuate defect (Bjerrum scotoma). **E:** Central scotoma.

Due to this complicated anatomic arrangement, lesions within different parts of the visual pathway are associated with a variety of specific visual field defects.

Optic Nerve Lesions of the optic nerve always cause unilateral visual field defects (Fig. 26.4). Optic nerve lesions are generally also associated with decreased visual acuity, decreased color vision, and a relative afferent pupillary defect.

Optic nerve damage may cause *monocular blindness*, a *central scotoma* (blurring only in the center of vision), or a *centrocecal scotoma* (vision loss in the center of vision that extends to the blind spot).

Reflecting the organization of RGC axons within the retina (Fig. 26.5), visual field defects due to optic nerve damage often respect the horizontal meridian (midline). *Superior* and *inferior altitudinal defects* affect the entire upper or lower field of vision respectively. *Superior*

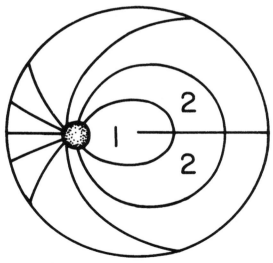

FIGURE 26.5 Retinal ganglion cell organization. Diagram of the fundus of the left eye. **(1)** The *papillomacular bundle* carries information from the center of the visual field. Lesions of the papillomacular bundle may result in a central scotoma. **(2)** The *arcuate bundles* arc around the papillomacular bundle. A lesion of an arcuate bundle may cause an arcuate defect or *Bjerrum scotoma*.

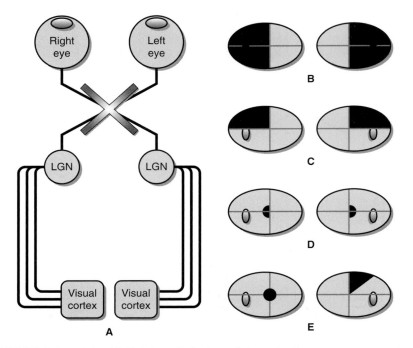

FIGURE 26.6 Chiasmal visual field defects. **A:** Lesions of the optic chiasm may cause a variety of visual field defects. **B:** Classically, a chiasmal lesion causes a *bitemporal hemianopia*. **C:** A *superior bitemporal hemianopia* may occur if the chiasm is compressed from below. **D:** A lesion of the posterior chiasm may result in a *central bitemporal hemianopia*. **E:** A lesion of the left optic nerve where it joins the chiasm may be associated with a *junctional scotoma*, a superior temporal defect on the side opposite the optic nerve visual field defect.

and *inferior arcuate defects* are curved scotomas that follow the anatomic organization of the arcuate bundles.

In general, these patterns of visual field loss are not specific for any particular type of optic neuropathy (see section Optic Neuropathy). Central scotomas, however, are commonly seen with optic neuritis. Bilateral centrocecal scotomas strongly suggest toxic–metabolic optic neuropathy. Inferior altitudinal defects are often associated with ischemic optic neuropathy. Arcuate defects (*Bjerrum scotomas*) can be seen in glaucoma.

Optic Chiasm   Chiasmal injury is classically associated with bitemporal visual field defects due to damage to crossing fibers that carry temporal visual field information from the nasal

retinas (Fig. 26.6). Retinal ganglion cells axons from either side (right or left) of the macula travel together through the optic nerve but separate at the optic chiasm. This divergence creates the hemianopic midline and is the reason that all chiasmal and retrochiasmal visual field defects respect the vertical meridian.

Though the chiasm may be affected by ischemia, infection, or demyelination, most symptomatic lesions of the chiasm are compressive. Pituitary macroadenomas are the most common cause of chiasmal compression, but other tumors (e.g., craniopharyngioma and meningioma) and aneurysms may also injure the chiasm.

Bitemporal hemianopias may be complete (with no vision temporal to fixation in either eye), but when compression is early or mild, the hemianopia may be denser superiorly (when the chiasm is compressed from below) or inferiorly (when the chiasm is compressed from above).

Because crossing macular fibers travel posteriorly, a lesion of the posterior chiasm may result in a *central bitemporal hemianopia*, sparing the more peripheral temporal fields.

Rarely, an anterior lesion at the junction of the optic nerve and the optic chiasm can injure crossing fibers from the opposite inferior retina (which loop forward into the optic nerve, forming *Wilbrand knee* before projecting posteriorly to the optic tract). As a result, the optic nerve visual field defect in one eye may be accompanied by a superior temporal scotoma in the other eye—the *junctional scotoma*.

Optic Tract   Each optic tract is comprised of uncrossed RGC axons from the temporal retina of the ipsilateral eye and crossed RGC axons from the nasal retina of the contralateral eye. The optic tract, therefore, carries visual information from both eyes but only from the contralateral hemifield (as opposed to the optic nerve, which carries information from both hemifields but only from one eye). Like the optic chiasm, the optic tract is most commonly injured by compression from a mass lesion.

A lesion of the optic tract results in a *homonymous hemianopia*—a loss of vision in the contralateral visual field of both eyes (Fig. 26.7). (For example, a left optic tract lesion will cause an inability to see to the right of midline in both eyes—a right homonymous hemianopia.) In fact, all retrochiasmal visual field defects are homonymous, meaning that the visual field defects will be in the same hemifield (left or right) of both eyes.

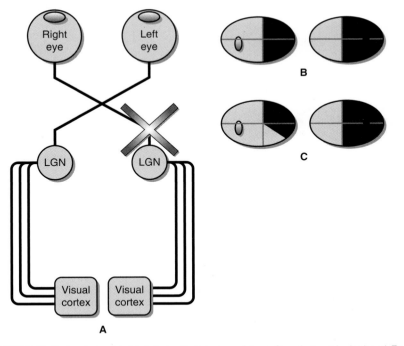

FIGURE 26.7 Optic tract visual field defects. **A:** A lesion of the left optic tract is depicted. **B:** A left optic tract lesion results in a right *homonymous hemianopia*. (Because the temporal field of the right eye is larger than the nasal field of the left eye, this homonymous hemianopia may be accompanied by a right relative afferent papillary defect.) **C:** Homonymous hemianopias due to tract lesions may be *incongruous*.

In order to distinguish a homonymous hemianopia due to a tract lesion from one caused by a lesion of visual cortex, it is important to check for a *relative afferent pupillary defect* and to assess the *congruity* of the visual field.

Although the optic tract primarily projects to the lateral geniculate nucleus of the thalamus (see below), some RGC axons are diverted from the tract to the posterior midbrain to control the pupillary light response (see section Pupil Anatomy and Function). Furthermore, because the temporal field is larger than the nasal field, a homonymous hemianopia causes relatively more visual field loss in one eye than the other. In the case of a lesion of the left optic tract, the resulting right homonymous hemianopia will cause a larger defect in the right eye than in the left eye and may therefore be accompanied by a right relative afferent pupillary defect.

Also, homonymous hemianopias caused by lesions of the optic tract are often *incongruous*, meaning that the density and shape of the visual field defects do not match completely. As a rule, visual field defect congruity increases as the visual pathway approaches the occipital lobe, with visual cortex lesions typically producing highly congruous visual field defects. Congruity can only be assessed if the homonymous hemianopia is incomplete.

Lateral Geniculate Nucleus   As with tract lesions, lesions of the lateral geniculate nucleus (LGN) of the thalamus will result in homonymous visual field defects (Fig. 26.8). Thalamic lesions associated with visual field defects are most commonly vascular.

Lateral (posterior) choroidal artery occlusion has been associated with a wedge-shaped homonymous scotoma along the horizontal

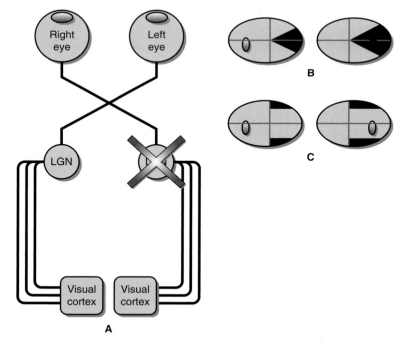

FIGURE 26.8 Lateral geniculate nucleus (LGN) visual field defects. **A:** A lesion of the left LGN may be associated with two different vascular lesions. **B:** Occlusion of the left lateral (posterior) choroidal artery may cause a right *horizontal sectoranopia*. **C:** Occlusion of the left anterior choroidal artery may result in a right *quadruple sectoranopia*.

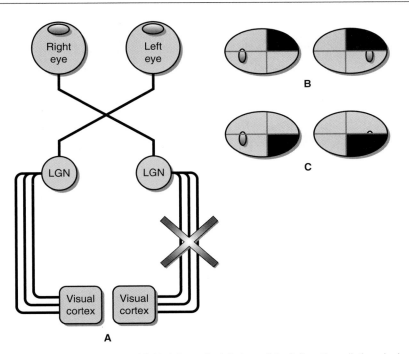

FIGURE 26.9 Optic radiation visual field defects. **A:** A lesion of the left optic radiations is depicted. **B:** A lesion in the left temporal lobe, affecting the inferior radiations (Meyer loop), will cause a right *superior quadrantanopia*, also known as a "pie in the sky" defect. **C:** A lesion in the left parietal lobe, affecting the superior radiations, will result in a right *inferior quadrantanopia*.

midline, sparing the upper and lower quadrants—a *horizontal sectoranopia*.

Anterior choroidal artery occlusion may result in the exact complement of the other geniculate syndrome, superior and inferior homonymous quadrantic defects that spare the area along the horizontal meridian—a *quadruple sectoranopia*.

Optic Radiations Axons radiating outward from the lateral geniculate nucleus toward primary visual cortex form two thin but wide bands that travel separately within the deep white matter of the cerebral hemispheres. Visual information from the upper visual field travels inferiorly through the temporal lobes, while information from the lower visual field travels superiorly through the parietal lobes. As a result of this separation, it is unusual for both sets of optic radiations to be injured simultaneously.

A lesion of a single set of optic radiations affects half of the contralateral hemifield, resulting in a homonymous *quadrantanopia* (Fig. 26.9). Temporal lobe lesions, including strokes, tumors, encephalitis, and demyelination, may damage the inferior radiations as they loop forward and then back toward the visual cortex, producing a *superior quadrantanopia*, also known as a "pie in the sky" defect. Similar lesions of the parietal lobe may damage the superior radiations, causing an *inferior quadrantanopia*.

Visual Cortex The visual pathway ends in the occipital lobe as the superior and inferior optic radiations converge on primary visual cortex (also known as *calcarine cortex* or *striate cortex*).

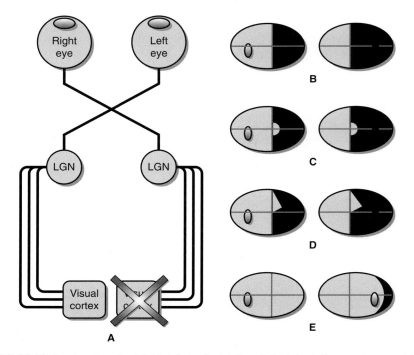

FIGURE 26.10 Visual cortex visual field defects. **A:** A left occipital lobe lesion may be associated with a variety of right homonymous hemianopias. **B:** Homonymous hemianopias without macular sparing are common. **C:** Homonymous hemianopias with macular sparing may occur. **D:** Incomplete homonymous hemianopias caused by occipital lobe lesions are highly congruous. **E:** A small lesion of the deep (anterior) visual cortex may result in a visual field defect that only involves the unpaired temporal crescent.

Lesions of the visual cortex, like lesions of the optic tract, frequently result in a contralateral *homonymous hemianopia* (Fig. 26.10). The most common causes of homonymous hemianopias due to an occipital lobe lesion are posterior cerebral artery infarction, hemorrhage, trauma, and tumor (Fig. 26.11). Rarely, patients present with homonymous hemianopias but no abnormalities on MRI, which raises the possibilies of Alzheimer disease or the Heidenhain variant of Creutzfeld–Jakob disease.

Homonymous hemianopias caused by visual cortex lesions are frequently complete. When incomplete, homonymous hemianopias tend to be congruous. Homonymous *quadrantanopias* can also be seen when damage to the visual cortex is limited.

Occasionally, central vision may be spared within the hemianopic field. The classic explanation for this *macular sparing* is collateral blood supply to the occipital lobe from a branch of the middle cerebral artery, though there are other possible explanations as well.

Rarely, a lesion may selectively affect only the deepest, most anterior part of the visual cortex, producing a visual field defect that is limited to the peripheral portion of the temporal field of the contralateral eye. Involvement of the *temporal crescent* is the only situation in which a retrochiamsal lesion results in a monocular visual field defect. (Sparing of the temporal crescent in the setting of a homonymous hemianopia is also possible.)

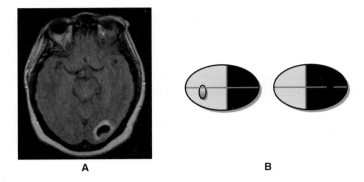

FIGURE 26.11 Occipital hemorrhage. **A:** Axial FLAIR MRI shows a left occipital lobe hemorrhage secondary to poorly controlled hypertension. **B:** The patient's only neurologic deficit was a complete right homonymous hemianopia.

Optic Neuropathy

Vision loss that is only present in one eye is generally either an ocular disorder affecting the structures of the eye itself (above) or an *optic neuropathy*, a lesion of the optic nerve. There are many different kinds of ischemic, inflammatory, infectious, infiltrative, demyelinating, and toxic–metabolic causes of optic neuropathy (only a few are discussed here), but in all cases of optic neuropathy, there should be decreased visual acuity, decreased color vision, a RAPD, and visual field defects.

Optic Neuritis   Optic neuritis is a specific demyelinating optic neuropathy, which may be idiopathic, but is strongly associated with multiple sclerosis (see Chapter 11). Optic neuritis typically occurs in young adults (ages 20 to 40) and is characterized by decreased vision in one eye that presents subacutely (over hours to days) accompanied by a relative afferent pupillary defect. Pain or discomfort exacerbated by eye movement is present more than 90% of the time. Patients with optic neuritis usually note poor color vision in the affected eye. The classic visual field defect associated with optic neuritis is a central scotoma, though other patterns are frequently seen. Funduscopic examination may reveal mild optic disc swelling or may be completely normal.

Optic neuritis is a clinical diagnosis; MRI of the orbits is not necessary when the presentation is classic (a young adult with subacute vision loss in one eye associated with decreased color vision and pain on eye movements). MRI of the brain, however, is useful as a way to identify patients at higher risk to go on to develop multiple sclerosis (MS). Patients with a single episode of optic neuritis who have demyelinating lesions on brain MRI are much more likely to go on to develop MS in the future than patients whose initial brain MRI shows no lesions.

The prognosis for recovery from optic neuritis is excellent. Most patients recover on their own. Intravenous corticosteroids may speed up the recovery of vision but do not provide any lasting benefit. Oral corticosteroids should not be used to treat optic neuritis due to an apparent increased risk of recurrence of optic neuritis.

■ **SPECIAL CLINICAL POINT: Optic neuritis should not be treated with oral corticosteroids, which provide no benefit and may increase the risk of recurrence.**

Ischemic Optic Neuropathy   Ischemia to the optic nerve head may result in sudden, painless loss of vision. Ischemic optic neuropathy may occur in adults over the age of 50, particularly those with vascular risk factors. Patients often wake up with vision loss. Decreased visual acuity, decreased color vision, a RAPD, and visual field defects (often altitudinal defects) are the norm. The optic disc is swollen (often with peripapillary hemorrhages) in *anterior ischemic optic neuropathy (AION)* but appears normal in *posterior ischemic optic neuropathy (PION)*. Anterior ischemic optic neuropathies are further subdivided into *arteritic AION* (caused by giant cell arteritis) and *nonarteritic AION (NAION)*. Ischemic optic neuropathy can usually be differentiated from optic neuritis by clinical features, such as the age of the patient, the acuity of the vision loss, the presence or absence of pain, and the presence or absence of disc swelling.

■ **SPECIAL CLINICAL POINT: In acute monocular vision loss, ischemic optic neuropathy is more likely that optic neuritis if (1) the vision loss presents very suddenly (within seconds or minutes), (2) the vision loss is completely painless, or (3) funduscopy reveals pronounced swelling of the optic disc with disc hemorrhages.**

Amaurosis Fugax

Transient, painless monocular vision loss (amaurosis fugax) lasting for minutes is highly suggestive of an embolic transient ischemic attack (TIA) related to internal carotid artery disease. Patients often describe the vision loss as a "shade coming down" over one eye. As with any other form of TIA, an urgent vascular workup is recommended, given a greatly increased risk of stroke in these patients (see Chapter 7).

Papilledema

Disc swelling secondary to increased intracranial pressure, unlike disc swelling from optic neuropathies, is often associated with surprisingly mild visual symptoms at first. Papilledema may be accompanied by headache, pulsatile tinnitus, transient visual obscurations, or horizontal double vision—all signs of increased

intracranial pressure. The workup of papilledema includes imaging (to rule out a mass lesion, hemorrhage, or hydrocephalus), lumbar puncture (to confirm the presence of increased intracranial pressure), and visual fields (to track any subclinical visual field loss).

The terms *pseudotumor cerebri* and *idiopathic intracranial hypertension* are sometimes used interchangably if no structural lesion is found on imaging, although the latter term should probably be reserved for cases in which no explanation for the increased intracranial pressure can be found. Known causes of "secondary" intracranial hypertension include a variety of medications (e.g., retinoids and tetracycline antibiotics), sleep apnea, cerebral venous thrombosis, and dural arteriovenous malformations. Patients with truly *idiopathic* intracranial hypertension are almost always young, overweight women who benefit from weight loss, but may require medical and surgical interventions to prevent vision loss.

Diplopia

Sometimes patients present complaining of "blurred vision" but actually have diplopia (double vision). The first question to ask in such a situation is, "Does the blurred vision go away if you close either eye?"

If the blurred or double vision resolves when either eye is closed, the patient has *binocular diploia* (only present when both eyes are open), a sign of ocular misalignment or *strabismus* (see section Vertical Double Vision and Horizontal Double Vision).

If the blurred vision goes away if one eye is covered but is still present when the other eye is covered, the patient has *monocular diplopia* (only present in one eye). For example, if the blurred or double vision goes away if the right eye is covered, but is present when the left eye is covered, the source of the monocular diplopia is the right eye.

Common causes of monocular diplopia include refractive error (cataract, astigmatism, keratoconus) or vitreoretinal disorders.

Occasionally monocular diplopia may be a functional (nonorganic) complaint. Monocular diplopia can be bilateral, in which case the double vision will be present in each eye when the opposite eye is covered.

■ **SPECIAL CLINICAL POINT: Monocular diplopia (double vision that is present when one eye is covered) is much more likely to be ophthalmologic or functional (nonorganic) than neurologic.**

HIGHER-ORDER VISUAL PROCESSING DISORDERS

Even after visual information reaches the occipital lobe, visual processing continues at a higher level within visual association cortex and in adjacent visual association areas, allowing a more complex "conscious" visual experience. Lesions within these cortical areas may be associated with a number of cognitive visual processing disturbances.

Cortical Vision Loss

Bilateral visual cortex lesions may cause total blindness. Because the problem lies within the occipital lobes, cortically blind patients have normal pupillary reactions and normal fundus examinations. Cortical blindness may be accompanied by *Anton syndrome*, *blindsight*, or *Charles Bonnet syndrome*. Unilateral visual cortex lesions may, under special circumstances, cause *alexia without agraphia*.

Anton Syndrome   Rarely, patients with cortical blindness actively deny that they are blind, confabulating answers to questions and behaving as though they can see. Their speech and behavior may be so convincing that the presence of Anton syndrome may be missed for some time. The cause of Anton syndrome is unknown.

Blindsight   Some cortically blind patients have the ability to respond to visual stimuli without any conscious perception of vision. They may be able to point to or identify objects by "guessing" while denying that they can see anything, or they may have the ability to detect the movement of an object without being able to perceive the object itself (the *Riddoch phenomenon*). The existence of blindsight seems to imply that there may be alternative visual pathways that bypass primary visual cortex, allowing unconscious visual perception.

Charles Bonnet syndrome   Vivid, complex visual hallucinations may develop in the setting of significant vision loss. Thought to be the brain's attempt to compensate for decreased visual stimulation, Charles Bonnet syndrome can occur in patients with glaucoma, macular degeneration, and bilateral optic neuropathy, as well as in cortically blind patients or in patients with homonymous hemianopias. Patients recognize that the hallucinations are not real but are often reluctant to admit their existence.

Alexia without Agraphia   A lesion of the left occipital lobe that extends to the posterior corpus callosum (splenium) may cause *alexia without agraphia*, a syndrome in which patients can write but are unable to read words, including words they have just written. It is thought that the lesion within the corpus callosum disconnects the right visual cortex from language areas in the left temporal lobe, leaving the patient unable to decipher the visual image of the text.

Disorders of Object Recognition

Lesions within temporo-occipital brain regions interrupt the ventral stream of visual processing (the "what pathway") resulting in problems recognizing objects and object characteristics.

Prosopagnosia   *Prosopagnosia*, the inability to recognize faces, is caused by a lesion of the right fusiform gyrus, located at the temporo-occipital junction. Patients with prosopagnosia have difficulty recognizing family members or celebrities by looking at their faces, but may be able to identify them by the sound of their voice or by distinctive hairstyles or clothing. Prosopagnosia may be accompanied by a left superior quadrantanopia due to involvement of the right inferior optic radiations (see section Visual Pathway and Visual Field Defects).

Cerebral Achromatopsia Bilateral lesions of the fusiform and lingual gyri in the temporo-occipital regions of both hemispheres can cause a loss of color perception—*achromatopsia*. Patients with cerebral achromatopsia see the world in black and white and shades of gray, and may also suffer from prosopagnosia and superior visual field defects.

Disorders of Visuospatial Processing

Lesions within parieto-occipital brain regions interrupt the dorsal stream of visual processing (the "where pathway") causing defects in spatial perception.

Visuospatial Neglect Parietal lesions can cause contralateral visuospatial neglect, in which patients ignore stimuli in their contralateral visual field. Visuospatial neglect seems to primarily occur following right parietal lesions (causing left visuospatial neglect). It is possible that the right hemisphere is specialized for attention and spatial processing, though it is also possible that it is harder to identify neglect in patients with left parietal lesions, due to coexisting aphasia.

Visuospatial neglect can be difficult to distinguish from a homonymous hemianopia but may be identified by abnormal *clock drawing* (see Chapter 1) or by *visual extinction* (the patient can count fingers in each visual quadrant, but when two sets of fingers are presented simultaneously, the patient ignores the fingers in the neglected hemifield).

Balint Syndrome Bilateral parieto-occipital lesions produce a clinical syndrome in which patients have special difficulty in directing their gaze in an orderly manner to scan a visual scene. The world for them is a fragmentary and disordered array of images, none organically articulated in a meaningful way. The classic triad of *Balint syndrome* includes (1) optic ataxia (a loss of hand–eye coordination), (2) ocular apraxia (difficulty directing voluntary eye movements), and (3) simultanagnosia (an inability to perceive multiple images within a complex visual scene).

PUPILLARY ABNORMALITIES

Pupil Anatomy and Function

The iris of the eye is an opaque diaphragm with an adjustable central opening—the pupil. The pupil can do only two things: it can constrict or it can dilate. Neither function is under voluntary control—pupillary control is autonomic. Ocular parasympathetics control pupillary constriction; ocular sympathetics control pupillary dilation.

Pupil Constriction The parasympathetic nervous system is responsible for pupillary constriction in response to light or a near target.

The afferent (sensory) arc of the parasympathetic light reflex is mediated by retinal ganglion cell axones that project (via the optic nerve, chiasm, and optic tract) to pretectal nuclei in the midbrain instead of to the lateral geniculate nucleus of the thalamus.

The parasympathetic efferent (motor) arc is mediated by (1) connections from the pretectal nuclei to the Edinger–Westphal subnuclei of the oculomotor complex, (2) preganglionic parasympathetic fibers projecting to the ciliary ganglion via the third nerve, and (3) postganglionic projections from the ciliary ganglion to the pupillary sphincter muscle.

Because of crossing of fibers in the optic chiasm and crossing of fibers between the midbrain pretectal nuclei and the Edinger–Westphal oculomotor subnuceli, light delivered to *one* eye causes equal reflexive contraction of *both* pupils. (The *direct response* is pupillary constriction in the stimulated eye; the *consensual response* is pupillary constriction in the opposite eye.)

■ **SPECIAL CLINICAL POINT: A unilateral optic nerve or optic tract lesion will never cause anisocoria (unequal pupils). Even if an optic nerve is completely transected, causing complete monocular blindness, both pupils will remain equal in size due to crossed light input from the intact right optic nerve.**

Constriction of the pupils to near stimulation is approximately as brisk and extensive as that to light, and is best elicited by having patients attempt to focus on their own thumb (not an examiner's finger) held about 2 or 3 cm from their nose.

Pupil Dilation   The sympathetic nervous system controls pupillary dilation, which occurs in the absence of parasympathetic stimulation (e.g., in the dark or when the parasympathetic pathways have been damaged) or when there are strong emotions (e.g., excitement, fear, or anger).

The afferent arc of the sympathetic system is not well defined, but presumably involves ascending sensory pathways and other limbic–diencephalic interfaces.

The sympathetic efferent (motor) arc is a three-neuron chain that includes: (1) *central* projections that descend from the hypothalamus into the brainstem and spinal cord, synapsing onto preganglionic neurons in the intermediolateral cell column of the spinal cord at around T1 (*ciliospinal center of Budge*), (2) *preganglionic* neurons projecting to the superior cervical ganglion (located behind the carotid bifurcation), and (3) *postganglionic* fibers from the superior cervical ganglion that climb within the sheath of the internal carotic artery to the cavernous sinus, then travel with other cranial nerves into the orbit to reach the iris dilator.

Pupil Dysfunction   The different types of pupillary dysfunction reflect these anatomic considerations. Lesions of the afferent visual pathways (including the optic nerve and optic tract) may

be associated with a *relative afferent pupillary defect*. Damage to the efferent sympathetic or parasympathetic pathways result in *anisocoria* (unequal pupils). Brainstem lesions affecting the posterior midbrain may interfere with one efferent parasympathetic pathway (light) but not the other (near), causing bilateral *light-near dissociation*.

Relative Afferent Pupillary Defect

The presence of a *relative afferent pupillary defect (RAPD)* or Marcus Gunn pupil implies a unilateral or asymmetric lesion between the retina and the midbrain (see section Evaluation of Vision Loss). Technically, pupillary function is normal in a RAPD (the asymmetric response to light accurately reflects a problem within the anterior visual pathway).

A pupil that paradoxically dilates to direct illumination may be seen in the most severe forms of optic neuropathy. More commonly, however, a RAPD may manifest more subtly as less early constriction in one eye than in the other during the swinging flashlight test. Pupillary constriction may not necessarily be completely abolished in a RAPD; asymmetry in pupil reaction to light is the critical feature.

Because the swinging flashlight technique is a comparative test that uses the fellow eye as an internal control, it may be difficult to interpret if both the left and right afferent pathways are equally affected, as in cases of bilateral optic neuropathy.

Hippus and Early Release   Some degree of rhythmic pupillary oscillation (alternating contraction and dilation) can be observed in many normal individuals during steady illumination of the eyes. Though the term *hippus* usually is reserved for those pupils that oscillate with fairly large amplitude, almost every pupil has small sinusoidal oscillations of size with steady illumination. High-amplitude oscillation is a curiosity but is not pathologic.

Frequently, the pupil may dilate slightly after initially constricting to a light stimulus.

This phenomenon of *early release* is normal and does not necessarily indicate an afferent defect. This slight redilatation should, however, be equal in amplitude between both eyes to qualify as a normal variant.

Anisocoria

Anisocoria (a difference in pupil size between the two eyes) is caused by lesions affecting the sympathetic or parasympathetic pupillary efferents. When examining a patient with pupils of unequal size, the first question to answer is which pupil is the abnormal one? Is it the smaller of the pupils or the larger of the two?

The answer can be determined by examining the pupils both in darkness and in light (Fig. 26.12). If the anisocoria remains proportional in both darkness and light, the patient likely has *physiologic anisocoria*. If the relative anisocoria increases in darkness, however, the smaller pupil is not dilating properly, implying a ocular sympathetic deficit, that is, *Horner syndrome*. If the anisocoria increases in light, the problem is that the larger pupil is not constricting. This implies an ocular parasympathetic deficit due to a *third nerve palsy*, *tonic pupil*, or *pharmacologic dilation*.

Physiologic Anisocoria   Approximately 15% of normal individuals have anisocoria of up to 1 mm without any lesion in either the sympathetic or parasympathetic systems. The difference in size remains proportional in bright and dim lighting, which serves to distinguish this benign anisocoria from pathologic states. The degree of anisocoria may vary or even switch sides over time.

Horner Syndrome   A lesion of the ocular sympathetic pathway leads to an inability to dilate the pupil and the classic triad of ipsilateral *miosis* (pupillary constriction), ipsilateral *ptosis* (eyelid drooping), and ipsilateral *anhidrosis* (lack of sweating on the face). Because the sympathetic efferent arc is a three-neuron chain, different causes of Horner syndrome may be grouped by whether the lesions affect the *central (first-order)*, *preganglionic (second-order)*, or *postganglionic (third-order)* neurons.

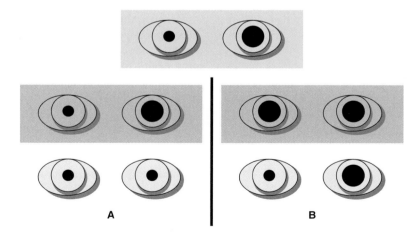

FIGURE 26.12 Anisocoria in light and darkness. **A:** When anisocoria is more obvious in the darkness than in the light, the smaller pupil is the pathologic one. In this case, the right pupil's failure to dilate suggests a right sympathetic deficit (i.e., *Horner syndrome*). **B:** When anisocoria is more obvious in the light than in the dark, the larger pupil is the pathologic one. In this case, the left pupil's failure to constrict in the light suggests a left parasympathetic deficit (i.e., *third nerve palsy, tonic pupil,* or *pharmacologic dilation*).

Central lesions (e.g., of the hypothalamus, brainstem, or cervical cord) are an uncommon cause of Horner syndrome, but are easily recognizable by associated cranial nerve, cerebellar, and sensorimotor long-tract findings. A classic cause of a central Horner syndrome is *Wallenberg syndrome (lateral medullary syndrome)*, in which Horner syndrome is accompanied by vertigo, dysphagia and dysarthria, ipsilateral facial numbness, and contralateral numbness in the arms and legs. Cervical cord injuries may also result in central Horner syndrome.

Preganglionic sympathetic fibers exit the spinal cord in the chest, and may be affected by lesions of the upper chest and the neck. Preganglionic Horner syndrome may result from cancer in the apex of the lung (Pancoast tumor), penetrating neck wounds, or as an iatrogenic complication of neck surgeries (e.g., anterior cervical discectomy).

Postganglionic lesions are commonly associated with pain in the ipsilateral orbit and eye. The combination of postganglionic Horner syndrome and ipsilateral headache or facial pain is known as *Raeder's paratrigeminal syndrome*, and may be a manifestation of internal carotid artery dissection or aneurysm, a cavernous sinus lesion, or (if no vascular or structural lesion can be found) a form of migraine or cluster headache.

In the orbit, the ocular sympathetics innervate small tarsal muscles in the upper and lower eyelids in addition to the iris dilator muscle. Damage to the ocular sympathetic pathway results in mild ptosis of the upper lid and mild elevation of the lower lid. The resulting narrowing of the palpebral fissure creates the illusion that the affected eye is sunken inward (*pseudoenophthalmos*).

The ptosis seen in Horner syndrome is mild (Figs. 26.13 and 26.14), and the function of levator palpebrae (innervated by the oculomotor nerve) remains normal. Complete unilateral ptosis (an inability to open the eye at all) is never seen in Horner syndrome and should raise the possibility of a third nerve palsy or myasthenia gravis instead.

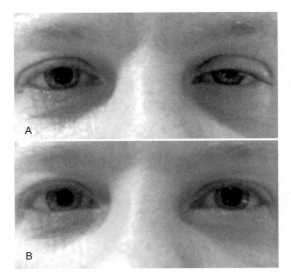

FIGURE 26.13 Horner syndrome. **A:** Left-sided ptosis and miosis developed after anterior cervical discectomy and fusion. **B:** After instillation of 0.5% apraclonidine, the anisocoria has reversed (the left pupil is now larger than the right) and the left-sided ptosis has resolved.

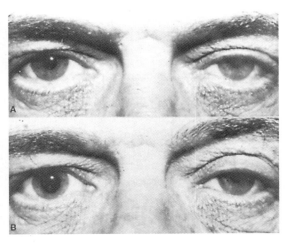

FIGURE 26.14 Raeder's paratrigeminal syndrome. **A:** Left-sided ptosis and miosis accompanying a left migrainous headache. **B:** The left pupil failed to dilate after instillation of 1% hydroxyamphetamine, confirming the diagnosis of a postganglionic (third-order) Horner syndrome.

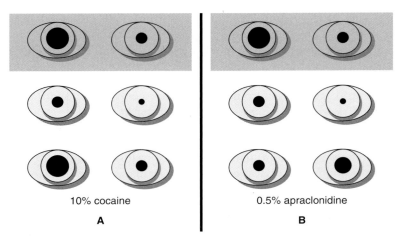

10% cocaine

A

0.5% apraclonidine

B

FIGURE 26.15 Pharmacologic testing in Horner syndrome. **A:** The anisocoria is greater in the darkness than in the light, suggesting a left ocular sympathetic deficit (failure to dilate). After administration of 10% cocaine eye drops (bottom), the right pupil dilates, but the left pupil remains small, confirming the diagnosis of Horner syndrome. **B:** In the same clinical setting, 0.5% apraclonidine eye drops cause dilation of the abnormal pupil, reversing the anisocoria and confirming the diagnosis of Horner syndrome.

■ **SPECIAL CLINICAL POINT: Sometimes Horner syndrome is congenital or long-standing and benign. A careful inspection of old photographs, which might reveal pre-existing ptosis and anisocoria, may help to avoid an unnecessary evaluation for tumor, dissection, or aneurysm. *Iris heterochromia*, a difference in the color of the two eyes (e.g., one blue, one brown), is another sign that can help identify a congenital Horner syndrome.**

Pharmacologic testing may be used to confirm a suspected diagnosis of Horner syndrome or when the clinical history and examination are equivocal. A drop of 10% cocaine can be placed into each eye and a second drop placed a minute later, or a single drop of 0.5% apraclonidine in each eye may be used. Any change in the size of the pupils should be noted at 30 and 60 minutes.

Cocaine blocks the reuptake of norepinephrine at the postganglionic nerve terminal, causing pupillary dilation under normal conditions. A lesion of any part of the three-neuron ocular sympathetic pathway will significantly reduce the amount of norepinephrine released at the nerve terminal, resulting in a failure of pupillary dilation if Horner syndrome is present. The cocaine test for Horner syndrome is therefore "positive" if the suspected pupil fails to dilate (Fig. 26.15). In a "negative" cocaine test, both pupils dilate fully, leaving no residual anisocoria.

Apraclonidine, an alpha-adrenergic agonist used in the treatment of glaucoma, is increasingly being used to confirm Horner syndrome when cocaine is not readily available. Apraclonidine has little effect on the size of normal pupils, but causes dilation in pupils affected by Horner syndrome due to denervation hypersensitivity (see Fig. 26.15). The apraclonidine test for Horner syndrome is "positive" if there is reversal of anisocoria (the formerly smaller pupil becomes the larger pupil). The ptosis associated with Horner syndrome may also resolve with apraclonidine testing (see Fig. 26.13). In a "negative" apraclonidine test, there will be no significant change in pupil size or ptosis.

Additional pharmacologic testing may aid in localization, distinguishing between different types of Horner syndrome. *Hydroxyamphetamine* stimulates the release of norepinephrine

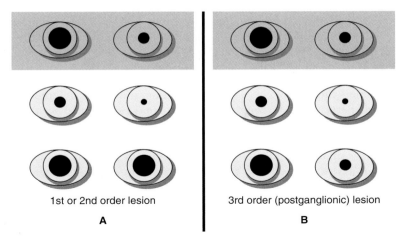

1st or 2nd order lesion

3rd order (postganglionic) lesion

A

B

FIGURE 26.16 Hydroxyamphetamine testing in Horner syndrome. **A:** Anisocoria, greater in the darkness than in the light, due to left Horner syndrome. After installation of 1% hydroxyamphetamine eye drops (bottom), both pupils dilate, indicating that the lesion is either first-order or second-order. **B:** A similar situation, except that after installation of 1% hydroxyamphetamine eye drops, the left pupil does not dilate, suggesting a third-order Horner syndrome.

from the postganglionic sympathetic neuron. As long as this postganglionic (third-order) neuron is intact, instillation of 1% hydroxyamphetamine will result in pupillary dilation. If, however, the postganglionic neuron has been injured (as in a third-order Horner syndrome), the affected pupil will fail to dilate in response to hydroxyamphetamine (see Fig. 26.14). In a "negative" hydroxyamphetamine test, both pupils will dilate. Assuming that Horner syndrome is present, the "negative" result indicates that the lesion is in either the central (first-order) or preganglionic (second-order) neuron, but further localization is not possible (Fig. 26.16).

■ **SPECIAL CLINICAL POINT: Although apraclonidine testing for Horner syndrome is becoming increasingly popular, it should be used with caution in children younger than 6 months old in whom respiratory depression and bradycardia may occur.**

The workup of Horner syndrome depends on the clinical history and the degree to which the sympathetic deficit can be localized on examination. Isolated, unexplained Horner syndrome that cannot be documented as old

and stable, may require chest and neck imaging with CT and MRI. If an aneurysm or dissection is suspected, vascular imaging with MRA, CTA, or even conventional angiography may be necessary.

Third Nerve Palsy Mydriasis (dilated pupil) may be a sign of compression of the third (oculomotor) nerve or other third nerve pathology (Fig. 26.17). It is theoretically possible for an aneurysm or other mass to compress the third

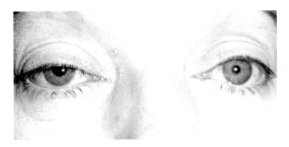

FIGURE 26.17 Partial right third nerve palsy. Right-sided ptosis and mydriasis (pupillary dilation) developed after herpes zoster ophthalmicus. The right eye is slightly abducted and depressed ("down and out") in primary position.

nerve in a way that only affects the pupil. Usually, however, a dilated pupil due to a lesion of the third nerve will be accompanied by ptosis and weakness of the extraocular muscles making the diagnosis fairly straightforward (see section Vertical Double Vision).

Whether the third nerve palsy is *complete* (complete ptosis and no ability to elevate, depress, or adduct the eye) or *partial*, if the pupil is *involved* (sluggish or dilated) at all, the patient should undergo a vascular workup that includes MR or CT angiography to rule out an aneurysm. If an aneurysm cannot be definitively ruled out noninvasively, then conventional angiography may be necessary.

In the past, patients with *partial, pupil-sparing third nerve palsies* were watched closely over time to see if the pupil eventually became involved. As noninvasive imaging techniques continue to improve, however, it may be reasonable to go ahead with MR or CT imaging in any case where an aneurysm is felt to be a possibility.

Perhaps the only time a patient with an oculomotor palsy does not clearly need be imaged is in the setting of a *complete, pupil-sparing third nerve palsy*, which, in a patient with clear vascular risk factors, is likely to be caused by microvascular ischemia.

Because the pupillary fibers travel along the outside of the third nerve, they can be spared by microvascular ischemia of the third nerve, which tends to damage the deeper axons within the third nerve bundle as opposed to more superficial ones.

■ **SPECIAL CLINICAL POINT: Microvascular third nerve palsies (sometimes called *diabetic third nerve palsies*) typically resolve over a 2 to 3-month period, requiring no treatment other than modification of any existing vascular risk factors.**

Unfortunately, sparing of the pupil does not guarantee that the etiology of the third nerve palsy is ischemic. If the patient is young (<50 years old) or has no history of smoking, hypertension, diabetes, or dyslipidemia, or if the patient's third nerve palsy does not significantly improve within a month or two, then a diagnosis of microvascular ischemia should be questioned.

In a critical care setting, large tumors or swelling following a large stroke or hemorrhage may cause uncal herniation, compressing the midbrain and the third nerve. A dilated pupil ("blown") in this setting is known as *Hutchinson pupil* and is a sign of impending catastrophe, requiring emergent intervention.

■ **SPECIAL CLINICAL POINT: A "blown pupil" in an obtunded patient may be a sign of impending transtentorial herniation and should be treated as a medical emergency.**

Tonic Pupil (Adie's Pupil)   The *tonic pupil* or *Adie's pupil* is a dilated pupil that is poorly reactive to light but tonically constricts to a near target (Fig. 26.18). Patients often complain of glare and blurred vision. Some complain of discomfort when focusing at near. Tonic pupil is more common in women than in men. In some cases, the tonic pupil is accompanied by areflexia—the combination of these two features is known as *Adie syndrome*.

The pupil is often large at first, but slowly constricts over time. Under magnification, the pupil is often irregular with segmental contraction and atrophy of the pupillary ruff.

Tonic pupils are a postganglionic parasympathetic lesion, possibly secondary to a viral infection of the ciliary ganglion. Due to this parasympathetic denervation, the iris develops cholinergic supersensitivity. Although a tonic pupil can often be distinguished from other causes of mydriasis (third nerve palsy or pharmacologic dilation) by its clinical features, dilute (0.1%) pilocarpine may be used to confirm the diagnosis.

The normal pupil serves as an internal control in this test. One drop of 0.1% pilocarpine is placed in both eyes, and a second drop is applied 10 minutes later. The pupil size is measured at 30 and 60 minutes. While this dose of pilocarpine is too weak to influence the normal pupil, the tonic

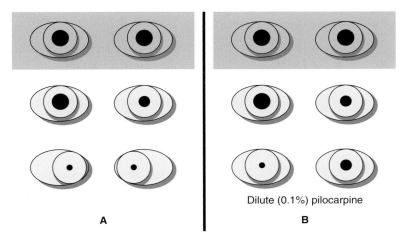

Dilute (0.1%) pilocarpine

A   B

FIGURE 26.18 Tonic pupil (Adie's pupil). **A:** The anisocoria is more obvious in the light because the right pupil fails to constrict. Both pupils constrict with convergence (bottom). This unilateral light-near dissociation distinguishes the tonic pupil from a third nerve palsy or pharmacologically dilated pupil. **B:** The diagnosis of tonic pupil can be confirmed by instillation of dilute (0.1%) pilocarpine. The tonic right pupil constricts due to denervation hypersensitivity.

pupil will constrict due to the presence of denervation supersensitivity (Figs. 26.18 and 26.19).

Pharmacologic Dilation   Atropine, scopolamine, and ipratropium are just a few of the anticholinergic compounds (muscarinic antagonists) that can get into the eye and cause mydriasis (pupillary dilation) and anisocoria.

Atropine is used to treat certain cardiac arrhythmias and as a long-acting cycloplegic agent for some eye problems. Scopolamine is administered by transdermal patch for the prevention of motion sickness. Aerosolized ipratropium is used as a bronchodilator in patients with chronic obstructive pulmonary disease. *Datura stramonium* (also known as *jimson weed*, *angel's trumpet*, and *thorn apple*) may grow as a weed in the garden or yard.

Medical personnel may be exposed to atropine at work. A poorly placed nebulizer mask may blow aerosolized ipratropium into a patient's eye. Travelers may forget to wash their hands after placing a scopolomine patch on their skin. Gardeners may accidentally rub their eyes while weeding. In rare instances,

people may intentionally place atropinic drugs into their eyes to feign a medical problem.

A pharmacologically dilated pupil is often very large and will not be associated with any eye movement abnormalities or ptosis. There will be no reaction to either light or a near target. If there is any question about the diagnosis, pharmacologic testing with 1% pilocarpine can be used—a pharmacologically dilated pupil will fail to contrict, while a tonic pupil or a dilated pupil due to a third nerve palsy will constrict (Fig. 26.19).

Bilateral Light-Near Dissociation

Light-near dissociation may be noted unilaterally in the case of a tonic pupil (see section Anisocoria), but when the phenomenon is bilateral, involvement of the posterior midbrain is likely. A lesion of the posterior (dorsal) midbrain may damage the pretectal nuclei, interrupting the pupillary light pathway, but may spare the near pathway, which projects farther forward to the Edinger–Westphal subnucleus of the oculomotor (III) complex.

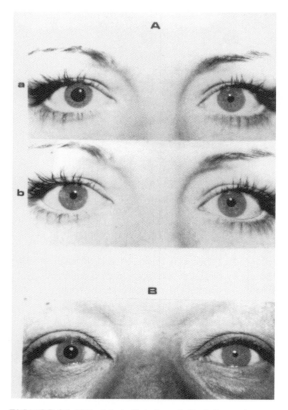

FIGURE 26.19 Isolated, dilated pupil. **A:** Adie syndrome. **(a)** The right pupil is dilated and unreactive to light. There is no ptosis or extraocular muscle weakness. **(b)** The right pupil constricts more than the left after instillation of 0.1% pilocarpine in both eyes, confirming denervation supersensitivity. **B:** Atropinized pupil. The dilated right pupil failed to constrict after instillation of 1% pilocarpine, indicating pharmacologic dilation.

Bilateral light-near dissociation is seen with *Argyll Robertson pupils* and in *Parinaud syndrome* (Fig. 26.20).

Argyll Robertson Pupils   Argyll Robertson pupils (syphilitic pupils) are typically small, irregular, and unreactive to light stimulation, with a preserved ability to constrict with accommodation. (The pupils "accommodate but do not react".) The phenomenon is most commonly bilateral but may be unilateral when first observed, becoming bilateral over time. Argyll

Robertson pupils are thought to be caused by damage to the pretectal area surrounding the sylvian aqueduct in the posterior midbrain secondary to neurosyphilis.

■ **SPECIAL CLINICAL POINT: Observation of small, unreactive pupils that accommodate should trigger detailed history-taking and serologic studies to establish or preclude past syphilitic infection.**

Parinaud Syndrome   Compressive lesions of the dorsal midbrain may cause pupillary paralysis with medium to large pupils that do not react to light, but do constrict with accommodation. In *Parinaud syndrome*, this light-near dissociation is accompanied by supranuclear vertical gaze palsy, lid retraction, and convergence–retraction nystagmus (see section Conjugate Gaze Abnormalities). Parinaud syndrome is classically associated with tumors of the pineal gland (located just behind the midbrain) or obstructive hydrocephalus, but may be caused by any type of lesion that affects the posterior midbrain.

ABNORMAL EYE MOVEMENTS

Eye movements are an important component of visual function. Humans have sharp, high-resolution vision only in a small area (2 to 3 degrees) in the center of our visual field. Although motion perception is good in the periphery, our ability to perceive fine spatial details declines rapidly the farther the image is from fixation. Eye movements, therefore, are necessary to allow us to scan our enviroment thoroughly without constant head motion.

Abnormal eye movements may be conjugate (the visual axes of the two eyes remain parallel and aligned) or dysconjugate (the eyes no longer move together). Dysconjugate eye movements create strabismus (misalignment of the eyes) which results in diplopia (double vision) that may be vertical or horizontal. *Conjugate gaze abnormalities*, *vertical double vision*, and *horizontal double vision* will be discussed separately below.

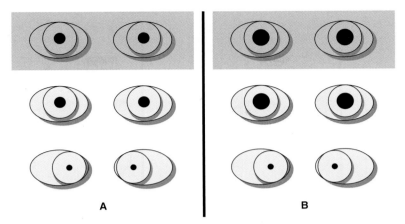

FIGURE 26.20 Bilateral light-near dissociation. **A:** Argyll Robertson pupils are typically small and unreactive to light, but constrict when gaze is focused on a near target (bottom). **B:** A similar pattern of light-near dissociation is seen in Parinaud syndrome without the characteristic miosis seen with syphilitic pupils.

Conjugate Gaze Abnormalities

A simplified sense of the anatomic differences between voluntary (cortically based) eye movements and reflexive (vestibulo-ocular) eye movements is necessary to understand conjugate gaze disorders such as *horizontal gaze palsy* and *supranuclear vertical gaze palsy*. In each of these disorders, the eyes remain aligned but have limited movement.

Voluntary horizontal eye movements are controlled by the frontal eye fields (FEF) in the cerebral cortex. Each FEF is responsible for horizontal gaze in the contralateral direction, sending projections down into the brainstem and across to the contralateral sixth (abducens) nerve nucleus, which acts as the horizontal gaze center. For example, the right FEF projects down to the left sixth nerve nucleus, which projects both to the right third nerve (which controls the right medial rectus muscle) and directly to the left lateral rectus muscle via the left sixth nerve to generate left gaze (Fig. 26.21).

Left gaze may also be generated reflexively by head movement through the *vestibulo-ocular reflex (VOR)*. Head movement toward the right stimulates the right vestibular nucleus, which sends projections across and up the brainstem to the left sixth nerve nucleus, which generates compensatory leftward eye movements (Fig. 26.21).

Analogous pathways exist for voluntary and reflexive vertical eye movements, which will not be discussed in detail here, except to note that while horizontal gaze is generated primarily in the pons, vertical gaze is primarily controlled by the midbrain.

Horizontal Gaze Palsy   Horizontal gaze palsies (an inability to look to one side) may occur with lesions in the ipsilateral pons or in the contralateral frontal lobe. In both cases, patients may tend to look away from the side of the gaze palsy. For example, patients with a *left gaze palsy* may be noted to have a *right gaze preference*.

A pontine lesion that damages the sixth (abducens) nerve nucleus (whether an infarct, hemorrhage, demyelination, or tumor) may cause an ipsilateral *horizontal gaze palsy* in which both voluntary and reflexive movements to that side are abolished. For example, a

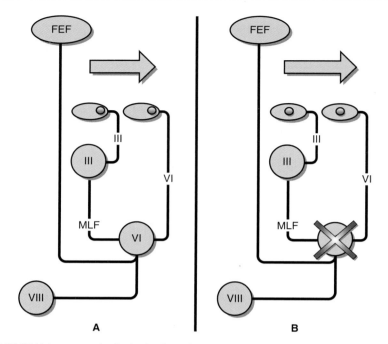

FIGURE 26.21 Voluntary and reflexive horizontal eye movements. **A:** A simplified diagram illustrating the connections between the right frontal eye fields (FEF) and the right vestibular (VIII) nucleus to the left abducens (VI) nucleus. The left abducens (VI) nucleus sends projections to the right oculomotor (III) nucleus (which in turn projects to the right medial rectus muscle) via the medial longitudinal fasciculus (MLF) and to the left lateral rectus muscle via the abducens (VI) nerve. **B:** A lesion of the left abducens (VI) nucleus results in a left horizontal gaze palsy. The eyes will not cross midline to the left either voluntarily or reflexively.

lesion of the left sixth nerve nucleus will result in an inability to look to the left regardless of whether the stimulus is a voluntary attempt to look left (from the right FEF) or a reflexive signal from the right vestibular nucleus during an attempted oculocephalic ("doll's eyes") maneuver (see Fig. 26.22).

These dorsal pontine lesions may be accompanied by other brainstem signs, including an ipsilateral facial (VII) nerve palsy (*Bell palsy*) or contralateral hemiparesis. For example, a left gaze palsy caused by a left pontine lesion may be accompanied by a left Bell palsy and right-sided weakness.

An horizontal gaze palsy may also occur after injury (most commonly a stroke) to the frontal eye fields (FEF) in the contralateral cerebral hemisphere. Unlike gaze palsies caused by

lesions within the pons, gaze palsies caused by frontal lobe lesions can be overcome by the *vestibulo-ocular reflex* (see Fig. 26.22). Gaze palsies from frontal lobe lesions may be accompanied by other neurologic signs referrable to the cerebral hemispheres. For example, a left gaze palsy caused by a right FEF lesion may be accompanied by left-sided weakness and numbness, a left homonymous hemianopia, or left visuospatial neglect, depending on how extensive the cerebral lesion might be.

■ **SPECIAL CLINICAL POINT: An infarct affecting the right frontal eye fields may cause a right gaze preference; the patient is said to be "looking toward the stroke." Excitation of the frontal eye fields produces the opposite effect, and therefore a seizure in the right frontal lobe may drive gaze to the left, in which**

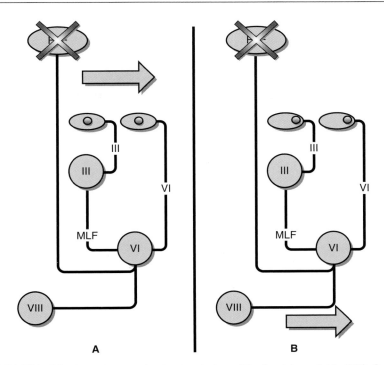

FIGURE 26.22 Left horizontal gaze palsy due to a lesion of the frontal eye fields (FEF). **A:** A right FEF lesion results in an inability to voluntarily move the eyes to the left. **B:** The vestibulo-ocular reflex is spared, allowing the eyes to cross midline during oculocephalic ("doll's eyes") testing.

case the patient is said to be "looking away from the seizure."

Supranuclear Vertical Gaze Palsy   Brainstem structures that mediate vertical gaze are situated in the midbrain tectum and pretectal areas above the level of the third and fourth cranial nerve nuclei. Lesions in this supranuclear midbrain region may result in impaired voluntary upgaze and downgaze. If infranuclear connections between the pontine vestibular nuclei and the midbrain oculomotor nuclei are intact, however, the *vestibulo-ocular reflex* will be preserved, allowing the eyes to move vertically in response to head movement (as in vertical oculocephalic testing). The preservation of these reflexive vertical eye movements when voluntary vertical gaze is impaired is the defining characteristic of *supranuclear vertical gaze palsy*.

In patients over the age of 50, a supranuclear vertical gaze palsy may develop in association with axial rigidity and other progressive parkinsonian symptoms. This neurodegenerative disorder is known as *progressive supranuclear palsy (PSP)* or *Steele–Richardson–Olszewski syndrome*. Downgaze is affected early in PSP, and, consequently, patients with PSP may be described as "messy eaters."

Compressive lesions of the posterior midbrain, affecting the posterior commissure, may cause a supranuclear vertical gaze palsy that predominantly affects upgaze (unlike PSP, in which downgaze is usually affected first). Other features of the *dorsal midbrain syndrome*, or *Parinaud syndrome*, include eyelid retraction, light-near dissociation (see section Bilateral Light-Near Dissociation), convergence–retraction nystagmus (rhythmic backward movements of the globes into the orbits on attempted upgaze), and lid retraction.

■ **SPECIAL CLINICAL POINT: Parinaud syndrome, the combination of (1) light-near dissociation, (2) supranuclear vertical gaze palsy, (3) lid retraction, and (4) convergence–retraction nystagmus, implies a lesion of the dorsal midbrain.**

Other rare disorders that may be associated with supranuclear vertical gaze palsy include Whipple's disease, Niemann–Pick disease, and anti-Ma2/Ta paraneoplastic limbic encephalitis.

Vertical Double Vision

Binocular diplopia in which the two images are separated vertically or diagonally suggests a problem with the *third nerve*, the *fourth nerve*, or the brainstem (*skew deviation*).

Third Nerve Palsy The third (oculomotor) nerve innervates the levator palpebrae, the pupil sphincter, and the superior rectus, inferior rectus, medial rectus, and inferior oblique muscles. A lesion of the third nerve typically causes ptosis, pupillary dilation, and an inability to elevate, depress, or adduct the eye (Fig. 26.23).

The third nerve originates from a cluster of oculomotor subnuclei within in the midbrain. Because of a mixture of crossed and uncrossed fibers, a unilateral lesion of the oculomotor nucleus may cause bilateral ptosis and failure of elevation of both eyes. Nuclear third nerve palsies are extremely rare and are caused primarily by small infarctions of medial penetrating vessels from the basilar artery.

Other midbrain lesions may cause a disruption of the fibers emerging from the third cranial nerve nuclei. These fascicular third nerve palsies are generally accompanied by additional signs and symptoms associated with adjacent midbrain structures. For example, a third nerve palsy accompanied by contralateral ataxia implies involvement of cerebellar projections to the red nucleus (*Claude syndrome*) while a third nerve palsy accompanied by

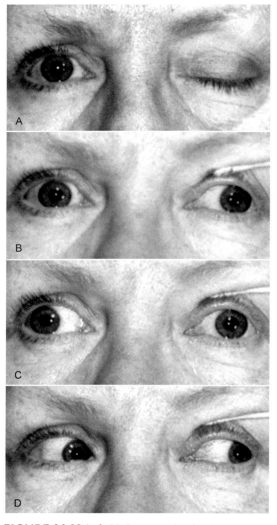

FIGURE 26.23 Left third nerve palsy due to ophthalmoplegic migraine. **A:** There is complete ptosis of the left eyelid. **B:** When the eyelid is lifted, the left eye is abducted and depressed ("down and out"). There is a small amount of left pupillary dilation (mydriasis). **C:** The left eye does not adduct on attempted right gaze. **D:** Abduction is normal in left gaze.

contralateral hemiplegia suggests involvement of the cerebral peduncle (*Weber syndrome*).

The third nerve exits the midbrain between the posterior cerebral artery and the superior cerebellar artery. It courses forward through the subarachnoid space toward the cavernous sinus, running parallel to the posterior communicating artery (PCoA). Like other cranial nerves, the third nerve may be damaged by inflammation, ischemia, or infection, but is additionally vulnerable to compression by PCoA aneurysms at the junction of the PCoA and the internal carotid artery.

Aberrant regeneration of the third nerve may rarely occur. When present, it is highly suggestive of a compressive lesion of the third nerve, as aberrant regeneration of the third nerve is not seen following microvascular ischemia. Eyelid elevation or pupillary constriction in attempted downgaze or adduction (Fig. 26.24) should trigger an urgent evaluation for possible aneurysm or tumor.

■ **SPECIAL CLINICAL POINT: Aberrant regeneration of the third nerve is a sign of compression of the oculomotor nerve (from aneurysm or tumor) and is never associated with microvascular or diabetic third nerve palsies.**

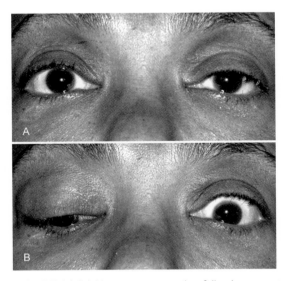

FIGURE 26.24 Aberrant regeneration following aneurysmal third nerve palsy. **A:** In primary position, there is ptosis of the left eyelid and subtle left hypotropia. **B:** In attempted downgaze, the left eyelid elevates (pseudo-von Graefe sign).

Pupillary involvement in aneurysmal third nerve palsies is common but is not invariably present, particularly when the third nerve palsy is mild or partial. The distinction between pupil-involving and pupil-sparing third nerve palsies has already been discussed (see section Anisocoria).

When the third nerve palsy is injured within the cavernous sinus, it is generally accompanied by additional cranial neuropathies (involving cranial nerves IV, V_1, V_2, or VI). The differential diagnosis of lesions of the cavernous sinus is broad and includes inflammatory disorders (e.g., Tolosa–Hunt syndrome), aneurysms of the cavernous internal carotid artery, and tumors (e.g., meningiomas).

■ **SPECIAL CLINICAL POINT: In the setting of a third nerve palsy, fourth nerve function can be tested by having the patient abduct the eye (assuming that the abducens nerve is intact) then look downward. If the fourth nerve is intact, intorsion will be noted on attempted downgaze. If the eye does not rotate, then the patient may have both a third and a fourth nerve palsy, suggesting a possible cavernous sinus lesion.**

Fourth Nerve Palsy   The fourth (trochlear) nerve innervates the superior oblique muscle. Lesions affecting this cranial nerve limit the eye's ability to depress and intort. This limitation of eye movement may be difficult to appreciate visually but causes the affected eye to be too high (hypertropic), resulting in vertical double vision.

The Parks–Bielschowsky test for fourth nerve palsy has three steps. First, determine which eye is higher (hypertropic). Second, determine whether the hypertropia is worse in right or left gaze. Third, determine whether the hypertropia is worse with right head tilt or left head tilt.

■ **SPECIAL CLINICAL POINT: With a right fourth nerve palsy, the right eye will be hypertropic. The hypertropia and double vision will worsen in left gaze and right head tilt. With a left fourth nerve palsy, the left eye will be hypertropic. The hypertropia and double vision will worsen in right gaze and left head tilt.**

The presence of a head tilt may be helpful. Because head tilt toward the lesion causes increased diplopia, the patient may habitually tilt the head away from the lesion. For example, in the setting of a right fourth nerve palsy, the patient may prefer to tilt the head to the left.

If a fourth nerve palsy is suspected, it may be helpful to show the patient a straight horizontal line and ask the patient to describe the double image seen. Because the superior oblique muscle contributes to intorsion, the image from the paretic eye will be tilted as well as displaced vertically. The arrowhead formed by the two lines will "point to" the side of the fourth nerve palsy (Fig. 26.25).

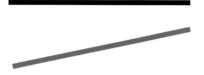

FIGURE 26.25 Right fourth nerve palsy. Because the right eye is hypertropic and extorted, the second image lies below and is tilted relative to the horizontal line. The angle formed by the two lines points to the right—the side of the cranial nerve palsy.

The fourth cranial nerve is unique in that it exits from the brainstem dorsally and crosses to the other side before encircling the brainstem on the way to the cavernous sinus. (The fourth nerve has the longest intracranial course of all cranial nerves.) This renders it particularly susceptible to trauma in which forces are brought to bear on the dorsal midbrain. Fourth cranial nerve palsies can occur secondary to microvascular ischemia, often associated with diabetes and long-standing hypertension. Tumors in the region of the midbrain tectum also occasionally can present with fourth cranial nerve palsies.

Occasionally, new double vision may represent "decompensation" of long-standing or congenital fourth nerve palsies that were never previously symptomatic, making it important to check childhood photographs to search for a head tilt that might indicate a long-standing condition.

Skew Deviation   Vertical misalignment of the eyes that does not fit the pattern of either a third or fourth cranial nerve palsy can occur with brainstem lesions. This skew deviation may be associated with other brainstem signs, including an ocular tilt reaction in which the skew deviation is accompanied by head tilt and torsion of the eyes. Neurologic consultation and MR imaging with attention to the brainstem should be requested for any patient with binocular vertical double vision that can not be attributed to a third or fourth cranial nerve palsy.

Horizontal Double Vision

Lateral gaze requires the coordination of the lateral rectus muscle (innervated by the sixth cranial nerve) of one eye with the medial rectus muscle (innervated by the third cranial nerve) of the other eye. For example, in order to look to the left, both the left lateral rectus muscle (controlled by the left abducens nerve) and the right medial rectus muscle (controlled by the right oculomotor nerve) must act together. The brainstem circuitry responsible for horizontal gaze lies primarily within the pons.

The sixth (abducens) nerve nucleus lies medial and dorsal in the brainstem within the pons. Large cells within the abducens nucleus innervate the lateral rectus muscle directly via the sixth cranial nerve, while a small cell population projects via the medial longitudinal fasciculus (MLF) to the contralateral third (oculomotor) nerve nucleus, which in turn projects to the medial rectus muscle.

Binocular horizontal double vision generally suggests either a lesion of the *abducens (VI) nerve* itself or a lesion of the MLF resulting in an *internuclear ophthalmoplegia (INO)* (Fig. 26.26).

Sixth Nerve Palsy   A lesion of the sixth (abducens) nerve results in the inability to abduct the ipsilateral eye, causing binocular, horizontal double vision that is worse when looking toward the lesion. For example, an injury to the left sixth nerve will impair abduction of the left

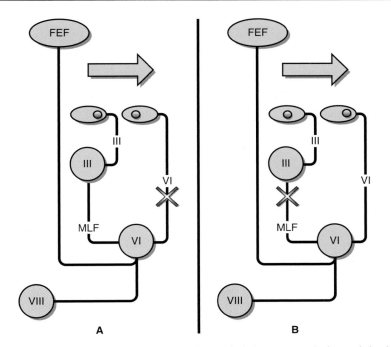

FIGURE 26.26 Horizontal diplopia. **A:** A lesion of the left sixth nerve results in no abduction of the left eye on attempted left gaze. **B:** A lesion of the right medial longitudinal fasciculus (MLF) results in no adduction of the right eye on attempted left gaze (internuclear ophthalmoplegia). Both lesions can cause binocular, horizontal diplopia in left gaze.

eye, which will cause the eyes to be turned toward each other (esotropia). The associated diplopia will be worse in attempted left gaze and at distance (Fig. 26.27).

Sixth cranial nerve palsies caused by microvascular ischemia are common, particularly in patients with vascular risk factors, but the complete differential diagnosis is broad. Fascicular lesions may occur within the pons due to hemorrhage, infarction, demyelination, or neoplasia (e.g., pontine gliomas or metastatic tumors). The sixth nerve also may be affected by inflammatory or infiltrating lesions of the cavernous sinuses or of the leptomeninges (e.g., Tolosa–Hunt syndrome, Lyme disease, or carcinomatous meningitis). Sixth nerve palsies may occur as a false-localizing sign in the setting of increased intracranial pressure (see section Papilledema), and have occasionally been documented as a transient phenomenon following lumbar puncture.

Internuclear Ophthalmoplegia (INO) As discussed above, the sixth (abducens) nerve nucleus and the contralateral third (oculomotor) nerve nucleus communicate via the medial longitudinal fasciculus (MLF) in the brainstem in order to generate conjugate horizontal gaze. A lesion of the MLF between these two nuclei interrupts this connection between the two nuclei, causing an *internuclear ophthalmoplegia*, characterized by an inability to fully adduct the eye on the same side as the lesion. In the case of a lesion of the right MLF, for example, the right eye will adduct poorly, causing double vision in attempted left gaze (Fig. 26.28). Slowing of adduction ("adduction lag") and a dissociated abducting nystagmus are also features of INO.

In young adults, the most common cause of an isolated INO is a small demyelinating plaque due to multiple sclerosis (see Chapter 11). In

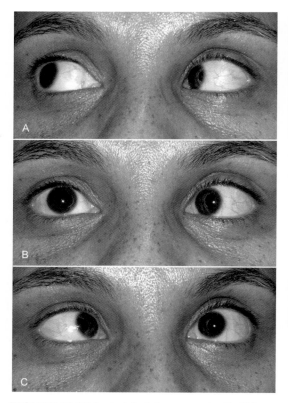

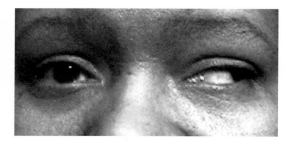

FIGURE 26.28 Right internuclear ophthalmoplegia (INO). In attempted left gaze, the right eye does not adduct, signifying a lesion of the right medial longitudinal fasciculus (MLF) in this patient with multiple sclerosis.

FIGURE 26.27 Acute left sixth nerve palsy. **A:** Right gaze is normal. **B:** In primary position, the patient is esotropic. **C:** In attempted left gaze, the left eye is unable to abduct.

older patients or patients with vascular risk factors, a small stroke should be suspected. Tumors and vascular malformations may also cause INO.

■ **SPECIAL CLINICAL POINT: An isolated, bilateral internuclear ophthalmoplegia (INO) is highly suggestive of multiple sclerosis.**

One-and-a-Half Syndrome   The combination of a horizontal gaze palsy and internuclear ophthalmoplegia is known as *one-and-a-half syndrome*. It implies a lesion of both the sixth (abducens) nerve nucleus and the adjacent ipsilateral MLF. The result of such a lesion (whether caused by infarction, hemorrhage, demyelination, or tumor) is an inability to look toward the side of the lesion and an inability to

adduct away from the lesion. Only abduction of the contralateral eye is spared.

Extraocular Pathology   Disorders of extraocular muscles or of the neuromuscular junction may mimic any form of eye movement disorder described above. Myasthenia gravis and thyroid eye disease should be considered in any patient who complains of double vision.

Myasthenia Gravis   Myasthenia gravis may cause weakness of the eyelid or extraocular muscles that may resemble a peripheral cranial nerve palsy or internuclear ophthalmoplegia. Fluctuating findings or a clear history of worsening later in the day or when fatigued may suggest myasthenia (see Chapter 17). As a rule there should be no pupillary involvement. If myasthenia gravis is suspected, referral to a neurologist for evaluation is recommended.

■ **SPECIAL CLINICAL POINT: Fluctuating double vision or double vision that worsens toward the end of the day suggests possibile myasthenia gravis.**

Thyroid Eye Disease   Hyperthyroidism (most commonly caused by Graves disease) can be associated with an autoimmune reaction that causes swelling of the orbital soft tissues. Enlargement and fibrosis of the extraocular muscles (inferior rectus and medial rectus muscles are the most commonly affected) may lead to a limitation of eye movements and double vision.

When thyroid eye disease is severe, there can be marked proptosis, periorbital edema, conjunctival injection, lid retraction, and possibly vision loss from compression of the optic nerve. CT scanning of the orbits may be helpful in identifying extraocular muscle enlargement when thyroid eye disease is suspected.

NYSTAGMUS/VERTIGO/OSCILLOPSIA

Rhythmic, conjugate movements of the eyes (nystagmus) generally signify vestibular or cerebellar dysfunction (see Chapter 20). Nystagmus may be associated with a subjective sense of movement (vertigo) or "shaking" of the visual world (oscillopsia). There are many different specific types of nystagmus, but they can be divided into two main categories: *jerk nystagmus* and *pendular nystagmus*.

Jerk Nystagmus

Jerk nystagmus is the more commonly seen type of nystagmus, characterized by a slow phase followed by a corrective quick phase. Jerk nystagmus is named for this quick component, for example, "right beating" or "up beating." There are two main types of jerk nystagmus: *gaze-evoked nystagmus* and *vestibular nystagmus*. *Brun's nystagmus* and *downbeat nystagmus* are other specific types of jerk nystagmus.

Gaze-Evoked Nystagmus   Coarse nystagmus that changes direction depending on the direction of gaze (e.g., right beating in right gaze, left beating in left gaze, up beating in up gaze, etc.) is gaze-evoked nystagmus. Gaze-evoked nystagmus is a gaze-holding problem and implies cerebellar dysfunction. Alcohol intoxication, anti-epileptic medications, cerebellar degenerative disorders, and cerebellar disorders may all be associated with gaze-evoked nystagmus. A few beats of symmetric gaze-evoked nystagmus in extreme gaze is normal and is known as end-point nystagmus. Unilateral gaze-evoked nystagmus signifies a unilateral, ipsilateral, cerebellar lesion (stroke, hemorrhage, or tumor).

In other words, unilateral right-beating gaze-evoked nystagmus suggests a lesion of the right cerebellar hemisphere.

Vestibular Nystagmus   A rapid, mixed horizontal-torsional jerk nystagmus that is unidirectional (e.g., right beating regardless of gaze) suggests vestibular dysfunction. Vestibular nystagmus beats away from the side of the dysfunction. For example, right-beating vestibular nystagmus is seen with left vestibular lesions. According to Alexander's Law, vestibular nystagmus is greatest in the direction it is beating (e.g., right-beating vestibular nystagmus is most prominent in right gaze). Vestibular nystagmus may be caused by either peripheral or central lesions (see Chapter 20).

Brun's Nystagmus   The combination of gaze-evoked nystagmus and vestibular nystagmus is known as *Brun's nystagmus*, which signifies a lesion of the cerebellopontine angle. For example, a patient with a coarse right-beating horizontal nystagmus in right gaze (right-beating gaze-evoked nystagmus implying a right cerebellar lesion) and a quick left-beating horizontal-torsional nystagmus in left gaze (left-beating vestibular nystagmus implying a right vestibular lesion) should be evaluated for a possible lesion of the right cerebellopontine angle (e.g., acoustic neuroma).

Downbeat Nystagmus   A specific type nystagmus can be seen with lesions at the cervicomedullary junction (e.g., Chiari malformation). This downbeating nystagmus is most prominent in upgaze and lateral downgaze. Downbeat nystagmus can also be seen with hypomagnesemia and lithium toxicity.

Pendular Nystagmus

Less common than jerk nystagmus, pendular nystagmus is characterized by back and forth slow phases. This type of nystagmus may be horizontal, vertical, or torsional (rotational), depending on the plane of the nystagmus. There are several notable types of pendular nystagmus.

See-saw Nystagmus   In pendular see-saw nystagmus, one eye moves upward and intorts while the other eye moves downward and extorts, back and forth, like two children on a see-saw. This rare form of nystagmus strongly suggests a midbrain or parasellar lesion (e.g., pituitary adenoma or craniopharyngioma) and often coexists with bitemporal hemianopia.

Oculopalatal Myoclonus   Pendular nystagmus (typically vertical) associated with rhythmic contractions of the soft palate implies a lesion within the brainstem. This oculopalatal myoclonus typically evolves weeks to months following a brainstem hemorrhage or stroke. It is thought to be caused by injury to the central tegmental tract lying within the Triangle of Guillain–Mollaret (whose corners are the red nucleus, inferior olive, and dentate gyrus).

Oculomasticatory Myorrhythmia   Slow, pendular convergence of the eyes associated with synchronous contraction of muscles of the jaw and face is highly suggestive of, if not pathognomonic for, Whipple's disease.

Always Remember

- Visual acuity, color vision, the presence or absence of an afferent pupillary defect (RAPD), the appearance of the optic discs, and visual fields must all be evaluated to determine the cause of vision loss.
- Higher-order visual processing problems provide insight into the organization of specialized cortical regions.
- The different causes of anisocoria can be sorted out on examination, but pharmacologic testing may help to confirm the diagnosis.
- Patterns of abnormal eye movements and diploia allow fairly precise lesion localization.
- The many types of nystagmus fall into a limited number of categories, each associated with specific pathology.

QUESTIONS AND DISCUSSION

1. A 58-year-old man presents with a history of pain in the left orbit. He denies double vision. The pain is described as intense and "boring" in quality without throbbing. He has no previous neurologic or ophthalmologic history. You have been monitoring him for 5 years for fairly well-controlled adult-onset diabetes mellitus treated with diet restriction alone. There is complete left eyelid ptosis, and the left eye is depressed and abducted ("down and out"). The pupil is 8 mm and fixed (no constriction to light or near). The patient is able to elevate and depress the eye through only about 10% of the expected range. There is no adduction past midline, but the left eye abducts fully. Which of the following is the most likely diagnosis?
   A. Myasthenia gravis
   B. Thyroid eye disease
   C. Third nerve palsy resulting from an intracranial aneurysm
   D. Third nerve palsy secondary to diabetes mellitus

The correct answer is C. Thyroid eye disease and myasthenia gravis can cause a variety of eye movement problems, and myasthenia gravis may present with ptosis. Pupillary involvement, however, would not accompany either. The combination of ptosis, and impaired adduction, elevation and depression suggests a third (oculomotor) nerve palsy. Diabetes is often associated with a pupil-sparing ischemic or microvascular third nerve palsy, but involvement of the pupil in this case strongly suggests the possibility of aneurysmal compression of the third nerve.

2. An 18-year-old student, brought in by her mother, reported that she had transiently gone blind in her right eye. The episode occurred in school and lasted 20 minutes. She noted that the right half of a large word on the blackboard seemed to be

missing and that "everything seemed to be shimmering and wavy." Other than a mild headache, she noted no other symptoms. She is in good general health, and the neurologic examination is normal. Which of the following would be the most appropriate next step for this patient?

A. Cerebral angiography
B. Carotid duplex examination
C. CT or MRI of the brain with contrast
D. Reassurance and a follow-up visit in 1 month or sooner should symptoms recur

The correct answer is D. Patients frequently interpret a homonymous hemianopia as vision loss in one eye or the other. In this case, the patient's inability to see the right half of a word written on the blackboard strongly suggests a right homonymous hemianopia, not monocular vision loss. For this reason, a vascular workup in search of a focal lesion of the right carotid artery or ophthalmic artery would not be indicated. The patient's symptoms are highly suggestive of migraine. Given her classic presentation and her young age, the likelihood of a structural lesion is small. Neuroimaging can be deferred unless her symptoms worsen or progress. Return visits are advisable, however, to ensure against missing progressive symptoms.

3. A 62-year-old man presents for a routine examination. He has no head or neck symptoms, but an examination reveals 1 to 2 mm of left ptosis. In a well-lighted examination room, the pupils appear to be equal in size at 2 mm. The patient denies awareness of the lid droop and denies head or neck trauma. Which of the following would be the most useful next step?

A. Chest x-ray
B. MRI/MRA of the head and neck
C. Examination of the pupils in a dim room
D. Pharmacologic testing

The correct answer is C. The pupils should be examined in darkness, since pupillary anisocoria due to Horner syndrome may be difficult

to see in even moderate illumination. If anisocoria is more noticeable in the darkness than in the light, a reasonable next step would be pharmacologic testing with either 10% cocaine or 0.5% apraclonidine to confirm ocular sympathetic dysfunction. Imaging studies may be useful once a diagnosis of Horner syndrome has been made in order to help determine its etiology.

4. A 30-year-old woman presents complaining of vertigo and "bouncing vision." She is on no medications. Her past medical history is unremarkable. On examination she has a rapid horizontal and torsional nystagmus on right gaze and a coarse, purely horizontal nystagmus in left gaze. What is the most likely diagnosis?

A. Acoustic neuroma
B. Cerebellar hemorrhage
C. Vestibular neuronitis
D. Chiari malformation

The correct answer is A. The patient has a combination of vestibular and gaze-evoked nystagmus, known as Brun's nystagmus, which is highly suggestive of a lesion at the cerebellopontine angle. Cerebellar hemorrhage would be associated with more severe symptoms and a unilateral gaze-evoked nystagmus. Vestibular neuronitis would produce a vestibular nystagmus. Chiari malformation is commonly a cause of downbeat nystagmus.

SUGGESTED READING

Asbury AK, Aldridge H, Hershberg R, et al. Oculomotor palsy in diabetes mellitus: a clinicopathologic study. *Brain.* 1970;93:555.

Giles CL, Henderson JW. Horner's syndrome: an analysis of 216 cases. *Am J Ophthalmol.* 1958;46:289.

Goodwin J. Disorders of higher cortical visual function. *Curr Neurol Neurosci Rep.* 2002;2(5):418–422.

Keitner JL, Johnson CA, Spurr JO, et al. Baseline visual field profile of optic neuritis: the experience of the Optic Neuritis Treatment Trial. *Arch Ophthalmol.* 1993;111:231.

Leigh RJ, Zee DS. *The Neurology of Eye Movements*. 3rd ed. Philadelphia, PA: FA Davis; 1999.

Liu GT, Volpe NJ, Galetta SL. *Neuro-Ophthalmology: Diagnosis and Management*. Philadelphia, PA: W. B. Saunders Company; 2001.

Loewenfeld IE. *The Pupil: Anatomy, Physiology, and Clinical Applications*. Ames/Detroit, MI: Iowa State University Press/Wayne State University Press; 1993.

Miller NR, Newman NJ, eds. *Walsh and Hoyt's Clinical Neuro-Ophthalmology*. 5th ed. Baltimore, MD: Williams & Wilkins; 1998.

Rucker CW. The causes of paralysis of the third, fourth and sixth cranial nerves. *Am J Ophthalmol*. 1966;61:1294.

Thompson HS, ed. *Topics in Neuro-Ophthalmology*. Baltimore, MD: Williams & Wilkins; 1979:104–113.

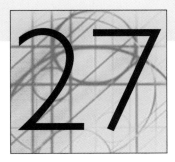

27 Principles of Neuro-rehabilitation

DAVID S. KUSHNER

key points

• Disablement involves the complex relationship between disease, impairment, disability, and handicap.

• Functional disabilities are targeted in neurorehabilitation.

• Neurorehabilitation encompasses medical, physical, social, educational, and vocational interventions provided in institutional or community settings.

• Ongoing and thorough patient assessment is crucial throughout the neurorehabilitation process.

• Rehabilitation goals and the management plan are regularly assessed and modified when necessary to maximize patient potential.

• Patients having disabilities due to an acute, chronic, or progressive neurologic condition may benefit from neurorehabilitation.

The World Health Organization has described disablement in terms of disease, impairment, disability, and handicap (Table 27.1). In this conceptual model, disease is an underlying condition or pathologic process that results in an impairment. *Impairment* is an abnormality in physical or psychological capacity. *Disability* is the limitation an impairment places on an individual's ability to perform necessary routine daily functional activities. *Handicap* is the social disadvantage that results from disabilities that prevent an individual from fulfilling his or her expected role in society.

TABLE 27.1	**Aspects of Disablement**

Disease: a condition or pathologic process that may result in an impairment

Impairment: an abnormality in physical or psychological capacity

Disability: limitations in function resulting from an impairment

Handicap: social disadvantages that result from disabilities

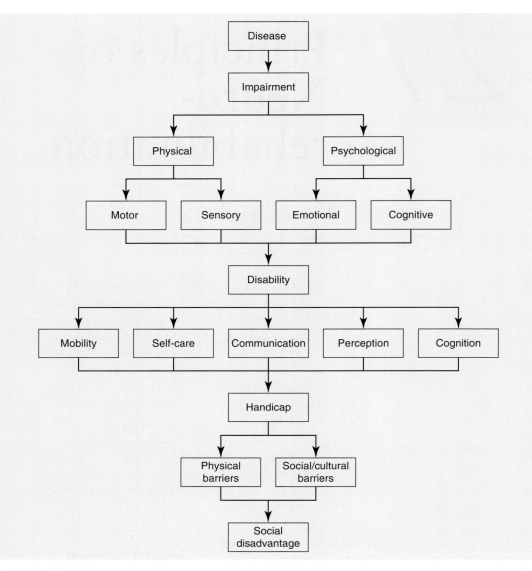

FIGURE 27.1 Process of disablement.

Handicap is influenced in a society by physical barriers, social and cultural factors, and the attitudes of those involved (Fig. 27.1).

■ **SPECIAL CLINICAL POINT: A host of neurologic conditions that may be developmental, hereditary, infectious, autoimmune, metabolic, degenerative, vascular, neoplastic, or traumatic exist that can result in static or progressive impairments.**

Neurologic disorders can occur at any point in an individual's lifetime and the pathology may involve any part of the nervous system, from the central nervous system (CNS) (including the brain or spinal cord) to the peripheral nervous system and the muscle (resulting in impairments such as disorders of strength, endurance, balance, coordination, mobility, cognition, perception, communication, swallowing, and sensation). The same neurologic impairments can vary in intensity among individuals depending on the pathologic cause or the region of the nervous system affected. Similarly, the prognosis may differ with similar impairments but with different pathologic processes at work. For example, hemiparesis resulting directly from an area of brain infarction would be less likely to resolve than would hemiparesis resulting from demyelination or edema involving the same region of the brain.

Disabilities that may result from neurologic impairments can involve mobility, self-care, communication, cognition, and perception. Deficits of mobility may include problem with bed mobility, transfers, and ambulation. Deficits of self-care may include problems with any of the routine daily functions of an individual from ordinary self-care tasks, including grooming, toileting, bathing, dressing, and feeding, to the more complex tasks of independent living, including financial management, shopping, home making, and the ability to use a telephone or drive a car. Pathology at different sites of the nervous system can result in similar functional disability manifestations between individuals. For example, disorders affecting balance, coordination, cognition, or strength all may separately result in the inability of an individual to walk or to effectively perform routine self-care activities.

■ **SPECIAL CLINICAL POINT: In neurorehabilitation, functional disabilities are the focus of medical, restorative, adaptive, environmental, and social interventions.**

Neurorehabilitation encompasses medical, physical, social, educational, and vocational interventions that can be provided in a variety of institutional and community settings. Professionals include specialized physicians, nurses, therapists, psychologists, social workers, dietitians, and orthotists. Goals include the prevention of secondary complications, treatment to reduce neurologic impairments, compensatory strategies for residual disabilities, patient and caretaker education, and maintenance of function (Table 27.2). Anyone with neurologic impairments can benefit from neurorehabilitation, but the setting, approach, and

TABLE 27.2	Goals of Neurorehabilitation

Treatments to reduce neurologic impairments
Compensatory strategies for residual disabilities
Prevention of secondary complications
Maintenance of function
Patient/caretaker education

limitations of treatment will vary with the type and extent of the disabilities. The objective is to match patient needs with capabilities of available programs. This chapter will focus on principles of neurorehabilitation, including a broad overview of the role of ongoing patient assessment, acute-care intervention, the determination of rehabilitation need and an appropriate setting, the rehabilitation management plan, and issues pertaining to community transition and neurorehabilitation outcomes. In addition, case presentations will be given in the Questions and Discussion section to explore potential benefits and limitations of neurorehabilitation in a variety of neurologic conditions.

ROLE OF ASSESSMENT IN NEUROREHABILITATION

Ongoing and thorough patient assessment is a crucial aspect of the neurorehabilitation process. The goals of assessment change over the clinical course of rehabilitation from the acute hospitalization, to the transfer to a rehabilitation facility or program, to the transition back to the community. Initial concerns often include patient survival, level of consciousness, and response to acute treatments. Later concerns focus on specific neurologic impairments and a patient's functional abilities.

■ **SPECIAL CLINICAL POINT: Patient evaluation throughout the neurorehabilitation process involves clinical examinations and well-validated standardized measures performed by various members of the interdisciplinary team of rehabilitation specialists.**

This team often is composed of the physician (neurologist or physiatrist), nurses, a social worker, therapists (including physical, occupational, speech, and recreational/vocational), and a psychologist.

The non-neurologist primary care physician will likely benefit from a neurorehabilitation consultation for evaluation of all patients admitted to the hospital with acute neurologic impairments resulting in functional deficits. In addition, patients with chronic medical or neurologic conditions with functional deficits that may be related to deconditioning weakness, reduced joint mobility, or progression of the condition also may benefit from rehabilitation. In principle, a neurorehabilitation evaluation should be obtained for all hospitalized or ambulatory clinic patients with functional decline in any routine daily functions including mobility; transfers; ambulation; or the ability to dress, bathe, feed, groom, speak, or carry out previously routine duties such as vocational or homemaking responsibilities.

The objectives of neurorehabilitation assessment during the acute hospital admission include documentation of the diagnosis, the impairments, and the disabilities as well as identification of treatment needs. Subsequent reevaluation focuses on response to acute-care treatments and any changes in neurologic or medical status. Once patients are medically stable, the evaluation is geared toward identifying those who will benefit from further rehabilitation intervention and determining the appropriate rehabilitation setting. Recommendation may be made for referral to an interdisciplinary rehabilitation program, in an inpatient or an outpatient facility, or for selected individual rehabilitation services in an ambulatory care setting.

On admission to a neurorehabilitation program, assessment is performed to help develop a rehabilitation management plan with realistic goals and to document a baseline level of function for monitoring progress. Periodic weekly or biweekly reassessment during the rehabilitation program allows patient progress to be monitored, treatment regimens to be adjusted when necessary to maximize patient potential, and discharge planning to be facilitated. Objectives of assessment after discharge include the evaluation of patient adaptation to the home environment and community setting, the determination of the need for further rehabilitation services, and the assessment of caregiver burden and needs.

Standardized assessment instruments in neurorehabilitation complement the neurologic examination in evaluating functional recovery. Standardized measurement scales facilitate reliable documentation of severity of functional disabilities, help to increase consistency of treatment decisions, facilitate communication between therapists, and provide a reliable basis for monitoring progress. Scales exist to measure many areas of neurologic function, such as consciousness, cognition, perception, communication, strength, mobility, balance, coordination, somatosensation, and affective function. For example, the Rancho Los Amigos Cognitive Scale often is used to document levels of cognitive recovery following a traumatic brain injury, and the Functional Independence Measure Scale often is used to assess levels of independence in areas of basic daily function. In addition, many other scales exist to help measure and quantify specific functional impairments and disabilities. Limitations of various standardized measurement scales often are counterbalanced by use of other scales and the neurologic examination.

Another important aspect of patient assessment in neurorehabilitation is the clarification of the complex relationship that exists between disease, impairment or severity of objective deficits, and disability or the impact of disease on function in any individual patient.

Specific neurologic impairments may play a role in multiple functional disabilities. For example, a patient's inability to adequately self-feed, dress, or propel a wheelchair could separately result from impairments in strength, endurance, cognition, comprehension, perception, sensation, coordination, balance, lack of motivation, or the presence of pain or fatigue. Furthermore, individual impairments may have multiple possible etiologies. For example, fatigue may result directly from a neurologic disease process or it may indirectly result from depression, sedative side effects of various medications, or a lack of adequate sleep. Similarly, a patient's inability to effectively concentrate and attend to therapies may result from impairments of cognition or perception resulting directly from neurologic disease or indirectly from depression, the side effects of medications, or the distraction of pain. Thus, the role of assessment in neurorehabilitation includes clarification of etiologies contributing to a patient's disabilities so that appropriate therapeutic interventions may be undertaken at any point during the rehabilitation process. In addition, certain treatments may be contraindicated or recovery may be limited by comorbid chronic conditions such as cardiovascular disease, chronic pulmonary disease, cancer, musculoskeletal disorders, or psychiatric conditions. Evaluation and treatment of poorly controlled comorbid medical conditions also will improve neurorehabilitation outcomes.

Neurorehabilitation During Acute Care

■ SPECIAL CLINICAL POINT:
Neurorehabilitation intervention should begin following an acute hospitalization once a neurologic diagnosis has been established and life-threatening problems are controlled. Highest priorities are the prevention of secondary complications, maintenance of general health functions, early mobilization, and resumption of self-care activities (Table 27.3).

Immediate neurorehabilitation concerns include the maintenance of homeostasis and the prevention of complications that could result from the particular neurologic condition. Maintenance of homeostasis is a priority in all neurologic patients in the acute-care hospital setting. Routine continuous monitoring of basic health functions can help to prevent further disability. Included in any rehabilitation program are efforts to ensure regulation and adequacy of nutrition and hydration, bladder and bowel function, and sleep. In addition, measures usually are undertaken to pre-

TABLE 27.3	Neurorehabilitation during Acute Care

Prevention of secondary complications
Deep vein thrombosis/pulmonary embolism
Skin breakdown
Joint contractures/dislocations/subluxations
Pneumonia
Falls
Autonomic dysfunction
Malnutrition/dehydration

Maintenance of homeostasis
Normalization of sleep
Normalization of bowel/bladder function
Normalization of nutritional states
Promotion of early mobilization and return to self-care

vent deep vein thrombosis (DVT), pulmonary embolism, skin ulcerations, orthostasis, development of joint contractures, and pneumonia, which all may result from impaired mobility. In those patients with disorders of swallowing or cognition, efforts also are undertaken to prevent malnutrition and dehydration. The prevention of recurrent stroke is a concern in those individuals with acute cerebrovascular disorders. Autonomic dysreflexia is of concern in individuals with spinal cord injury or disorders. Autonomic dysfunction including cardiovascular dysfunction is of concern in patients with the acute Guillain–Barré syndrome (acute demyelinating polyneuropathies). In addition, efforts to prevent falls and accidental fractures or joint dislocations are undertaken in all patients who may be at risk.

Maintenance of Homeostasis

Dehydration and malnutrition may be consequences of neurologic disorders resulting in dysphagia, inability to self-feed, confusion, or inability to communicate hunger or thirst. Reduction of risk may include monitoring daily intake of liquids and calories, weekly determinations of body weight, and supervision with meals. A formal dysphagia assessment may be indicated in certain patients (see Management of Dysphasia and Aspiration, below).

Bladder dysfunction is another possible consequence of neurologic disease. Bladder dysfunction may result from neurologic conditions causing bladder hypertonicity, bladder hypotonicity, and areflexia or hyperactivity of the internal or external sphincters. Often, a urologic consultation and urodynamic testing is necessary. Treatment may involve a program of bladder training that may include intermittent bladder catheterization, certain medications, and toileting at regular intervals. Use of indwelling Foley catheters is avoided with the exceptions of urinary retention that cannot otherwise be controlled, in patients with extensive skin ulcerations, or if incontinence interferes with fluid and electrolyte balance monitoring.

Bowel dysfunction, and particularly constipation or fecal impaction, may occur in neurologic disease as a result of immobility, inadequate nutrition (food or fluid), cognitive impairment, neurogenic bowel, and even depression or anxiety. Treatment measures include the assurance of adequate intake of fluids and fiber, establishment of a regular toileting schedule, and judicious use of stool softeners or laxatives.

Insomnia may occur as a direct result of a neurologic disorder, or it may result indirectly from comorbidities including depression, agitation, anxiety, the side effects of medications, muscle spasms, pain, inability to move in bed, urinary frequency or incontinence, or interruptions related to the hospital environment. Inadequate sleep can result in daytime drowsiness and inability to fully benefit from rehabilitation therapies. Goals of management include determination and treatment of a specific etiology if one exists; alteration of the environment if necessary to reduce disturbances of sleep; adjustment of type, timing, and dose of offending medications; and if all else fails, limited judicious use of hypnotic medications.

Prevention of Deep Vein Thrombosis

Acute prolonged immobility, and particularly the paralysis of one or both legs, places an individual at risk for deep vein thrombosis (DVT) and pulmonary embolism. Randomized trials have shown effective risk reduction with use of subcutaneous low-dose heparin or low-molecular-weight heparin products. In addition, warfarin, intermittent pneumatic compression, early mobilization, and elastic stockings have been shown to be effective. Management of DVT risk in neurorehabilitation often includes early mobilization; elastic stockings; and, in the absence of contraindications, mini-dose subcutaneous heparin.

Prevention of Skin Breakdown

Risk factors for skin breakdown include impaired cognition, poor mobility, incontinence, spasticity, and obesity. Steps to maintain skin integrity in those at risk include systemic daily inspection, gentle routine skin cleansing, protection from moisture, maintenance of hydration and nutrition, efforts to improve patient mobility, frequent turning and repositioning of immobile patients, and avoidance of skin pressure or friction. Prior to discharge from the acute-care hospital setting, patients or caretakers should be educated on skin care issues.

Prevention of Joint Contractures

A patient's potential for functional recovery may be limited by the restriction of movement or pain that results from joint contractures. The joints of spastic paretic limbs are most at risk for contractures. Simple prolonged disuse of an extremity also can result in contractures. For example, a comatose individual with spastic hemiparesis is at risk for bilateral plantar flexion contractures, with one plantar flexion contracture related to spasticity and the other related to simple disuse. Spasticity often develops in individuals with so-called "upper motor neuron lesions" that result from disorders involving the brain or spinal cord. Spasticity may involve one extremity (monoparesis) to all four extremities (quadriparesis), depending on the underlying pathologic process.

■ **SPECIAL CLINICAL POINT: Routine prevention of contractures often includes antispastic limb positioning, frequent range-of-motion exercises with passive or active stretching, and splinting or bracing where necessary.**

Other treatment options to further limit the effects of spasticity or reduce early contractures may include medications, progressive casting, surgical correction (i.e., tendon release procedures), motor point blocks, botulinum toxin injections, or an intrathecal baclofen pump. Antispasticity medications exist with various sites of action, ranging from effects at the CNS to effects at the muscle. Patients with early contractures in a monoparesis or hemiparesis pattern may benefit from botulinum toxin injections of involved muscles. Patients with spastic quadriparesis may benefit from placement of an intrathecal baclofen pump. In general, botulinum toxin or intrathecal baclofen may be indicated if reduction of spasticity/early contractures will improve functional independence, hygiene, or comfort or will decrease the risk of skin breakdown.

Prevention of Pneumonia

Pneumonia is a common complication of neurologic illness. Risk factors include depressed cognition, swallowing disorders, and impaired mobility. Risk reduction programs include efforts toward early mobilization as well as prevention of aspiration through modification of diet, alteration of means of nutrition intake if necessary, and proper positioning during feedings. Prolonged bed rest can result in poor aeration of the lungs, atelectasis, and a greater likelihood for development of pneumonia. Early patient mobilization can minimize this risk.

Management of Dysphagia and Aspiration Dysphagia occurs in certain neurologic conditions and may lead to aspiration pneumonia. Swallowing dysfunction can occur as a result of impaired cognition or from incoordination or weakness of the muscles of deglutition. Thus, swallowing is assessed prior to oral feedings in those patients who may be at risk (patients with strokes, brain injuries, neuromuscular diseases, etc.). Signs of possible dysphagia include dysarthria, confusion, frequent coughing, choking on fluids, nasal regurgitation, and pneumonia. Currently, the gold standard of diagnosis is a modified barium swallow study, which can help clarify the phase of swallowing that may be impaired. Goals of dysphagia management include the prevention of aspiration, dehydration, and malnutrition and the restoration of the ability to chew and swallow safely. Treatment includes oral motor exercises, compensatory feeding strategies, modification of food textures, or alternative methods of feeding such as nasogastric tubes or percutaneous endoscopic gastrostomy tubes.

Prevention of Falls, Fractures, and Dislocations

A goal of neurorehabilitation intervention includes ensuring patient safety by preventing falls. The risk of falls is increased in patients with sensorimotor deficits, confusion, or difficulty with communication. Methods to prevent falls vary with the type and severity of the disabilities.

■ **SPECIAL CLINICAL POINT: A fall risk reduction program may include supervision of high-risk patients, toileting at regular intervals, supervision of transfers and ambulation, adapted nurse call systems, and patient and family education.**

The use of restraints is avoided whenever possible because restraints may lead to other injuries or cause greater agitation in those already restless.

Another concern is prevention of shoulder dislocations in patients with paretic upper extremities. There is a tendency for subluxation to occur at the shoulder joint capsule as a result of the gravitational pull from the weight of a paretic arm. Preventive measures include maintenance of normal scapulohumeral positioning through physical measures, use of lap trays on wheelchairs, use of pull sheets during bed positioning, and avoidance of excessive range-of-motion exercises. Caution must be taken with lap trays because improper use can lead to nerve injuries or wrist flexion contractures; furthermore, sling arm supports may promote upper-extremity flexion contractures if used improperly. The differential diagnosis for shoulder pain in those with paretic upper extremities also includes rotator cuff tears, adhesive capsulitis, bicipital tendonitis, reflex sympathetic dystrophy, arthritis, and previous injuries.

Prevention in Specific Neurologic Disorders

Patients who have had an ischemic stroke are at substantial risk for a recurrent stroke. Often, the acute-care team will determine the need for carotid endarterectomy or anticoagulation with warfarin, ticlopidine, or aspirin. Neurorehabilitation can help with patient and family education regarding potential modifiable risk factors including hypertension, diabetes mellitus, cigarette smoking, alcohol consumption, drug abuse, obesity, high serum cholesterol, coronary artery disease, left ventricular hypertrophy, and atrial fibrillation.

Spinal cord injuries and disorders can result in a potential for autonomic dysreflexia. This is more likely with high-level cord pathology. Autonomic dysreflexia manifests as precipitous drops or elevations in blood pressure or pulse, often accompanied by a pounding headache, hyperventilation, and flushing or sweating above the level of the lesion. The cause is usually a noxious stimulus involving a numb portion of the body detectable only to the autonomic nervous system. Possible causes may include a full bladder, a fecal impaction, tight-fitting clothing or shoes, a skin irritation, a DVT, or an infection. Prevention includes a routine bowel and bladder program, daily skin inspection, and careful dressing. Treatment of

acute autonomic dysreflexia includes blood pressure stabilization as well as determination and correction of the etiology.

Autonomic dysfunction also may occur in the setting of acute demyelinating polyneuropathy (Guillain–Barré syndrome). Autonomic symptoms including sinus tachycardia, bradycardia, facial flushing, hypotension, or hypertension; profuse diaphoresis; or even anhydrosis can occur. In addition, urinary retention also may occur in some patients. The autonomic dysfunction associated with acute demyelinating polyneuropathies often remits after a few weeks. Treatment is supportive and expectant.

Early Mobilization and Return to Self-Care

Another goal of acute neurorehabilitation intervention is early patient mobilization and the encouragement of self-care activities.

■ **SPECIAL CLINICAL POINT: Early mobilization helps to prevent DVT, skin breakdowns, pneumonia, joint contractures, and constipation; it promotes early ambulation, better orthostatic tolerance, and performance of basic activities of daily living.**

Early participation in self-care activities can help to increase strength, endurance, awareness, communication, problem solving, and social activity. Mobilization and the encouragement of self-care is beneficial as soon as a patient's medical and neurologic condition is stabilized, and, if possible, within 1 to 2 days of admission to the hospital. Early mobilization is delayed or approached with caution in patients with coma, obtundation, evolving neurologic signs, intracranial hemorrhage, DVT, or persistent orthostasis.

Mobilization may be passive or active at first, depending on a patient's condition. It will progress variably from ability to move in bed, to sitting in bed, to sitting up, to transferring, to operating a wheelchair, to standing and bearing weight, and eventually to walking. Basic self-care activities, including feeding, grooming, toileting, bathing, and dressing, are encouraged as soon as possible. Training in compensatory strategies and use of adaptive devices is offered to any patient with persistent disability with any aspect of mobility or self-care.

Discharge from Acute Care

Ideally, acute-care discharge planning should begin shortly after admission. Objectives of rehabilitation involvement in the discharge process include determining need for further rehabilitation services, helping to select the best discharge environment, educating the patient and caretakers regarding pertinent issues, and ensuring continuity of care. Patients or caretakers should be instructed on the effects and prognosis of the neurologic condition, the prevention of potential complications, and the need and rationale for further treatments. The patient and family are included in the discharge decision-making process whenever possible.

Determination of Rehabilitation Need and Setting

▪ **SPECIAL CLINICAL POINT: A patient's medical condition and the extent of functional disabilities are the most important determinants of need for neurorehabilitation services and the choice of an appropriate rehabilitation setting.**

The neurologic condition, medical comorbidities, ability to tolerate physical activity, and ability to learn are all important considerations. Rehabilitation services can be provided in a variety of programs and settings following discharge from acute care. Neurorehabilitation may continue in an inpatient rehabilitation hospital or the rehabilitation unit of an acute-care hospital, in a nursing home, in the patient's home, or in an outpatient facility. Determination of an appropriate program is based on patient needs and capabilities.

Rehabilitation Program Criteria

Referrals for neurorehabilitation programs usually are made on patients in an acute-care hospital setting, but patients with chronic stable impairments and disabilities also may be referred from ambulatory care settings. The rehabilitation specialist physician often will be consulted to help facilitate the evaluation and transfer process. Determination of the most appropriate rehabilitation setting is based on strict criteria.

Threshold criteria for admission to any active rehabilitation program include medical stability, one or more persistent disabilities, the ability to learn, and the endurance to sit supported at least 1 hr/day. More debilitated patients may benefit from rehabilitation services at home or in a supported living setting. Candidates for intense interdisciplinary inpatient rehabilitation require total to moderate assistance in either mobility or self-care function and are able to tolerate at least 3 hours of active daily therapy. Candidates for outpatient rehabilitation programs include patients with limited mild functional deficits who are otherwise able to live independently and those requiring supervision to minimal assistance with mobility or self-care. Patients having complex medical problems are candidates for inpatient programs with 24-hour medical supervision.

In general, the inability to learn that results from a fixed static lesion is a contraindication to active neurorehabilitation. However, some patients may have cognitive deficits that are temporary and that have the potential to clear over time as a lesion resolves (e.g., some cases of brain swelling, multiple sclerosis, or traumatic brain injury). In such cases, a trial admission to an active rehabilitation program is warranted. Also, some patients who are unable to learn still may benefit from a course of passive rehabilitation, such as those with severe spasticity who recently may have received botulinum toxin injections or an intrathecal baclofen pump. In cases such as those, vigorous passive range-of-motion exercises may further help to reduce early contractures to allow better hygiene, to help decrease pain and discomfort, and to prevent skin breakdown. In addition, families and caretakers of such patients can benefit from education regarding pertinent care issues, including a program of passive range-of-motion exercises as well as other preventive care.

Programs And Settings

Freestanding rehabilitation hospitals and rehabilitation units in acute-care hospitals usually offer intense comprehensive programs staffed by a full range of rehabilitation professionals. A physician certified in neurorehabilitation or psychiatry is available at all times for patient management issues. General practitioners and specialist medical consultants are generally available as needed. Weekly interdisciplinary team care plan conferences are held and attended by the physician, nurse, and therapists to establish goals, to develop a plan to achieve goals, to assess patient progress, to identify barriers to progress, and to facilitate revision of goals and the management plan when necessary. These programs are active and require greater physical and cognitive effort from patients than would be necessary in other rehabilitation settings.

Rehabilitation programs also exist at nursing facilities, which also may be hospital based or freestanding. Staff, rehabilitation services, and physician coverage vary between facilities. Usually, supportive care and low-level rehabilitation services (so-called "subacute rehabilitation programs") are offered. Programs may provide 1 hour of selected rehabilitation services 5 days a week, or they may provide comprehensive therapies that may include physical, occupational, speech, psychology, and recreational therapies several hours per day. Interdisciplinary team care plan conferences usually are held every 2 weeks. These programs can accommodate patients who have the potential to later become suitable candidates for further rehabilitation at an inpatient hospital, at home, or in an outpatient rehabilitation program.

Outpatient rehabilitation facilities also may be hospital based or freestanding and can provide selected rehabilitation therapies or comprehensive programs. Services and intensity vary with patient needs from 1 hour to several hours of therapy per day, from 1 to 5 days per week. Team care plan conferences often are held monthly to review patient progress. These programs allow a patient to reintegrate into home life while providing necessary therapies, rehabilitation equipment, social contact, and peer support.

Home rehabilitation programs vary in capabilities from comprehensive services to selected rehabilitation therapies. These programs are designed for patients who are medically stable. Advantages include that skills will be learned and applied at home where they are most necessary, and some patients may function better in a familiar environment. Disadvantages include absence of peer support (fellow patients), limited availability of specialized rehabilitation equipment, and increased burden on caregivers.

REHABILITATION MANAGEMENT PLAN

On admission to a neurorehabilitation program, a patient management plan is formulated by the rehabilitation physician and the therapy team. The rehabilitation management plan includes a clear description of a patient's impairments, disabilities, and strengths; explicit short- and long-term functional goals; and specification of treatment strategies to achieve goals and to prevent secondary complications. The objective is to devise short-term and long-term goals that are realistic in terms of patient potential. Overly ambitious goals can set a patient up for failure, and overly modest goals can limit a patient's potential for recovery.

■ **SPECIAL CLINICAL POINT: A rehabilitation management care plan is reevaluated on a regular basis on the basis of patient progress, and it may be adjusted as needed to suit patient needs (Table 27.4).**

Typically, in an intense multidisciplinary inpatient program, the management plan and patient progress are reviewed on a weekly basis; in less intense rehabilitation programs, the care

TABLE 27.4	Impairments, Disabilities, and Treatments

Impaired mobility/self-care	*Management of impaired mobility*
Abnormal muscle strength/tone	Remediation/facilitation (volitional movement present):
Loss of joint range of motion	Traditional exercises
Psychomotor delay	Resistive training
Abnormal muscle synergy/sequencing	Forced sensory stimulation
Abnormal coordination/balance	Compensatory strategies (volitional movement absent):
Loss of endurance	Use of unaffected limbs
Sensory impairments/pain	Use of orthotics or braces
Abnormalities of cognition	Use of adaptive equipment
	Task-specific retraining (motor apraxias):
	Components of above strategies
	Environmental cues to enhance performance
	Pharmacologic interventions
Impaired cognition	*Management of impaired cognition/perception*
Poor concentration/attention	Identify/treat causal factors (e.g., sedation)
Disorientation	Cognitive retraining
Impaired memory, perception, executive function	Substitution of intact abilities
Fatigue/apathy/sedation	Compensatory strategies
Emotional dysfunction	Pharmacologic interventions
Distracters (pain, diplopia, anxiety, etc.)	
Impaired communication	*Management of communication disorders*
Aphasias	Aphasias:
	Enhancement of comprehension/expression
	Compensatory strategies
	Adjustment issues
	Caregiver/patient communication issues
Right-hemispheric language disorders	Right-hemisphere language disorders:
	Increase awareness of deficits
	Reinstate pragmatics of communication
	Compensatory strategies
Dysarthrias	Dysarthrias:
	Oral motor exercises
	Manipulation of vocalization/articulation/ respiration/prosody

plan is reviewed monthly. Pharmacologic interventions in neurorehabilitation vary on the basis of a patient's condition (Table 27.5).

Management of Impaired Mobility

Disabilities involving mobility may result from impairment that can include muscle weakness, abnormal muscle tone, loss of joint range of motion, delayed response time, abnormal muscle synergy patterns, abnormal muscle contraction sequencing (motor apraxia), abnormal coordination or balance, lack of endurance, pain, and sensory impairments (especially proprioception). Prior to treatment, the specific cause of motor dysfunction and impaired mobility must be determined. Options for treatment may include a program of remediation/ facilitation, compensation, or task-specific motor retraining.

TABLE 27.5 | **Pharmacologic Treatments in Neurorehabilitation**

Medication Class	Reasons
Antispasticity medications	Tone reduction/contracture prevention; analgesia
Analgesics	Pain relief
Psychostimulants	Enhancement of concentration, attention, arousal
Antidepressants	Depression relief; improvement of motivation; pain relief
Antipsychotics	Enhancement of reality testing; reduction of agitation/hallucinations/delusions
Cholinergics	Improvement of memory/cognition
Anticonvulsants	Management of seizures/mood disorders/pain
Antithrombotics	Prevention of deep vein thrombosis/stroke/pulmonary embolism
Dopaminergics	Enhancement of arousal/cognition; improvement of mobility in patients with Parkinson disease

Some degree of volitional movement is required in an affected limb for remediation/facilitation to be effective. This approach includes traditional exercises, resistive training, and forced sensory stimulation modalities to improve limb strength and function.

In the compensation approach, the goal is to improve a patient's level of functional independence in performing self-care activities by teaching compensatory strategies that involve the unaffected limbs. The compensation approach can result in learned nonuse of an impaired limb and therefore is reserved for patients with a poor prognosis for recovery of sensorimotor function or those whose motor recovery has reached a plateau.

A program of task-specific motor retraining involves some components of both remediation/facilitation and compensation and use of environmental cues to assist in enhancement of performance of specific tasks. This approach may be helpful for patients with motor apraxias.

The effectiveness of these functional approaches may be enhanced by treatment of specific causes of impaired mobility, such as spasticity, contractures, or chronic pain, and use of orthotic devices, braces, and adaptive equipment when necessary. Adjunct modalities that also may aid in functional recovery include biofeedback, functional electrical stimulation, and various computerized retraining devices.

In summary, patients with some voluntary motor control are encouraged to use an affected limb in functional tasks. Patients unable to use an affected limb are taught compensatory strategies. Adaptive devices are used if more natural methods are not available or cannot be learned, and orthotic devices or braces are indicated if joint or limb stabilization will help improve function or ambulation.

Management of Impaired Cognition

Limitations in cognition or perception are important in planning and conducting rehabilitation efforts, in preparing for functional safety on discharge, and in predicting a patient's ability to resume vocational activities. Cognitive deficits may involve difficulties of concentration, attention, orientation, memory, perception, and executive function.

Causes may include specific brain lesions and environmental or nonenvironmental distractors. Nonenvironmental distractors may include chronic pain, vertigo, lack of motivation, diplopia, visual loss, hearing loss, fatigue, impulsiveness, the side effects of medications, the effect of emotional disturbances (e.g., depression, anxiety, or agitation), or intermittent seizures such as nonconvulsive seizures or brief absence or psychomotor seizures. Environmental distractors can include aspects of the hospital routine that may prevent adequate sleep at night such as late medications or busy or noisy therapy areas.

Prior to treatment, specific etiologies are identified and a relevant management plan is devised. A cognitive remediation program often includes the efforts of an occupational therapist, a speech therapist, and a psychologist. Treatments emphasize cognitive retraining, substitution of intact abilities, and compensatory strategies. Irreversible cognitive deficits that absolutely preclude learning are a contraindication to active neurorehabilitation (see Rehabilitation Program Criteria, above).

Management of Communication Disorders

Impairments of speech and language may include aphasias, disorders of pragmatics (right-hemisphere communication disorders), and difficulties related to dysarthria. Management varies with etiology and often involves the services of a speech therapist and a psychologist. Treatment of aphasia targets problems of comprehension or expression. Specific goals variably include improving ability to speak, comprehend, read, or write; developing strategies to compensate for persistent problems; addressing associated adjustment issues; and teaching caregivers to communicate with the patient. Goals of treatment for right-hemisphere language disorders (i.e., right-hemispheric strokes with left hemineglect) include increasing the awareness of deficits, reinstating the pragmatics of communication, and providing appropriate compensatory strategies. Treatment goals for dysarthria include improving intelligibility of speech through special exercises and compensatory strategies such as manipulation of respiration, phonation, resonation, articulation, and prosody.

Management of Emotional Dysfunction

Emotional disturbances such as depression, anxiety, apathy, mania, agitation, delusions, hallucinations, personality changes, and obsessive–compulsive behavior may occur in association with certain neurologic conditions.

The etiology of emotional dysfunction complicating a neurologic condition may be multifactorial. Possible causes include organic brain damage, exacerbation of a preexisting psychiatric condition or personality disorder, the side effects of medications, acute medical conditions (e.g., electrolyte disturbances, hypothyroidism, or hyperthyroidism), chronic pain, environmental factors (e.g., interruption of sleep), or a reaction to functional loss.

Emotional dysfunction can adversely affect participation in active rehabilitation and long-term outcomes. Effective treatment depends on an accurate diagnosis of etiology. A psychiatry consultation may be indicated.

Management may include psychotherapy, a brief course of a psychoactive medication, a program of maladaptive behavior modification, and addressing specific etiologies. A behavior modification program will involve the interdisciplinary team in redirecting and discouraging socially inappropriate behaviors while encouraging appropriate conduct.

Management of Chronic Pain

The physiologic and psychological causes and effects of chronic pain are quite complex. Pain occurs in many forms and may involve any portion of the body. The stimulus for pain may arise at the level of the peripheral nerves, the autonomic nervous system, or the CNS.

Etiologies may include static or progressive disorders involving soft tissues, joints, bones, the viscera (internal organs), the peripheral nerves or nerve roots, and the CNS. Pain could result from pathology related to the postoperative state, trauma, burns, and a host of other conditions including degenerative, inflammatory, infectious, metabolic, or neoplastic disorders.

Environmental factors may interact with internal factors to result in pain. For example, individuals with muscle spasticity, contractures, or decubitus skin ulcers often experience pain when being moved or repositioned. Also, the perception of pain may be modified by certain psychological factors, which can contribute to the onset, severity, exacerbation, and maintenance of chronic pain.

It is known that chronic anxiety or depression can adversely influence the subjective experience of pain, and similarly chronic pain can result in the onset of chronic anxiety or depression. The pattern of behavior resulting from chronic pain may include irritability, anger, dysphoric moods, loss of self-confidence or self-esteem, poor treatment compliance, and deterioration of important social relationships (possibly including the doctor–patient relationship).

The subjective experience of chronic pain may also adversely affect cognitive functioning and overall functional recovery outcomes. Concentration, attention, mental alertness, and capacity to perform complex neuropsychological tasks may be reduced by the direct distraction of pain or may be indirectly impaired by associated fatigue, sleep deprivation, depression, anxiety, poor motivation, or the effects of analgesics. In addition, physical capacity, including mobility and the ability to perform self-care activities, may be diminished by chronic pain.

■ **SPECIAL CLINICAL POINT: The treatment of chronic pain involves the identification and correction of causal factors whenever possible. A course of opioid or nonopioid analgesic, anxiolytic, or antidepressant medications may be useful. Long-term use of narcotic or anxiolytic medications should be avoided with few exceptions (e.g., cancer pain).**

Often, a psychological evaluation and course of psychotherapy may be beneficial for adjustment issues and associated affective dysfunction. If there are prominent signs of affective dysfunction, a psychiatry consultation may be necessary. Pain and other somatic complaints rooted in emotional dysfunction may be refractive to traditional treatments but responsive to psychopharmacologic intervention.

Physical modalities that may be helpful in a pain management program include thermotherapy (hot packs, ultrasound, analgesic creams), cryotherapy (cold packs), transcuta-

neous electrical nerve stimulation, massage, progressive joint mobilization, acupressure or acupuncture, biofeedback, relaxation exercises, and movement education regarding proper body mechanics. Consultation with an anesthesia or pain specialist for local anesthesia, regional blocks, epidural analgesics, or sympathetic nerve blocks may be helpful to break a cycle of pain. Refractive cases may require a surgical consultation. For example, orthopaedic surgeons may be able to replace painful degenerative joints. Neurosurgeons may be able to correct or ablate sources of chronic neuropathic pain. Finally, compensation issues also should be considered in certain cases as a possible source of chronic pain.

Discharge Planning

Discharge planning is an integral part of a rehabilitation management plan and involves the interdisciplinary team, the patient, and the family or caregivers. Objectives include the education of the patient or caregivers and the determination of the best living environment if other than home, family or caregiver capabilities, home accessibility, special equipment needs, disability entitlements, the ability to return to work or to school, driving issues including handicap parking needs, need for further rehabilitation therapies such as vocational rehabilitation, and necessary community services including appropriate medical follow-up.

Discharge occurs when reasonable treatment goals have been achieved. Reasonable treatment goals can include the progression from one level of functional dependence to a more independent level that is realistic for that patient. For example, discharge may be indicated when a patient who initially required total assistance in certain mobility or self-care activities progresses to a level of moderate or minimal assistance or supervision. In general, inpatients are discharged from intense comprehensive rehabilitation programs when they progress to a level of minimal assistance in mobility, which may include proficiency in wheelchair operation or progression to ambulation with the physical assistance of another person with use of an assistive device, and have the ability to assist caregivers with transfers.

Discharge from an outpatient program often occurs when a level of supervision to independence is reached in mobility and self-care activities. Absence of patient progress in mobility or self-care function on two successive care plan evaluations suggests a functional plateau and a need to reconsider the treatment regimen or the rehabilitation setting. Interdisciplinary care plan conferences are held weekly in intense comprehensive inpatient programs and bimonthly to monthly in outpatient or subacute rehabilitation programs. These meetings are held to allow interdisciplinary team members the chance to update one another on patient progress and potential problems. The care plan meetings facilitate the formulation of individualized rehabilitation management plans, modifications of existing plans, and the discharge planning process.

A crucial aspect of the discharge planning process is the determination of the best living environment and family caregiver capabilities. Therapeutic weekend day passes often are encouraged during a comprehensive inpatient rehabilitation program to allow a patient and caregivers the opportunity to test their abilities at home and in the community. Thus, problem areas of community transition may be identified, allowing therapists to focus special attention prior to discharge. In addition, some programs allow therapists to perform home consultations to determine potential safety hazards and special home equipment needs (e.g., wheelchair ramps, grab bars), to help patients and caregivers rehearse the daily routine, and to assess accessibility of community facilities that still may be used by the patient following discharge. Whether a patient is discharged to home or to an alternative living facility depends in part on patient or caregiver preferences and a realistic assessment of patient or caregiver capabilities. For example, an elderly, chroni-

cally ill spouse may not be able to care for the patient unless full-time help is available at home. Also, patients who previously lived independently may no longer be able to do so. In addition, some patients may require temporary placement in a transitional living program in preparation for more independent living. In other cases, the availability of home health care services including a home health aide and a visiting nurse may allow a patient to be discharged to the home setting.

Another important objective of the discharge planning process is patient or caregiver education and training regarding pertinent care issues and community transition. This includes prevention of complications, necessary techniques such as safe car transfers, home exercises, proper use of necessary adaptive equipment or braces, routine care needs such as bladder catheterization or the use of alternative feeding devices, instruction on medication administration or potential side effects, information regarding specific precautions such as driving or the use of machinery, information regarding sexual issues, information regarding available community services that may include vocational or recreational programs and support groups, and instructions regarding discharge follow-up and continued therapy needs.

The importance of continuity of care is emphasized. Usually, the team case manager will assist the patient and caregivers in arranging for necessary community services such as home health care and outpatient therapies. In addition, arrangements are made for important medical follow-up that often includes the primary medical physician, the neurorehabilitation specialist, and all other treating specialist physicians.

Prior to discharge, a patient's functional baseline is documented to help monitor subsequent progress and maintenance of function. Also, disability entitlements are addressed, such as handicapped parking needs, certification of disabilities, and clarification of a patient's ability to return to work or school. If necessary, arrangements are made for special education or vocational programs. Whenever possible, adaptive equipment or strategies are offered to allow individuals the ability to return to work or school.

Neurorehabilitation Follow-Up And Community Transition

Gaps in medical follow-up increase risks for institutionalization of patients with certain disabilities. Therefore, routine medical follow-up is encouraged following discharge from a neurorehabilitation program. The frequency of recommended follow-up varies with patient needs. Responsibility for coordination of outpatient medical care, rehabilitation services, and determination of further rehabilitation needs rests with the primary care physician, who may be the previous treating family physician, internist, pediatrician, or rehabilitation specialist.

Goals of follow-up include assessment of a patient's health status, safety at home and in the community, and maintenance of function. In addition, if applicable, the follow-up physician should assess the adequacy of family or caregiver interventions. Areas of concern include medical, physical, cognitive, emotional, and social function. Problems may develop once an individual begins to attempt resumption of previous community activities and social relationships. This is when the full impact of disabilities resulting from a neurologic condition may become apparent to the patient or the family.

Changes in traditional family roles also may have profound consequences on the patient or the family members. Support groups and psychotherapy may be useful in certain situations. Also, the ability of a family member or caretaker to provide effective care for a patient with severe disabilities must be reevaluated constantly. Even committed caregivers may reach a point of desperation when providing continuous support without relief.

Another concern is a patient's ability to maintain functional levels previously achieved during a rehabilitation program. Loss of function may occur secondary to exacerbation of medical comorbid conditions or the neurologic disorder or from lack of stimulation, lack of self-confidence, physical barriers to activity, or inadvertent suppression of initiation by overprotective caregivers.

The need for continued or additional rehabilitation services also must be considered. Further outpatient rehabilitation needs vary with a patient's progress in an existing program and the extent of remaining disabilities. Goals of further rehabilitation services may include encouragement of recreational activities and the return to work, school, or driving.

Specific rehabilitation programs exist to assess the capacity to perform certain activities such as the ability to drive or to return to work-related physical activities. Work-capacity assessments are available. In addition, driving programs for handicapped people exist to assess driving safety as well as to teach adaptive strategies. The ability to drive is influenced by an individual's impairments, including visual/spatial and cognitive function. Adaptive driving instruction programs are available for appropriate patients.

Another follow-up concern includes sexual function issues. Adaptive strategies, devices, and counseling can enhance sexual function in patients with disabilities and can even allow sexual reproduction for patients with spinal cord injuries.

In summary, in an attempt to maximize the quality of life and functional independence, neurorehabilitation outpatient follow-up concerns include medical, physical, cognitive, emotional, and social aspects of patient function during the transition back into the community.

When to Refer a Patient to a Neurorehabilitation Specialist

The most common disease processes for which neurorehabilitation interventions are warranted include stroke, multiple sclerosis, traumatic brain injury, and postoperative conditions following neurosurgery. In addition, all individuals with an acute (e.g., stroke), chronic (e.g., multiple sclerosis), or progressive (e.g., Parkinson disease) neurologic disorder may benefit at least to some degree from neurorehabilitation treatment to enhance function and to improve the quality of life.

The primary care physician is the usual gatekeeper for patient referrals to the neurorehabilitation specialist. Patient referrals to a neurorehabilitation specialist can be made at any point during an individual's disease process, from the time of the acute hospitalization to the time following discharge to home care. As previously outlined in this chapter, neurorehabilitation can be carried out in a variety of settings, ranging from inpatient to outpatient care settings. Early patient referrals for neurorehabilitation treatment can enhance functional outcomes. For example, studies have shown that beginning rehabilitation as early as possible after a stroke produces better results than if rehabilitation treatment was started later. However, the primary care physician should never consider it too late to refer a patient for an evaluation with a neurorehabilitation specialist to determine whether there may be helpful physical, pharmacologic, or adaptive interventions that may improve function and quality of life for that individual.

Primary care physicians always should be aware that patients with impairments and disabilities resulting from neurologic conditions may benefit at least to some degree from neurorehabilitation interventions. Also, it is important that primary care physicians closely monitor their outpatients with neurologic conditions for any deterioration in function either related to the disease process, aging, or other intercurrent illnesses because these patients also may benefit from further neurorehabilitation interventions.

■ **SPECIAL CLINICAL POINT: Ideally, primary care physicians should request a neurorehabilitation evaluation for all their patients with impairments or disabilities related to a neurologic condition who have not yet undergone rehabilitation treatment and for those patients who have undergone rehabilitation treatment** but who have experienced a decline in their level of functional independence.

Special Challenges for Hospitalized Patients

Hospitalizations for intercurrent illnesses pose special challenges to individuals with neurologic conditions who may have been undergoing rehabilitation treatment. Functional decline commonly results from an acute intercurrent illness in patients who already have chronic impairments due to a neurologic disorder or disease. For example, individuals with a history of stroke, multiple sclerosis, Parkinson disease, spinal cord injury, or brain injury who may require hospital treatment for an intercurrent illness such as pneumonia, heart disease, or urosepsis usually will experience a setback in their functional status. In addition, the more prolonged a hospitalization for an intercurrent illness may be, the more profound will be the setback in that individual's functional recovery.

Aspects of a rehospitalization that are counterproductive to the functional recovery process include a number of factors. Prolonged bed rest and immobility are among the single most damaging factors. The risks associated with bed rest and immobility were discussed at length earlier in this chapter and include the possibility for the development of DVT, joint contractures, skin breakdown, pneumonia, deconditioning weakness, and orthostatic intolerance. Impaired nutritional status resulting from an intercurrent illness may also negatively affect motor function recovery and lead to muscle wasting and worsened weakness. Infections such as pneumonia or urinary tract infections may result in exacerbations of confusion in patients with brain injuries or encephalopathies.

Hospitalizations for a second stroke or hospitalizations for exacerbations of multiple sclerosis can have obvious detrimental effects in a patient who had been undergoing rehabilitation treatment. Measures to prevent the complications of immobility should be instituted in all patients with neurologic conditions who may require a hospitalization for an intercurrent illness. In addition, early rehabilitation interventions by rehabilitation specialists and therapists during the rehospitalizations are critical to enhance functional recovery once the patient is stabilized.

Neurorehabilitation Outcomes

The effectiveness of a medical treatment may be measured in terms of biologic or functional changes in an individual and cost efficiency. The biologic effectiveness of a medical treatment can be assessed in terms of changes in an impairment rating such as the degree of sensory loss, spasticity, or weakness. The functional effectiveness of a medical treatment may be measured by changes in disability or handicap scores. The cost efficiency of a medical treatment may be measured in terms of relative monetary savings or losses to the payer in relation to the outcome, which may include length of hospital stay or an individual's ability to return to work, school, or independent living. Variables that may complicate the assessment of a specific medical treatment outcome on an individual may include age, sex, social factors such as prior education, coexistent chronic medical or psychological problems, the effects of other treatments, and patient compliance.

Numerous prior and ongoing outcome studies exist regarding the effectiveness of neurorehabilitation in terms of various neurologic impairments, disabilities, handicaps, and cost efficiency. The goal of these studies has been to determine the most effective and cost-efficient neurorehabilitation approaches for a host of specific neurologic impairments or disorders, while considering possible individual variables. Already, a number of specific neurorehabilitation interventions have been shown to be effective for a variety of impairments (e.g., various speech therapy language exercises for certain aphasias or dysphasias and various occupational therapy and physical therapy interventions for certain problems of mobility). In addition, the multidisciplinary rehabilitation team approach has been shown to be effective in a variety of neurologic

disorders such as stroke and traumatic brain and spinal cord injury. National collaborative rehabilitation outcome studies should continue to provide useful data for determination of model systems of care for a host of neurologic conditions and disorders.

Always Remember

- Disablement is best understood in terms of the complex relationship between disease, impairment, disability, and handicap.
- Neurorehabilitation targets disabilities resulting from disease-related impairments to reduce handicaps.
- The neurorehabilitation process encompasses medical, physical, social, education, and vocational interventions that can be provided in a variety of institutional or community settings.
- Ongoing and thorough patient assessment is a crucial aspect of the neurorehabilitation process from the acute hospitalization, to the transfer to a rehabilitation facility or program, to the transition back to the community.
- Short- and long-term rehabilitation goals and a management plan are formulated and regularly revised as needed to maximize patient potential at all stages of recovery.
- Neurorehabilitation evaluation is warranted for all patients having disabilities related to an acute, chronic, or progressive neurologic condition who have not yet undergone rehabilitation treatment and for those having new functional deficits.
- The neurorehabilitation plan always involves the patient and key caregiver, so that goals of the effort fit with the short-term and long-term goals of the family.

QUESTIONS AND DISCUSSION

1. A 51-year-old woman with a history of multiple substance abuse developed difficulty swallowing. Two days later, she developed an acute onset of paraplegia and

was admitted for an evaluation. She was diagnosed with an extensive retropharyngeal abscess with compression of the cervical spinal cord. She underwent surgical drainage of the abscess and was prescribed broad-spectrum intravenous antibiotics. One month later, she presents for neurorehabilitation with incomplete quadriplegia with four-fifths strength in both arms and two-fifths strength in both legs. A low cervical sensory level is present, below which there is partial pinprick and light touch sensation to the toes. An indwelling Foley catheter is in place, and there is a small area of superficial skin breakdown at the sacrum involving only the epidermis. Which of the following statements is correct?

A. Urologic consultation is unnecessary at this point.

B. The indwelling Foley catheter should not be removed while localized skin breakdown is present.

C. Short-term rehabilitation goals should include strengthening of deconditioned muscles.

D. The long-term prognosis for recovery of ambulation is poor.

The correct answer is C. The indwelling Foley catheter should be removed on admission, and a program of bladder training should be started. Initially, bladder catheterizations should be performed at least every 6 hours, and postvoid residuals should be monitored closely. Bladder catheterization frequency may be tapered as postvoid residuals diminish. A urology consultation may be helpful in determining medications that may hasten recovery of bladder function. Superficial skin breakdown is not a contraindication to removal of the Foley catheter. However, if the area of skin ulceration penetrated through the dermis into the soft tissue or muscle, then Foley catheter removal might be contraindicated. Moisture from urine incontinence can contribute to further skin ulceration.

Short-term neurorehabilitation goals in this patient would include patient and family education, prevention of secondary complications, strengthening of deconditioned muscles, and provision of compensatory strategies to overcome functional disabilities. Long-term prognosis for recovery of ambulation in this patient is fair because there is already some movement and sensation present in both legs.

2. A previously healthy 49-year-old man developed progressive weakness that started in his legs following a flulike illness. A workup included a lumbar puncture, which demonstrated an elevated protein, and an electromyographic nerve conduction study that showed nerve demyelination with axonal involvement. He was diagnosed with Guillain–Barré syndrome and underwent a course of plasmapheresis. On admission for neurorehabilitation 2 months later, he presents with flaccid quadriplegia, with the ability to shrug his shoulders. Proprioception is intact down to the ankles but is absent at the toes. Reflexes are absent. Bulbar muscles are not involved. Which of the following statements is correct?

A. Dysautonomia may develop months into his recovery

B. The patient is at risk of developing pneumonia.

C. Ambulation should be set as a long-term neurorehabilitation goal.

D. After 2 months, quadriplegia is likely permanent.

The correct answer is B. He is at risk for complications of immobility including pneumonia, contractures, DVT, and skin breakdown. In addition, he is at risk for orthostasis and dysautonomia. The latter is a rare complication of Guillain–Barré syndrome that occurs most often during the acute illness rather than the convalescence.

Ambulation would be an unrealistic long-term rehabilitation goal at the time of his admission because he is presenting as a flaccid quadriplegic. However, many patients with acute demyelinating polyneuropathies present for rehabilitation with flaccid quadriplegia 1 to 2 months after onset of their illness and later recover the ability to ambulate. Therefore, ambulation would not be an impossibility in this patient.

Short-term rehabilitation goals here would include patient education, prevention of secondary complications, and gradual mobilization with passive range-of-motion exercises to help strengthen deconditioned muscles and prevent development of contractures. Motor recovery may be delayed in this patient because his polyneuropathy involves both demyelination and axonal nerve damage. Motor recovery occurs more rapidly in those individuals with only demyelination.

3. A 70-year-old woman underwent a coronary artery bypass graft and suffered a left-hemispheric stroke 3 days later. Her hospital stay was complicated by pneumonia. Three weeks later, she is transferred for neurorehabilitation with a nasogastric feeding tube in place, expressive aphasia, a flaccid right arm, and two-fifths strength present in the right leg. She is able to follow simple commands. Mood and affect are flat to tearful. Which of the following statements is correct?
   A. The patient should be taught compensatory strategies.
   B. The nasogastric feeding tube should be removed, and a trial pureed diet with thickened liquids should be started.
   C. Bracing and splinting should be avoided to encourage mobility.
   D. The patient's expressive aphasia will significantly impede rehabilitation.

The correct answer is A. Short-term rehabilitation goals in this patient should include compensatory strategies to overcome functional disabilities, bracing and splinting to enhance function and prevent contractures, prevention of secondary complications, and patient and family education.

There is a nasogastric feeding tube in place that should not be removed until a swallowing study is performed to evaluate for aspiration. Previous history of pneumonia is suggestive of aspiration. A modified barium swallow study can be performed to document safety in all phases of swallowing with various food textures. Compensatory swallowing strategies are available for certain types of dysphagia, but a temporary alternative means of feeding may be necessary in patients at high risk for aspiration.

Gradual recovery of some functional abilities is likely in this patient. Prognosis for functional recovery is best in those with the ability to comprehend and learn. Rehabilitation is still possible, although more difficult, in patients with receptive aphasias or hemineglect.

4. A 14-year-old boy was involved in a motor vehicle accident. He remained comatose for 5 days following admission. He was found to have a left ankle fracture and diffuse axonal brain injury. Three weeks later, on transfer for neurorehabilitation, he is restless and agitated with poor concentration and attention. He is nonverbal but attempts to follow some simple commands. There is diminished movement on the left side. A nasogastric feeding tube is in place due to dysphagia and risk for aspiration, and the left ankle is in a cast. Which of the following statements is correct?
   A. The patient is at risk of elopement from the rehabilitation facility.
   B. Cognitive improvement at this point is unlikely.
   C. Restraints should be avoided to prevent agitation.
   D. One-to-one supervision is necessary to ensure safety.

The correct answer is D. This young man is confused, restless, and agitated, which places him at risk for falls and inadvertent removal of the nasogastric tube. Elopement from the facility is less likely because he is hemiparetic and confused.

Initial measures to ensure safety may include one-to-one supervision, a low bed, and a right-hand mitt restraint. Redirection alone is unlikely to be successful because he is confused with poor attention and concentration. Although restraints could result in further agitation, a right-hand mitt will be necessary to help prevent the otherwise likely removed of the nasogastric feeding tube. A low bed will limit the risk for serious injury should this patient fall out of bed. Medications may be effective if one-to-one supervision fails to ensure safety and to redirect impulsive or aggressive behavior.

Cognitive improvement is expected. Cognitive function most likely will improve in patients with traumatic brain injuries in which coma lasted 13 days or less. These individuals generally will have selective impairments on neuropsychological testing at 1 year following injury. Those individuals in a coma lasting 2 weeks to 29 days are more likely to have impairments in all areas of cognitive function at 1 year following trauma. More than one-half of those individuals with coma lasting more than 29 days will remain severely impaired in all areas of cognitive function 1 year following injury.

SUGGESTED READING

Braddom RL, ed. *Physical Medicine and Rehabilitation*. Philadelphia: Saunders Elsevier; 2007.

Delisa JA, ed. *Physical Medicine and Rehabilitation: Principles and Practice*. 4th ed. Philadelphia: Lippincott Williams & Wilkins; 2005.

Dikmen S, Machamer JE. Neurobehavioral outcomes and their determinants. *J Head Trauma Rehabil*. 1995;10:74–86.

Dobkin BH. Impairments, disabilities, and bases for neurological rehabilitation after stroke. *J Stroke Cerebrovasc Dis*. 1997;6:221–226.

Gordon J. Assumptions underlying physical therapy intervention: theoretical and historical perspectives. In: Carr J, Shepherd RB, Gordon J, et al, eds. *Movement Science Foundations for Physical Therapy in Rehabilitation*. Rockville, MD: Aspen; 1987.

Granger CV, Black T, Braun SL. Quality and outcome measures for medical rehabilitation. In: Delisa JA, ed. *Rehabilitation Medicine. Principles and Practice*. 4th ed. Philadelphia: Lippincott Williams & Wilkins; 2005: 151–164.

Granger CV, Hamilton BB. UDS report: the uniform data system for medical rehabilitation report on the first admissions for 1990. *Am J Phys Med Rehabil*. 1992;71:108–113.

Gresham GE, Duncan PW, Stason WB, et al. Post-stroke rehabilitation: clinical practice guideline. Rockville, MD: U.S. Department of Health and Human Services, Agency for Healthcare Policy and Research; 1995.

Hamilton BB, Laughlin JA, Granger CV, et al. Interrater agreement of the seven level functional independence measures (FIM). *Arch Phys Med Rehabil*. 1991;72:790.

Hobart JC. Evidence-based measurement: which disability scale for neurologic rehabilitation? *Neurology*. 2001; 57(4):639–644.

Kesselring J. Neurorehabilitation: a bridge between basic science and clinical practice. *Eur J Neurol*. 2001; 8(3):221–225.

Kushner D. Neurorehabilitation. In: Evans RW, ed. *Saunders Manual of Neurologic Practice*. Philadelphia: WB Saunders; 2003.

Kushner D. Neurorehabilitation of brain injuries. In: Evans RW, ed. *Saunders Manual of Neurologic Practice*. Philadelphia: WB Saunders; 2003.

Macdonell RA. Neurologic disability and neurologic rehabilitation. *Med J Aust*. 2001;174(12):653–658.

Taub E, Uswatte G. New treatments in neurorehabilitation founded on basic research. *Nat Rev Neurosci*. 2002;3(3):228–236.

Thompson AJ. Neurological rehabilitation: from mechanisms to management. *J Neurol Neurosurg Psychiatry*. 2000;69(6):718–722.

Umphred DA, ed. *Neurological Rehabilitation*. St. Louis: CV Mosby; 1990.

Wade DT. *Measurement in Neurological Rehabilitation*. Oxford: Oxford University Press; 1992.

World Health Organization. *International Classification of Functioning, Disability and Health*: ICF. Geneva: WHO; 2001.

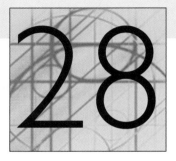

28

Medicolegal Issues in the Care of Patients with Neurologic Illness

MARIA R. SCHIMER AND
LOIS MARGARET NORA

---

key points

- Excellent communication skills, including the ability to listen effectively, are among the most important risk management skills that the physician can employ.

- Treating physicians have a legal duty to their patients to possess a reasonable degree of skill and knowledge, to use care and diligence in exercising this skill and knowledge, to employ approved methods in general use, and to use their best judgment.

- Informed consent is a process that has essential legal requirements including a legally and clinically competent patient, who is given adequate and understandable information about the proposed medical intervention by the treating physician and who voluntarily agrees to the intervention.

- Competent patients, or their surrogate decision makers, may withdraw their consent for a medical intervention.

- When determining death using neurologic criteria, the clinical evaluation should be done by experienced examiners who adhere to the recognized practice

> parameters and follow institutional requirements to establish the diagnosis.
>
> • Documenting advice and directives that are given to a patient with neurologic disease who wishes to drive is an important risk management strategy. All states have Department of Motor Vehicle Web sites that can provide information helpful in determining driving regulations for patients who are impaired for any reason.

n recent years, legal aspects of medical practice have become increasingly visible and important, particularly in the care of patients with neurologic disease. Although some physicians are intimidated by medicolegal issues, knowledge of legal aspects of medical practice can give the clinician a greater sense of mastery and may reduce the defensive practice of medicine and thus promote better patient care.

Three important types of law affect medical practice: case law, statutory law, and administrative law. Case law (also known as the common law) is developed by both the state and the federal courts (the judicial system) through the resolution of various criminal and civil matters. The decisions of these courts form a body of law that is binding within a given jurisdiction because of a legal doctrine known as *stare decisis*, or the doctrine of precedent, which requires courts to follow earlier court decisions when the same legal question arises again. A court's jurisdiction is the geographic or subject matter area over which that court has decision-making authority. Within any jurisdiction, courts are divided into trial courts and appellate courts.

Physicians are often most concerned with the law developed by the judicial system because this is where the majority of law in the area of medical malpractice arises. The law which is developed in this area has a substantial impact on malpractice insurance premiums for physicians. Medical malpractice is generally a civil action heard in a court that is part of a state court system. However, if the alleged malpractice occurred in a federal facility (e.g., a Veterans Administration hospital), the matter is heard in a federal court because of the provisions of the Federal Tort Claims Act.

Most medical malpractice actions allege that the physician (Defendant) was negligent in the care of the patient (Plaintiff).

■ **SPECIAL CLINICAL POINT: To win a lawsuit alleging professional negligence, the Plaintiff must demonstrate by a "preponderance of the evidence" (greater or stronger evidence) (a) that the physician had a duty of care to the patient, (b) that the physician breached that duty, (c) that the breach proximately caused injury to the Plaintiff, and (d) that the injury resulted in damage to the Plaintiff.**

Duty arises at the beginning of a patient–physician relationship and continues until the relationship is appropriately concluded through proper written notification to the patient by the physician or patient withdrawal from the relationship. Generally, a patient–physician relationship arises when a physician first sees a patient in a patient care setting and agrees to be the patient's physician. The concept of duty in this context has several components including the duties to (a) possess a reasonable degree of skill and knowledge, (b) use reasonable care and diligence in exercising this skill and knowledge, (c) employ approved methods in general use, and (d) use his or her best judgment.

■ **SPECIAL CLINICAL POINT: The injury alleged must have been caused by some particular thing that the Defendant either did or** failed to do which a physician of ordinary skill, care, and diligence would or would not have done under like or similar circumstances. It must then be proven that the injury was directly and proximately caused by the Defendant's action or inaction; attorneys often call this the "but for" test. Expert medical testimony is provided by another physician who, through experience and education, has developed sufficient skill and knowledge in a particular area of medicine to be able to form and give an opinion that will assist the judge or jury in deciding the case.

The second body of law affecting a physician's medical practice is statutory law. Statutory law is the body of law developed by local, state, or federal legislative bodies; this body of law applies to persons within the jurisdictional bounds of those legislative bodies. Examples of such statutory laws include the federal and state statutes concerning medical malpractice, abortion, advance directives (living wills and health care powers of attorney), and termination of treatment. Laws must be consistent with the United States Constitution, which is the most fundamental and organic source of law, and with the individual state's constitution. When a statute is unclear or when it is in conflict with the Constitution (federal or state) or another statute, the judicial system is employed to clarify or interpret the statute or to resolve conflicts.

■ **SPECIAL CLINICAL POINT: Administrative law is a body of law with three distinct components: the enabling legislation that creates the governmental agency and gives it its powers; the rules and regulations that are promulgated by the agency in accordance with the power granted to it; and the body of opinions, reports, and orders that the agency issues.**

An example of an agency that regulates some aspects of clinical practice is the U.S. Food and Drug Administration (FDA). Among other areas of authority, the FDA regulates pharmaceuticals and medical devices. Another agency, the Office for Human Research Protections (OHRP), has regulatory authority over much of the research involving patients.

The Health Insurance Portability and Accountability Act (HIPAA) is an example of a federal law that is administered by the Office of Civil Rights at the Department of Health and Human Services through multiple administrative regulations. These regulations dramatically affect the patient care environment and expand upon the longstanding responsibilities of physicians to honor patient confidentiality. For example, the HIPAA privacy rules regulate the gathering of information from patients, electronic sharing and storage of information in the medical record, and communication of such information with patients' family members and others. HIPAA rules impose substantial penalties for noncompliance by physicians and organizations.

The remainder of this chapter addresses three specific areas at the intersection between medical and legal matters and the care of patients with neurologic illness. These areas are (a) informed consent, a legal principle that affirms patient self-determination; (b) the use of neurologic criteria to declare death; and (c) the licensing of drivers with neurologic disorders, with a focus on seizure disorders.

INFORMED CONSENT

Informed consent is a fundamental legal concept based on medical ethics. The purpose of obtaining informed consent is to promote the autonomy of the patient in medical decision making. Informed consent involves two distinct legal rights of the patient: the right to obtain information and the right to make a decision. The informed consent process, which is best thought of as shared decision making, requires that the treating physician disclose sufficient information to enable the patient to evaluate a procedure before consenting to it.

■ **SPECIAL CLINICAL POINT: Informed consent is predicated on several important assumptions. These assumptions are that the patient (a) is competent, (b) is free from duress,**

(c) has received the disclosure of necessary information from the treating physician in a manner that renders the information understandable, and (d) has voluntarily given permission or made a choice.

To give informed consent, a patient must be competent. The President's Commission for the Study of Ethical Problems in Medicine and Biomedical and Behavioral Research wrote that competence involves the possession of a set of values and goals, the ability to communicate and understand information, and the ability to reason and deliberate about one's choices. Although this is an excellent standard by which to measure competence, the clinical practitioner often deals with situations in which the patient's abilities fluctuate over time and vary depending on the functional domain. It is helpful to understand the construct that the patient must be *both* legally and clinically competent to provide informed consent for a medical intervention.

Adults are presumed to be legally competent unless they have been declared legally incompetent by a court of law. When a person has been declared incompetent by the court, the court names a guardian who stands in the place of the incompetent person (ward) for all purposes set forth in the guardianship documents. Although many well-meaning family members confuse the two, the practitioner must be careful to distinguish between documents signifying that a person is under guardianship and those signifying that a person has given another person the power to act for him or her in the event of incompetence, that is, a health care power of attorney. A physician's failure to secure consent before providing treatment may result in charges of battery (criminal, civil, or both) and malpractice.

■ **SPECIAL CLINICAL POINT: The general rule is that a competent adult may consent to, refuse to consent to, or withdraw consent for treatment in any form.**

Generally, minors are not considered legally competent. Consent for the treatment of minors must, in most cases, be sought from their guardians, usually their parents. However, there are exceptions. A minor who has been legally emancipated is considered legally competent to make medical decisions. In addition, minors may be legally competent for certain interventions but not for others. For example, in some states adolescents are considered legally competent to make reproductive health decisions, even though they lack legal competence to make other medical care decisions.

■ **SPECIAL CLINICAL POINT: Legal competence, by itself, is not enough. A person must also be clinically competent.**

Clinical competence implies that the patient can understand information, formulate a decision, and communicate that decision. Assistive devices (e.g., hearing aids, glasses, or communication devices) can be helpful in maintaining a patient's clinical competence. Clinical competence is a medical decision. In some situations, a person may be legally competent but not clinically competent. Dementia, encephalopathy, and other conditions may render the patient incapable of providing informed consent for a variable period.

In situations where it is impossible to secure consent from the patient because the patient is incompetent, the physician must consult a surrogate decision maker for the patient. This person is often the patient's next of kin. The decision maker may also be a person appointed earlier by the patient through a written advance directive, or a court-appointed guardian.

■ **SPECIAL CLINICAL POINT: Two distinct legal standards have been established for surrogate decision makers. These standards are the *substituted judgment* standard and the *best interest* standard.**

The substituted judgment standard requires the surrogate decision maker to review the patient's known beliefs, previous actions, statements, and any available documentation, to determine what decision the patient would have made. Put simply, the surrogate decision maker must "put himself or herself in the place of the patient." The best interest standard requires the surrogate decision maker to look at all of the facts and circumstances surrounding the case and to attempt to identify the action that, in the minds of most persons in the jurisdiction, would be in the best interest of the incompetent patient.

The second requirement for informed consent is that adequate information be provided to the patient in an understandable fashion. Information provided to the patient should include the nature and purpose of the proposed intervention, its risks and anticipated benefits, alternatives to the proposed interventions, prognosis without the intervention, and prognosis with alternative interventions. The patient should be told of the right to refuse and to withdraw consent at any time.

■ **SPECIAL CLINICAL POINT: Although other health care personnel may be involved in obtaining consent, the physician remains responsible for ensuring the provision of adequate information and for the other aspects of the informed consent process.**

The adequacy of information provided to a patient can be an issue in malpractice suits. Two legal standards of information disclosure are recognized: the professional standard and the material risk standard. The professional standard requires the physician to give the patient information that other physicians of the same specialty, in the same community, would give to patients considering the same intervention. At trial, expert testimony is necessary to determine the nature and extent of this information. This is the more traditional of the two standards and is currently preferred in most jurisdictions.

The material risk standard requires the physician to provide any information that a reasonable person in the patient's position would want disclosed or would use in making a consent decision. Advocates of this standard identify its emphasis on the patient's need for information. Opponents point to its retrospective application

as a serious disadvantage. The most appropriate approach is probably a hybrid of the two standards.

■ **SPECIAL CLINICAL POINT: Physicians should communicate those risks that occur often enough or that are so severe, even if they occur infrequently, that a patient would usually wish to know of them.**

For example, patients should be advised of the possibility of hirsutism and gingival hyperplasia with phenytoin use, and they should be given information about spinal headaches before undergoing lumbar puncture. In addition, if a physician is aware of a particular characteristic of a patient that would make a potential adverse effect more important to that patient, this adverse effect should be communicated, even if the physician would not have discussed it with other patients. For example, potential teratogenic effects of medications should be discussed with female patients who may become pregnant.

The third requirement of informed consent is that the patient must give consent voluntarily. Coercion and duress invalidate consent. A physician should provide patients with advice and guidance regarding proposed therapies, but this must be done in a noncoercive manner. No explicit or implicit threat of loss of medical or nursing care should be linked to a decision.

The consent discussion should be documented in the patient record. A patient-signed consent document is not required for valid consent, but it provides at least some evidence of decision making by the patient. Although prepared consent forms can be helpful, the value of these documents should not be overestimated. Courts and juries are often suspicious of complicated consent documents that appear to be written more to protect the physician than to inform the patient.

Care must be taken that interventions remain within the scope of the consent given by the patient. Consent should be secured for a given procedure, for other procedures that are within the scope of that procedure, and for procedures that can or should be reasonably expected. Consent usually is given to a particular person and to those working with that person. The physician should not overextend the consent to procedures that are not logically associated with the consent or to personnel not reasonably anticipated by the patient.

■ **SPECIAL CLINICAL POINT: In emergency situations, the guidelines for informed consent do not strictly follow the standard informed consent principles.**

When a patient is unconscious or incompetent (by reason of mental impairment) and has sustained injuries that are likely to result in the imminent loss of life, and no surrogate decision maker is available, the health care professionals caring for the person are required to act in accordance with reasonable medical standards to save the patient's life.

It is also important to recognize that a competent patient may "waive" the right to informed consent by "letting the doctor decide" what course of action to take in a given situation. For example, the patient may say, "I am not a physician. I trust you; that is why I came here. Do what you think is best." Some would argue that this is not a waiver at all, but rather a conscious decision on the part of the patient to let another make a critical judgment. Although courts recognize the right of a patient to waive informed consent, physicians should make sure that waiver decisions are carefully documented, and they should have the patient put the waiver in writing.

Therapeutic privilege is another exception to informed consent. This exception is used when the physician determines that an informed consent discussion will prove so detrimental to the patient's health that it should not be undertaken. For example, some physicians have used this exception to justify not disclosing the risk of tardive dyskinesia when neuroleptic medications are prescribed to certain patients who, they fear, will refuse a potentially beneficial medication because of a severe, but unlikely, side effect.

Physicians must be extremely cautious in their use of therapeutic privilege. Courts may not be sympathetic to physicians' defending their use of therapeutic privilege when confronted by an uninformed patient who has suffered severe adverse effects. If a physician believes that the use of therapeutic privilege is absolutely necessary, involving the patient's family in the decision may be beneficial, but this involvement must not violate the patient's privacy. Complete disclosure to the patient at the earliest opportunity is also advisable. The physician should maintain contemporaneous and clear documentation of the reasons for the decision.

■ **SPECIAL CLINICAL POINT: The right of a competent patient to give informed consent carries with it an obvious recognition of the patient's right of informed refusal. Patients have a legal right to refuse interventions, even if the refusal will result in the patient's death.**

Physicians must inform patients of potential problems related to refusing a potential intervention, and this action should also be documented. Education and persuasion of the patient are two important tools available to the physician when a patient refuses consent. When a physician is confronted by a patient refusal that may result in serious adverse consequences for the patient and the physician is uncertain whether the refusal is the result of a patient's inability to perceive the nature and extent of his or her clinical predicament (e.g., where the patient is in a state of early to mid-stage dementia), a psychological or psychiatric consult may be helpful.

Informed refusal is not an absolute right. Certain exceptions to the patient's right to refuse an intervention have been recognized, and judicial intervention is possible in certain situations. Courts will not permit the use of informed refusal as a means of committing suicide and may override a patient's refusal if such an action is deemed necessary for the protection of innocent third parties. The court may modify a patient's refusal to protect the standards of the medical profession or of an institution.

Legal proceedings against physicians for failure to obtain informed consent may take two forms. First, a physician may be sued for battery, the intentional touching of a person (the patient) by another (the physician) without consent. Because battery is generally an intentional tort, punitive damages (monetary damages meant to punish the physician, not merely to recompense the patient) may be available if a physician is found liable. Except in extreme cases in which no consent was obtained or in which misrepresentation or fraud was used to obtain the consent, it is unlikely that battery will be alleged. The fact that malpractice insurance coverage is usually not available for intentional torts also may limit the use of a battery action by Plaintiffs.

Second, and more commonly, failure to obtain informed consent can lead to a medical malpractice (negligence) suit. To win, the Plaintiff must demonstrate by a preponderance of the evidence that (a) the injury sustained was a known risk of the therapy, (b) the physician failed to meet the applicable standard of care regarding information about the risk that caused the injury, and (c) the patient would not have consented to the therapy if the information had been provided. If these things are proved, the Plaintiff can succeed, even if the sustained injury (and damage) was a known complication of the intervention and did not result through any fault of the physician.

■ **SPECIAL CLINICAL POINT:** Five primary guiding principles should maximize effective informed consent:

- **Physicians remain responsible for informed consent even when others are involved in obtaining it.**
- **Information given to patients should be adequate and understandable.**
- **Patients must be legally and clinically competent, and their consent to interventions must be given voluntarily.**

- **Informed consent is a process; written documentation is evidence of the process.**
- **The better the quality of the process and documentation of the process, the more likely the physician is to prevail in any legal action against him or her.**

In the case of legal incompetence, guardians should be approached for consent. When a patient is legally competent but clinically incompetent, medical care may proceed if consent is given by a surrogate decision maker who is employing the correct standard for decision making. In a limited number of circumstances, intervention by the courts may be necessary in determining nonemergency care for incompetent patients. In most emergency situations, reasonable medical care should be rendered to preserve life and limb.

In the case of informed refusal, care must be taken to inform the patient of the risks of refusal. If the patient, in the judgment of the treating physician, does not appreciate the nature and extent of his or her clinical predicament, an appropriate mental health professional should be consulted. However, if the patient is both legally and clinically competent, informed refusal (even though life threatening) is the patient's right, except in very limited circumstances. Patients whose informed refusal may result in death remain entitled to receive excellent medical and nursing care until the end of life (e.g., palliative and supportive care). Documentation in such circumstance is essential.

DECLARING DEATH BY USING NEUROLOGIC CRITERIA (BRAIN DEATH)

Traditionally, death was defined clinically by the absence of cardiac and pulmonary functioning. Today, medical and technologic advances make artificial ventilation, continued cardiac rhythm, and the continued oxygenation of many of the body's tissues possible after the death of the entire brain.

The concept that death might be defined using neurologic criteria was first articulated by the Harvard criteria in 1968. A 1977 National Institutes of Health Collaborative Study and a 1982 President's Commission for the Study of Ethical Problems in Medicine and Biomedical and Behavioral Research further explored the issues. In 1980, the United States Uniform Determination of Death Act codified the use of neurologic criteria (brain death) as an acceptable method of determining death. In the United States, there has been gradual and substantial acceptance of the use of brain death criteria as an appropriate means of determining the death has occurred. Practice parameters and diagnosis guidelines for using neurologic criteria to declare death have been developed.

All 50 states currently define death either as the irreversible cessation of circulation and respiratory functioning or as the irreversible cessation of all functions of the entire brain, including the brain stem. These definitions do not imply that there are two types of death but rather two methods of determining death.

Two elements are crucial to the determination of brain death: (a) total cessation of functioning of the entire brain (including the brainstem) and (b) irreversibility of the condition. Potential legal difficulties related to brain death can be avoided by a rigorous medical approach to establishing the condition and distinguishing it from other neurologic conditions. Clear and considerate communication with family members and loved ones of the brain-dead patient contributes to optimal care and the avoidance of legal problems.

■ **SPECIAL CLINICAL POINT: The diagnosis of brain death should be made by a physician experienced in this process, usually a neurologist, neurosurgeon, or critical care specialist. Any physician with a real or perceived conflict of interest in the diagnosis (e.g., a member of a transplant team or a relative of a potential organ recipient) should not be involved in making this diagnosis.**

The brain death discussion in this chapter is focused on adult patients. Pediatric experts should be consulted when the brain death of a child must be determined.

The diagnosis of brain death is established in three interrelated steps. First, an irreversible cause must be established, and certain conditions that can mimic brain death but are reversible must be excluded. Second, an extensive neurologic evaluation of the patient must be carefully performed. Third, ancillary laboratory tests may be used to confirm the diagnosis and the prognosis. Rigorous attention to these three steps will ensure that complete cessation of brain functioning and its irreversibility are established. Physicians should also be aware of institution-specific requirements related to diagnosing brain death. Surprisingly, the requirements for making this diagnosis vary widely across institutions; for example, some institutions require the completion of a formal check list or the performance of specific ancillary tests.

The reason for the patient's condition must be known. In general, brain death should not be diagnosed if the cause is not clear. Common causes of brain death are head trauma, intracerebral hemorrhage, and anoxia during cardiopulmonary arrest. Careful history-taking, a detailed examination, and various laboratory tests and imaging studies (e.g., magnetic resonance imaging) may be helpful in determining the cause of brain death.

Medical conditions that can mimic brain death must be ruled out before brain death is diagnosed. These medical conditions include hypothermia, metabolic dysfunction, and drug intoxication. In the setting of hypothermia, the core body temperature must be corrected before the diagnosis can be made. Barbiturate and anesthetic agents are the drugs most frequently implicated in this setting, but multiple other medications, including tricyclic antidepressants, may also be involved. When a medical condition exists that can mimic brain death, the condition should be corrected before the diagnosis is made. If correcting the condition is impossible, ancillary tests demonstrating the lack of cerebral circulation are necessary.

The second component of the brain death evaluation is the clinical examination. The complexity of the neurologic examination for establishing brain death mandates that the examiner be experienced. The clinical examination establishes the total absence of brain (cerebral and brain stem) function and helps rule out those conditions that may mimic brain death. These conditions may be medical, as discussed above; neurologic conditions that are sometimes misdiagnosed as brain death include locked-in syndrome and the vegetative state. There have been unfortunate instances when patients in vegetative states have been wrongly declared brain dead; this underscores the importance of qualified, experienced examiners making the diagnosis and rigorously adhering to established criteria.

The patient must be unresponsive to any external stimuli, including pain. Any form of purposeful response, seizure activity, or decorticate posturing is inconsistent with the diagnosis of brain death. All activities mediated by the cortex and the brain stem, including reflexes, must be absent. Pupils are usually midpoint. The light reflex must be absent. Other brain stem reflexes, including doll's eyes, caloric, corneal, gag, swallow, and cough reflexes, must be absent.

The brain stem controls respiration, and the evaluation of brain death should include formal apnea testing to rule out the ability of the brain stem to maintain respiration. Formal apnea testing should be performed only by physicians familiar with and experienced in performing this test. The patient must be pre-oxygenated before apnea testing and should receive oxygen during the test. The ventilator is disconnected long enough for the $PaCO_2$ to increase to at least 60 mm Hg. When the $PaCO_2$ is at this level, no spontaneous attempts at respiration should be evident before it can be determined with confidence that the patient has no spontaneous respiration.

Although brain stem reflexes are completely absent with brain death, certain spinal-mediated reflexes can be preserved. The presence of these reflexes does not preclude the diagnosis, but to the inexperienced eye some of these reflex activities may imply brain activity. It is very important that the health care team have a common understanding about what these reflex movements may look like, what they represent, and that they are neither purposeful activity nor mediated by the brain. This common understanding also will allow the health care team to most effectively communicate these facts to the family members.

The third component of a brain death evaluation is laboratory testing and imaging studies. These tests can help rule out conditions that mimic brain death, confirm the neurologic examination, and establish irreversibility of the condition. Although laboratory tests are usually considered optional, confirmatory laboratory tests are mandatory in some situations, for example, when specific components of clinical testing cannot be reliably evaluated, when a cause for the diagnosis is not established, and when local regulations require such testing.

The electroencephalogram (EEG) has been used as part of brain death evaluation for many years. Great care must be taken to ensure adequate technical quality of these studies. Cerebral blood flow studies can be very helpful in the diagnosing of brain death and are often easier to complete than EEG studies. Blood flow studies that demonstrate no intracranial circulation for at least 10 minutes provide compelling and conclusive evidence of irreversible brain death.

It is crucial to allow adequate time for complete evaluation and serial observations of the patient during the determination of brain death. Repeated clinical examinations are recommended. The time required for reaching the diagnosis will vary depending on the cause of the patient's condition, the clinical expertise of the examiner, and the use of various diagnostic tests. Some states and certain institutions may have local rules about reexamination. Pressure for organ harvesting and other concerns should not prevent the careful and thorough processes necessary for reaching the diagnosis.

■ **SPECIAL CLINICAL POINT: One of the most frequent errors in the clinical setting, as well as in the published literature about brain death, is the suggestion that the brain-dead patient is somehow still alive.**

This suggestion is usually made inadvertently when a health care provider refers to the brain as "dead" but to the body as "alive." For example, a family member may be told that the "patient is dead [because of brain death], but we are keeping him [or her] alive [because of the desire for organ donation]." This information is confusing to the family and is made more so by the chest movements that result from the ventilator and by the cardiac rhythm that continues to appear on the monitor. The situation becomes even more complicated if activities around the bedside stimulate some form of spinal reflex response.

It is extremely important to communicate that neurologic criteria can be used to diagnose death and that brain death is death. Families must be helped to understand that their loved one is dead. Continued pharmacologic and technologic support should be described in terms of perfusing organs (particularly when the specific organs are being considered for donation) rather than as keeping the patient alive. Pharmacologic and technologic support should be discontinued as soon as feasible after the diagnosis of brain death. Allowing families to say their goodbyes before discontinuation of machinery may be appropriate; extended technologic support of a dead body is not.

It must be recognized that some persons, and some religious traditions, debate the validity of using neurologic criteria to diagnose death. The situation is made more complicated because studies have shown that physicians often lack a rigorous approach to completing all steps in making a diagnosis of death using neurologic criteria. Care must be taken when

a patient or a patient's family has religious or cultural objections to the use of neurologic criteria to diagnose death. Several states have created laws that either preclude the use of neurologic criteria to diagnose death when there are religious objections to these criteria or mandate procedures for accommodating such objections.

Often brain death is diagnosed in conjunction with a decision that the patient or decedent may serve as an organ donor. Although organ harvesting is possible in the absence of familial consent (e.g., with a valid donor card), physicians usually will not harvest organs without this consent. Such restraint is appropriate from a risk management perspective. When organ donation is a possibility, it should be discussed with the family early in the care process by persons who are uninvolved, and who will remain uninvolved, in the diagnostic and treatment decisions. Organ procurement programs have specially trained professionals work with families to facilitate the organ donation decision. In no event should undue pressure be exerted to convince family members to consent to organ harvesting.

When organ harvesting is not being considered, there may be less inclination to declare the patient brain dead and to discontinue mechanical perfusion of the remaining organs, particularly if the family does not wish to discontinue the use of a ventilator. Nonetheless, this course of action must be weighed against the ethics of using limited medical resources (including nursing and ancillary support staff) to support a corpse.

LICENSING OF DRIVERS

Driving a car is an important life activity for most adults, and limitations on driving exert important occupational and social impacts. Physicians often become engaged in discussions about whether patients with neurologic diseases—including epilepsy, movement disorders, and dementia—should drive. This discussion will focus on licensing of drivers (noncommercial) with seizure disorders because this is a common issue and the discussion has parallels with other neurologic conditions.

Most patients with controlled seizures can drive safely and without incident. However, some types of seizures pose a risk of injury and death to the patient who is driving, to passengers, and to others on the road. It is part of good medical practice for physicians to inform patients with seizures about any recommended lifestyle, recreational, or occupational limitations related to the seizure disorder. It is common to recommend that patients abstain from driving after a seizure, particularly if the seizure involves an alteration in consciousness or a loss of motor control.

Several questions of legal interest are related to the management of the patient with seizures who wishes to drive. What are the Department of Motor Vehicle (DOMV) requirements in the state in which the patient is obtaining a license? How does the physician participate in the patient's obtaining and maintaining a license? How should the physician document the advice given to patients about their driving activities? If a person with an active seizure disorder drives against medical advice, how does the physician balance the duty to maintain patient confidentiality with the duty to warn others about behavior that places the patient and others in danger?

Most states require a mandatory seizure-free interval before licensing is allowed. These mandatory seizure-free periods range from 3 to 18 months; 6 months is the most common interval. Some states do not require a mandatory seizure-free interval before licensure; instead, decisions are based on individualized determinations. In such states, important findings considered in each decision include the length of time since the last seizure, the type of seizure, precipitants, and other factors reasonably expected to affect the applicant's ability to control a motor vehicle. Additionally, these states

commonly require a physician statement, indicating that the patient's condition is under sufficient control to permit the safe operation of a motor vehicle. Most states either require periodic medical updates or give the DOMV the discretion to require such an update from the licensed person.

Restricted licenses are available in many states. Examples include licenses that permit the person to drive only in an emergency, to only to and from work, or to drive only during daylight hours. These restricted licenses may allow patients to drive even though they cannot meet the statutory seizure-free interval.

■ **SPECIAL CLINICAL POINT: The physician should make individualized medical judgments about necessary driving limitations for each patient, and state requirements should be considered in formulating any recommendations that the physician makes to the patients.**

If a restricted license or some other exception to the state rules appears appropriate, the physician can work with the patient and the state agency. Any recommendations about driving restrictions and other occupational and recreational limits should be carefully documented in the patient's chart. One effective method of documentation is to have the patient record his understanding of the physician's advice and to incorporate this document into the chart. This process encourages discussion between the patient and the physician, and it also provides clear evidence of the patient's involvement and understanding.

The physician may find that direct interaction with the state's DOMV or similar agency is necessary. In several states, physicians are required to report patients with seizure disorders to the DOMV or another state agency. Mandatory reporting is, however, uncommon and is considered unwise for many reasons. It infantilizes the patient, diminishes patient responsibility, and interposes a third party into the patient–physician relationship. Nonetheless, when such requirements exist, physicians must comply with them. Physicians who do not comply can be penalized by the state and could be held liable if third parties are injured as a result of a seizure of unreported seizure disorders. Even when the physician is immunized from suit for providing such information to the state, the patient should still be told that the information will be transmitted.

In general, no information about a patient's medical condition should be released without the express consent of the patient. Many states require that the physician complete initial and periodic reports on persons with seizures who drive. Physicians must fill out these forms honestly and usually are immune from suit for doing so. Office staff should be aware that complying with a state DOMV request neither violates nor lessens the responsibility of maintaining the patient's expectations of confidentiality.

Physicians should be aware of the procedures for obtaining a driver license in their state. Typically, applicants for initial or renewal licensure complete forms developed by the DOMV. These forms may specifically inquire about a seizure or epilepsy. However, in some jurisdictions, the questions are more general—asking about disorders characterized by "lapses of consciousness" or "episodes of marked confusion" that may be recurrent—and as such encompass epilepsy and other medical conditions. When a seizure disorder (or other medical problem) is identified, DOMV personnel may act on available information or may ask for additional input.

Once adequate information is available, DOMV personnel may grant the license, refuse it, or refer the question to a medical advisory panel, a group of experts who advise the state about the correct procedures to follow and about individual cases. If DOMV personnel refuse to grant a license, the applicant may be able to appeal to the medical advisory panel, and this body may contact the physician for more information. On the basis of the panel's recommendation, the applicant may subsequently may be granted or denied licensure. In all states, the denial of a license can be appealed.

Perhaps the most difficult problem that the physician faces occurs when a patient with poorly controlled seizures persists in driving despite medical advice. In states with mandatory reporting, the physician is not only allowed to report such behavior but may be required to do so. A model driver licensing statute developed by the Epilepsy Foundation of American proposes that physicians be immunized from suit for reporting, in good faith, patients with seizures who drive despite loss of consciousness or loss of bodily control. Many states have incorporated such language into their law. Although the law is not settled in all jurisdictions, it seems unlikely that a court would find a physician liable for breaching confidentiality if the physician notified the state when a patient refused to comply with medical advice and continued driving despite ongoing seizures that made such driving unsafe.

Physicians may be liable to persons other than their own patients. Most physicians are aware of the Tarasoff case in which a health professional was found liable for not notifying a specifically identified potential victim that a patient was threatening her. Plaintiffs have attempted to hold physicians liable for injuries suffered in automobile accidents with defendant patients. Plaintiffs have sought to hold physicians liable under a number of theories, including telling patients that they could drive, failing to warn patients that they could not drive, failing to warn a patient about the adverse effects of medications, and failing to comply with statutory requirements. The law is not settled in this area.

Additional information about the status of state and federal laws in this ever-changing area can be found at www.epilepsyfoundation.org. In addition, information for individual states can be accessed through individual state's DOMV Web sites. A case history and recommendations for the physician are considered in Figure 28.1.

Two weeks ago, a 22-year-old college student had a first seizure following a period of substantial sleep deprivation (while preparing for college final exams) and heavy alcohol intake (after the last exam was completed). Today, he is in his family doctor's office and mentions that he drove to the physician's office in his new car. What should the family physician do? What are the key issues to consider? Will a neurologist help?

Make a medical judgment about what, if any, driving restrictions you believe are appropriate for this patient. Issues to consider may include: the type of seizure; whether or not the patient is on medication; neurologic examination; other medical conditions. A neurologist may be helpful in considering this issue. The patient asks if you will report him to the state authorities? How will you respond?

Be aware that all states have laws about patients who drive and have episodes involving altered consciousness and loss of motor control. Know the specific rules about driver licensing for your state. Check the Epilepsy Foundation of America Web site or the Department of Motor Vehicles Web site for your state to make sure that you are aware of the latest rules for your state. After checking your state's requirements, if they seem overly stringent, what are your medical options?

Advise the patient of your own medical advice regarding driving. Also, advise the patient of the relevant state rules regarding driving. From a risk management perspective, you should not give the patient any advice or directives that are less restrictive than the state law. If you believe that a less restrictive option is indicated in this patient, you can offer to participate in a special petition to the relevant DOMV medical board but you must stress that the state restrictions must be followed. The patient accepts this advice, but still wants to know if you are obligated to report him to the authorities and even if you are not obligated, will you file a report to the driving bureau.

Advise the patient of any state reporting requirements that you, as the physician, must follow. These may include mandatory reporting of the patient (with or without the patient's consent) and completing inquiry forms from the DOMV. Be honest with your patient and tell him exactly what you will do. Are there any other safeguards that you should complete before the patient leaves?

Document your advice to the patient in the chart. Ideally, have the patient document his understanding of your advice and make this part of the chart. Another potential option is to document your advice and have the patient sign the chart page. If the patient drove himself to the office, ensure that the patient has an opportunity to call family or friends for a ride home. After the patient leaves, you will need to complete state or local documentation requirements if there are any. If your medical judgment is that less restrictive rules about driving should be applied to this patient's case, you can participate in the patient's initiated request to the state for official review and assignment of less restrictive rules.

FIGURE 28.1 Legal approach to a new patient with seizures who is driving.

Always Remember

- The most important risk management practices for any physician are to maintain clinical competence and to employ excellent communication.
- While many neurologic diseases can be effectively managed by the primary care physician, the diagnosis of death using neurologic criteria should only be made by a physician knowledgeable in the techniques and experienced in making the diagnosis. In order to avoid misdiagnosis, rigorous adherence to practice parameters and any institution-specific guidelines should occur.
- While informed consent forms can be helpful in documenting a consent discussion, these forms cannot, and should never, replace a dialogue between the patient and the physician about the medical intervention that is being considered; the potential benefits and risks of the intervention; the alternatives to the intervention (including doing nothing) and the potential benefits and risks of those alternatives; and a decision on the part of the patient.
- Physicians who have patients with seizure disorders, and other illnesses that can impact awareness or motor control, must be aware of their state's licensing rules and comply with those rules.

QUESTIONS AND DISCUSSION

1. For informed consent to be valid:
   A. Without exception, it must be given after information is supplied to the patient in an understandable fashion.
   B. It must be given voluntarily.
   C. It must be accompanied by a witnessed form.
   D. The person providing consent does not have to be competent.

The correct answer is B. Answer A is correct ordinarily, but there are exceptions, namely when the patient has waived the information provision or when the physician has used the therapeutic privilege exception (which should be used only cautiously). Answer C is incorrect—although informed consent should be documented, a specific form and witnessing is not absolutely necessary. Informed consent forms may be useful in demonstrating consent, but they are not foolproof, and if they are not "user friendly," they actually can do more harm than good. In all cases, informed consent is invalid if the person giving the consent is incompetent.

2. An adult patient is competent to provide consent unless he has been judged incompetent in legal proceedings. True or false?

The above statement is false. A patient must be both clinically and legally competent to provide informed consent. An adult patient is presumed to be legally competent unless he has been found incompetent in judicial proceedings. Clinical competence is a medical decision. A patient may be clinically incompetent although legally competent.

3. A 50-year-old man is found collapsed on a city street by paramedics who initiate cardiopulmonary resuscitation and take him to the hospital. One hour later, he is in the emergency room on a ventilator, totally unresponsive to all stimuli and without brain stem reflexes. He has a completed donor card. The most appropriate action at this time is:
   A. To pronounce brain death and call the transplant team to come in and recover the organs
   B. To call the family to see if they agree with the organ donation
   C. To observe the patient in the emergency department for 2 more hours to ensure that there is no change in the examination
   D. To transfer the patient to an intensive care setting for further evaluation and workup

The correct answer is D. There is no clear etiology for this patient's clinical condition; there is no indication that conditions that can produce this clinical picture, but that might be reversible (e.g., drug overdose), have been ruled out. It is unlikely that a complete examination to establish death (using neurologic criteria) has occurred in this setting. This patient should receive additional evaluation prior to being declared dead.

Although the family's consent for organ retrieval is not absolutely necessary in the presence of a valid organ donor card, most physicians wish to obtain consent of next of kin prior to organ retrieval.

4. In a state with mandatory reporting of persons with seizure disorders, the physician has a duty to inform the patient's family and employer of the diagnosis. True or false?

The above statement is false. Mandatory reporting requirements apply only to the specific state agency mentioned in the statute. Disclosure to any other person or institution is precluded by the physician's duty to maintain patient confidences.

5. Actions to be taken when a patient with uncontrolled seizures continues to operate a motor vehicle include the following:
   A. Educate the patient about the risks to himself and others.
   B. Carefully document discussions with the patient about driving and have the patient document his understanding of the discussion in the record as well.
   C. In states with mandatory reporting, conform to the requirements of the applicable statute.
   D. In cases in which patient education has been ineffective and the patient continues to place himself or herself and others at risk by driving despite poor control of seizures, inform the patient of the need to report to the state Department of Motor Vehicles, and do so.
   E. All are correct.

The correct answer is E. Patient education is an important aspect of handling driving restrictions because of uncontrolled seizures. When a patient with uncontrolled seizures persists in driving despite warnings of the risk to self and others, the physician should inform the patient of the need to report to the state. Some states provide immunity for the physician who reports in these instances. Although not all states provide immunities, it is unlikely that a suit for breach of confidentiality would be successful. In some states, a physician may be found liable for failing to report dangerous behavior on the part of the patient.

SUGGESTED READING

A definition of irreversible coma: report of the Ad Hoc Committee of the Harvard Medical School to examine the definition of brain death. *JAMA*. 1968;205:337.

AAA Foundation for Traffic Safety. Medical Fitness to Drive and a Voluntary State Reporting Law. AAA Foundation for Traffic Safety. October 2008. Available at: http://www.aaafoundation.org/pdf/MedicalFitnesstoDriveReport.pdf. Accessed January 2009.

American Academy of Neurology, American Epilepsy Society, and Epilepsy Foundation of America. Consensus statements, sample statutory provisions, and model regulations regarding driver licensing and epilepsy. *Epilepsia*. 1994;35:696–705.

American Medical Association. Patient Physician Relationship Topics, "Informed Consent". Available at: http://www.ama-assn.org/ama/pub/physician-resources/legal-topics/patient-physician-relationship-top/informed-consent.shtml. Accessed January 2009.

Bernat JL. The whole-brain concept of death remains optimum public policy. *J Law Med Ethics*. 2006;34:35–43.

Breitowitz YA. The brain death controversy in Jewish law. Jewish Law Articles. Examining Halacha, Jewish Issues and Secular Law. Available at: http://www.jlaw.com/Articles/ brain.html. Accessed January 2009.

Campbell GH, Lutsep HL. Driving and neurological disease. February 2007. Available at: emedicine.medscape.com/article/1147487. Accessed January 2009.

Canadian Neurocritical Care Group. Guidelines for the diagnosis of brain death. *Can J Neurol Sci*. 2000;26:64–66.

Cruzan v Director, Missouri Department of Health, 497 U.S. 261; 110 S. Ct. 2841 (1990).

Epilepsy Foundation of America. Driver's licensing overview. Available at: http://www.epilepsyfoundation. org/living/wellness/transportation/driverlicensing.cfm. Accessed January 2009.

Epilepsy Foundation of America. State Driving Laws Database. Available at: http://www.epilepsyfoundation.org/ living/wellness/transportation/drivinglaws.cfm. Accessed January 2009.

Shemie S, Pollack MM, Morioka M, et al. Diagnosis of brain death in children. *Lancet Neurol.* 2007;6:87–92.

Hyman v Jewish Chronic Disease Hospital, 251 N.Y. 2d 818 (1964), 206 N.E. 2d 338 (1965).

Jain S, DeGeorgia M. Brain death-associated reflexes and automatisms. *Neurocrit Care.* 2005;3:122–126.

Lustig BA. Theoretical and clinical concerns about brain death: the debate continues. *J Med Philos.* 2001; 26(5):447.

Matter of Eichner, 52 N.Y.2d 363, 420 N.E.2d 64, 438 N.Y.S.2d 266 (1981).

Matter of Fosmire, 75 N.Y.2d 218, 551 N.E.2d 77, 551 N.Y.S.2d 876 (1990).

Matter of K.L., 1 N.Y.3d 362, 806 N.E.2d 480, 774 N.Y.S. 2d 472 (2004).

Matter of Storar, 52 N.Y.2d 363, 420 N.E.2d 64, 438 N.Y.S.2d 266 (1981).

National Institutes of Health. A collaborative study: an appraisal of the criteria of cerebral death—a summary statement. *JAMA.* 1977;237:982.

N.J. Stat Sec. 26:6A-1 "New Jersey Declaration of Death Act" (2008) and N.J.A.C. 10:8-2.3 "Advance Directives to Make Health Care Decisions, Do Not Resuscitate Orders (DNR Orders), and Declaration of Death" (2008).

Odrobina JL. 2004 John M. Manos Writing Competition on Evidence: The Lingering Questions of a Supreme Court Decision: The Confines of the Psychotherapist–Patient Privilege, 52 Clev. St. L. Rev. 551 (2004).

Ohio Revised Code Section 1337.12, "Durable Power of Attorney for Health Care" (2008) and Ohio Revised Code Chapter 2133; "Modified Uniform Rights of the Terminally Ill Act and the DNR Identification and Do-Not-Resuscitate Order Law" (2008).

President's Commission for the Study of Ethical Problems in Medicine and Biomedical and Behavioral Research. Defining death: a report on the medical, legal and ethical issues in the determination of death, 1981.

Quality Standards Committee. American Academy of Neurology. Practice parameters for determining brain death in adults (summary statement). *Neurology.* 1995;45:1012–1014.

Schiavo v Schiavo, 544 U.S. 957, 125 S.Ct. 1722 (2005).

Schloendorff v Society of New York Hospitals, 211 N.Y. 125, 105 N.E. 2d 92 (1914).

Shaner DM, Orr MD, Drought T, et al. Really, most sincerely dead. Policy and procedure in the diagnosis of death by neurologic criteria. *Neurology.* 2004; 62:1683–1686.

Strachan v John F. Kennedy Memorial Hospital, 583 A. 2d 346 (N. J. 1988).

The Health Insurance Portability and Accountability Act of 1996, Public Law 104-191 (HIPAA), Privacy Rule. Available at: http://www.hhs.gov/ocr/privacy/index. html. Accessed January 2009.

Uniform Determination of Death Act, Drafted by the National Conference of Commissioners on Uniform State Laws 1980, Approved by the American Medical Association, October 19, 1980, Approved by the American Bar Association, February 19, 1981.

Wijdicks E. The diagnosis of brain death. *N Engl J Med.* 2001;344:1215.

Wijdicks EFM. Brain death worldwide: accepted fact but no global consensus in diagnostic criteria. *Neurology.* 2002;58:20–25.

Wolfe S. Law & bioethics: from values to violence. *J Law Med Ethics.* 2004;32:293.

Index

Page numbers followed by *f* indicate figures; those followed by *t* indicate tabular material.

A

Abducens nerve (CN VI), 544
  coma and, 95, 96
  eye muscles and, 7
Abductor dysphonia, 243
Abnormal sensory weighting
  falls associated with, 435
Abscess
  brain, 494–495
    clinical features, 494
    laboratory findings, 494
    management and prognosis, 495
    in posterior temporal lobe, 495*f*
    symptoms, 494
    treatment of, 495
Absence epilepsy
  children and, 145
Abulia
  TBI and, 338
Academy of Neurology, 295
ACD. *See* Alcoholic cerebellar degeneration
Acetazolamide
  Ménière disease and, 421
Acetylcholine receptor (AChR), 359
Acetylcholinesterase (AchE)
  AD and, 298, 299
AchE. *See* Acetylcholinesterase
Achilles tendon reflex, 11
AChR. *See* Acetylcholine receptor
Acid maltase deficiency
  McArdle disease and, 346*t*, 365
Acoustic nerve (cranial nerve VIII), 8–9
  assessment of, 9
  dysfunction of, 9
  testing methods, 9
Acoustic neuroma
  neighborhood signs and, 424
Acquired hepatocerebral degeneration (AHCD)
  alcoholism and, 475–476
  diagnosis, 475
  pathophysiology of, 475
  symptoms and signs, 475

  treatment of, 476
  versus Wilson disease, 475
Acquired immunodeficiency syndrome (AIDS), 504
  dementia and, 291
Acute alteration of mental status, 69–74
  causes of, 71
  cerebellar stroke and, 70–71
  characterizations of, 69
  delirium and, 69
  diagnostic testing for, 73
  herpes simplex encephalitis and, 69–70
  intracranial hematoma and, 70
  metabolic encephalopathies and, 71
  neuroimaging and, 73
  neurologic examination and, 73
  patient history and, 72
  treatment of, 73–74
Acute bacterial meningitis, 489–491
  diagnosis of, 489
  risk factors, 491
  treatment of, 489, 490–491
    seizures, 490
Acute demyelinating polyneuropathy
  neurorehabilitation intervention and, 558
Acute disseminated encephalomyelitis (ADEM), 200
Acute epidural hematoma, 70
  CT brain scan and, 70
Acute hospitalization
  TBI and, 330
Acute intermittent porphyria
  Guillain-Barré syndrome *vs.*, 81, 82, 82*t*
Acute intracranial hypertension
  causes of
    herniation risks and, 75, 75*t*
    cranium components of, 74
    symptoms and signs of, 75, 76
    treatment of, 76–77
Acute ischemic stroke
  hierarchy of, 110, 110*t*
  interventional therapy for rt-PA and, 109
Acute necrotizing hemorrhagic encephalopathy
  (ANHE), 200

Acute neuroleptic-induced dystonia
    anticholinergics and, 458
    neuroleptic therapy and, 458
    risk factors for, 458
Acute optic neuritis, 519
Acute peripheral vestibulopathy
    as cause of vertigo, 419–420
    pharmacologic treatments for, 420f
Acute spinal cord compression
    causes of, 77, 77t
    diagnosis of, 78
    symptoms of, 77–78
    treatment of, 78–79
Acute subdural hematomas, 70
Acyclovir
    herpes simplex encephalitis and, 69
    side effects of, 448
        encephalitis, 493
    viral meningitis and, 489
AD. *See* Alzheimer's disease
ADC. *See* Apparent diffusion coefficient
ADD. *See* Attentional deficit disorder
Additives
    neurotoxic effects of, 464–466
ADEAR. *See* Alzheimer's Disease Education and
        Referral Center
ADEM. *See* Acute disseminated encephalomyelitis
Adenocarcinoma
    brain metastases and, 505
Adenosine receptors
    caffeine and, 464
ADHD. *See* Attention deficit hyperactivity
        disorder
Adie's pupil, 536–537, 537f
Administrative law
    health care and, 574
Adrenergic drugs
    neurologic effects of, 456
Adrenergic receptors
    three types of, 456
Adult-onset craniocervical dystonia, 247
Adult-onset primary dystonia, 247
Adults
    precipitants of SE in, 65
Advanced-sleep-phase syndrome, 170
AED. *See* Antiepileptic drug
Afebrile seizure, 143
Affect
    mania and, 3
Aging
    falls increases with, 428

Agitation
    TBI and, 336–338, 337f
AHCD. *See* Acquired hepatocerebral degeneration
AHI. *See* Apnea-hypopnea index
AICA. *See* Anterior inferior cerebellar artery
AIDS (acquired immunodeficiency syndrome)
    ICH and, 118
AION. *See* Anterior ischemic optic neuropathy
Akathisia
    anti dopaminergic agents and, 458
Akinesia
    Parkinson's disease and, 231
Akinetic rigid syndrome, 226
Akinetic seizures, 144
Albuterol
    neurologic complications and, 456
Alcohol abuse
    due to cirrhosis, 474
Alcoholic cerebellar degeneration (ACD)
    alcoholism and, 478
    cerebellar abnormalities in, 478
Alcoholic dementia
    alcoholism and, 478–479
Alcoholic myopathy
    versus alcoholic neuropathy, 481
    alcoholism and, 480–482
    as cause of muscle disease, 481
    clinical syndrome of, 481
    diagnosis, 481
    neurologic examination of, 481–482
    risk factors, 481
    treatment of, 482
Alcoholic neuropathy
    alcoholism and, 479–480
    due to thiamine deficiency, 480
    neurologic examination of, 479
    prognosis, 480
    signs and symptoms, 479
    treatment of, 480
    variant of, 480
Alcohol intoxication, 470
    acute alteration in mental status and, 71–72
    cluster headache and, 131
    coma and, 93t, 94
    dementia and, 291
    early morning awakening, 170
    hypnotic drugs and, 165
    toxic myopathies and, 366
Alcohol intoxification
    ET and, 255, 258
Aldolase, 354

Alexander's law
    for vestibular nystagmus, 547
Alexia without agraphia
    in cortical blindness, 529
Alkaline phosphatase, 406
Almotriptan
    migraine and, 134
Alpha agonist midodrine
    orthostatic hypotension and, 414
Alpha EEG arousal, 175
Alpha-fetoprotein, 507
Alpha receptors
    prazosin and, 453
Alprazolam
    ET and, 258, 259
    MS and, 217
    sleep and, 164
ALS. *See* Amyotrophic lateral sclerosis
Alternative therapies
    MS and, 218
    sleep cycle and, 166
Alveolar hypoventilation syndrome
    OSA and, 174
Alzheimer, A.
    dementia and, 287
Alzheimer's Association, 301
Alzheimer's disease, 287, 320, 526
    alternative treatments for, 300
    ancillary tests, 294–295
    clinical symptoms of, 292–294
    community resources for, 301–302
    diagnosis of, 293–294
    epidemiology of, 292
    hospitalized patients and, 302, 303
    MCI and, 288
    neurologic examination and, 293–294
    pathology of, 295–297
    prognosis, 302
    treatment of, 298–301, 298*f*
        pharmacologic, 300–301
Alzheimer's Disease Education and Referral Center
        (ADEAR), 301
Amantadine
    HD and, 265
    Parkinson's disease and, 228
    side effects of, 448
    sleep–wake cycle and, 331, 331*t*
    TD syndrome and, 283
Amaurosis fugax, 528
AmBisome, 492
Ambulation

disequilibrium and, 423
gait examination with, 15
American Academy of Neurology
    concussive injury and, 339
    laboratory and, 40
    Parkinson's therapy and, 229
American Congress of Rehabilitation Medicine,
        338, 339*f*
Amikacin
    side effects of, 447
Aminoglycoside antibiotics
    disequilibrium and, 424
    neurotoxic effects of, 447
Aminoglycosides hearing loss, 447
Aminophylline
    bronchoconstriction and, 456
Amiodarone
    neurotoxic effect of, 452
Amitriptyline (Elavil), 339
    early morning awakening and, 170
    MS and, 217
Ammonia, 6
Amniocentesis
    Becker dystrophy, 362
Amphetamines
    ICH and, 118
    narcolepsy and, 180
Amphotericin B
    systemic fungal infection and, 447
Amsler grid
    MS and, 202
Amyotrophic lateral sclerosis (ALS), 351*f*,
        358–359, 385
    cause of, 358
    family history of, 358–359
    pseudobulbar affect in, 359
    weakness and, 358
Anaerobic bacteria
    in brain abscesses, 494
Analgesics
    rebound headache and, 130, 130*t*
Anaplastic astrocytoma
    radiation therapy and, 501
    therapeutic agents for, 501
Anesthesia
    hypersomnia and, 184
    malignant hyperthermia and, 366
    MS and, 217
    treatment of refractory SE and, 68
Aneurysmal rupture, 120
    complications of, 121*t*

Aneurysmal sac
  cerebral aneurysms and, 121
Aneurysmal subarachnoid hemorrhage
  epidemiology and, 120
Angiography
  catheter, 36–37
  magnetic resonance, 36
Angiotensin-converting enzyme inhibitors
  neurologic effect of, 454
  RAA axis for, 454
ANHE. *See* Acute necrotizing hemorrhagic
      encephalopathy
Anisocoria, 532–537
  Horner syndrome, 532–535, 533*f*
  in light and darkness, 532, 532*f*
  pharmacologic dilation, 537
  physiologic, 532
  third nerve palsy mydriasis, 535–536, 535*f*
  tonic pupil, 536–537, 537*f*
"Ankle jerk." *See* Achilles tendon reflex
Anosagnosia, 24
Anoxia
  comatose patient and, 100
Anoxic injury
  and TBI, 326
Antacids, aluminum
  neurologic symptoms from, 456
Antacids, magnesium
  neurologic symptoms from, 456
Antalgic gait, 27
Anterior horn cells, 355, 359
Anterior inferior cerebellar artery (AICA)
  vertigo and, 422
Anterior ischemic optic neuropathy (AION), 528
Anterocollis, 248
Antiacidity agents
  neurologic effects of, 456
Antianginal agents
  neurologic effect of, 451
Antiarrhythmics
  neurologic effect of, 451–452
Antibiotics
  aminoglycosides, 447
  antifungal agents, 447
  antituberculous drugs, 447–448
  antiviral drugs, 448
  bacterial meningitis and, 489, 490*t*
  brain abscess and, 495
  cephalosporins, 447
  penicillins, 447
Antibody testing, 386

Anticholinergics
  acute neuroleptic-induced dystonia, 458
  dystonia and, 252
Anticoagulant therapy
  in ischemic stroke, 116
  TEE and, 112
Anticonvulsants
  disequilibrium and, 424
  in vestibular dysfunction, 424
Antidepressant agents
  neurologic effects of, 459–461
Antidiarrheals
  neurologic effects of, 455–456
Antidopaminergics, RLS and, 171
Antiemetics
  neurologic effects of, 455
Antiepileptic drugs (AED)
  discontinuing, 153
  individual, 151–152
  levels of, 150–151
  for management of HSE, 70
  properties of, 150*t*
  SE and, 66
  seizures and, 148
Antifungal agents
  neurologic effect of, 447
Antiinflammatory agents
  hormones, 463–464
  neurologic effects of, 461–466
  nonsteroidal agents, 463
  salicylate compounds, 461–462
  steroids, 462–463
  vitamins and additives, 464–466
Antineuronal specific antibodies, 512, 513*t*
Antiretroviral medications
  neurologic effect of, 449
Antituberculous drugs
  neurologic effect of, 447–448
Antiviral drugs
  neurologic effect of, 448
Anton syndrome
  in cortical blindness, 529
Anxiety
  MS and, 217
Anxiolytics
  neurotoxic effects of, 459
Aortic stenosis
  exercise-related presyncope and, 415
Aphasia, 3, 22
Apnea
  coma and, 94

Apnea-hypopnea index (AHI)
    sleep apnea severity and, 175
Apnea testing
    brain death and, 580
Apneustic respiration
    coma and, 94
Apolipoprotein e4 allele
    AD and, 288, 292
Apoptic cell death
    HD and, 264
Apparent diffusion coefficient (ADC), 35
Appearance and behavior
    mental status examination and, 2
Apraclonidine
    for glaucoma, 534
Aqueductal stenosis, 50f
Arbovirus
    encephalitis and, 496
Areflexia
    Adie's pupil and, 536, 537f
    Guillain–Barré syndrome and, 12, 81
Argyll Robertson pupils, 538
Aripiprazole
    TD syndrome, 281
Arrhythmia
    cardiac presyncope and, 415
Arteriovenous malformations (AVMs), 34, 106
    embryonal development and, 121–122
Arthritis
    medication side effects of, 463
Artificial hyperventilation, 413
Aseptic meningitis
    ibuprofen and, 463
Asomatagnosia, 24
Aspiration
    management of
        neurologic illness and, 557
Aspirin
    ischemic stroke and, 116
    stroke prevention and, 115
Assistive device
    fall prevention by, 441–442
Asterixis
    in hepatic encephalopathy, 474
Asthma
    propranolol and, 257
Astrocytoma, 500–502
    chemotherapy for, 501
    clinical presentation, 500–501
    diagnosis, 501
    Kernohan grading system of, 500
    radiation therapy for, 501

temozolomide for, 501–502
    treatment of, 501–502
Asymmetric extensor toe signs
    coma and, 98
Ataxia, 14
    acquired causes of, 433
    AED and, 151
    falling associated with, 432–433
        medical treatment for, 439
    gait disorders and, 28
    inherited causes of, 432–433
    midline cerebellar dysfunction and, 14
    phenytoin and, 151
    in vertigo, 417
Ataxic gait, 15
Ataxic respirations
    coma and, 94–95
Atherosclerosis
    ischemic stroke and, 114
Atherosclerotic plaque
    ischemic stroke risk and, 114
Atonic seizures, 144
ATP7B
    WD and, 269
Atrophy of muscles, 351–352
Atropine
    for cardiac arrhythmias, 537
    pupillary size and, 95
Attentional deficit disorder (ADD), 461
Attention deficit hyperactivity disorder (ADHD)
    GTS and, 275, 278
Auditory toxicity
    drugs and, 447
Auras, 144
Autoimmune disease
    MS and, 196
Autoimmune process
    systemic cancer and, 512, 512t
Automatisms
    TLE and, 310
Autonomic dysfunction
    neurorehabilitation intervention and, 558
Autonomic dysreflexia
    neurorehabilitation intervention and, 558
Autonomic neuropathies
    orthostatic hypotension and, 414
Autosomal recessive disorder, 366
AVMs. See Arteriovenous malformations
Avonex
    MS and, 209, 210, 211, 212
Axial dystonia, 243
Axon

and TBI, 326
Azathioprine
  MG and, 360
Azithromycin
  neurotoxicity and, 449

B
Babinski's sign, 10, 12
  HD and, 260
  MS and, 202
Backward spelling
  for working memory testing, 3
Baclofen
  dystonia and, 253
  spasticity treatment and, 214t, 215, 439
Bacterial endocarditis
  blood cultures and, 112
  as complication of tumor therapy, 510
Bacterial meningitis, 489–491
  focal neurologic signs of, 489
  infecting organisms in
    initial antibiotic therapy for, 490t
Bacteroides fragilis
  brain abscess and, 494
BAEP. See Brainstem auditory evoked potential
BAER. See Brainstem auditory evoked response
Balance disorders, 27
Balance Evaluation Systems Test (BESTest), 440
Balance systems
  constraints on, 434, 434t
  falling associated with, 434–437
Balance tests, 15, 440
Balance training
  fall prevention by, 440
Balint syndrome, 530
Barbiturates, 150, 153
  neurologic effects of, 461
Barotrauma
  perilymph fistula syndrome and, 421
Basal ganglia
  dystonic movements and, 243
  GTS and, 276
  HD and, 264
  postural stability, 14
Basal skull fracture, 94
Basilar migraine
  in vertigo, 423
Basiliximab
  neurologic effect of, 450
Battle's sign
  coma and, 94

Becker dystrophy, 361–362
Behavior
  mental status examination and, 2
Behavioral disorders
  GTS and, 275
  severe
    TBI and, 341
Behavioral neurology
  anatomic lesions of, 311–312
  etiology of, 312
  overview, 307–308
  Papez circuit, 308–309, 308f
  refer neurologists, 312–313
  TLE and, 309–311
Behavioral sequelae
  of TBI, 325
Behavioral therapies, insomnia and, 161–162
Bell palsy, 8, 386, 540
Benign paroxysmal positional vertigo (BPPV),
    418–419, 433
  treatment of, 418
Benzodiazepines, 333
  acute alteration in mental status and, 74
  alcohol and
    acute alteration in mental status and, 72
  disadvantage of, 68
  dystonia and, 253
  liver function and, 166
  neurologic effects of, 459
  SE and, 65, 66, 68
  sleep and, 162
  for spasticity, 439
  in vestibular dysfunction, 424
Berg Balance Scale, 439–440
BESTest. See Balance Evaluation Systems Test
Beta-blockers
  head injuries and, 335
  migraine and, 135
  MS and, 216
  side effects of, 258
  TBI and, 337
Beta human chorionic gonadotropin, 507
Beta interferons (IFNα)
  MS and, 210–211, 210t
Betaseron
  MS and, 209, 210
Bevacizumab, 511
Bilateral decerebrate posturing
  coma and, 98
Bilateral light-near dissociation, 537–538
  Argyll Robertson pupils, 538
  Parinaud syndrome, 538

Bilevel positive airway pressure (BiPAP), 80
   sleep apnea and, 178
Bilevel positive airway pressure in spontaneous-timed
      mode (BPAP-ST)
   central sleep apnea and, 178
Biofeedback
   primary headaches and, 133
Biopsy
   of brain tissue, 39
   muscle, 39–40, 357
      oculopharyngeal dystrophy, 363
   nerve, 39–40, 357
   skin, 40
Biopterin
   DRD and, 251
BiPAP. *See* Bilevel positive airway pressure
Bitemporal hemianopias, 6, 522–523
Bitter orange *(Citrus aurantium)*
   ephedrine and, 183
Bladder dysfunction
   MS and, 203–204
      treatment of, 215–216
   neurorehabilitation and, 556
Blepharospasm, 243, 247
   features aggravating, 247
   GTS and, 273
   myectomy of orbicularis oculi for, 253
   toxic injection for, 253
Blepharospasm–oromandibular dystonia syndrome.
      See Meige syndrome
Blindsight
   in cortical blindness, 529
Blinking
   coma and, 95
Blood–brain barrier
   levodopa and, 227
Blood pressure
   stroke and, 107, 114
Blood urea nitrogen (BUN)
   comatose patient and, 99
Bony spine pain, 402
Borrelia burgdorferi, 491
Botulinum toxin (BoNT)
   dystonia and, 253
   focal dystonias and, 253, 254
   GTS and, 278
   injections of
      spasticity, 439
      TD syndrome, 283
   migraine and, 136
Botulinum toxin A (Botox)

cervical dystonia and, 253
   ET and, 259
Botulinum toxin B
   cervical dystonia and, 253
Botulism
   Guillain-Barré syndrome *vs.*, 82, 82*t*
Bowel dysfunction
   MS and, 204
      treatment in, 216
   neurorehabilitation and, 556
BPAP. *See* Bilevel positive airway pressure
BPPV. *See* Benign paroxysmal positional vertigo
Brachial dystonia, 243
Brachial plexus, 376
   terminal nerves of, 378
Bradykinesia
   levodopa induced dyskinesia v., 231
   Parkinson's disease and, 225
Brain
   evaluation of, 47
   MS, 204, 205*t*
Brain abscess, 494–495
   clinical features, 494
   dementia and, 291
   laboratory findings, 494
   management and prognosis, 495
   in posterior temporal lobe, 495*f*
   symptoms, 494
   treatment of, 495
Brain biopsy, 39
Brain death
   aspects determining, 578–581
   diagnosis of, 578–581
   laws governing, 578–581
Brain hemorrhage
   low platelet count and, 118
Brain herniation
   mass lesions associated with, 75, 75*t*
Brain injury. *See also* Traumatic brain injury
   low-level, 331
   postacute hospitalization, 331
   primary generalized epilepsies and, 144–145
   RLA and, 328
   severity of, 329*f*
Brain metastases, 507*f*
   chemotherapy for, 506–507
   diagnosis of, 506
   radiation therapy for, 506
   risk factors, 505
   signs and symptoms, 506
   treatment of, 506–507

Brain scan. *See also* Computed tomography imaging; Magnetic resonance imaging
   AD and, 294
Brainstem auditory evoked potential (BAEP), 38
Brainstem auditory evoked response (BAER), 38
   MS and, 208
Brainstem lesions
   characteristics of, 24
Brainstem reflexes
   brain death and, 580
Brain tumor
   dementia and, 290
Breathing
   sleep apnea and, 175, 177
Bretylium
   neurologic effect of, 452
Bromocriptine
   Parkinson's disease and, 227
   Parkinson's therapy and, 229
   sleep–wake cycle and, 331, 331*t*
   TD syndrome, 283
Brun's nystagmus, 547
BuChE. *See* Butyrylcholinesterase
Bulbar dysfunction
   pneumonia, 370
BUN. *See* Blood urea nitrogen
Bupropion
   MS and, 217
Butyrophenones
   HD and, 265
Butyrylcholinesterase (BuChE)
   AD and, 299

C
Caffeine
   herbal medicinal products with, 183
   neurotoxic effects of, 464–465
Caffein–halothane contracture test
   for malignant hyperthermia, 366
CAG. *See* Cytosin–adenin–guanine
CAG trinucleotide repeat
   huntingtin protein and, 263, 264
Calcium channel blockers
   GTS and, 278
   migraine and, 135
   neurologic effect of, 453
Cancer, 499
   challenges for, 513
   metastatic complications of systemic

intracranial metastases, 504–507, 505*f*
   leptomeningeal metastases, 507–509
   spinal metastases, 509–510
nonmetastatic complications
   cerebrovascular, 510–511
   metabolic and nutritional, 511
   paraneoplastic syndromes, 511–512, 513*t*
primary CNS lymphoma, 504
primary CNS tumors
   astrocytoma, 500–502
   ependymoma, 502–503
   meningiomas, 503
   oligodendroglioma, 502
radiation therapy, complications from, 512–513
Cane
   fall prevention by, 441–442
Carbamazepine, 340
   dystonia and, 252–253
   seizures and, 151
Carbidopa
   Parkinson's disease and, 227
Carbidopa-levodopa (Sinemet)
   complications of, 230–232
   dosage of, 238
   Parkinson's disease and, 229, 232
   RLS and, 168
   side effects of, 168
   sleep-related eating disorders and, 186
   toxicity associated with, 230*t*
Carcinoembryonic antigen, 507
Carcinomatous meningitis, 506
Cardiac arrhythmias
   seizures *vs.*, 149
   status epilepticus and, 65
Cardiac complications
   neuromuscular disorder and, 370
Cardiac conduction block
   DMI and, 363
Cardiac conduction disturbances
   in myotonic dystrophy, 370
Cardiac drugs
   angiotensin-converting enzyme inhibitors, 454
   antianginal agents, 451
   antiarrhythmics, 451–452
   cholesterol-lowering agents, 454
   diuretics, 452–453
   glycosides, 450–451
   sympatholytics, 453
   vasodilators, 453
Cardiac dysrhythmias
   phenytoin IV and, 66

Cardiac evaluation
  embolism and, 112
Cardiac presyncope, 415
Cardiogenic attacks
  seizures vs., 149
Cardiogenic stroke, 106
Cardiovascular diseases and OSA, 174
Carnitine deficiency
  symptoms of, 366
Carnitine palmitoyl transferase deficiency
      (CPT II), 365
Carotid dissection syndromes
  secondary headache disorders and, 137
Carotid endarterectomy
  stroke prevention and, 113, 115
Carotid ischemia
  vertebrobasilar distribution ischemia vs., 113, 113t
Carotid sinus hypersensitivity
  as cause of presyncope, 415
Carotid syndromes
  headache and, 137
Carpal tunnel syndrome (CTS), 380, 392
Case law, 573
Cataplexy, 179
  tricyclic antidepressants and, 183
Catathrenia, 186
Catechol-O-methyltransferase (COMT)
  Parkinson's disease and, 227
Catechol-O-methyltransferase (COMT) inhibitors
  Parkinson's disease and, 230, 232
Catheter angiography, 36–37
Catnip (Nepeta cataria)
  sleep cycle and, 166–167
Cauda equina syndrome, 402
  surgical consultation, 406
CBF. See Cerebral blood flow
CBGD. See Corticobasal ganglionic degeneration
Celecoxib
  AD and, 300
Centers for Medicare and Medicaid Services,
      295, 297
Central herniation syndrome, 75
Central integration, abnormalities of
  in disequilibrium, 424
Central nervous system (CNS), 45, 91, 375
  lesions
    MS and, 204
  MS and, 192
  secondary dystonia and, 251
  status epilepticus, 63–65
    causes of, 64, 65

complications of, 68
convulsive, 64
CT brain scan and, 68
defined, 64
morbidity, 64
mortality rate, 64
nonconvulsive, 64
patient history and, 68
precipitants of, 65
refractory, 68
treatment of, 65–69, 66t, 67t
type of, 64
WD and, 268
Central neurogenic hyperventilation
  coma and, 94
Central pontine myelinolysis (CPM)
  alcoholism and, 477
  signs and symptoms, 477
  treatment of, 477
Central scotoma, 521
Central sleep apnea
  respiratory control and, 174
  treatment of, 178
  v. OSA, 174
Central vertigo, 416–417, 416t, 421
  associated with brainstem, 417
  causes of
    basilar migraine, 423
    cerebellar hemorrhage, 422–423
    lateral medullary ischemia, 422
    lateral pontine ischemia, 422
    multiple sclerosis, 423
    transient ischemic attack, 422
  cerebellar signs in, 417
Centrocecal scotoma, 521
  MS and, 202
Cephalosporins
  neurologic effect of, 447
Cerebellar hemorrhage
  in vertigo, 422–423
Cerebellar kinetic tremor, 256–257
Cerebellar outflow rubral tremor, 257
Cerebellar stroke, 70–71
  acute alteration of mental status and, 70–71
  management of, difficulties in, 70–71
Cerebellar tremor
  types of, 256–257
Cerebellum
  disorders of
    ataxic gait and, 27
  metastasis of, 507f

Cerebral achromatopsia, 530
Cerebral aneurysm
   anterior circulation and, 120
Cerebral aneurysm, ruptured
   clinical manifestations of, 120–121
   complications of, 121*t*
Cerebral arteriography
   aneurysm and, 120, 120*f*
Cerebral blood flow (CBF)
   intracranial hypertension and, 74
Cerebral dysfunction
   acute alteration in mental status and, 71
Cerebral hypoperfusion
   intracranial hypertension and, 74
Cerebral infarction
   consciousness and, 91
   secondary dystonia and, 251
Cerebral perfusion pressure (CPP)
   intracranial hypertension and, 74
Cerebral somatostatin
   dystonia and, 252
Cerebral vascular accident (CVA)
   pallidotomy and, 233
Cerebral venous occlusion
   headache and, 137
   secondary headache disorders and, 137
Cerebrospinal fluid (CSF), 65, 332, 389
   Alzheimer's disease and, 288
   CNS infections and, 496
   inflammation and
      PP-MS and, 198
   lumbar puncture and, 70
   neoplastic meningitis and, 507–508
Cerebrospinal fluid (CSF) pressure
   secondary headache disorders and, 137
Cerebrospinal fluid rhinorrhea
   coma and, 94
Cerebrovascular complications
   as result of malignancy, 510–511
Ceruloplasmin
   WD and, 268
Ceruloplasmin level
   WD and, 269
Cervical dystonia, 243, 248–249, 248*f*, 249*f*
   BoNT and, 253
   characterization of, 248, 248*f*
   ET v., 256
   factors that exacerbate, 248–249
Cervical neck fracture
   coma and, 94
Cervical spine, 400*f*

Channelopathies, 363
   affecting skeletal muscle, 364
Charcot-Marie-Tooth disease, 381, 387
Charles Bonnet syndrome
   in cortical blindness, 529
Chelation therapy
   Parkinson's disease and, 236
   WD and, 272
Chemotherapy
   neurotoxicity of, 512*t*
Cheyne–Stokes respiration
   coma and, 94, 99*t*
CHI. *See* Closed-head injury
Chiari malformation
   MS v., 209
Chiasmal injury, 522–523, 522*f*
Childhood-onset dystonia, 242
Children
   anticholinergics and, 252
   delayed-onset dystonia in, 251
   disorders of arousal and, 185
   DM and, 363, 364
   DUD and, 362
   epilepsy syndromes in, 145
   hypnotic drugs and, 165–166
   neuroleptics and
      tics and, 278
   neuromuscular disease and, 367–368
   phenytoin and, 151
   seizure and, 144, 146
      EEG diagnoses of, 148
   with type 2 SMA, 368
Cholesterol-lowering agents
   neurologic effects of, 454
Cholinergic crisis, 79
Cholinesterase inhibitors
   AD and, 299
Chorea, 242, 464
   HD and, 260, 261, 265
   Parkinson's disease and, 230, 231
   TD syndrome and, 283
Chorea, 11
Choreiform movement disorders, 251, 285
   HD and, 260
   Parkinson's disease and, 237
   TD syndrome and, 280, 283
Chorionic villus biopsy
   Becker dystrophy, 362
Chromosome
   disorder and, 358
Chromosome 5, 358

Chromosome 19
    AD and, 292
Chronic active hepatitis
    WD and, 267
Chronic daily headache
    clinical subtypes of, 130
Chronic disulfiram therapy, 461
Chronic inflammatory demyelinating polyradicu-
        loneuropathy (CIDP), 39, 390
Chronic insomnia, 160
Chronic migraine, 129
    comorbid conditions with, 129
Chronic obstructive lung disease
    propranolol and, 257
Chronic paroxysmal hemicrania (CPH)
    indomethacin and, 137
    treatment of, 137
Chronotherapy, 161
CIDP. See Chronic inflammatory demyelinating
        polyradiculoneuropathy
Cimetidine (Tagamet)
    neurologic effects of, 456
Cinnarizine
    neurologic effect of, 453
Ciprofloxacin, 491
Circadian rhythm sleep disorders, 160
Cirrhosis
    alcohol abuse due to, 474
    WD and, 267
Cisplatin, 511
Citalopram
    MS and, 217
CJD. See Creutzfeldt-Jakob disease
Clarithromycin
    neurologic effect of, 449
Claude syndrome, 542
Clinical competence
    medical decision of, 575
Clofibrate
    neurologic effects of, 454
Clomipramine
    cataplectic attacks and, 183
Clonazepam
    dystonia and, 253
    ET and, 258, 259
    GTS and, 278
    RBD and, 186
    sleep-related eating disorders and, 186
Clonidine
    adverse effects of, 278
    GTS and, 278

    neurologic effect of, 453
    TD syndrome and, 283
Clopidogrel
    stroke prevention and, 115
Closed-head injury (CHI), 330
Clozapine, 238
    dystonia and, 253
    ET and, 259
    GTS and, 277
    HD and, 265, 266
    HD related psychosis, 266
    neurologic effects of, 457–458
    Parkinson's disease and, 231
    TD syndrome and, 279, 281, 282, 283
Cluster breathing
    coma and, 94
Cluster headache
    clinical features of, 131
    migraine headache vs., 131, 131t
    treatment for, 136–137
        acute, 136t
        preventive, 136, 136t, 137
CNPase. See Cyclic nucleotide
        3′-phosphohydrolase
CNS. See Central nervous system
CNS infections, 486–496
    brain abscess, 494–495
    encephalitis, 492–494
    identification of, antibiotic therapy for, 490t
    meningitis, 487–492
    prion diseases, 495–496
    spinal fluid profiles in, 488t
CNS lymphoma, primary, 504
CNS tumors, primary
    astrocytoma, 500–502
    ependymoma, 502–503
    meningiomas, 503
    oligodendroglioma, 502
Cocaine, 534
    ICH and, 118
Coccyx, 399
Cochlear nerve, 8
Coenzyme Q10
    HD and, 265
Cognition
    abnormalities of, 4–5
Cognitive domains, primary
    executive function, 3
    memory, 3–4
    perceptual disturbances, 4
    speech and language, 2–3

Cognitive function
 old age and, 287
Cognitive therapy
 insomnia and, 162
 primary headaches and, 133
Cogwheel rigidity
 Parkinson's disease and, 225, 232
Collagen vascular disease
 inflammatory myopathy and, 364
Color desaturation, in eye, 517
Color vision test, 517–518
Coma. *See also* Hepatic coma
 anatomy of, 91
 causes of, 92*t*, 93*t*
 clinical examination with, 93–99
 emergency treatment for, 99
 etiology of, 91–93, 92*t*, 93*t*
 laboratory evaluation of, 99, 100*t*
 patient history and, 93
 pentobarbital and, 330
 prognosis of, 102
 states of, 90
 treatment of, 99–101
Coma recovery score, 331
Comatose patient
 treatment of, 101*t*
Comatose patient, 2
Communicating hydrocephalus, 49
Complete blood count (CBC)
 comatose patient and, 99
 SAH and, 109
 sleep apnea and, 175
Complex motor tics, 273
Complex partial seizures, 144
 phases of, 146
Complex sleep apnea, 174
Complex vocal tics
 GTS and, 273
Computed tomographic angiography (CTA), 36, 46
 infarct evaluation and, 59, 60*f*
Computed tomography (CT), 34–35
 advanced techniques for, 46
 contrast agents used in, 46–17
 infarct evaluation and, 56–60
 versus MRI, 44–46, 45*f*
 in pregnant patients, 46
Computed tomography (CT) imaging
 acute epidural hematoma and, 70
 acute spinal cord compression and, 78
 acute stroke evaluation and, 110
 AD and, 294

aneurysm and, 120, 120*f*
 rapture of, 120–121
 comatose patient and, 100
 DBS and, 259
 rt-PA and, 109, 115, 116*t*
 SAH and, 109
 SE and, 68
 VaD and, 296
 WD and, 270
Computed tomography (CT) scan
 intraparenchymal hemorrhage on, 326
 spine and, 405
 TBI and, 326
COMT. *See* Catechol-O-methyltransferase
Concussive injury, sports-related grade of, 339–340
Conduction velocity (CV), 383
 motor responses with, 383*f*
Congenital muscular dystrophy
 symptoms of, 346*t*
Congenital myopathies, 367
Conjugate gaze abnormalities
 horizontal gaze palsies, 539–541, 540*f*, 541*f*
 supranuclear vertical gaze palsy, 541–542
Conjugate vision pathways, 95, 96*f*
Consciousness, defined, 90
Constipation
 MS and, 204, 216
Content
 abnormalities of, 4
Context-specific instability, 436
Continuous positive airway pressure (CPAP)
 hypersomnia and, 184
 OSA and, 177
Contractures
 rehabilitation and neuromuscular diseases and, 368
Contrast agents
 gadolinium-based, 47
 versus noncontrast agents, 46–47
Contusion, hemorrhagic
 TBI and, 325
Convulsions
 temporal lobe injury and, 146
Coordination, 14–15
 neurologic examination and, 1, 1*t*
 pediatric neurology and, 16
Copaxone
 MS and, 210*t*, 211
Copper
 WD and, 266, 268, 269

Coprolalia
  GTS and, 273
Copropraxia
  GTS and, 273
Cord infarct, 402
Cortical sensory functions
  sensory examination and, 14
Cortical vision loss, 529
Corticobasal ganglionic degeneration (CBGD)
  as cause of parkinsonism in falling, 432
Corticospinal tracts
  lesions of, 24
Corticosteroids
  acute intracranial hypertension and, 76
  acute spinal cord compression and, 78
  for brain metastases, 506
  comatose patient and, 100
  complications of, 511t
  for dermatomyositis, 365
  MS and, 213, 214–215
  myasthenic crisis and, 80
  use in cancer, 511
Counseling
  sleep disorders and, 161
COX. *See* Cytochrome c oxidase
CPH. *See* Chronic paroxysmal hemicrania
CPK. *See* Creatinine phosphokinase
CPM. *See* Central pontine myelinolysis
CPP. *See* Cerebral perfusion pressure
CPT II. *See* Carnitine palmitoyl transferase
    deficiency
Cramps, occupational, 250
Cranial dystonia, 247–248
Cranial nerve(s)
  functions of, 5–6, 5t
  neurologic examination, 1, 1t
  pediatric neurology and, 16
Cranial nerve VIII. *See* Acoustic nerve
Cranial neuropathy, 21, 21t
C-reactive protein (CRP), 406
C-reactive protein (CRP) level
  stroke and, 113
Creatinine phosphokinase (CPK), 84
Creutzfeldt-Jakob disease (CJD), 37, 292, 298,
    495–496, 526
  variant of, –496
CRP. *See* C-reactive protein
Crural dystonia, 243
  clinical presentation in, 246
Cryptococcal meningitis
  dementia and, 291

Cryptococcus neoformans, 491
CSF. *See* Cerebrospinal fluid
CSF analysis
  MS and, 206–208
CT. *See* Computed tomography imaging
CTA. *See* Computed tomographic angiography
CT imaging. *See* Computed tomography imaging
CT myelogram, 405
CTS. *See* Carpal tunnel syndrome
Cumulative cardiotoxicity
  mitoxantrone and, 211
Cup test
  tremor and, 255
Cutaneous root distribution
  sequential nature of, 377
Cutaneous sensation
  pathways for, 25–26
CV. *See* Conduction velocity
CVA. *See* Cerebral vascular accident
Cyclic nucleotide 3′-phosphohydrolase (CNPase)
  MS and, 195
Cyclosporine
  neurologic effect of, 449–450
Cytochrome c oxidase (COX), 366
Cytosin–adenin–guanine (CAG), 358
Cytotoxic edema, 51f
  versus vasogenic edema, 50–51

D
Daclizumab
  neurologic effect of, 450
DAI. *See* Diffuse axonal injury
DAP. *See* 3,4-diaminopyridine
Dapsone, 387
Datura stramonium, 537
DBS. *See* Deep brain stimulation
DDAVP. *See* Desamino-D-arginine vasopressin
Death
  physicians and, 371
Decerebrate (extensor) posturing
  coma and, 98
  midbrain dysfunction and, 98
Decorticate posturing
  coma and, 98
Deep brain stimulation (DBS)
  dystonia and, 253
  ET and, 259
  Parkinson's disease and, 233
Deep hemispheric lesions, 24
Deep tendon reflexes (DTRs), 11–12

grading, 11–12, 11t
neurologic examination of, 1, 1t
pediatric neurology and, 16
segmental innervation of, 11t
Deep vein thrombosis
neurorehabilitation and, 556
Defibrillator
cardiac complications and, 370
Deformities
neuromuscular disorder and, 354, 354f
Degenerative osteoarthritis
cervical dystonia and, 249
Dehydration
neurorehabilitation and, 555–556
Delayed-onset dystonia
children and, 251
Delayed postural response latencies, 434
Delayed sleep-phase syndrome, 160
Delayed-type hypersensitivity (DTH) reaction
MS and, 197
Delayed word recall
for long-term memory testing, 3
Delirium, 69
acute alteration of mental status and, 69
dementia vs., 290
diagnosis of, 69
differential diagnosis of, 69
drug toxicity and, 291
hyperactive, 69
hypoactive, 69
subtypes of, 69
treatment of, 73–74
Delusions, 4
Demand pacemaker
neuromuscular disorder and cardiac
complications in, 370
Dementia
alcoholic, 478–479
algorithm, approach to memory concern,
289, 289f
brain tumor and, 290
causes of, 290
defined, 288
delirium vs., 290
depression and, 290
differential diagnosis of, 289
laboratory aids in, 294t
evaluation for, 288
HD and, 260
neurologic examination and, 290
Parkinson's disease and, 234–235

patient history and, 289
of pellagra, 472–473
treatment of, 298, 298f
Dementia with Lewy bodies (DLB), 291, 296–297
diagnosis of, 297
Demyelination
MS and, 194, 194f, 195
Dental structures
headache and, 137
secondary headache disorders and, 137, 137t
Department of Motor Vehicle (DOMV)
seizures and, 582–583
Depression, 341
dementia and, 290
dystonia and, 252
early morning awakening and, 170
MS and, 203
treatment of, 216–217
reserpine and, 283
seizures and, 146
sign of, 3
St. John's wort (Hypericum perforatum) and, 166
WD and, 267
"Dermatitis" of pellagra, 473
Dermatomyositis (DM), 40, 364–365
PM v., 364
Dermatomyositis (DM), juvenile
symptoms of, 364–365
Desamino-D-arginine vasopressin (DDAVP)
sleep-related enuresis and, 186
Desmopressin
MS and, 216
Devic disease, 199–200
Dexamethasone, 490, 492
acute intracranial hypertension and, 76
Dextroamphetamine
narcolepsy and, 180
Diabetes mellitus
propranolol and, 257
stroke and, 106
Diabetes mellitus, neuropathy with, 390–392
natural history of, 391
nerve dysfunction of, 390
pathogenesis of, 391
Diagnostic and Statistical Manual of Mental
Disorders, 4th edition (DSM IV), 69
Diagnostic testing
acute alteration of mental status and, 73
secondary headache disorders and, 137–138,
137t
3,4-diaminopyridine (DAP), 361

Diazepam
    dystonia and, 253
    MS and, 217
    SE and, 66
    sleep and, 164
Didanosine
    neurologic effect of, 449
Diet
    epilepsy and, 153
    MS and, 218
    Parkinson's disease and, 232
Diffuse axonal injury (DAI), 325
Diffuse brain injury
    seizures and, 146
Diffusion-weighted imaging (DWI), 35, 44
    acute stroke evaluation and, 111
Digit span
    for measurement of working memory, 3
Diphenhydramine, 335
Diphenoxylateatropine (Lomotil)
    neurologic effects of, 455–456
Diphtheric neuropathy
    Guillain-Barré syndrome vs., 82, 82t
Diplopia, 79, 528–529
    horizontal, 545f
Disablement
    aspects of, 551t
    neurologic conditions and, 552–553
    process of, 552f
Discharge planning
    neurorehabilitation and, 564–566
Disc herniation, 400–401
    at L4-5, 401f
Disease-modifying therapy
    Parkinson's disease and, 234–235
Disequilibrium
    causes of
        abnormalities of central integration, 424
        abnormalities of motor response, 424–425
        loss of proprioception, 423–424
        vestibular dysfunction, 424
        visual dysfunction, 423
Dislocations
    prevention of
        neurorehabilitation intervention and, 557–558
Disorders of arousal
    parasomnias and, 185
Disorders of partial arousal
    parasomnias and, 184
Disorders of sleep-stage transition
    parasomnias and, 184

Distal axonal projections, 375
Disulfiram, 387
    neurologic effects of, 461
Diuretics
    as cause of orthostasis, 414
    neurologic effect of, 452–453
    stroke prevention and, 114
Dix–Hallpike positional test, 418, 418f
Dizziness
    categories of, 412–413
    disequilibrium, 413
    overview, 412
    presyncope, 412–413
        causes of, 413–415
    as symptom of cerebrovascular disease, 412
    vertigo. See Vertigo
DLB. See Dementia with Lewy bodies
DM. See Dermatomyositis
DM1. See Myotonic dystrophy 1
DNA tests
    myotonia congenita and, 364
Docusate sodium (Colace)
    neurologic effects of, 455
DOMV. See Department of Motor Vehicle
Donepezil
    AD and, 299
    GTS and, 278
Dopamine
    DRD and, 252
    GTS and, 276
    loss of, 239
    Parkinson's disease and, 227, 228, 229
    TD syndrome and, 280–281
Dopamine agonists
    HD and, 265
    Parkinson's disease and, 228t, 229
    RLS and, 168
    TD syndrome and, 280, 283
    tics syndrome and, 277
Dopamine receptor
    drug-induced Parkinsonism, 233–234
    TD syndrome and, 280, 281, 282
Dopaminergic therapy
    choreiform movement, 237
    psychiatric side effects of, 231
Dopaminergic ventrotegmental area (VTA)
    sleep and, 156, 157
Dopamine transporter single-photon emission
        computed tomography (SPECT)
    DRD and, 251
Dopa-responsive dystonia (DRD)

clinical features of, 250–251
genetic links of, 251
Downbeat nystagmus, 547
D-penicillamine
WD and, 270
Driving restrictions
epilepsy and, 583
Droperidol
neuroleptic malignant syndrome and, 171
Drowsiness, 90
medicinal and toxic contributions to, 184
Drugs
acute alteration in mental status and, 71
anesthetic
malignant hyperthermia, 366
antidepressants
early morning awakening and, 170
antidopaminergics
RLS and, 171
antiepileptic
TBI and, 340
antiplatelet
stroke prevention and, 115
antipsychotics
TD syndrome, 279, 281, 282, 283
antithrombotics
stroke prevention and, 114
cardiac. *See* Cardiac drugs
GABA-agonist
TD syndrome, 283
immunosuppressive
MS and, 213
neurotoxic effects of, 446–466
overdose of
coma prognosis in, 102
sleep and, 160
sleep apnea and, 176
sleep inducing
choice of, 162–164, 163*t*–164*t*
toxic myopathies and, 367
transplant. *See* Transplant drugs
Drug screen
comatose patient and, 99
Drug therapy
MS and, 213–218, 214*t*
urinary retention in, 215–216
DTH. *See* Delayed-type hypersensitivity reaction
DTRs. *See* Deep tendon reflexes
Duchenne dystrophy (DUD), 352
Duchenne muscular dystrophy, 350*f*, 354, 361–362
DUD. *See* Duchenne dystrophy

DWI. *See* Diffusion-weighted imaging
Dynorphin
GTS and, 276
Dysarthria
treatment goals for, 563
WD and, 267
Dysarthric speech, 2
Dysautonomia
head injury and, 335
Dysdiadochokinesia, 14
Dysesthesias, 377
Dyskinesias, 239
drug-induced, 238
drug-related
levodopa and, 230, 231
Parkinson's disease and, 229
involuntary movements in, 242
Parkinson's disease and, 232
Dysphagia
management of
neurologic illness and, 557
MG and, 359
neuroleptic malignant syndrome and, 84
Dyspnea, 371
propranolol and, 257
Dystonia, 242. *See also* Early-onset dystonia
classification of, 244–245, 244*t*–245*t*, 246*t*
drug-induced, 251
ET v., 256
genes and, 245
HD and, 260
hospitalized patients, challenges for, 254
neurochemistry of, 251–252
neurologist referral for, 254
pathology of, 251–252
treatment of, 252–254, 252*t*
types of, 243
Dystonia-plus syndrome, 245
Dystonic cramps, 249
Dystonic movements, 242, 243
pathophysiology of, 243
Dystonic postures, 237, 238
Dystonic tics
GTS and, 273
DYT1 dystonia, 246–247. *See also* Crural dystonia
pathophysiology of, 246–247
DYT6 dystonia, 247
DYT1 gene, 246, 247
DYT6 gene, 247
DYT7 gene, 247
DYT13 gene, 247

E
EAE. *See* Experimental allergic encephalomyelitis
Early morning awakening
    drugs for, 170
Early-onset dystonia, 244
    clinical spectrum of, 246–247
Eating disorders
    sleep and, 186
Edema
    from infarction and gliosis/encephalomalacia,
        57
    mass effect and, 48
Edrophonium (Tensilon)
    MG and, 360
EEG. *See* Electroencephalogram; Electroen-
        cephalography
Ehlers–Danlos syndrome type IV
    aneurysmal rupture and, 120
EKG. *See* Electrocardiograms
Eldercare Locator, 301
Elderly
    advanced-sleep-phase syndrome, 170
    hypnotic drugs and, 166
Elderly patients
    chronic subdural hematomas in, 70
Electrical potentials, 356
Electrocardiograms (EKG)
    DMI and, 363
Electroencephalogram (EEG)
    comatose patient and, 101
    HSE and, 70
    metabolic encephalopathy and, 73
    nonconvulsive SE and, 64
    of NREM sleep, 157
    of REM sleep, 158
    SE and, 65, 68
    seizures and, 143, 147
Electroencephalography (EEG), 37
Electromyogram (EMG), 157
Electromyogram/Nerve conduction studies
        (EMG/NCS)
    of muscles and nerve, 406
Electromyography (EMG), 37–38, 382
    BoNT injections using, 254
    degree of nerve injury, 386
    disryption of, 385
    single motor unit action potentials, 357*f*
    using electrodes, 385
Electro-oculogram (EOG), 157
Eletriptan
    migraine and, 134

Embolic stroke
    thrombotic stroke *vs.*, 109, 109*t*
Embolism
    cardiac evaluation and, 112
Embryonal development
    AVM and, 121–122
Emergency room (ER)
    stroke presenting in, 107
EMG. *See* Electromyogram; Electromyography
EMG biofeedback for insomnia, 161
EMG/NCS. *See* Electromyogram/Nerve conduction
        studies
Emotional disturbances
    neurorehabilitation and, 563
Encephalitis, 492–494
    causes of, 492
    clinical features, 493
    laboratory findings, 493
    management and prognosis, 493–494
Encephalopathy, 20–21, 21*t*, 69. *See also* Delirium
Endocrine encephalopathy
    acute alteration in mental status and, 71
End-of-life care
    physician and, 371
Endolymphatic hydrops, 421
Endovascular coiling
    cerebral aneurysms and, 121
Entacapone
    Parkinson's disease and, 228
    Parkinson's therapy and, 230
Enteroviruses, 488
Enuresis, sleep-related, 186
Enzyme elevation, for muscle necrosis, 354–355
EOG. *See* Electro-oculogram
Ependymoma, 502–503
    treatment of, 503
EPH. *See* Episodic paroxysmal hemicrania
Ephedra
    weight loss and, 183
Epidural abscess
    acute spinal cord compression and, 78
Epidural hematomas, 55, 55*f*
    location of, 53–54
Epilepsy
    AED and, 150–152, 153
    diagnosing, 147–148
    differential diagnosis of, 148
    licensing of drivers with
        legal considerations of, 581–583
    neurologist referral and, 154
    patients with, challenges for managing, 153, 154

posttraumatic head injury and, 340
treatment of, 148–150, 149t
surgical therapies for, 152–153
women and, 153
Epilepsy syndromes, 144–147
Epileptic aura, 309
Epileptic seizures
status epilepticus and, 63
Episodic paroxysmal hemicrania (EPH)
indomethacin and, 137
treatment of, 137
Epley maneuver, 418, 419f
EPS. See Extrapyramidal symptomatology
Equipment, special
rehabilitation and neuromuscular diseases
and, 369
ER. See Emergency room
Ergotamine tartrate
rebound headache and, 130, 130t
Ergot derivatives
migraine and, 134
Erythrocyte sedimentation rate
stroke-like symptoms and, 112
Erythromycin, 448
Escitalopram
MS and, 217
Esotropia ("crossed eyes"), 7
Essential tremor (ET), 242, 284, 285
classification of, 254
clinical features of, 254–256
differential diagnosis of, 255t, 256–257
dystonia and, 249
genetics and, 256
hospitalized patients, challenges for, 260
neurologist referral for, 259–260
Parkinson's disease v., 256
pathology of, 256
pathophysiology of, 256
patient evaluation and, 257
treatment of, 257–259, 258t
Estrogen
migraine and, 129
Eszopiclone, insomnia and, 165
ET. See Essential tremor
Evoked potentials, 38
MS and, 208
Excitotoxicity
HD and, 264
Excitotoxic neuronal injury, 64
Executive cognitive deficits
associated with falls, 436

Executive function
mental status examination and, 3–4
Experimental allergic encephalomyelitis (EAE)
MS and, 196
Expressive aphasia, 3
Extra-axial lesions, 52, 52f
intra-axial lesions versus, 51–53, 52f
Extraocular pathology, 546
Extrapyramidal symptomatology (EPS)
GTS and, 278
Eye movements, 538
coma and, 95, 96, 97
conjugate gaze abnormalities, 539–542
examination, 7
horizontal double vision, 544–547
vertical double vision, 542–544

F
Facial diplegia, 389
Facial masking
Parkinson's disease and, 223, 224f, 225f
Facial nerve (CN VII)
integrity of, 8
Facial weakness, 8
Facioscapulohumeral (FSH) dystrophy, 362
mutation with chromosome 4, 362
symptoms of, 362
Fall(s), 427–442
aging and, 428
associated with ataxia, 432–433
medical treatment for, 439
autonomic dysfunction, 431
balance problems associated with, 434–437
definitions, 427
diagnosing cause of, 429–434, 430f
due to medication side effects, 431
economic cost in U.S., 428
incidence in neurologic patients, 428–429, 428f
multifactorial, 437–438
overview, 427–428
associated with Parkinsonism, 431–432
medical treatment for, 438–439
prevention of
neurorehabilitation intervention and, 557–558
psychotropic medications for, 429
risk factors for, 429, 429t
extrinsic, 429
intrinsic, 429
associated with spasticity, 432
medical treatment for, 439

Fall(s) (*Continued*)
  Tinetti's definition of, 427–428
  treatment to prevent
    medical treatment, 438–439
    rehabilitation, 439–442
    associated with vestibular system disorders, 433
      medical treatment for, 439
    associated with weakness, 433–434
      medical treatment for, 439
Famotidine (Pepcid)
  neurologic effects of, 456
Fascicles, 376
Fasciculations, 353
Fatigue
  MS and, 203
    treatment of, 217
FDA. *See* Food and Drug Administration
FDG-PET. *See* Fluorodeoxyglucose- positron
    emission tomography
Federal Tort Claims Act, 573
FEF. *See* Frontal eye fields
Female hormones
  neurotoxic effects of, 463–464
Fentanyl
  neuroleptic malignant syndrome and, 171
Fetal malformations
  AED and, 153
Fetal tissue implants (mesencephalon)
  Parkinson's disease and, 233
Fever
  MS and, 217
Fibrillation potentials, 356, 357f
Fibromyalgia, 327
Finger to nose test, 14
  MS and, 206
  tremor and, 254
FLAIR. *See* Fluid-attenuated inversion recovery
FLAIR sequence, 44, 450
Flight of ideas, 4
Fluconazole, 492
Fluent aphasia, 308
  etiology of, 314–315
  evaluation of, 313
  for hospitalized patients, 315
  language difficulty, 314
  overview, 313
  refer neurologists, 315
  treatment of, 315
  types of, 314t
Fluid-attenuated inversion recovery (FLAIR), 35
  MS and, 205, 206

Flunarizine
  neurologic effect of, 453
Fluorodeoxyglucose- positron emission
    tomography (FDG-PET)
  AD and, 295
Fluoxetine
  GTS and, 278
  MS and, 216
  serotonin uptake and, 183
  sleep apnea syndromes and, 176
  sleep-related eating disorders and, 186
Flurazepam, 164
Flycatcher's tongue
  TD syndrome and, 279
FMRI. *See* Function magnetic resonance imagery
Focal cervical dystonia, 247
Focal cortical contusion
  TBI and, 325, 326f
Focal dystonia, 244
  DBS and, 253
Focal epilepsy, 146, 153
Focal neuropathies, 392–393
  carpal tunnel syndrome, 392
  peroneal neuropathy, 393
  ulnar neuropathy, 392–393
Focal orbital pain
  cluster headache and, 131
Focal seizures, 144, 145
Folate
  AED and, 152
Folstein Mini-Mental Status Examination
  acute alteration of mental status and, 73
Food and Drug Administration (FDA), 165,
    473, 574
  AD and, 298
  botox and, 253
  medical and law, 574
Foot dorsiflexion weakness
  gait disorders and, 27
Forced vital capacity (FVC), 80
Foster Kennedy syndrome, 519
FOUR (Full Outline of UnResponsiveness) score,
    98, 99t
"4-4-4" rule, 6
Fourth nerve palsy
  in vertical double vision, 543–544, 544f
Fractures
  prevention of
    neurorehabilitation intervention and,
      557–558
Fragile X tremor–ataxia syndrome, 433

Free radicals
    HD and, 264, 265
Frontal eye fields (FEF), 539
Frontal lobe disorders, 27
Frontal lobes
    damage of, 4
Frontotemporal dementia (FTD), 291, 297–298
    neurologic examination and, 297
    pharmacologic treatment of, 297
    prion diseases, 297–298
Frozen shoulder
    rehabilitation and neuromuscular diseases
        and, 368
FSH. *See* Facioscapulohumeral dystrophy
FTD. *See* Frontotemporal dementia
Full Outline of UnResponsiveness (FOUR) score,
    98, 99*t*
Fulminant hepatitis
    WD and, 267, 272
Function magnetic resonance imagery
    (fMRI), 321
Fungal meningitis, 491–492
FVC. *See* Forced vital capacity

G
GABA. *See* Gamma-aminobutyric acid
Gabapentin, 480
    ET and, 259
    RLS and, 168
    seizures and, 151–152
    side effects of, 168
    SUNCT syndrome, 137
GAD. *See* Glutamic acid decarboxylase
Gadolinium, 35
Gadolinium diethylenetriaminepentaacetic acid
    (GdDTPA)
    MS and, 206
Gadolinium dye, 405
Gadolinium-enhancing lesions
    MS and, 199
Gadolinium MRI
    of brain and spinal cord, 508, 508*f*
Gag reflex, 9
Gait
    HD and, 260, 261, 265
    proximal weakness and, 350
    unstable, with head motion
        falls associated with, 436
Gait disorders, 27–28
    non-neurologic causes of, 27

Gait examination
    clinical assessment in, 14–15
    neurological examination and, 1, 1*t*
Gait spasticity, 15
Gait testing, 15
Gait training
    fall prevention by, 441
Galantamine
    AD and, 299
Galveston Orientation and Amnesia Test (GOAT)
    PTA and, 329
Gamma-amino-butyric acid (GABA), 151
    dystonia and, 252
    sleep and, 156
    TBI and, 338
    TD syndrome and, 281
Gamma-amino-butyric acid (GABA) levels
    HD and, 264
Gastroesophageal reflux
    insomnia and, 171
Gastrointestinal agents, 454
    antiacidity agents, 456
    antidiarrheals, 455–456
    antiemetics, 455
    laxatives, 455
    neurotoxic effects of, 454–456
Gastrostomy feeding tube
    oculopharyngeal dystrophy and, 363
Gastrostomy tube, 370
Gaze-evoked nystagmus, 416, 547
GBS. *See* Guillain-Barré syndrome
GCG. *See* Polyalanine triplet
GCS. *See* Glasgow Coma Scale
GdDTPA. *See* Gadolinium diethylenetriaminepen-
    taacetic acid
Generalized dystonia, 244
Gene test
    HD and, 261, 262
Genetic canine narcolepsy
    genes in, 180
Genetic mapping
    ET and, 256
Genetics
    Becker dystrophy and, 361–362
    carnitine deficiency and, 366
    congenital muscular dystrophy and, 346*t*
    CPT II and, 365
    DM and, 363
    dystonia and, 245
    HD and, 261–263
    LGMD and, 362

Genetics (*Continued*)
  malignant hyperthermia and, 366
  McArdle disease and, 365
  mitochondrial myopathies and, 366
  MS and, 196
  muscle biopsy and, 357
  myotonia congenita and, 364
  narcolepsy and, 180
  oculopharyngeal muscular dystrophy and,
    362–363
  SMA and, 358
Genetic testing
  AD and, 295
Genomic imprinting
  GTS and, 276
Gentamycin
  neurologic effect of, 447
GFAP. *See* Glial fibrillary acidic protein
Gilles de la Tourette syndrome (GTS),
    242, 284
  associated behavioral disturbances in,
    274–275
  diagnosis of, 275
  differential diagnosis of, 275
  environmental factors in, 276
  genetics and, 275–276
  hospitalized patients, challenges for, 279
  maternal influences on, 276
  neurologist referral for, 279
  pathophysiology of, 275–276
  tics and, 273–274
  treatment for, 276–279, 277*t*
Ginkgo biloba
  AD and, 300
  Parkinson's disease and, 236
Ginseng (*Panax ginseng*—Korean ginseng)
  ephedrine and, 183
Glabellar reflex, abnormal, 4
Glasgow Coma Scale (GCS), 33, 98, 99*t*
  acute alteration of mental status and, 73
  scoring sheet, 327*f*
  TBI and, 326
Glatiramer acetate (Copaxone)
  MS and, 211
Glial fibrillary acidic protein (GFAP), 500
Glioblastoma multiforme, 502
Gliosis
  HD and, 263, 264
Gliosis/encephalomalacia, 48
Global aphasia
  coma *vs.*, 91

Globus pallidus
  dystonia and, 243, 253
  GTS and, 276
  HD and, 264
Glossopharyngeal nerve (CN IX), 9
Glutamate antagonists
  HD and, 264, 265
Glutamatergic agents
  TD syndrome and, 283
Glutamic acid decarboxylase (GAD)
  HD and, 264
Glycogen
  skeletal muscle and autosomal recessive disorders
    and, 365
Glycogen storage diseases
  CPT II v., 365
Glycoprotein
  myelin-associated, 387
Glycosides
  neurologic effect of, 450–451
GOAT. *See* Galveston Orientation and Amnesia Test
Gotu cola (*Centella asiatica*)
  sleep cycle and, 167
Gowers maneuver, 350, 350*f*
  weakness and, 350
Grand mal seizure
  causes of, 143
Graphesthesia, 14
Guanfacine
  GTS and, 278
Guillain-Barré syndrome (GBS), 21, 38, 81–83,
    381, 389–390, 402, 407, 480
  acute intermittent porphyria *vs.*, 81, 82, 82*t*
  botulism *vs.*, 82, 82*t*
  clinical presentation of, 81
  differential diagnosis of, 81–82, 82*t*
  diphtheric neuropathy *vs.*, 82, 82*t*
  IVIG and, 83
  mortality rate, 81
  origin of, 390
  patient history and, 81
  poliomyelitis *vs.*, 82, 82*t*
  recovery of, 390
  tick-bite paralysis *vs.*, 82, 82*t*
  treatment of, 82–83
Guillain–Mollaret triangle, 548

H
Haemophilus influenzae, 487, 489
Hallucinations, 4

Hallucinosis
  Parkinson's disease and, 232
Halmagyi head thrust test, 417
Haloperidol
  acute alteration in mental status and, 74
  dystonia and, 246t
  HD and, 265
  side effects of, 277
  tics syndrome and, 277
Halothane
  malignant hyperthermia of, 366
Hand
  cutaneous innervation of, 378f
Hatchet face, 363
HD. See Huntington's disease
HD (Huntington's disease) gene, 261
Headache. See also Tension-type headache
  aneurysmal rupture and, 120
  case studies and, 124–125
  hospital care and, 133t
  hospitalization for
    criteria for, 138, 139t
    inpatient care with, 139, 139t
  intracranial hypertension and, 76
  treatment of, 138
Headaches
  mild TBI and, 339
  refractory, 340
Head injury. See also Brain injury; Traumatic brain
      injury
  hospitalized patient with special challenges of,
      332–335
  seizure prophylaxis and, 330
  vocational programmes and, 332
Head motion
  unstable gait with, 436
Head thrust test, 417
Head titubation, 257
Health care
  administrative law and, 574
Health Insurance Portability and Accountability
      Act (HIPAA)
  medical law and, 574
Hearing loss
  in peripheral vestibular lesions, 417
Heel-to-shin testing, 14
Hemicrania continua
  indomethacin and, 137
Hemidystonia, 244
Hemiparesis, 22
  intracranial hypertension and, 75

Hemiparetic gait, 15
Hemiplegia, 22
Hemispatial neglect
  sensory examination and, 14
Hemispheric motor cortex lesions
  etiology of, 23–24
Hemorrhage
  intracranial, 53–56
  risk of, 56
  types of, 53
Heparin
  ICH and, 119
Hepatic encephalopathy
  acute alteration in mental status and, 71
  alcoholism and, 474–475
  asterixis in, 474
  diagnosis, 474
  etiology of, 474
  treatment of, 474–475
Hepatic WD
  diagnosing, 269
  presentations of, 267
Hepatitis WD, 267
Herbal medicinal products
  caffeine and, 183
Hereditary-degenerative syndromes, 245
Herniation
  and mass effect, 47–49, 48f
Herniation syndromes
  types of
    intracranial hypertension and, 75
Herpes encephalitis, 308
Herpes simplex encephalitis (HSE), 69–70,
      319–321
  acute alteration of mental status and, 69–70
  AED therapy for treatment of, 70
  bizarre behavioral and, 319
  diagnostic testing for, 69–70
  for hospitalized patients, 320
  overview, 319
  refer neurologists, 320
  treatment of, 320
Herpes simplex type 1 virus, 492
Herpes simplex virus (HSV)-1, 69
Heterozygotes
  WD and, 269
High postural tone, 434
HIPAA. See Health Insurance Portability and
      Accountability Act
Hippus, 531
HIV. See Human immunodeficiency virus

HIV infection
  antiretrovirals for, 449
HIV testing
  stroke-like symptoms and, 112
HMG-CoA reductase inhibitors
  neurologic effects of, 454
Homonymous hemianopia, 6, 523, 526, 526f
Horizontal double vision, 544–547
  extraocular pathology, 546
  hyperthyroidism in, 546–547
  internuclear ophthalmoplegia, 545–546
  myasthenia gravis, 546
  one-and-a-half syndrome, 546
  sixth nerve palsy, 544–545, 545f
Horizontal gaze palsies, 539–541, 540f, 541f
Horizontal oculocephalic maneuvers
  coma and, 97
Horizontal sectoranopia, 525
Hormones
  neurotoxic effects of, 463–464
Horner syndrome, in anisocoria, 532–535, 533f
  apraclonidine test for, 534
  hydroxyamphetamine testing for, 534–535, 535f
  pharmacologic testing in, 534, 534f
  postganglionic lesions in, 533
  preganglionic sympathetic fibers, 533
  ptosis in, 533
  Raeder's paratrigeminal syndrome, 533, 533f
Hospitalization
  GCS and, 330
Hounsfield units (HU), 44
H₂ receptor antagonists
  neurologic effects of, 456
HSE. See Herpes simplex encephalitis
HSV-1. See Herpes simplex virus
HU. See Hounsfield units
Human immunodeficiency virus (HIV), 381, 504
  dementia and, 291
Human leukocyte antigen (HLA) allele
  narcoleptics and, 179
Huntingtin protein
  CAG trinucleotide repeat and, 264
Huntington disease (HD), 242
  characteristics of, 260
  clinical features of, 260–261
  differential diagnosis of, 262t
  genetics of, 261–263
  hospitalized patients, challenges for, 266
  neurochemistry of, 263–264
  neurologist referral for, 266
  pathogenesis of, 263–264

pathology of, 263–264
treatment of
  disease-modifying agents in, 265
  symptomatic therapy in, 265–266
Hydralazine
  neurologic effect of, 453
Hydrocephalus, 49, 50f
  evaluation of, 49
  versus volume loss, 49–50
Hydrocephalus, late onset
  TBI and, 335–336
Hydroxyamphetamine
  in Horner syndrome, 534–535, 535f
Hyperactive delirium, 69
Hyperactive reflexes, 11
Hypercoagulable state
  evaluation for, 112
"Hyperdense MCA sign," 57
Hyperesthesia, 377
Hyperpnea
  Cheyne–Stokes respiration and, 94
Hyperreflexia
  acute alteration of mental status and, 73
  MS and, 206
Hypersomnia
  hospitalized patients, special challenges for, 184
  sleep specialist and, referral to, 184
Hypersomnolence, 334
  sleep disorders associated with, 172
Hypertension
  MS and, 216
  OSA and, 174
Hyperthermia
  neuroleptic malignant syndrome and, 84
Hyperthyroidism
  ET and, 257
  in eye disease, 546–547
Hypertrophy, 352–353
Hyperventilation
  intracranial pressure and, 76
Hyperventilation syndrome
  as cause of presyncope, 413–414
  symptoms of, 413
Hypnosedative agents
  neurologic effects of, 461
Hypnosis
  epilepsy and, 153
Hypnotic drugs for insomnia
  children and, 165–166
  efficacy of, 162
  half-life of, 164, 165

Hypoactive delirium, 69
Hypocretin-containing neurons, narcolepsy and, 180
Hypoesthesia, 377
Hypofibrinogenemia
    ICH and, 118
Hypoglossal nerve (CN XII), 9–10
Hypoglycemia
    as cause of presyncope, 415
    comatose patient and, 100
Hypokalemia
    MS and, 214
Hyponatremia
    acute alteration in mental status and, 72
    TBI and, 335
Hypoparathyroidism, 367
Hypotension
    phenobarbital IV and, 68
    phenytoin IV and, 66
    SE and, 68
Hypothalamus, sleep and, 156, 157
Hypothermia
    comatose patient and, 100
Hypothyroidism
    dementia and, 291
Hypotonia, 354
Hypoventilation, 174
Hypoxia
    delayed-onset dystonia and, 251

I
IBM. See Inclusion body myositis
ICH. See Intracerebral hemorrhage
ICP. See Intracranial pressure
ICSD-2. See International Classification of Sleep
        Disorders-2
ICU. See Intensive care unit
Idiopathic dystonia
    secondary dystonia v., 251
Idiopathic insomnia, 159
Idiopathic intracranial hypertension, 528
IgM. See Immunoglobulin M
Illusions, 4
Imaging
    of spine, 53
Imipramine
    cataplectic attacks and, 183
Immunoglobulin M (IgM), 387
Immunosuppressives, transplant, 450
Inclusion body myositis (IBM), 351
    muscles biopsy and, 365

Indian sida (Sida cordifolia), ephedrine and,
        183
Indomethacin
    CPH and, 137
    EPH and, 137
    hemicrania continua and, 137
    neurotoxic effects of, 463
Infantile hypotonia, 354
Infant(s)
    hypotonia, 354
Infarcts
    acute cerebral, 57f, 58f
    evaluation of, 56
        and vascular imaging, 56–60
    recent versus chronic MCA, 58f
    treatment, 56
Infections
    common sites of neuromuscular disorders
        and, 370
    neuromuscular disorders and, 370
Inferior arcuate defects, 522
Inflammatory myopathies, 364
    muscles and, 353
Informed consent, 574–578
INH. See Isoniazid
Inherited disease, 285
Inherited syndrome
    DYT1 dystonia and, 246
INO. See Internuclear ophthalmoplegia
INR. See International normalization ratio
Insomnia
    hospitalized patients, special challenges for,
        171–172
    medical conditions and, 171
    neurorehabilitation and, 556
    pattern of, 160
    sleep disorders associated with, 159–160
    sleep specialist and, 171
    treatment of, 161–162, 164–165
"Insular ribbon sign," 57
Intensive care unit (ICU), 65
Internal capsule lesions
    characteristics of, 24
International Classification of Sleep Disorders-2
        (ICSD-2), 159
    division of sleep disorders in, 159
International Headache Society's (IHS)
    classification of headaches and, 128, 128t
    criteria for MOH, 130t
International normalization ratio (INR)
    SAH and, 109

Internuclear ophthalmoplegia (INO), 97, 544, 545–546
   MS and, 202
Intra-arterial cerebral arteriography
   extracranial circulation and, 111
Intra-arterial mechanical thrombectomy, 56
Intra-arterial thrombolytic therapy, 56
Intra-axial lesions, 51, 52f
   versus extra-axial lesions, 51–53, 52f
Intracerebral hemorrhage (ICH)
   causes of, 117, 117t
   clinical approach to, 117–118
   CT scan and, 118
   treatment for, 118–119
Intracranial aneurysm, 120
Intracranial hematoma
   acute alteration of mental status and, 70
Intracranial hemorrhage, 53–56
Intracranial hypertension. See Acute intracranial hypertension
Intracranial metastases, 504–507, 505f
   diagnosis of, 506
   risk factors, 505
   signs and symptoms, 506
   treatment of, 506–507
Intracranial pressure (ICP). See also Acute intracranial hypertension
   hyperventilation and, 76
   measurements of, 76
Intramedullary spine lesions, 54f
   differential diagnosis of, 53
Intraparenchymal hemorrhage
   differential diagnosis of, 55–56, 56f
   etiology for, 55
   location of, 53
   pallidotomy and, 233
Intrathecal baclofen
   dystonia and, 253
Intrathecal immunoglobulin (Ig) synthesis
   MS and, 206–208
Intravenous immune globulins (IVIG), 390
   GBS and, 83
   myasthenic crisis and, 80–81
Intravenous (IV) benzodiazepine administration, 65
Intravenous methylprednisolone (IVMP)
   MS and, 214, 215
Intravenous TPA, 56
Involuntary movements
   TD syndrome and, 282
Iron deficiency, RLS and, 167, 168
Ischemic optic neuropathy, 527–528

Ischemic stroke, 105
   hematologic factors associated with, 112
   hemorrhagic transformation of, 116, 117f
   prevention of
      neurorehabilitation intervention and, 558
   treatment of, 114–117
Ischemic stroke syndromes
   associated with vertigo, 422
Isoniazid (INH)
   neurotoxic effects of, 447
Itraconazole, 492
IVIG. See Intravenous immune globulins
IVMP. See Intravenous methylprednisolone

J
Jacobus Pharmaceutical Company, 361
Jaw jerk reflex, 7, 8
Jaw strength
   testing of, 7–8
Jerk nystagmus, 547
   Brun's nystagmus, 547
   downbeat nystagmus, 547
   gaze-evoked nystagmus, 547
   vestibular nystagmus, 547
JFK Coma Recovery Score
   brain injury and, 331
Joint contractures
   prevention of
      neurologic illness and, 556–557
Judgment
   mental status and, 4
Junctional scotoma, 523
Juvenile myoclonic epilepsy, 145

K
Kanamycin
   neurologic effect of, 447
Kava kava (Piper methysticum), insomnia and, 166
Kayser–Fleischer (KF) ring
   WD and, 267, 268, 268f, 269
Kearns-Sayre syndrome (KSS)
   syncope and, 369
Kennedy disease, 358
Kernohan grading system, 500
Ketoconazole
   AD and, 299
Ketogenic diet
   epilepsy and, 153
Kinetic tremor, 235, 257

Kleine–Levin syndrome, sleepiness and, 184
Kluver–Bucy syndrome, 320
Knee extensor weakness, 350
"Knee jerk." *See* Patellar reflex
Knee reflex, 404
Korsakoff psychosis, 316
Korsakoff syndrome
    dementia and, 291
Kyphoscoliosis
    poliomyelitis and, 175
    rehabilitation and neuromuscular diseases
        and, 361

L
Laboratory testings
    neuromuscular diseases and, 406
Lactulose
    WD and, 272
Lacunar-type stroke
    indications of, 114
Lambert– Eaton myasthenic syndrome (LEMS), 361
    immunomodulatory treatments for, 361
Lamotrigine
    seizures and, 149, 152
    SUNCT syndrome and, 137
Landry–Guillain–Barré syndrome, 381
Language
    mental status examination and, 2–3
Large artery thrombotic stroke, 106
Laryngeal dystonia, 243
Late-onset dystonia, 244
Lateral geniculate nucleus (LGN), 520
    visual field defects in, 524–525, 525f
Lateral medullary infarction, 422
    as cause of vertigo, 422
Lateral pontine ischemia
    as cause of vertigo, 422
Laterocollis, 248
Lavender *(Lavandula angustifolia)*, sleep cycle
        and, 167
Lawsuits. *See* Medical malpractice suits
Laxatives
    MS and, 216
    neurologic effects of, 455
LDN. *See* Low-dose naltrexone
Leber optic neuropathy
    dystonia and, 245t
LEMS. *See* Lambert–Eaton myasthenic syndrome
Lenticular nuclei
    WD and, 268

Leptomeningeal metastases, 507–509
    symptoms and signs, 507
Lethargy, 90
Leukoencephalopathy, 513
Level of consciousness
    alterations in, 21–22
    mental status examination and, 2
Levels of consciousness
    assessment of, 90
Levetiracetam, 340
    seizures and, 152
Levodopa
    DLB and, 297
    DRD and, 250, 251
    dystonia and, 252, 252t
    Parkinson's disease and, 227, 228, 229, 233
    TD syndrome and, 283
Levodopa-carbidopa, 239
    sleep–wake cycle and, 331, 331t
Lewy bodies
    Parkinson's disease and, 226
LGMD. *See* Limb girdle muscular dystrophy
LGN. *See* Lateral geniculate nucleus
Lhermitte's sign, 26
    MS and, 203
Licensing of drivers, 581–583
Lidocaine-induced CNS toxicity, 451
Ligaments pain, 400
Limb girdle muscular dystrophy (LGMD)
    symptoms of, 362
Limbs
    cutaneous innervation of, 380t
Lingual dystonia, 243
Lipid metabolism
    disorders of, 365–366
Lipohyalinosis
    lacunar-type stroke, 114
Lithium carbonate
    neurologic effects of, 460–461
Liver failure, 272
Liver function tests
    comatose patient and, 99
Liver transplant, 272
Lobar hematoma, 118
    surgery and, 119
Lobar hemorrhage
    aneurysms *vs.*, 118
Localization-related epilepsies, 145
LOH. *See* "Loss of heterozygosity"
Long-term memory
    testing, 3

Loop diuretics
    neurologic effect of, 452
Loosening of associations, 4
Lorazepam
    SE and, 66
    sleep and, 164
"Loss of heterozygosity" (LOH), 502
Loss of proprioception
    in disequilibrium, 423–424
Low back pain
    anatomy of, 398–400
    causes of new-onset, 407t
    epidemiology of, 398
    examination for, 403
        motor, 403
        sensory, 404
        vibratory, 404
    neurologic examination for, 403–404
    psychosocial factors, 403
    structural causes of
        ligament pain, 400
        muscle pain, 400
        referred pain, 402–403
    treatment of, 406–408
        conservative, 407–408
        4 to 6 week, 408
Low-dose naltrexone (LDN)
    MS and, 218
Lower motor neuron lesions
    symptoms of, 24–25
Lower motor neuron signs, 10
LP. See Lumbar puncture
L5 radiculopathy, 403
Lumbar puncture (LP), 36
    AD and, 294
    CSF evaluation for, 38, 70
    SAH and, 109
    technique for, 39
Lumbosacral spine, 400f
    anatomic landmarks of, 399
Lupus erythematosus syndrome, 451
Lymphomatous meningitis, 506

M
Macrocytosis
    AED and, 151
Macular sparing, 526
MAG. See Myelin-associated glycoprotein
Magnesium
    PLMs and, 170
    in thiamine metabolism, 471

Magnetic resonance angiography (MRA), 36, 46
    acute stroke evaluation and, 111
    infarct evaluation and, 59, 59f
Magnetic resonance imaging (MRI), 35
    acute spinal cord compression and, 78
    AD and, 294
    advanced techniques for, 46
    comatose patient and, 100
    contrast agents used in, 46–47
    versus CT, 44–46, 45f
    GTS and, 276
    herpes simplex encephalitis and, 69–70
    infarct evaluation and, 56–60
    mitoxantrone and, 211
    MS and, 193, 204–206, 205t, 206f, 207f, 212, 213, 213f
        pathologic correlations with, 195–196
    PP-MS and, 198
    in pregnant patients, 46
    VaD and, 296
    WD and, 270, 271f
Magnetic resonance venography (MRV), 36
Major histocompatibility complex (MHC)
    MS and, 210
Malignant hyperthermia, 366
Malnutrition
    neurorehabilitation and, 555–556
Mandibular branch (V_2), of trigeminal nerve, 7, 8f
Mania
    sign of, 3
Mannitol
    acute intracranial hypertension and, 76
MAO-B. See Monoamine oxidase B
MAO inhibitors. See Monoamine oxidase inhibitors
MAP. See Mean arterial blood pressure
Marburg disease, 199
Marchiafava–Bignami disease (MBD)
    alcoholism and, 477–478
    callosal atrophy in, 478
    clinical variations of, 477–478
    diagnosis, 477
    extracallosal lesions in, 478
Marcus Gunn pupil, 518
    MS and, 202
Marfan syndrome
    aneurysmal rupture and, 120
Mass effect
    and herniation, 47–49, 48f
Maxillary branch (V_2), of trigeminal nerve, 7, 8f
MBD. See Marchiafava-Bignami disease

MBP. *See* Myelin basic protein
McArdle disease, 365
  acid maltase deficiency and, 346*t*, 365
  symptoms of, 365
Mc-Donald diagnostic criteria
  MS and, 204, 205*t*
MCI. *See* Mild cognitive impairment
Mean arterial blood pressure (MAP)
  intracranial hypertension and, 74
Meclizine
  for vestibular-based dizziness, 439
Medial longitudinal fasciculus (MLF), 544, 545
Medical malpractice suits, 573–574
Medical Research Council (MRC)
  grading of muscle strength, 10*t*
Medication overuse headache (MOH)
  features of, 130, 130*t*
  IHS criteria for, 130*t*
  treatment of, 133–134, 133*t*
Medulla
  ET and, 256
  sleep and, 156
Meige syndrome, 247–248, 284
  ET and, 249, 256
Melatonin
  pineal gland and, 157
  sleep cycle and, 166
Memantine
  AD and, 299
Memory
  components of, 3
  mental status examination and, 3–4
  MS and, 203
Ménière disease
  as cause of vertigo, 420–421
  symptoms, 421
  vestibular dysfunction and, 433
Meningeal carcinomatosis, 506
Meningiomas, 503
  chemotherapy for, 503
  focal motor seizures and, 145
  radiotherapy for, 503
  symptoms, 503
  treatment for, 503
Meningitis, 487–492
  acute bacterial, 489–491
  etiology of, 487
  features of, 487
  laboratory findings, 487–488, 488*f*
  spirochete, 491
  tuberculous and fungal, 491–492
  viral, 488–489

Meningovascular syphilis
  ICH and, 118
Menstruation-associated hypersomnia, sleepiness
    and, 184
Mental status, 1
  appearance and, 2
  and cognition, 1–5
  diagnostic process and, 21–22
  neurologic examination, 1, 1*t*
  pediatric neurology and, 15
Metabolic abnormalities
  as result of malignancy, 511
Metabolic depression
  coma and, 91, 92
Metabolic encephalopathies, 92
  acquired hepatocerebral degeneration, 475–476
  acute alteration of mental status and, 71
  alcoholism and, 474–477
  decerebrate posturing and, 98
  EEG and, 73
  hepatic encephalopathy, 474–475
  pancreatic encephalopathy, 476–477
Metabolic myopathies, 365–366
  glycogen storage diseases, 365
  lipid metabolism, disorder of, 365–366
  mitochondrial myopathies, 366
Metabolic profile
  SAH and, 109
Metallothionein levels
  WD and, 270, 271
Metastases
  intracranial, 504–507, 505*f*
  leptomeningeal, 507–509
  spinal, 509–510
Methamphetamine, narcolepsy and, 180
Methaqualone
  neurologic effects of, 461
Methazolamide
  ET and, 259
Methylphenidate (MPH)
  ADHD and, 278
  narcolepsy and, 180
  OCD and, 275
  sleep–wake cycle and, 331, 331*t*
Methylprednisolone
  acute intracranial hypertension and, 76
Metoclopramide
  Parkinson's disease and, 236
Metoclopramide (Reglan)
  neurologic effects of, 455
Metoprolol
  ET and, 257–258

Mexiletine
    dystonia and, 253
MG. *See* Myasthenia gravis
MHC. *See* Major histocompatibility complex
Microelectrode recordings
    dystonia and, 243
Midazolam
    SE and, 68
Migraine
    basilar, in vertigo, 423
Migraine headache
    acute treatment of, 134–135, 134t
    categories of medications, 134t, 135t
    classification of, 128–129
    clinical symptoms of, 129
    cluster headache *vs.*, 131, 131t
    comorbid conditions associated with, 129
    defined, 128
    pathogenesis of, 129, 129t
    pharmacologic treatment of, 134
    preventive treatment of, 135–136, 135t
Migraine with aura
    characterizations of, 128
Migraine without aura, 128
Mild cognitive impairment (MCI), 288
    AD and, 288
    AIDS and, 291
    causes of, 289
    clinical evaluation of, 288
Mild TBI, 338–340
Miller–Fisher syndrome, 389
Mini-mental status examination (MMSE), 4–5
Mini-mental status examination (MMSE) scores
    MCI and, 288
Mirtazapine
    ET and, 259
Mitochondrial DNA
    mitochondrial myopathies and, 366
Mitochondrial dysfunction, 367
    HD, 264
Mitochondrial myopathies, 366
Mitoxantrone (Novantrone)
    MS and, 211
Mixed apnea, 172
Miyoshi myopathy, 362
MLF. *See* Medial longitudinal fasciculus
MMSE. *See* Mini-mental status examination
MMSE scores. *See* Mini-mental status examination
        scores
MND. *See* Motor neuron disease
MoCA. *See* Montreal Cognitive Assessment

Modafinil
    mechanism of action, 181
    narcolepsy and, 180, 181
    stimulants v., 181
MOG. *See* Myelin oligodendrocyte protein
MOH. *See* Medication overuse headache
Monoamine oxidase B (MAO-B)
    Parkinson's disease and, 227
Monoamine oxidase (MAO) inhibitors
    neurologic effects of, 460
Monocular blindness, 521
Mononeuropathy multiplex, 380
Monoparesis, 22
Monoplegia, 22
Monozygotic twins
    MS and, 196
Montreal Cognitive Assessment (MoCA),
        5, 73
Mood
    depression and, 3
Mood disorder
    epilepsy and, 146
Mortality rate
    of Guillain–Barré syndrome, 81
    of myasthenic crisis, 79
    of NMS, 85
    of status epilepticus, 64
Motoneuron, 375
Motor cortex
    dystonia and, 243–244
Motor dysfunction
    MS and, 202
Motor examination
    motor system dysfunctions and, 10–11
    pediatric neurology and, 16
Motor fluctuations
    Parkinson's disease and, 232
Motor nerve
    response of, 382–383
Motor neuron diseases (MND), 297, 358–359
Motor neuron lesions
    lower, symptoms of, 24–25
    upper, symptoms of, 23–24
Motor response, abnormalities of
    in disequilibrium, 424–425
Motor strength, 403
Motor task
    writer's cramp and, 250
Motor tics
    GTS and, 273
Motor unit potentials, 356, 357f

Motor-vehicle accidents (MVA), 325
Movement-related vertigo (MRV), 421
Moyamoya disease
   angiography and, 112
MPH. *See* Methylphenidate
MRA. *See* Magnetic resonance angiography
MRC. *See* Medical Research Council
MRI. *See* Magnetic resonance imaging
   with gadolinium
      of spine, 405
   of L4-5 disc, 401*f*
   without gadolinium dye
      of spine, 405
MRV. *See* Magnetic resonance venography;
      Movement-related vertigo; Venography
MS. *See* Multiple sclerosis
MSA. *See* Multiple system atrophy
MSLT. *See* Multiple Sleep Latency test
Multifocal brain injury
   seizures and, 146
Multifocal dystonia, 244
Multiple motor tics, 274
Multiple sclerosis (MS), 527. *See also* National
      Multiple Sclerosis Society; Progressive-re-
      lapsing multiple sclerosis; Relapsing-remit-
      ting multiple sclerosis; Secondary
      progressive multiple sclerosis
   alternative therapies and, 218
   brain abnormality
      MRI criteria for, 204, 205*t*
   case studies, 219–220
   cerebellar signs of, 202–203
   clinical patterns of, 197–199, 197*t*
   cognitive symptoms of, 203
   combination therapy in, 213
   corticosteroids and, 213, 214–215
   diagnosis of, 204–209
      errors in, 208–209, 208*t*, 209*t*
   disease course of, 197–199, 197*t*
   disease-modifying therapies for, 209–212, 210*t*
   epidemiologic studies, 193, 193*f*
   etiology and immunopathogenesis and,
      196–197
   experimental immunomodulatory
      approaches, 218
   fatigue treatment in, 217
   genetics and, 196
   history of, 192–193
   hospitalized patients with, 217–218
   immunology of, 196–197
   Mc-Donald diagnostic criteria, 204, 205*t*

MRI and
   pathologic correlations with, 195–196
neurobehavioral manifestations of,
   216–217
pathology of, 193–196, 194*f*
precipitation factors of, 200
prognosis, 199
psychiatric manifestations of, 203
sensory symptoms of, 203
spasticity treatment for, 214*t*, 215
symptoms of, 200–204, 200t, 201t
therapy in, 209–219, 210*t*
variants of, 199–200
in vertigo, 423
Multiple sclerosis (MS) plaque
   pathogenesis of, 194–195, 194*f*
Multiple Sleep Latency test (MSLT), 179
Multiple system atrophy (MSA), 226
   as cause of parkinsonism in falling, 432
Muscle atrophy, 351–352
   motor neuron disease and, 350*f*
   weakness and, 351
Muscle biopsy. *See* Biopsy, muscle
Muscle bulk examination, 10
Muscle contraction
   electrical-activity generated by, 384
Muscle cramp, 353
Muscle disease
   alcoholic myopathy as cause of, 481
Muscle hypertrophy, 10
Muscle injury
   alcoholism and, 481
Muscle movements
   innervation of, 379, 379t
   speed and dexterity examination, 11
Muscle necrosis, 354
Muscle pain, 353, 400
Muscles
   dystonia and, 243
Muscle spasm, 399
Muscle stiffness, 353
Muscle strength
   examination, 10
   grading of, 10–11, 10*t*
Muscle strength testing, 382
Muscle stretch reflexes. *See* Deep tendon reflexes
Muscle tone
   defined, 10
   examination, 10
Muscle twitching, 353
Muscle wasting, 10

Muscular dystrophies
  in adult, 368–369
  causes of, 361–362
  in children, 367–368
  diagnosis of, 361
Muscular weakness
  central nervous system and, 22–23
Mutant Huntingtin
  CAG trinucleotide repeat and, 263, 264
MVA. *See* Motor-vehicle accidents
Myasthenia gravis (MG), 7, 350, 359–360, 546
  diagnosis of, 360
  drugs exacerbating, 79, 79*t*
  swallowing dysfunction in, 370
  treatment of, 360
Myasthenic crisis, 79–81
  mortality rate, 79
  treatment of, 80–81
Mycobacterium tuberculosis, 487
Mycophenolate mofetil
  neurologic effect of, 450
Myectomy of orbicularis oculi
  blepharospasm and, 253
Myelin, 376
  MS and, 195
Myelin-associated glycoprotein (MAG)
  MS and, 195
Myelin basic protein (MBP)
  MS and, 195
Myelin oligodendrocyte protein (MOG)
  MS and, 195
Myelography, 35–36
Myelopathies, 21, 21*t*. *See* Spinal cord lesions
  cervical dystonia and, 249
Myoclonic jerks
  AD and, 294
Myoclonic seizures, 144
Myoclonus, 242
  comatose patient and, 100
Myofascial pain, 399
Myoglobinuria, 354, 370–371
  CPT II v., 365–366
Myopathies, 21, 21*t*, 25
  toxic, 366–367
Myotonia, 353
Myotonia congenita, 364
Myotonic disorders, 363
Myotonic dystrophy
  facial appearance in, 352*f*
  syncope and, 369
  weakness and, 352*f*

Myotonic dystrophy 1 (DM1)
  symptoms of, 363

N
NAbs. *See* Neutralizing antibodies
NAD. *See* Nicotinamide adenine dinucleotide
NADP. *See* Nicotinamide adenine dinucleotide
    phosphate
NAION. *See* Nonarteritic AION
NAIP. *See* Neuronal apoptotic inhibitory protein
Naproxen
  AD and, 300
  neurotoxic effects of, 463
Narcolepsy
  diagnosing, 179
  questions about, 187, 188–189
  symptoms of, 179
  treatment of, 180–181, 181*t*, 182*t*, 183
  twin studies and, 180
Nasal obstruction, sleep apnea and, 178
Natalizumab (Tysabri)
  MS and, 211–212
National Adult Day Services Association, 301
National Center for Complementary and Alternative
    Medicine, 300
National Institute on Aging, 300, 301
National Institutes of Health (NIH) Stroke Scale
  neurologic examination and, 109
National Institutes of Mental Health, 300
National Multiple Sclerosis Society (NMSS)
  recommendation of, 212
National Traumatic Coma Data Bank, 331
Nausea
  due to clinical intoxication, 451
NCS. *See* Nerve conduction study
Needle EMG
  NCS and, 355
Neomycin
  neurologic effect of, 447
  WD and, 272
Neoplastic meningitis, 506
  diagnosis of, 506
  treatment of, 509
Neostigmine
  myasthenic crisis and, 80
Nephrogenic fibrosing dermopathy, 35
Nephrogenic systemic fibrosis (NSF), 35, 47
Nerve biopsy, 39–40, 386
Nerve conduction study (NCS), 37
Nerve root motor, and sensory findings, 404*t*

Nervous system
  ET and, 254
Neurocardiogenic presyncope. *See* Vasovagal
      presyncope
Neurocardiogenic (vasovagal) syncope
  seizures *vs.*, 148
Neurodiagnostic studies, 34*t*
Neurogenic claudication, 402
Neurogenic pain, 400
Neuroimaging
  acute alteration of mental status and, 73
Neuroimaging tests, 34–36
  computed tomography (CT), 34–35
  magnetic resonance imaging, 35
  myelography, 34–35
Neuroleptic agents
  acute, subacute, and chronic side effects of,
      457*t*
  neurologic effects of, 457–459
Neuroleptic-induced parkinsonism, 458
Neuroleptic-induced (tardive dystonia), 251
Neuroleptic malignant syndrome (NMS),
      83–86, 458
  acute alteration in mental status and, 74
  causes of, 83, 83*t*
  diagnosis of, 86
  differential diagnosis of, 84
  features of, 84
    cardiovascular complications and, 85
    respiratory complications and, 85
  metabolic factors and, 84
  mortality rate, 85
  risk factors, 458
  RLS and, 171
  treatment of, 84–86
Neuroleptics, 285
  acute alteration in mental status and, 74
  TD syndrome and, 281, 282, 283
  tics and, 278
Neurologic diagnosis
  elements of, 21
  patient history and, 20
  role of temporal course of neurologic illness in,
      28–29
  symptoms and, 20
Neurologic disorders, 552–553
  involuntary movements and, 242
Neurologic dysfunction
  descriptive terms in, 20–21, 21*t*
Neurologic examination
  acute alteration of mental status and, 73

AD and, 293–294
  coma and, 94
  coordination and gait, 14–15
  cranial nerves, 5–10
  dementia and, 290
  DTRs, 11–12
  FTD and, 297
  mental status and cognition, 1–5
  motor function, 10–11
  organization of, 1, 1*t*
  pediatric neurology and, 15–16
    coordination, 16
    cranial nerves, 16
    DTRs, 16
    mental status, 15
    motor examination, 16
    sensory system, 16
  primary generalized epilepsies and, 144
  rt-PA and, 109
  sensory examination, 12–14
  TBI and, 330, 339
Neurologist
  dystonia and, 254
  ET referral to, 259–260
  GTS referral to, 279
  HD and, 266
  MS referral to, 209
  Parkinson's disease referral to, 235
  referral to, 102
  referring to
    epilepsy and, 154
    stroke management and, 122
  TD syndrome and, 284
  WD and, 273
Neurology, pediatric, 15–16
  coordination examination in, 16
  cranial nerves examination in, 16
  mental status examination in, 15
  motor examination in, 16
  reflex examination in, 16
  sensory examination in, 16
Neuromuscular diseases
  algorithm for, 356*f*
  challenges in the hospitalized patient,
      370–371
  clinical presentations of, 344–352
  electrodiagnostic studies, 355–357, 371
  enzyme elevation in, 354–355
  gene abnormalities in, 345*t*–347*t*
  motor neuron diseases, 358–359
  nerve and muscle biopsy, 357

Neuromuscular diseases (*Continued*)
  outpatient treatment principles, 367–369
  overview, 344
  pharmacologic treatments in, 348t–349t
  refer to neurologist, 371–372
Neuromuscular disorders
  differential diagnosis for patients with, 354
  findings and helpful tests in, 355t
  hospitalized patient, special challenges in,
      370–371
  scoliosis in, 354f
  specific issues in, 357–359
Neuromuscular junction
  myasthenia gravis in, 38
Neuromyelitis optica (NMO), 199–200
Neuronal apoptotic inhibitory protein (NAIP), 358
Neuron-specific enolase (NSE), 102
Neuropathic disorder
  myopathic disorder v., 354
Neuropathic injury
  indications of, 377
Neuropathies
  characteristics of, 21, 21t
Neurophysiologic tests, 37–38
  electroencephalography (EEG), 37
  electromyography (EMG), 37–38
Neuroprotection
  MS and, 218
Neuroprotective therapy
  Parkinson's disease and, 234
Neuropsychologic testing
  TBI and, 340
Neuroradiology, 43–60
  contrast *versus* noncontrast, 46–47
  CT *versus* MRI, 44–46
  cytotoxic *versus* vasogenic edema, 50–51
  herniation and mass effect, 47–49, 48f
  hydrocephalus *versus* volume loss, 49–50, 52f
  infarct evaluation and vascular imaging, 56–60
  intra-axial *versus* extra-axial lesions, 51–53, 52f
  intracranial hemorrhage, 53–56
  overview, 43
  spine imaging, 53
Neurorehabilitation, 551
  acute care, 555, 555t
  assessment role in, 553–555
  chronic pain in, 563–564
  communication disorders in, 563
  discussion questions about, 568–571
  emotional dysfunction in, 563
  follow-up and
    community transition and, 565

  goals of, 553t
  homeostasis maintenance and, 555
  hospitalization following
    special challenges in, 567–568
  outcomes of, 568
  pharmacologic treatments in, 562t
Neurorehabilitation intervention
  acute-care discharge and, 559
  determination of rehabilitation setting and, 559
  management plan for, 560–561, 561t
  return to self-care, 558–559
Neurorehabilitation specialist
  patient referral to, 566–567
Neurotoxicology, 446
Neutralizing antibodies (NAbs)
  MS and, 210, 211
Niacin deficiency
  pellagra and, 473
Nicotinamide adenine dinucleotide (NAD)
  role of, 473
Nicotinamide adenine dinucleotide phosphate
      (NADP)
  role of, 473
Nicotine
  neurotoxic effects of, 465
Nicotine patches
  GTS and, 278
Niemann–Pick disease, 542
Nightmare, REM sleep and, 185
Nigral neuron
  parkinsonism and, 235
NIMV. *See* Non-invasive mechanical ventilation
Nitrate therapy
  neurologic effect of, 451
Nitrofurantoin therapy
  neurologic effect of, 448, 449
Nitroglycerin
  neurologic effect of, 451
Nizatidine (Axid)
  neurologic effects of, 456
NMDA. *See* N-methyl-D-aspartate
N-methyl-D-aspartate (NMDA), 299
NMO. *See* Neuromyelitis optica
NMO-IgG. *See* NMO serum biomarker
NMO serum biomarker (NMO-IgG), 199–200
NMS. *See* Neuroleptic malignant syndrome
NMSS. *See* National Multiple Sclerosis Society
Nociceptive (pain) fibers, 398
Nonarteritic AION (NAION), 528
Nonbenzodiazepine hypnotics, advantages of,
      165, 166
Non-Hodgkin lymphoma, 504

Non-invasive mechanical ventilation (NIMV)
central sleep apnea and, 178
Nonmetastatic complications
cerebrovascular, 510–511
metabolic and nutritional, 511
paraneoplastic syndromes, 511–512, 513*t*
Nonnucleoside reverse transcriptase inhibitors
neurologic side effects of, 449
Nonspecific back pain, 399
Nonspecific degenerative disease, 399
Nonsteroidal anti-inflammatory agents (NSAIDs),
335, 407
MS and, 211
neurotoxic effects of, 463
Noradrenergic antagonists
TD syndrome and, 283
Norepinephrine
dystonia and, 252
Normal pressure hydrocephalus (NPH)
dementia and, 290
Nortriptyline, cataplectic attacks and, 183
Novantrone
MS and, 210*t*, 211
NPH. *See* Normal pressure hydrocephalus
NREM sleep
stages of, 157–158, 159*f*
NSAIDs. *See* Nonsteroidal antiinflammatory drugs
NSE. *See* Neuron-specific enolase
NSF. *See* Nephrogenic systemic fibrosis
Nuchal rigidity
coma and, 93*t*, 94
Nucleoside reverse transcriptase inhibitors
neurologic side effects of, 449
"Numbness"
symptom of, 25
Nutrient arteries, 376
Nystagmus, 7, 416. *See also* Vertigo
AED and, 151
end point, 416
gaze-evoked, 416
jerk, 547
MS and, 202
pendular, 547–548
vestibular, 416

O

Obesity, sleep apnea and, 173
Obsessions, 4
Obsessive-compulsive disorder
GTS and, 275, 276, 278
HD and, 260

Obstructive hydrocephalus, 49
Obstructive sleep apnea (OSA), 172–175, 173*f*
cardiovascular diseases and, 174
causes of, 175
chronic obstructive pulmonary disease (COPD)
and, 174
diagnosis of, 174, 175
question about, 189–190
sleep architecture of, 176*f*
symptoms of, 173–174
treatment of, 177
CPAP in, 177
surgical techniques in, 178
v. central sleep apnea, 174
waking respiratory functions and, 174
Occipital focus, 144
Occipital nerve blocks
cluster headaches and, 136, 136*t*, 137
primary headaches, 132, 132*t*
Occupational therapy
ET and, 259
OCD. *See* Obsessive-compulsive disorder
OCT. *See* Optical coherence tomography scan
Ocular bobbing, 97
Ocular dysmetria
MS and, 202
Oculocephalic responses
metabolic encephalopathy, 102
Oculomasticatory myorrhythmia, 548
Oculomotor nerve (CN III), 7
lesion of, 7
Oculomotor syndromes
MS and, 202
Oculopalatal myoclonus, 548
Oculopharyngeal dystrophy
symptoms of, 362–363
Oculovestibular responses
coma and, 97, 98
metabolic encephalopathy, 102
Office for Human Research Protections (OHRP),
574
OHRP. *See* Office for Human Research Protections
Olanzapine
HD-related psychosis, 266
neurologic effects of, 458
TD syndrome and, 281, 282
tics and, 278
Olfaction
loss of, 6
Olfactory nerve (CN I)
olfaction and, 6
Oligodendrocyte, 502

Oligodendroglioma, 502
    management of, 502
One-and-a-half syndrome, 546
ONTT. *See* Optic Neuritis Treatment Trial
Ophthalmic branch (V$_1$), of trigeminal nerve, 7, 8f
Ophthalmoparesis, 351
Ophthalmoscopy, 518
Opiate
    GTS and, 278
Oppenheim dystonia, 246
Optical coherence tomography (OCT) scan
    MS and, 202
Optic atrophy, 7
Optic chiasm, 520
    visual field defects in, 522–523, 522f
Optic disc appearance, 518–520, 519f
Optic disc pallor, 519
Optic disc swelling, 519
    in papilledema, 519
Optic nerve (CN II), 6–7
    lesion of, 6
    lesions of, 521, 521f
Optic neuritis, 527
    clinical diagnosis of, 527
    MS and, 200, 202, 215
    prognosis for, 527
Optic Neuritis Treatment Trial (ONTT)
    MS and, 215
Optic neuropathy, 519, 527–528
    in pseudo-Foster Kennedy syndrome, 520
Optic radiations, 520
    visual field defects in, 525, 525f
Optic tracts, 520
    visual field defects in, 523–524, 523f
Oral contraceptive
    epilepsy and, 153
Oral contraceptives
    neurotoxic effects of, 463–464
Oral trail making
    assessment of, 3–4
Orbital MRI, 35
Orexin in waking, 156
Organ donation
    brain death and, 581
Organ harvesting
    brain death and, 581
Orobuccolingual (OBL) dyskinesia
    TD syndrome and, 279–280
Oromandibular dystonia, 243, 248
    BoNT and, 254

Orthostatic hypotension
    as cause of presyncope, 414
    patient evaluation for, 414
    symptoms, 414
OSA. *See* Obstructive sleep apnea
Osmotic agents
    acute alteration in mental status and, 76
Osmotic demyelination syndrome, 477
Osteomyelitis, 402
Otorrhea
    coma and, 94
Overlap syndrome, 174, 177
Oxazepam, sleep and, 164
Oxcarbazepine
    seizures and, 152
Oxybutynin
    urinary urgency and, 214t, 216
Oxybutynin chloride, sleep-related enuresis and, 186
Oxygen, sleep apnea and, 176
Oxygenation
    evaluation of, SE and, 65

P
PABP2 gene, 363
Pain
    acute spinal cord compression and, 77
    bony spine, 402
    in ligaments, 400
    management of
        rehabilitation and, 563–564
    MS and, 203
        treatment in, 215
    in muscles, 400
    nervous system structures and, 25–27
    neurogenic, 401
    radicular
        cervical processes and, 26
    referred, from abdominal, 402–403
Pain sensation
    sensory examination and, 13
Pallidotomy
    complication from
        Parkinson's disease and, 233
Palmar grasp reflex, presence of, 4
Palmomental reflex, presence of, 4
Palpitations
    neuromuscular disorder with, 369
Pancreatic encephalopathy
    alcoholism and, 476–477
    diagnosis, 476

pathophysiology of, 476
treatment of, 476–477
PANDAS. *See* Pediatric autoimmune neuropsychi-
atric disorders associated with streptococcal
infection
Panic attacks
seizures *vs.*, 148
Papez circuit
behavioral neurology and, 308–309, 308*f*
Papez loop, 3
Papilledema, 528
in optic disc swelling, 519
Paramedian pontine reticular formation (PPRF)
coma and, 95, 96
Paraneoplastic syndromes, 511–512, 513*t*
Paraparesis, 22
Paraplegia, 22
Parasomnias
pathophysiologic mechanism of, 184–186
specialist referral for, 186
Parcopa, RLS and, 168
Paresis, 22
Paresthesias
MS and, 203
Parinaud syndrome, 538
Parkinsonism, 226–227
dopamine system and, 234
drug-induced
anticholinergics, 280
diagnosis of, 234
Parkinson's disease v., 233–234
falling associated with, 431–432
medical treatment for, 438–439
neuroleptic-induced, 458
Parkinson's disease (PD)
basal ganglia dysfunction of, 27
case studies of, 237–240
as cause of parkinsonism in falling, 431
clinical features of, 222–226, 223*f*, 224*f*
complementary therapies for, 235–236
DBS surgery and, 233, 239–240
disease-modifying therapy and, 234–235
ET v., 255, 255*t*, 256, 257, 259
hospitalized patients and
challenges of, 236
Lewy bodies and, 296
mechanisms of, 226–228
neurologist referral for, 235
resting tremor and, 254
surgery and, 233
treatment for, 228–230, 228*t*

Parkinson's disease with dopaminergic adverse
events, 237
Parks–Bielschowsky test
for fourth nerve palsy, 543
Paroxetine, serotonin uptake and, 183
Paroxysmal hemicrania, 186
Partial thromboplastin time (PTT)
comatose patient and, 99
SAH and, 109
Patellar reflex, 11
Patient history
acute alteration of mental status and, 72
dementia and, 289
Guillain-Barré syndrome and, 81
SE and, 68
stroke and, 106
Patrick sign, 403
PCNSL. *See* Primary CNS lymphoma
PCoA. *See* Posterior communicating artery
PCR. *See* Polymerase chain reaction
PD. *See* Parkinson's disease
Pediatric autoimmune neuropsychiatric disorders
associated with streptococcal infection
(PANDAS)
GTS and, 276
Pediatric neurology. *See* Neurology, pediatric
Pellagra encephalopathy
alcoholism and, 472–473
treatment of, 473
Wernicke encephalopathy *versus*, 473
Pendular nystagmus, 547–548
oculomasticatory myorrhythmia, 548
oculopalatal myoclonus, 548
sea-saw, 548
Penicillamine therapy, 270, 272*t*
adverse effects of
WD and, 270
Penicillins
neurologic effect of, 447
Pentobarbital coma, 330
Perceptual disturbances
mental status examination and, 4
Perfusion–diffusion mismatch, 111
Pergolide
Parkinson's disease and, 227, 229
Perilymph fistula
as cause of vertigo, 421
Perindopril
stroke prevention and, 114
Periodic, lateralized, epileptiform discharges
(PLEDs), 70

Periodic limb movement (PLM) disorder, 157
Peripheral nerve lesions
    sensory symptoms of, 26
Peripheral nerves
    anatomy of, 376
Peripheral nervous system (PNS), 375
    disorder of, 388*t*
    manifestations of chronic alcoholism,
        479–482
    myasthenic crisis, 79–81
Peripheral neuropathy
    alcoholim and, 387
    anticonvulsants used for, 387
    clinical features of, 375–376
    with diabetes mellitus, 390–392
    diagnosis of, 382–389
    drug treatment of, 389*t*
    future prospectives, 393
    pathology of, 381–382
    patterns of abnormality, 380–381
    questions and discussion with,
        394–396
    symptoms and signs of, 377
Peripheral vertigo, 416–417, 416*t*
    causes of
        acute peripheral vestibulopathy,
            419–420
        BPPV, 418–419
        Ménière disease, 420–421
        perilymph fistula, 421
    hearing loss in, 417
    tinnitus in, 417
Peroneal neuropathy, 393
Personality disorders, sleep and, 160
PET. *See* Positron emission tomography
Phalen's sign, 392
Pharmacologic therapy
    primary headaches, 132, 132*t*
Pharyngeal dystonia, 243
Pharyngeal weakness
    neuromuscular diseases and, 369
Phenobarbital IV
    SE and, 68
Phenothiazines
    HD and, 265
Phenytoin
    ataxia and, 151
    children and, 151
    phosphenytoin *vs.*, 67–68
    SE and, 66
Phobias, 4

Phosphenytoin
    phenytoin IV *vs.*, 67–68
    SE and, 66, 67–68
Physical examination
    acute alteration of mental status and, 72
Physical therapy
    MS and, 218
Physiologic anisocoria, 532
Physostigmine
    neurologic effects of, 460
PICA. *See* Posterior inferior cere bellar artery
Pick disease, 297, 320
Pimozide
    GTS and, 277, 278
    side effects of, 278
Pineal gland, melatonin and, 157
Pinpoint pupils, 95
PION. *See* Posterior ischemic optic neuropathy
Pituitary macroadenomas, 522
Plantar response
    assessment of, 12
Plasma
    ICH and, 119
Plasma homocysteine level
    stroke and, 113
Plasmapheresis, 360, 390
    myasthenic crisis and, 80
Platelet count
    SAH and, 109
PLEDs. *See* Periodic, lateralized, epileptiform
        discharges
Plegia, 22
Plexopathies, 381
PLM. *See* Periodic limb movement disorder
PLMs of wakefulness (PLMW), 167
PLMW. *See* PLMs of wakefulness
PLP. *See* Proteolipid protein
PM. *See* Polymyositis
PMR. *See* Polymyalgia rheumatica
Pneumonia
    with bulbar dysfunction, 370
    neurorehabilitation and, 557
PNS. *See* Peripheral nervous system
Poliomyelitis
    Guillain-Barré syndrome *vs.*, 82, 82*t*
    sleep apneas and, 175
Poliovirus infection, 359
Polyalanine triplet (GCG), 363
Polycystic kidney disease
    aneurysm rupture and, 120
Polycythemia, complete blood count and, 175

Polymerase chain reaction (PCR)
  herpes simplex encephalitis and, 320
Polymyalgia rheumatica (PMR), 364
Polymyositis (PM), 354, 364–365
Polymyxins
  neurologic effect of, 447
Polyneuropathies, 25, 448
Polyradiculopathies, 25
Polysomnogram (PSMG), 157, 158f, 175, 176f
  sleep and, 157, 158f
  sleep apneas and, 175, 176f
Polysomnographic finding
  for endogenous v. bipolar depression, 170
Polysomnography, 334
Poor verticality
  falls associated with, 436
Popeye arms, 352
Posaconazole, 492
Positive sharp waves, 356, 385
Positron emission tomography (PET), 513
  dementia and, 294
  ET and, 171
  GTS and, 276
Postacute hospitalization
  TBI and, 331–332
Postanoxic coma
  prognosis of, 102
Postconcussive syndrome, 338
Posterior communicating artery (PCoA), 543
Posterior inferior cere bellar artery (PICA), 422
Posterior ischemic optic neuropathy (PION),
    519, 528
Posterior reversible encephalopathy syndrome
    (PRES), 511
Postpolio syndrome, 359
  sleep apnea and, 175
Posttraumatic amnesia (PTA)
  TBI and, 328
Posttraumatic cephalgia
  mild TBI and, 340
Posttraumatic epilepsy, 340
Posttraumatic hemidystonia, 251
Postural adjustments
  small anticipatory, 435
Postural reflexes
  Parkinson's disease and, 225–226, 226f,
    238–239
Postural responses
  associated with falls, 434–437
Postural tremor, 254, 285
  ET v., 256

Potassium-sparing diuretics
  neurologic effect of, 453
PP-MS. See Primary progressive multiple sclerosis
Pramipexole
  dyskinesia and, 239
  Parkinson's disease and, 227, 229, 232
Pramipexole (Mirapex)
  doses, 168
  RLS and, 168
Prazosin
  neurologic effect of, 453
Prednisone
  AD and, 300
  cluster headache and, 137, 137t
  MS and, 214
  myasthenic crisis and, 80
  recommended dosage of, 137t
Prednisone therapy
  for MG, 360
Pregabalin
  seizures and, 151–152
Pregabalin, 480
Pregnancy
  AED and, 153
  hypnotic drugs and, 165
  MS and, 200
  RLS and, 167
  WD and, 272
Premature awakening, 160, 170
Prenatal testing
  HD and, 263
PRES. See Posterior reversible encephalopathy
    syndrome
Presyncope, 412–413
  cardiac, 415
  carotid sinus hypersensitivity and, 415
  causes of, 413–415
  hyperventilation syndrome and, 413–414
  hypoglycemia and, 415
  orthostatic hypotension and, 414
  vasovagal/vasodepressor, 414
Primary brain injury
  coma secondary to, 92t
Primary CNS lymphoma (PCNSL), 504
Primary CNS neoplasm
  ICH and, 118
Primary dystonias
  classification of, 244–245
  epidemiology of, 242–244
Primary generalized epilepsy
  case reviews for, 154

Primary headaches
  classifications of, 128–129, 128*t*
  treatment of, 132, 132*t*
    nonpharmacologic, 132–133
Primary hemorrhage stroke, 106
Primary inherited dystonias, 245–247
Primary intracerebral hemorrhage (ICH), 105
Primary memory. *See* Working memory
Primary progressive aphasia, 297
Primary progressive multiple sclerosis (PP-MS)
  clinical symptoms of, 198
Primary torsion dystonia, 246
Primidone
  ET and, 258, 258*t*
  side effects of, 258
Primitive coma, 90
Prion diseases, 297–298, 495–496
Prions, defined, 486
PR-MS. *See* Progressive-relapsing multiple
    sclerosis
Procainamide
  neurologic effect of, 451
Procarin
  MS and, 218
Prochlorperazine (Compazine)
  neurologic effects of, 455
Prodrome, 128
Progressive-relapsing multiple sclerosis
    (PR-MS)
  clinical symptoms of, 198–199
Progressive sinus bradycardia, OSA and, 174
Progressive supranuclear palsy (PSP), 226,
    238, 541
  as cause of parkinsonism in falling, 432
  posture and, 238–239
Promethazine (Phenergan)
  neurologic effects of, 455
Pronator drift
  testing for, 11
Propofol-infusion syndrome, 68
Propranolol, 285
  ET and, 257, 258, 258*t*
  TD syndrome, 283
Proprioception
  assessment of, 15
Prosopagnosia, 529–530
Proteolipid protein (PLP)
  MS and, 195
Prothrombin time (PT)
  comatose patient and, 99
  SAH and, 109

Protriptyline
  cataplectic attacks and, 183
  sleep apnea syndromes and, 176
Pseudobulbar syndrome
  MS and, 217
Pseudohypertrophy of claves, 353*f*
Pseudoprogression, 513
Pseudoseizures
  EEG in, 37
  seizures *vs.*
    AED treatment and, 148
Pseudotumor cerebri, 528
PSMG. *See* Polysomnogram
PSP. *See* Progressive supranuclear palsy
Psychiatric drugs
  antidepressant agents, 459–461
  anxiolytics, 459
  hypnosedative, 461
  neuroleptic agents, 457–459
  neurotoxic effects of, 457–461
Psychiatric symptoms
  MS and, 203
  WD and, 267, 269
Psychogenic seizures
  AED treatment and, 148
Psychogenic unresponsiveness (hysterical coma),
    90
Psychomotor epilepsy, 309
Psychophysiologic insomnia, 159
Psychosis, drug-induced
  Parkinson's disease and, 231
Psychotherapy
  primary headaches and, 136
PT. *See* Prothrombin time
PTA. *See* Posttraumatic amnesia
Ptosis, 79, 351
PTT. *See* Partial thromboplastin time
Pulmonary function studies, primary hypertension
    and, 175
Punch biopsy
  of skin, 386
Pupil constriction, 530–531
Pupil dilation, 531
Pupil dysfunction, 531
Pupillary abnormalities, 530–538
  anisocoria, 532–537
  bilateral light-near dissociation, 537–538
  pupil constriction, 530–531
  pupil dilation, 531
  pupil dysfunction, 531
  relative afferent pupillary defect, 531–532

Pupillary response
  coma and, 95
Pyridostigmine, 360
  MG and, 360
  myasthenic crisis and, 80
Pyridoxine, 466
  WD and, 270
Pyrimethamine
  neurologic effect of, 448

Q

Quadrantanopia, 525, 525f
Quadrantanopias, 6
Quadruple sectoranopia, 525
QuantiFERON–TB Gold test, 491
Quetiapine, 457
  HD and, 265
  HD related psychosis, 266
  Parkinson's disease and, 231
  TD syndrome and, 281, 282
  tics and, 278
Quinidine
  neurologic effect of, 451

R

RAA axis. *See* Renin-angiotensin-aldosterone axis
Rabies encephalitis, 494
Raccoon eyes
  coma and, 94
Radiation necrosis, 513
Radiation therapy
  complications from, 512–513
  late effects of, 513
Radicular pain
  cervical processes and, 26
Radiculopathy
  cervical dystonia and, 249
  characteristics of, 21, 21t
Radionuclide bone scan, 406
Radiotherapy
  AVM and, 122
Raeder's paratrigeminal syndrome, 533, 533f
Ramelteon, insomnia and, 165
Ramipril
  stroke prevention and, 114
Rancho Los Amigos Scale (RLAS)
  brain injury and, 326
    cognitive function after TBI, 328
Range-of-motion exercises
  neuromuscular diseases and, 368, 370

Ranitidine (Zantac)
  neurologic effects of, 456
RAPD. *See* Relative afferent pupillary defect
Rasagiline
  Parkinson's therapy and, 230
Rash, skin
  AED and, 151
  lamotrigine
    seizures and, 152
RBC. *See* Red blood cell
Rebif
  MS and, 209, 210
Rebound, 168
Rebound headache. *See* Medication overuse
    headache
Receptive aphasia, 3
Recombinant tissue plasminogen activator
    (rt-PA), 106
  acute ischemic stroke interventional therapy
    and, 107
  case studies and, 123–125
  complications with, 117
  contraindications for, 109
  indications *vs.* contraindications for, 115, 116t
Rectal exam, 404
Red blood cell (RBC), 70
Referred pain, from abdominal, 402–403
Reflexes
  HD and, 260
Rehabilitation
  children and neuromuscular disease and,
    367–368
  determining need for, 559
  discharge planning and, 564–566
  program criteria for, 559–560
Rehabilitation, fall prevention by
  assistive devices use, 441–442
  balance training, 440
  fall risk assessment, 439–440
  gait training, 441
  strength training, 440–441
Rehabilitation programs
  home, 560
  management plan for, 560–561, 561t
    impaired cognition and, 562–563
    impaired mobility and, 561, 562
  nursing facilities with, 560
  outpatient, 560
  settings for, 560
Rehabilitative therapies
  epilepsy and, 153

Relapsing progressive multiple sclerosis, 199
Relapsing-remitting multiple sclerosis (RR-MS)
  clinical symptoms of, 197–198
Relative afferent pupillary defect (RAPD), 6, 518
  in optic tracts, 524
  in pupillary abnormalities, 531–532
Remacemide
  HD and, 265
Remission
  cervical dystonia and, 248
REM sleep, 158
  hypnosedatives and, 162
  narcolepsy and, 179
Remyelination
  MS and, 218
Renal dialysis
  rhabdomyolysis and, 371
Renal failure
  status epilepticus and, 64
Renin–angiotensin–aldosterone (RAA) axis, 454
Rescue therapy
  for SE patients, 65
Reserpine
  depression and, 283
  dystonia and, 252
  GTS and, 278
  HD and, 265
  side effects of, 252
  TD syndrome and, 283
Respiratory agents
  adrenergic drugs, 456
  neurotoxic effects of, 456–457
  xanthine bronchodilators, 456–457
Respiratory depression, 370
  neuromuscular disorders and, 370
Respiratory patterns
  coma and, 94
Resting tremor, 254
  WD and, 266
Restless legs syndrome (RLS), 167–170
  causes of, 167
  diagnosis for, 167
  pathophysiology of, 167–168
  prevalence of, 167
  treatment of, 168–170, 169t
Reticular-activating system in waking, 156
Retinal gangion cell (RGC), 520
Retrobulbar neuritis
  MS and, 202
Retrocollis, 248
RGC. See Retinal gangion cell

Rhabdomyolysis, 370–371
  status epilepticus and, 64
Riddoch phenomenon
  in cortical blindness, 529
Rifampin, 491
Rifaximin
  used in hepatic encephalopathy, 475
Right hemispheral destructive lesion, 103
Rigidity
  HD and, 260
Riluzole
  HD and, 265
Rinne test
  for acoustic nerve, 9
Risperidone
  GTS and, 277, 278
  HD and, 265
  HD-related psychosis, 266
Risperidone, 457
  neurologic effects of, 458
Rivastigmine
  AD and, 299
RLAS. See Rancho Los Amigos Scale
Romberg test, 15
Rooting reflex, 4
Ropinirole (Requip)
  doses, 168
  RLS and, 168
Rotigotine
  Parkinson's disease and, 229
RR-MS. See Relapsing-remitting multiple sclerosis
Rt-PA. See Recombinant tissue plasminogen
      activator
Ryanodine receptor gene, 366

S
Sacroiliac joint pain, 402
SAH. See Subarachnoid hemorrhage
Salicylate compounds
  neurotoxic effects of, 461–462
"Salicylate jag," 462
SCA. See Spinocerebellar ataxias
Scapular winging
  weakness and, 350, 350f
Schizophrenia, 309
  psychotic bizarre behaviors of, 310
  TD syndrome and, 281
  TLE behavior and, 310t
Schwann cells, 375, 376
Sciatica, 401

SCN. *See* Suprachiasmatic nucleus
Scoliosis
    in chronic infantile spinal muscular atrophy
        and, 354*f*
Scopolamine
    neurologic effects of, 455
SCUs. *See* Special care units
SDH. *See* Succinate dehydrogenase
SE. *See* Status epilepticus
Sea-saw nystagmus, 548
Secondary dystonia, 243
    diagnosis of, 251
    etiology of, 244*t*, 245
Secondary headaches
    classification of, 128–129, 128*t*
    conditions that produce, 128*t*
    diagnostic testing and, 127–128, 127*t*
Secondary memory. *See* Long-term memory
Secondary progressive multiple sclerosis (SP-MS)
    clinical symptoms of, 198
Sedatives
    comatose patient and, 101
Segawa dystonia, 242
Segmental dystonia, 244
Seizure disorders
    sleep and, 186
Seizure(s)
    AED treatment and, 148
    dietary therapy for, 153
    DOMV requirements for, 582–583
    in pediatric patients, 450–451
    rehabilitative therapies for, 153
    surgical therapies for, 152–153
    treatment of, 149, 149*t*
    types of, 143–144
    WD and, 267
    Westphal variant and, 260
Selective neuronal degeneration
    HD and, 264
Selective serotonin reuptake inhibitors (SSRIs)
    CNS side effects of, 460
    migraine and, 136
    MS and, 216
    OCD and, 278
    TBI and, 335
Selegiline
    GTS and, 278
    narcolepsy and, 181
    Parkinson's therapy and, 229–230
Sensation
    cutaneous, pathways for, 25–26

"Sensory ataxia," 439
Sensory disturbance
    MS and, 203
Sensory exam, 404
Sensory feedback
    loss of, 435
Sensory system
    evaluation of, 12
    nerves
        peripheral distribution, 12–13, 13*f*
    neurologic examination of, 1, 1*t*
    pediatric neurology and, 16
    syndromes
        nervous system structures and, 25–27
Sensory tics
    GTS and, 273
Sensory weighting
    abnormal, 435–436
    falls associated with, 435
Serologic testing
    MS and, 208
Serotonin reuptake inhibitors (SSRI), 338, 408
Sertraline
    serotonin uptake and, 183
Serum creatine kinase (CK)
    Becker dystrophy and, 361
    muscle necrosis and, 354
    PM and, 364
Severe metabolic coma
    drugs and, 97
Severe orthostatic hypotension, 235
Sexual dysfunction
    MS and, 204
        treatment in, 216
Short tau inversion recovery (STIR) images
    MS and, 205
Short-term memory loss
    MS and, 203
Shoulder girdle, 377
Shy–Drager syndrome, 414
SIADH. *See* Syndrome of inappropriate antidiuretic
        hormone
Siberian ginseng *(Eleutherococcus senticosus)*
    ephedrine and, 183
Sildenafil
    MS and, 214*t*, 216
Simple motor tics
    GTS and, 273
Simple partial seizures, 144, 145
Simple vocal tics
    GTS and, 273

Single-photon emission computed tomography
    (SPECT), 513
    dementia and, 294
    DRD and, 251
    GTS and, 276
Sirolimus
    neurologic effect of, 450
Sixth nerve palsy
    in horizontal double vision, 544–545, 545f
Skeletal muscle
    channelopathies affecting, 364
    mitochondrial myopathies and, 366
Skew deviation
    in vertical double vision, 544
Skin biopsy, 40
Skin breakdown
    prevention of, 556
Skull flap, 330
Sleep
    insufficient, 183–184
    laboratories, use of, 157
    neurochemistry of, 157
    stages of, 157–159, 158f, 159f
    structures facilitating, 156
Sleep apnea syndrome, 172
    diagnosis of, 175
    drugs for, 176
    evaluation of, 175
    frequent awakenings and, 171
    hypnotic drugs and, 165
    oral appliances for, 178
    postpolio syndrome and, 175
    question about, 188–189
    treatment of, 176–179, 177t
    types of, 172
        central, 172, 174
        mixed, 172
        obstructive, 172–175, 173f
Sleep architecture
    of obstructive sleep apnea syndrome, 176f
    REM and, 157–158, 159f
Sleep attacks, 168
    in narcolepsy, 179
Sleep-disordered breathing, 160
Sleep disorders
    classification of, 159
    questions about, 187–190
    tests available for, 157
Sleep fragmentation, causes of, 171
Sleep hygiene, 161
Sleepiness, syndromes causing, 184

Sleep latency, drugs and, 162, 163t, 164t
Sleep maintenance, 164
Sleep-maintenance insomnia, 160
    temazepam and, 164
Sleep-onset delay, 160–161
    circadian rhythm and, 160–161
    drug induced, 160
    insomnia and, 160
    psychological factors in, 160
    treatment of, 161–162
Sleep-onset insomnia, 160
    triazolam and, 164
Sleep paralysis, 179
Sleep-phase syndrome, 160
Sleep position, sleep apnea syndrome and,
    176–177
Sleep restriction, 162
Sleep-state misperception, 159
Sleep terror, 185
Sleep–wake cycle
    agitation and, 336
Sleep– wake cycle disturbance (SWCD), 332
SLR. See Straight leg raise test
SMA. See Spinal muscular atrophies
Small artery thrombotic (lacunar) stroke,
    105
"Small-fiber" nerves, 12
SMN. See Survival motor neuron gene
Smoking
    cessation
        aneurysm and, 120
Snoring, UPPP and, 178
Snort arousals in obstructive sleep apnea, 173
Snout reflex, 4
Sodium oxybate
    cataplexy and, 181, 183
    narcolepsy and, 181
Somato-sensory evoked potential (SSEP), 38
    MS and, 208
Somatostatin
    HD and, 264
Somnambulism, 185, 186
Somnolence
    medical causes of, 184
    question about, 188
Spasm, 400
Spasmodic dysphonia, 243
    BoNT and, 253–254
Spasmodic movement, 248, 249
Spasmodic torticollis. See Cervical dystonia
Spasms. See Spasticity

Spasticity
  falling associated with, 432
    medical treatment for, 439
  MS and, 206
    treatment of, 214*t*, 215
  TBI and, 338
Special care units (SCUs)
  AD and, 301
SPECT. *See* Single-photon emission computed
    tomography
Speech
  mental status examination and, 2–3
Speech therapy, 315, 320
  WD and, 272
Sphenoid sinus disease
  secondary headache disorders and, 137
Sphenoid sinuses
  headache and, 137
Spinal accessory nerve (CN XI), 9
Spinal cord compression, 402. *See* Acute spinal
    cord compression
Spinal cord injury
  neurorehabilitation intervention and, 558
Spinal cord lesions, 26
  MS and, 212–213, 213*f*
Spinal deformities, 402
Spinal metastases, 509–510
  treatment of, 510
Spinal muscular atrophies (SMA), 358
Spinal reflex response
  brain death and, 581
Spinal stenosis, 401
Spine
  CT scan, 405
  MRI with gadolinium, 405
  MRI without gadolinium dye, 405
  x-rays of, 405
Spine imaging, 53
Spine lesions, 53, 54*f*
Spinocerebellar ataxias (SCA), 235
Spirochete meningitis, 491
SP-MS. *See* Secondary progressive multiple sclerosis
Spondylolysis, 402
Sports-related concussive injury
  mild TBI and, 339–340
Sprain, 400
SSEP. *See* Somato-sensory evoked potential
SSRI. *See* Selective serotonin reuptake inhibitors
St. John's wort *(Hypericum perforatum)*, 166
Stability
  asymmetrical limits of, 435

Staphylococcus aureus, 494
Stare decisis, 573
Statins
  stroke prevention and, 114
Status epilepticus (SE), 63–65
  causes of, 64, 65
  complications of, 68
  convulsive, 64
  CT brain scan and, 68
  defined, 64
  morbidity, 64
  mortality rate, 64
  nonconvulsive, 64
  patient history and, 68
  precipitants of, 65
  refractory, 68
    anesthesia for treatment of, 68
    EEG monitoring and, 68
  treatment of, 65–69, 66*t*, 67*t*
  type of, 64
Statutory law, 574
Stavudine, 449
Steele–Richardson–Olszewski syndrome, 541
Stem cells
  MS and, 218
Stereognosis, 14
Stereotactic techniques
  ET and, 259
Stereotypy, 242
Steroid myopathy, 463
Steroids
  cluster headache and, 136
  neurotoxic effects of, 462–463
Stimulus control therapy, 162
STIR. *See* Short tau inversion recovery images
Stokes–Adams attacks
  seizures *vs.*, 148
Straight leg raise (SLR) test, 403
Strain, 399, 400
Strength training
  fall prevention by, 440–441
Streptococcus pneumoniae, 487, 489
Streptomycin
  neurologic effect of, 447
Stress
  tics syndrome and, 274, 275, 279
Striatal dopamine receptor
  Parkinson's disease and, 235
Stroke
  case studies and, 123–125
  clinical evaluation, 108–110

Stroke (*Continued*)
  diagnostic evaluation, 110–113
  epidemiology of, 105–108
  patient challenges with, 122–123
  prevention
    pharmacologic treatment for, 114–115, 115*t*
  primary etiologies for, 106*t*
  recurrent
    predictors of, 107
  risk factors for, 107*t*
Stroke management
  standard measures for, 116, 117, 117*t*
Stupor, 90
Stuporous patient, 2
Subacute meningitis
  evaluation of, 492*t*
Subarachnoid hemorrhage (SAH), 105, 120–122
  cause of, 55
  CT brain scan and, 109
  location of, 53
  with suprasellar cistern, 55, 55*f*
Subdural hematomas, 55, 55*f*
  location of, 53, 54
Subfalcine herniation, 47, 48, 48*f*
Substantia nigra, 239
  Parkinson's disease and, 226
Subthalamic nucleus
  DSB and, 233
Subwakefulness, 172
Succinate dehydrogenase (SDH), 366
Succinylcholine, 366
  malignant hyperthermia, 366
Sucralfate
  neurologic effects of, 456
Sulfonamide
  neurologic effect of, 448
Sumatriptan
  migraine and, 134
SUNCT syndrome
  treatment of, 137
Sunflower cataract
  WD and, 268
Superior arcuate defects, 522
Superoxide dismutase (SOD1) gene mutation
  on chromosome 21, 359
Superselective vascular catheterization
  AVM and, 122
Suprachiasmatic nucleus (SCN)
  circadian sleep rhythm and, 157
Supranuclear vertical gaze palsy, 541–542

Surgery
  cerebral aneurysms and, 121
  dystonia and, 253
  ET and, 259
  hypersomnia and, 184
  malignant hyperthermia, 366
  Parkinson's disease and, 233
Surgery DBS
  Parkinson's disease and, 239–240
Survival motor neuron (SMN) gene, 358
Swallowing dysfunction
  neuromuscular disorder and, 370
SWCD. *See* Sleep– wake cycle disturbance
Swinging flashlight test
  for vision loss, 518, 518*f*
Sydenham chorea. *See also* Chorea
  GTS and, 276
Sydenham's chorea, 464
Symmetric polyneuropathy, 380
Sympatholytics, 453
Syncope
  due to clinical intoxication, 451
  neuromucular disorders with, 369
Syndrome of inappropriate antidiuretic hormone
    (SIADH), 335
Syphilis serology
  stroke-like symptoms and, 112
Systemic depression
  coma and, 91, 92

T
Tacrine
  AD and, 298
Tacrolimus, 450
  neurologic effect of, 450
Tardive dyskinesia (TD), 242
  classification of, 279
  clinical features of, 279–280
  hospitalized patients, challenges for, 284
  pathophysiology of, 280–281
  prevention of, 281–282
  treatment of, 282–283
Tardive dyskinesia (TD) syndrome, 237, 238
TBI. *See* Traumatic brain injury
TCAs. *See* Tricyclic antidepressants
TCD. *See* Transcranial Doppler
TD syndrome. *See* Tardive dyskinesia
TEE. *See* Transesophageal echocardiography
Temazepam, sleep and, 164

Temozolomide
for astrocytoma, 501–502
Temperature sensation
sensory examination and, 13
Temporal arteritis, 381
Temporal dispersion, 384
Temporal lobe epilepsy (TLE), 308,
309–311
drug used in, 312t
for hospitalized patients, 313
refer neurologists, 312–313
Temporal Lobe Foci, 309t
Temporal lobe herniation
coma and, 95
Temporal lobe injury
convulsions and, 146
Temporomandibular structures
headache and, 137
TENS. *See* Transcutaneous electrical nerve
stimulation; Transcutaneous electrical
nerve stimulator
Tension-type headache
classification of, 129
Tentorium cerebelli
intracranial hypertension and, 75
Terazosin
MS and, 216
Terminal insomnia, 160
Tetrabenazine
depression and, 283
GTS and, 278
HD and, 265–266
Meige syndrome and, 252
TD syndrome, 283
Tetracycline, 448
Tetrahydrobiopterin
DRD and, 251
Tetrathiomolybdate (TTM)
WD and, 272, 272t
Thalamic lesions, 26
Thalamotomy, dystonia and, 246t
Thalamus, sleep and, 156
Theophylline
neurologic effects of, 456–457
"The three Ds" of pellagra, 472–473
Thiamine deficiency
alcoholic neuropathy due to, 480
alcoholism and, 471
Thiamine diphosphate
role in enzyme pathways, 471

Thiazide diuretics
neurologic effect of, 452
in vertigo, 421
Third nerve palsy
mydriasis, 535–536, 535f
in vertical double vision, 542–543, 542f
Thomsen disease, 364
Thoracic cord compression, 77
Thoracic radiculopathies
causes of, 26
Thought blocking, 4
Thought form
abnormalities of, 4
Threshold values
and TBI, 329
Thrombocytopenia
differential diagnosis of, 118
as result of malignancy, 510
Thrombotic stroke
embolic stroke *vs.*, 109, 109t
Thrombus
occurrence of, 57
Thymectomy
in patients with MG, 360
Thymic tumors
in patients with MG, 360
Thyroid eye disease, 7
Thyroid function studies
ET and, 257
TIA. *See* Transient ischemic attack
Tiagabine
seizures and, 152
Tick-bite paralysis
Guillain-Barré syndrome *vs.*, 82, 82t
Tics syndrome, 242
characteristics of, 273–274
classification of, 273
clinical spectrum of, 274
etiology of, 275
GTS and, 273
medical therapy for, 277t
movement disorder v., 273
stress and, 279
Time of flight (TOF) technique, 47
Tinel's sign, 392
Tinetti's Balance and Gait Test, 440
Tinetti's definition of fall, 427–428
Tinnitus
in peripheral vestibular lesions, 417
Tissue biopsy, 39–40

Tissue plasminogen activator (TPA), 56
Tizanidine
    migraine and, 136
    spasticity treatment and, 214*t*, 215, 439
TLE. *See* Temporal lobe epilepsy
TMN. *See* Tuberomammillary histaminergic
        neurons
Tobramycin
    neurologic effect of, 447
Tocainide hydrochloride
    neurologic effect of, 451–452
Todd's paralysis, 431
TOF technique. *See* Time of flight technique
Tolcapone
    Parkinson's disease and, 228, 228*t*
    Parkinson's therapy and, 230, 232
Tolterodine
    urinary urgency and, 214*t*, 216
Tongue protrusion
    HD and, 261
Tonic–clonic epilepsy
    juvenile myoclonic epilepsy as, 145
Tonic–clonic seizures
    causes of, 143
Tonic pupil, 536–537, 537*f*
Tonsillar herniation, 47, 48, 48*f*
Topiramate
    adverse effects of, 259
    ET and, 259
    GTS and, 278
    seizures and, 151, 152
    SUNCT syndrome, 137
Torticollis, 243, 248
    GTS and, 273
    secondary dystonia v., 251
Toxic compounds
    toxic myopathies, 366–367
Toxic myopathies, 366–367
TPA. *See* Tissue plasminogen activator
Transcranial Doppler (TCD), 36
Transcutaneous electrical nerve stimulation
        (TENS), 408
Transcutaneous electrical nerve stimulator
        (TENS), 340
Transesophageal echocardiography (TEE)
    anticoagulant therapy and, 112
Transformed migraine, 129
Transient global amnesia, 308, 317–319
    consult neurologists, 319
    for hospitalized patients, 319
    memory testing during, 318

pathologic studies, 318
    treatment of, 318–319
Transient insomnia, 160
Transient ischemic attack (TIA), 528
    patient challanges with, 122–123
    routine studies performed with, 110, 110*t*
    stroke and, 107
Transient RBD, drug intoxications and, 185
Transient tic disorder, 274, 276
Transitional multiple sclerosis, 199
Transplant drugs
    cyclosporine, 449–450
    immunosuppressives, 450
Transplant immunosuppressives, 450
Transtentorial herniation, 47, 48, 48*f*
    sequelae of, 49*f*
Trauma
    coma and, 92*t*
Trauma, perinatal
    delayed-onset dystonia in, 251
Traumatic brain injury (TBI), 324
    abulia and, 338
    acute hospitalization, 330
    agitation, 336–338, 337*f*
    behavioral disorder/depression, 341
    discussion questions for, 341–343
    dysautonomia, 335
    epidemiology of, 324–325
    hyponatremia, 335
    late-onset hydrocephalus, 335–336
    neuropsychologic testing, 340
    neurostimulant agents for, 331
    overview, 324–325
    pathology of, 325–330
    postacute hospitalization, 331–332
    refer neurologists, 340–341
    spasticity and, 338
    SWCD, 332–335
Trazadone, 408
Tremor, 11, 237, 242
    botulinum toxin and, 249
    cervical dystonia and, 249
    DBS and, 259
    differential diagnosis of, 255*t*
    Parkinson's disease and, 223, 224
    voice, 255
Treponema pallidum, 487, 491
Triazolam, sleep and, 164
Tricyclic antidepressants (TCAs)
    cataplexy and, 183
    early morning awakening and, 170

migraine and, 136
MS and, 217
neurologic effects of, 459–460
sleep-related enuresis and, 186
Tricyclics
discontinuation of, side effects of, 183
Trientine
WD and, 270, 272t
Trigeminal autonomic cephalgias
characterization of, 132, 132t
Trigeminal cervical connection
headache and, 137
Trigeminal nerve (CN V)
distribution of, 7, 8f
functions of, 7–8
Trihexyphenidyl
dystonia and, 252
side effects of, 252
Trimethoprim
neurologic effect of, 448
Trimipramine, early morning awakening and,
170
Triple flexor response
coma and, 98
Triptans
medication overuse headache and, 130, 130t
migraine and, 134
Trochlear nerve (CN IV), 7
lesion of, 7
Truncal dystonia, 243
Tryptophan, 466
TTM. See Tetrathiomolybdate
Tuberculous meningitis, 491–492
treatment of, 491–492
Tuberomammillary histaminergic neurons
(TMN), 156
sleep and, 156
T1-weighted images, 35, 44, 45f
T2-weighted images, 35, 44, 45f
Type 2 diabetes and OSA, 174
Tyrosine hydroxylase
DRD and, 251
Tysabri
MS and, 210t, 211–212

U
UARS. See Upper airway resistance syndrome
Ulnar neuropathy, 392–393
Ultrasonography, 36
Uncal herniation syndrome, 75

United States Uniform Determination of Death Act
brain death and, 579
Upper airway patency, 174
Upper airway resistance syndrome (UARS), 174
Upper motor neuron lesions
symptoms of, 23–24
Upper motor neuron signs, 10
UPPP. See Uvulopalatopharyngoplasty
Uremic encephalopathy
acute alteration in mental status and, 71
Uremic neuropathies, 387
Urinary tract infections (UTIs)
antibiotics used in, 448
Urination
MS and, 204
UTIs. See Urinary tract infections
Uvulopalatopharyngoplasty (UPPP), 178

V
VaD. See Vascular dementia
Vagus nerve (CN X), 9
Valproate
seizures and, 149
side effects of
seizures and, 151
Valproate IV
SE and, 68
Variant of CJD (vCJD), 496
Vascular dementia (VaD), 291, 295–296
risk factors for, 295
Vascular endothelial growth factor (VEGF), 502
Vascular imaging, 36–37
catheter angiography, 36–37
computed tomographic angiography, 36
infarct evaluation and, 56–60
magnetic resonance angiography, 36
magnetic resonance venography, 36
ultrasonography, 36
Vasodilators
neurologic effect of, 453
Vasogenic edema, 52f
acute intracranial hypertension and, 76
cytotoxic edema versus, 50–51
Vasospasm
cerebral aneurysms and, 121
Vasovagal presyncope, 414
VCJD. See Variant of CJD
Vegetative state
locked-in syndrome, 90, 91
VEGF. See Vascular endothelial growth factor

Venlafaxine
  MS and, 217
Venography (MRV)
  acute stroke evaluation and, 111
Ventilation
  neuromuscular diseases and, 369
Ventricular trapping, 48*f*
Ventrolateral preoptic nucleus (VLPO)
  sleep and, 156
VEP. *See* Visual evoked potential
Verbal fluency
  assessment of, 3
Vertebral bodies
  compression fracture of, 402
Vertebral dissection syndromes
  headache and, 137
  secondary headache disorders and, 137
Vertebrobasilar distribution ischemia
  carotid ischemia *vs.*, 113, 113*t*
Vertical double vision, 542–544
  fourth nerve palsy, 543–544, 544*f*
  skew deviation, 544
  third nerve palsy, 542–543, 542*f*, 543*f*
Vertigo, 413
  associated with brainstem, 417
  ataxia in, 417
  central, 416–417, 421
    basilar migraine, 423
    cerebellar hemorrhage, 422–423
    lateral medullary ischemia, 422
    lateral pontine ischemia, 422
    multiple sclerosis, 423
    transient ischemic attack, 422
  cerebellar signs in, 417
  distinguishing peripheral and central, 416*t*
  Dix–Hallpike positional test for, 418, 418*f*
  Halmagyi head thrust test in, 417
  hearing loss in, 417
  mild TBI and, 339
  nystagmus and, 416
  peripheral, 416–417
    acute peripheral vestibulopathy, 419–420
    BPPV, 418–419
    Ménière disease, 420–421
    perilymph fistula, 421
  pharmacologic treatments for, 420*t*
  symptoms, 415
  tinnitus in, 417
Vestibular dysfunction
  in disequilibrium, 424

Vestibular nystagmus, 416, 547
Vestibular system disorders
  falling associated with, 433
    medical treatment for, 439
  Ménière disease and, 433
Vestibulocochlear nerve (CN VIII), 8–9
Vestibuloocular reflex (VOR), 417, 539, 540, 541
Vestibulotoxins, 424
VGCC. *See* Voltage-gated P/Q-type calcium
  channels
Vibratory exam, 404
Vincristine, 387
Viral meningitis, 488–489
Vision loss, 517–518
  cortical, 529
  evaluation of, 517–518
Visual acuity
  testing of, 6
Visual acuity test
  for vision loss, 517
Visual cortex
  radiations converge on, 520
  visual field defects in, 525–526, 526*f*
Visual disorders
  cortical vision loss, 529
  of object recognition, 529–530
  of visuospatial processing, 530
Visual dysfunction
  in disequilibrium, 423
Visual evoked potential (VEP), 38
  MS and, 208
Visual field defects, 6
  in lateral geniculate nucleus, 524–525, 525*f*
  in optic chiasm, 522–523, 522*f*
  optic nerve defects, 521*f*
  in optic radiations, 525, 525*f*
  in optic tracts, 523–524, 523*f*
  in visual cortex, 525–526, 526*f*
Visual fields, 520–527, 520*f*
  testing of, 6
Visual pathway. *See* Visual field
Visuospatial neglect, 530
Visuospatial processing
  mental status examination and, 3
Vitamin A, 465
Vitamin B$_6$, 466. *See* Pyridoxine
Vitamin B$_{12}$
  MS and, 218
Vitamin C therapy
  Parkinson's disease and, 234

Vitamin D, 465
  MS and, 200
Vitamin E
  HD and, 265
  TD syndrome and, 283
Vitamin E therapy
  Parkinson's disease and, 234
Vitamins
  neurotoxic effects of, 464–466
VLPO. *See* Ventrolateral preoptic nucleus
Vocal tics
  GTS and, 273
Voice tremor, 255
Voltage-gated P/Q-type calcium channels
      (VGCC), 361
Volume loss, 49
  hydrocephalus *versus*, 49–50
Voluntary conjugate gaze (PSP), 235
VOR. *See* Vestibuloocular reflex
Voriconazole, 492
VTA. *See* Dopaminergic ventrotegmental area

W

Wakefulness after sleep onset (WASO), 165
Wake-promoting hypocretin system in waking,
      156
"Walk and Talk" task, 436
Wallenberg syndrome, 533. *See* Lateral medullary
      infarction
Wallerian degeneration, 326
Warfarin
  ICH and, 119
  stroke prevention and, 115
Wartenburg sign, 392
WASO. *See* Wakefulness after sleep onset
Wax and wane
  GTS and, 274, 275
Weakness
  falling associated with, 433–434
    medical treatment for, 439
  MS and, 206
  neurologic diagnostic process and, 22–25
  shoulder girdle, 350, 351*f*
Weak postural responses, 434
Weber syndrome, 542
Weber test
  for acoustic nerve, 9
Weight loss
  HD and, 261

  herbal, 183
  sleep apnea and, 176
Wernicke aphasia, 3, 314–315
Wernicke encephalopathy, 308. *See* Wernicke–
Korsakoff syndrome
  acute alteration in mental status and, 72
  alcoholism and, 471–472
  dementia and, 291
  diagnosis of, 472
  versus pellagra, 473
  symptoms, 471
  treatment of, 472
Wernicke–Korsakoff syndrome, 479
  behavioral picture of, 316
  comatose patient and, 100
  diagnosis of, 316
  overview, 315–316
  refer neurologists, 317
  treatment of, 317
West Nile virus, 492
Westphal variant
  HD and, 260
Whipple's disease, 542, 548
WHO. *See* World Health Organization
Wilbrand knee, 523
Wilson disease (WD), 237, 238, 242
  AHCD *versus*, 475
  clinical manifestations of, 266–268
  diagnosis of, 269–270
  genetics of, 268–269
  neurologist referral for, 273
  neuropathology of, 268
  new-onset dystonia and, 251
  pathogenesis of, 268–269
  treatment of, 270–272, 272*t*
Women's Health Initiative Memory Study, 300
Working memory
  testing, 3
World Health Organization (WHO)
  definition of fall by, 427
  disablement and, 551, 551*t*
Writer's cramp
  cervical dystonia and, 249
  dystonia and, 249–250, 250*f*

X

Xanthine bronchodilators
  neurologic effects of, 456–457
X-linked dystrophin gene, 361

X-rays, 35
    acute spinal cord compression and, 78
    for spine, 405

Z
Zalcitabine
    neurologic effect of, 449
Zaleplon, insomnia and, 165
Zeitgebers, 157

Zinc acetate
    WD and, 270–272, 272t
Ziprasidone
    TD syndrome and, 282
    tics and, 278
Zolmitriptan
    migraine and, 134
Zolpidem, insomnia and, 165
Zonisamide
    seizures and, 149, 152